Public Health Nutrition

Edited on beha—

Michael J

John M K

Blackwell
Science

NS

© The Nutrition Society 2004

Blackwell Science Ltd, a Blackwell Publishing company
Editorial offices:
Blackwell Science Ltd, 9600 Garsington Road, Oxford OX4 2DQ, UK
   Tel: +44 (0) 1865 776868
Blackwell Publishing Professional, 2121 State Avenue, Ames, Iowa 50014-8300, USA
   Tel: +1 515 292 0140
Blackwell Science Asia Pty Ltd, 550 Swanston Street, Carlton, Victoria 3053, Australia
   Tel : +61 (0)3 8359 1011

First published 2004
Reprinted 2006

ISBN-10: 0-632-05627-4
ISBN-13: 978-0-632-05627-9

Library of Congress Cataloging-in-Publication Data
Public health nutrition / edited on behalf of The Nutrition Society by Michael J.
Gibney ... [et al.].
     p. cm.
   Includes bibliographical references and index.
   ISBN 0-632-05627 -4 (pbk. : alk. paper)
  1. Nutritionally induced diseases. 2. Nutrition. 3. Public health. I. Gibney,
Michael J, II. Nutrition Society (Great Britain)
RA645.N87P83 2004
616.3'9--dc22   2004010644

A catalogue record for this title is available from the British Library

Produced and typeset in Minion
by Gray Publishing, Tunbridge Wells, Kent
Printed and bound in India
by Gopsons Papers Ltd, Noida

For further information on Blackwell Publishing, visit our website:
www.blackwellpublishing.com

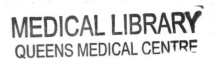

The Human Nutrition Textbook Series

The International Scientific Committee

Editor-in-Chief
Professor Michael J Gibney
Trinity College, Dublin, Ireland

Assistant Editor
Julie Dowsett
Trinity College, Dublin, Ireland

Professor Lenore Arab
University of North Carolina, USA

Professor Yvon Carpentier
Université Libre de Bruxelles, Belgium

Professor Marinos Elia
University of Southampton, UK

Professor Frans J Kok
Wageningen University, Netherlands

Professor Olle Ljungqvist
Ersta Hospital & Huddinge University Hospital, Sweden

Professor Ian A Macdonald
University of Nottingham, UK

Professor Barrie M Margetts
University of Southampton, UK

Professor Kerin O'Dea
Menzies School of Health Research, Darwin, Australia

Dr Helen M Roche
Trinity College, Dublin, Ireland

Professor Hester H Vorster
Potchefstroom, South Africa

Dr John M Kearney
Dublin Institute of Technology, Ireland

Textbook Editors

Introduction to Human Nutrition
Editor-in-Chief
Professor Michael J Gibney
Trinity College, Dublin, Ireland

Professor Hester H Vorster
Potchefstroom, South Africa

Professor Frans J Kok
Wageningen University,
Netherlands

Nutrition and Metabolism
Editor-in-Chief
Professor Michael J Gibney
Trinity College, Dublin, Ireland

Professor Ian A Macdonald
University of Nottingham, UK

Dr Helen M Roche
Trinity College, Dublin, Ireland

Public Health Nutrition
Editor-in-Chief
Professor Michael J Gibney
Trinity College, Dublin, Ireland

Professor Barrie M Margetts
University of Southampton, UK

Professor Lenore Arab
University of North Carolina, USA

Dr John Kearney
Dublin Institute of Technology, Ireland

Clinical Nutrition
Editor-in-Chief
Professor Michael J Gibney
Trinity College, Dublin, Ireland

Professor Marinos Elia
University of Southampton, UK

Professor Olle Ljungqvist
Ersta Hospital & Huddinge University Hospital, Sweden

Julie Dowsett
Trinity College, Dublin, Ireland

www.nutritiontexts.com

A unique feature of The Nutrition Society Textbook Series is that each chapter will have its own web pages, accessible at www.nutritiontexts.com. In the course of time, each will have downloadable teaching aids, suggestions for projects, updates on the content of each chapter and sample multiple choice questions. With input from teachers and students we will have a vibrant, informative and social website.

The Human Nutrition Textbook series comprises:

Introduction to Human Nutrition

Introduction to human nutrition: a global perspective on food and nutrition
Body composition
Energy metabolism
Nutrition and metabolism of proteins and amino acids
Digestion and metabolism of carbohydrates
Nutrition and metabolism of lipids
Dietary reference standards
The vitamins
Minerals and trace elements
Measuring food intake
Food composition
Food policy and regulatory issues
Nutrition research methodology
Food safety: a public health issue of growing importance
Food and nutrition: the global challenge

Public Health Nutrition

An overview of public health nutrition
Nutritional epidemiology
Assessment of nutritional status in individuals and populations
Assessment of physical activity
Public health nutrition strategies for intervention at the ecological level
Public health nutrition strategies for intervention at the individual level
Dietary guidelines
Food choice
Public health aspects of overnutrition
Public health aspects of undernutrition
Vitamin A deficiency
Iodine and iron-deficiency disorders
Iron-deficiency anemias
Fear of fatness and fad slimming diets
Nutrition and child development
Infant feeding
Adverse outcomes in pregnancy: the role of folate and related B-vitamins
Maternal nutrition, fetal programming and adult chronic disease
Cardiovascular disease
Diabetes mellitus
Cancer and diet
Disease prevention: osteoporosis and hip fracture

Nutrition and Metabolism

Core concepts of nutrition
Molecular nutrition
Integration of metabolism 1: Energy
Integration of metabolism 2: Protein and amino acids
Integration of metabolism 3: Macronutrients
Pregnancy and lactation
Growth and aging
Nutrition and the brain
The sensory systems: taste, smell, chemesthesis and vision
The gastrointestinal tract
The cardiovascular system
The skeletal system
The immune and inflammatory systems
Phytochemicals
The control of food intake
Overnutrition
Undernutrition
Exercise performance

Clinical Nutrition

General principles of clinical nutrition
Metabolic and nutritional assessment
Overnutrition
Undernutrition
Metabolic disorders
Eating disorders
Adverse reactions to foods
Nutritional support
Ethical and legal issues
Gastrointestinal tract
The liver
The pancreas
The kidney
Blood and bone marrow
The lung
Immune and inflammatory systems
Heart and blood vessels
The skeleton
Perioperative nutrition
Infectious diseases
Malignant diseases
Pediatric nutrition
Cystic fibrosis
Water and electrolytes
Clinical cases

Contents

Series Foreword

The early decades of the twentieth century were a period of intense research on constituents of food essential for normal growth and development, and saw the discovery of most of the vitamins, minerals, amino acids and essential fatty acids. In 1941, a group of leading physiologists, biochemists and medical scientists recognized that the emerging discipline of nutrition needed its own learned society and The Nutrition Society was established. Our mission was, and remains, *"to advance the scientific study of nutrition and its application to the maintenance of human and animal health".* The Nutrition Society is the largest learned society for nutrition in Europe and we have over 2000 members worldwide. You can find out more about the Society and how to become a member by visiting our website at www.nutsoc.org.uk

The ongoing revolution in biology initiated by large-scale genome mapping and facilitated by the development of reliable, simple-to-use molecular biological tools makes this a very exciting time to be working in nutrition. We now have the opportunity to obtain a much better understanding of how specific genes interact with nutritional intake and other lifestyle factors to influence gene expression in individual cells and tissues and, ultimately, affect our health. Knowledge of the polymorphisms in key genes carried by a patient will allow the prescription of more effective, and safe, dietary treatments. At the population level, molecular epidemiology is opening up much more incisive approaches to understanding the role of particular dietary patterns in disease causation. This excitement is reflected in the several scientific meetings that The Nutrition Society, often in collaboration with sister learned societies in Europe, organizes each year. We provide travel grants and other assistance to encourage students and young researchers to attend and participate in these meetings.

Throughout its history a primary objective of the Society has been to encourage nutrition research and to disseminate the results of such research. Our first journal, *The Proceedings of The Nutrition Society,* recorded, as it still does, the scientific presentations made to the Society. Shortly afterwards, *The British Journal of Nutrition* was established to provide a medium for the publication of primary research on all aspects of human and animal nutrition by scientists from around the world. Recognizing the needs of students and their teachers for authoritative reviews on topical issues in nutrition, the Society began publishing *Nutrition Research Reviews* in 1988. More recently, we launched *Public Health Nutrition,* the first international first journal dedicated to this important and growing area. All of these journals are available in electronic, as well as in the conventional paper form and we are exploring new opportunities to exploit the web to make the outcomes of nutritional research more quickly and more readily accessible.

To protect the public and to enhance the career prospects of nutritionists, The Nutrition Society is committed to ensuring that those who practice as nutritionists are properly trained and qualified. This is recognized by placing the names of suitably qualified individuals on our professional registers and by the award of the qualifications Registered Public Health Nutritionist (RPHNutr) and Registered Nutritionist (RNutr). Graduates with appropriate degrees but who do not yet have sufficient postgraduate experience can join our Associate Nutritionist registers. We undertake accreditation of university degree programs in public health nutrition and are developing accreditation processes for other nutrition degree programs.

Just as in research, having the best possible tools is an enormous advantage in teaching and learning. This is the reasoning behind the initiative to launch this series of human nutrition textbooks designed for use worldwide. The Society is deeply indebted to its former President, Professor Mike Gibney, for his foresight, and to him and his team of editors for their innovative approaches and hard work in bringing this major publishing exercise to successful fruition. Read, learn and enjoy.

John Mathers
President of The Nutrition Society

Preface

This book represents the third in a series of four for honors or masters level students of nutrition. The first book serves as a broad introduction, not just for nutrition students, but also for students of disciplines such as nursing, pharmacy, food science and agriculture. All the ensuing books are aimed at nutrition students. The second textbook, *Nutrition and Metabolism*, provides students with the biological basis of nutrition in health and disease. Thereafter, most students will make a choice to pursue either a clinical stream or a public health nutrition stream. The present book is focused on the latter, a subject that is growing in importance, taking into account the real potential to reduce the burden on noncommunicable chronic disease through diet. The Nutrition Society has championed the development of recognition of public health nutrition as a specialized discipline in the field, complementing the established specialty of clinical nutrition where the target audience is an individual patient on a one-to-one basis. In the case of public health nutrition the target audience is the population as a whole or specific subpopulations. The textbook is structured to begin with an overview taking students through a cycle of procedures, which should ideally be a feature of any program of public health nutrition. The first eight chapters of the book describe the skills needed in public health nutrition. The next six outline the major public health nutrition problems arising from overnutrition and from undernutrition. Maternal and child health issues are covered in the next four chapters, and some major diseases, cancer, diabetes, heart disease and osteoporosis, are dealt with in the final four chapters. As has been pointed out in the prefaces to the first two books in this series, there will be some overlap, but students will find the orientation different for similar subjects across texts. In some chapters, the public health nutrition element is accompanied by relevant material in clinical nutrition or in molecular nutrition, which will help students appreciate the links between all elements of nutrition.

The editors once again express their sincere thanks to their Assistant Editor Julie Dowsett and her heroic husband Greg.

Michael J Gibney
Editor-in-Chief

Contributors

Dr Faruk Ahmed
Nutrition Program – Division of International Health
School of Population Health
Public Health Building
Herston, Queensland, Australia

Dr Annie S Anderson
Centre for Public Health Nutrition Research
Department of Medicine
University of Dundee
Ninewells Hospital and Medical School
Dundee, UK

Professor Lenore Arab
Amgen, Inc.
Thousand Oaks
California, USA
Professor of Nutrition and Epidemiology
UNC School of Public Health
Chapel Hill, North Carolina, USA

Dr Helen Baker-Henningham
Centre of International Child Health
Institute of Child Health
London, UK

Professor David JP Barker
MRC Environmental Epidemiology Unit
Southampton General Hospital
Southampton, UK

Ms Jane Bentley
Department of Pediatrics and Child Health
University of Natal
Durban, South Africa

Dr Shirley AA Beresford
Department of Epidemiology
School of Public Health and Community Medicine
University of Washington
Seattle, Washington, USA

Professor Cyrus Cooper
Professor of Rheumatology
MRC Epidemiology Resource Centre
University of Southampton
Southampton General Hospital
Southampton, UK

Professor Anna Coutsoudis
Department of Pediatrics and Child Health
University of Natal
Durban, South Africa

Dr David N Cox
CSIRO Health Sciences and Nutrition
Adelaide, SA, Australia

Dr Ian Darnton-Hill
Nutrition Section, UNICEF
New York, USA

Dr Ulf Ekelund
Karolinska Institutet
Unit for Preventive Nutrition
Department of Biosciences at Novum
Huddinge, Sweden

Dr Mary AT Flynn
Coordinator, Nutrition and Active Living
Calgary Health Region
Adjunct Professor
Department of Agriculture and Nutritional Sciences
University of Alberta and
Department of Community Health Sciences
University of Calgary, Alberta, Canada

Professor Michael J Gibney
Department of Clinical Medicine
Trinity Centre for Health Sciences
St James' Hospital
Dublin, Ireland

Dr Keith M Godfrey
MRC Clinical Scientist
MRC Environmental Epidemiology Unit
Southampton General Hospital
Southampton, UK

Professor Sally Grantham-McGregor
Centre of International Child Health
Institute of Child Health
London, UK

Dr Nicholas Harvey
MRC Epidemiology Resource Centre
University of Southampton
Southampton General Hospital
Southampton, UK

Dr Pieter L Jooste
National Intervention Research Unit
Medical Research Council
Tygerberg, Cape Town, South Africa

Dr John M Kearney
Department of Biological Science
Dublin Institute of Technology
Dublin, Ireland

Dr Knut-Inge Klepp
Department of Nutrition
University of Oslo
Oslo, Norway

Professor Helene McNulty
School of Biomedical Sciences
University of Ulster at Coleraine
Londonderry, UK

Dr Mark Manary
Department of Pediatrics
Washington University
School of Medicine
St. Louis, Missouri, USA

Professor Jim Mann
Department of Human Nutrition
University of Otago
Dunedin, New Zealand

Professor Barrie M Margetts
Institute of Human Nutrition
University of Southampton
Southampton, UK

Dr Michael Nelson
Department of Nutrition and Dietetics
King's College London
London, UK

Dr Chandrakant S Pandav
Regional Coordinator
ICCIDD, South Asia and Pacific Region
New Delhi, India

Dr Ruth E Patterson
Research Associate Professor
Department of Epidemiology
University of Washington
Seattle, Washington, USA

Dr Pirjo Pietinen
National Public Health Institute
Mannerheimintie
Helsinki, Finland

Dr Ambady Ramachandran
Diabetes Research Centre and
M. V. Hospital for Diabetes
Royapuram, Chennai, India

Dr Kim D Reynolds
University of Southern California
Institute for Health Promotion and Disease
Prevention Research
Los Angeles, California, USA

Professor John Scott
Biochemistry Department
Trinity College
Dublin, Ireland

Dr Jacob C Seidell
Department for Nutrition and Health
Free University
Amsterdam, The Netherlands

Dr Michael Sjöström
Karolinska Institutet
Unit for Preventive Nutrition
Department of Biosciences at Novum
Huddinge, Sweden

Dr Chamukuttan Snehalatha
Diabetes Research Centre and M. V. Hospital for Diabetes
Royapuram, Chennai, India

Dr Noel W Solomons
Director
Center for Studies of Sensory Impairment
(CESSIAM)
Guatamala City, Guatamala

Dr Susan Steck-Scott
Department of Nutrition
University of North Carolina
Chapel Hill, North Carolina, USA

Dr Kamasamudram Vijayaraghavan
Senior Deputy Director
National Institute of Nutrition
Indian Council of Medical Research
Hyderbad, India

Dr Tommy LS Visscher
Department for Nutrition and Health
Free University
Amsterdam, The Netherlands

Dr Clive E West
Division of Human Nutrition and Epidemiology
Wageningen Agricultural University
Wageningen, The Netherlands

Dr Petro Wolmarans
National Research Programme for Nutritional Intervention
Medical Research Council
Tygerberg, South Africa

Dr Amy Yaroch
National Cancer Institute
Division of Cancer control and Population Sciences
Bethesda, Maryland, USA

Dr Agneta Yngve
Karolinska Institutet
Unit for Preventive Nutrition
Department of Biosciences at Novum
Huddinge, Sweden

1
An Overview of Public Health Nutrition

Barrie M Margetts

Key messages

- Public health nutrition is the promotion of good health through primary prevention of nutrition-related illness in the population.
- Public health nutrition builds on a foundation of biological and social sciences, depends on epidemiological evidence and involves the development and implementation of programs to improve and maintain health.
- Performance as a public health nutritionist requires a specific set of knowledge- and skill-based competencies

to implement all stages of the public health nutrition cycle.
- It is essential to develop appropriate knowledge, attitudes, understanding and professional skills to practice as a public health nutritionist.
- An appreciation and critical evaluation of the impact of research on the practice of public health nutrition also needs to be developed.

1.1 Introduction

The knowledge base underpinning the public health nutritionist professional is developed over years and built on a foundation of biology, biochemistry, physiology and basic nutritional sciences, as well as an understanding of social anthropology. The development of the foundations is not within the scope of this book. Many of these competencies are covered in the accompanying textbooks, particularly the *Introduction to Human Nutrition* and *Nutrition and Metabolism*. The aims of this book are to cover the skills needed in public health nutrition and to provide a coherent structure to enable the reader:

- to identify nutrition-related public health problems relevant at the local, regional, national and international levels
- to identify causes of these problems
- to develop strategies to deal with these problems
- to evaluate the impact of these strategies
- to understand the process whereby research-based evidence provides a basis for the development of public health policy

- ultimately, to improve nutrition-related health by applying evidence to action to solve problems.

Public health nutrition is about applying knowledge to the solution of nutrition-related health problems. Often when confronted with a problem, people do not know where to start, become lost in the detail, and sometimes miss the obvious and simple critical steps that will really make a difference. In this introductory chapter an attempt is made to provide a framework for the reader to think logically and systematically: to provide a template to proceed in a logical and systematic way. People often want to jump in with what they think is the solution to the problem confronting them; the aim here is to help readers to think before they jump. It is now fashionable to talk about an evidence-based approach to public health. All this really means is finding out what others already know, putting aside one's prejudices, assessing the situation objectively, and coming up with the best and most effective solution. It may seem obvious, but there is no need to fix that which is not broken. Rather, the effort should be to try to identify the key rate-limiting step (or major constraint to behavior) in the causal pathway and fix that. Our knowledge as to what the rate-limiting step is can never be perfect, so some judgment is required. However, the more systematically the evidence is gathered and reviewed, both in terms of the causal pathway and in terms of effective interventions, the more effective the effort will be in achieving the targeted health gains. The aim of this book is to give the student the knowledge and skills to think clearly about how to solve problems. The primary purpose of good nutrition is to maintain health and well-being. Nutrition is more than the food supply: it reflects the interaction between what we eat, and the metabolic demands of the body to maintain functional capacity. The basic, underlying and immediate causes of malnutrition are summarized in Figure 1.1. If nutrition is only thought of as the supply side of this balance this is likely to lead to a misunderstanding of the key

rate-limiting steps that link good nutrition to well-being. It is also important to consider the social as well as the biological context within which individuals live and interact in society. While it is beyond the scope of this text to cover all aspects of whole-body integrated metabolism, some understanding of the underlying mechanisms that link diet and style of living to health is required to understand whether the lifestyle changes that are being suggested to improve health make sense biologically. Inevitably, good nutrition-related health is about understanding the relationships between the biological and sociological context within which individuals live and interact in society. Where food supply is limited there is a clear biological imperative to obtain enough to eat; where supply is in excess, social imperatives that restrain or limit behavior come into play. In all societies, especially those in transition, there is a complex mix of problems of overnutrition

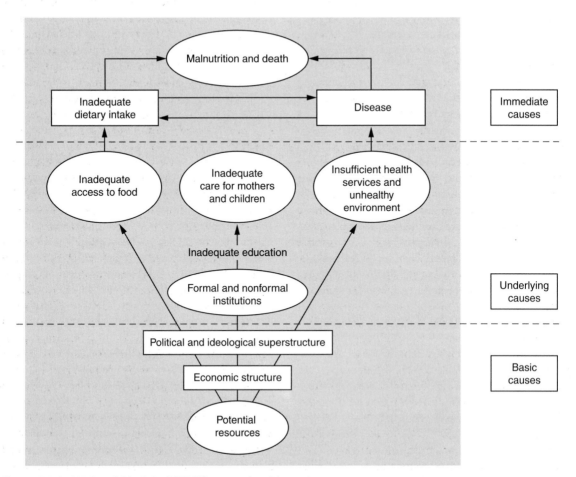

Figure 1.1 United Nations Children's Fund (UNICEF) conceptual model.

and undernutrition occurring in close proximity. The job of the public health nutritionist is to try to understand this complexity and to provide guidance as to what is best for most people. This book aims to help students in this task.

1.2 Organization of the book

There are 22 chapters in this book. The first eight chapters are designed to develop the skills required to understand how to identify and subsequently to develop approaches to address the major nutrition-related public health problems. Chapter 2 on nutritional epidemiology addresses the skills required for the design of appropriate studies, for conducting nutritional surveillance and the development of research protocols. It also reviews the analytical skills required in the use of nutritional and other relevant data and databases including the statistical issues, sampling study size and power, determination and application of appropriate statistical analytical techniques. Chapter 3 defines and describes the tools used to assess nutritional status at the individual and population levels. The emphasis in Chapter 3 is on assessment of dietary intake. Chapter 4 describes the methods and approaches used to assess physical activity. Nutritional status embraces an understanding of the dynamic between supply and demands, and increasingly it is becoming clear that, particularly in terms of understanding energy balance, it is essential to assess both intake and expenditure, and factors that affect both. Identifying the problem is only the first step in solving the problem; Chapters 5 and 6 describe the approaches to developing effective interventions in groups and individuals, respectively and Chapter 7 describes how to develop and present dietary guidelines that communicate dietary advice in the most sensible way possible, once it is clear what is the required or optimal nutritional pattern or profile. There is considerable overlap in the approaches used, broadly, the aim should be to use that approach which is most effective for most people, or different approaches for different groups if there appear to be different constraints in subgroups. Understanding the constraints on behavior and factors affecting food choice is the subject of Chapter 8.

Chapters 9–14 describe different aspects of malnutrition. Chapters 9 (overnutrition) and 10 (undernutrition) describe the development of aspects of what might be termed macronutrient malnutrition, while Chapters 11–13 describe specific micronutrient malnutrition deficiencies. Increasingly, it is becoming clear that undernutrition and overnutrition occur in different groups of people in the same countries, and that macronutrient and micronutrient imbalances can occur in the same people. Chapter 14 describes the complex area of eating disorders, which lead mainly to undernutrition of both macronutrients and micronutrients, but with different causes, and tending to affect different groups within a society, from those described in Chapters 9–13.

Chapters 15–18 describe different aspects of maternal and child health; Chapter 15 focuses on aspects of cognitive development, Chapter 16 focuses on the importance of infant feeding, Chapter 17 focuses on adverse outcomes of pregnancy in relation to folate and related B-group vitamins, and Chapter 18 describes the concepts that underpin fetal programming. Taken together, these chapters highlight the importance of achieving the optimal nutrient supply at the critical time to enhance and maintain function. This may be considered a key part, or first step of a life-course approach, recognizing that what happens after certain critical events is constrained by these earlier events and interacts with current behavior. Current health and well-being cannot be fully explained by current behavior alone, and early events (programming, early exposure) influence the way in which an individual and society react to what appears to be the same exposure. This may be described as explaining the sources of heterogeneity within a population, which may be also a mix of different levels of the expression of genes, gene–nutrient and nutrient–gene interactions.

Chapters 19–22 describe the main chronic disease that affect large numbers of people around the world; Chapter 19 describes cardiovascular diseases, Chapter 20 diabetes, Chapter 21 cancer and Chapter 22 osteoporosis. Already these chronic diseases affect more people in developing than in developed countries, and it is likely that this will increase as the nutrition transition continues in developing countries and rates of chronic diseases decline in developed countries.

There is no specific chapter on communicable or infectious diseases; the impact of these is covered extensively in the chapters on undernutrition. The aim has been to use major health problems as a way of illustrating approaches and ways of thinking that should help the reader to think about how to understand and address specific problems.

1.3 Definitions used in public health

Public health nutrition

A public health nutrition approach focuses on the promotion of good health (the maintenance of well-being or wellness, quality of life) through nutrition and the primary (and secondary) prevention of nutrition-related illness in the population. Public health nutrition is built on a foundation of basic and applied sciences, operates in a public health context, and uses the skills and knowledge of epidemiology and health promotion. The World Health Organization (WHO) defines health as a state of complete mental, physical and social well-being, and not merely the absence of disease or infirmity. Public health is defined as the collective action taken by society to protect and promote the health of entire populations. Alternatively, it can be defined as the art and science of preventing disease, promoting health and prolonging life through the organized efforts of society. Epidemiology provides a rigorous set of methods to study disease occurrence in human populations.

Public health

The approach to public health may be summarized as being either broad or narrow (Table 1.1).

The narrow approach

The narrow approach focuses on disease prevention and cost containment, with health defined as the absence of disease. The underlying theory is that the way in which individuals live their lives (what they eat, what they do, whether they smoke or drink or engage in risky behavior) is the main cause of disease, and that the motivation to change behavior is based on reducing risk at an individual level. The evidence base comes from clinical and molecular epidemiology; research is

undertaken that identifies differences in risk factors, and on the basis of that information, advice is given to the public that if they change their behavior they will reduce their risk of developing the disease (cancer or heart disease, etc.). This approach links an individual's own behavior to risk of disease. The burden of prevention and health promotion lies with the individual and it is seen as their responsibility to address their risk behavior. The approach is aimed at identifying immediate and obvious problems now and addressing them now. The disadvantage of the narrow approach is that it may miss fundamental threats within society that may be outside the individual's control (basic and underlying causes such as the wider socioeconomic factors, education and access to services, environmental factors, and the overarching values in society).

The broad approach

The broad approach defines health as more than the absence of disease. It considers well-being in terms of mental and physical health and also includes a sense of having some control over your life. The approach links public health science with policy: the action and structures agreed by society aimed at improving and maintaining health. The underlying theoretical model is sociocultural; it focuses on the wider environment and seeks to understand the factors that enable individuals to make healthy choices, or inhibit them. The motivating concern is about addressing the underlying sociostructural factors such as poverty, global issues and structures at a local, regional, national and international level that affect health. The evidence base for a broad approach comes from epidemiology as well as other approaches more suitable to exploring the sociostructural context. The broad approach takes a more long-term view of causes and solutions, addressing

Table 1.1 Different approaches to public health

Characteristics	Broad	Narrow
Major public health activities	Link public health science with policy	Cost-containment, disease prevention
Place of epidemiology	Balanced by other methods	Clinical and molecular epidemiology
Advantages	Long term, global	Short
Disadvantages	Risk of failure because of breadth	Miss fundamental threats
Define health	Foundations for health	Absence of disease
Underlying theory	Sociostructural	Lifestyle
Motivating concerns	Inequalities, poverty, global	Individual risks

structural issues in society that make it more difficult for individuals to make optimal choices. The disadvantage of a broad approach is that because the approach is so broad it may never address the key rate-limiting steps in a timely manner.

The broad public health approach has been taken up and developed by UNICEF into a conceptual model. The UNICEF model is now widely used, at least in research and development in developing countries[1] (this term is used in the sense of gross domestic product, rather than social and cultural development, and is not meant to imply a hierarchy or judgment about better or worse than a developed country) (see Figure 1.1). This conceptual model acknowledges that while the immediate causes of undernutrition may be a lack of food, often coupled with a high burden of infection, the provision of adequate education and health care has an important impact on health. The provision of these underlying factors is determined by basic causes such as the resources that are available in a society, and decisions about how these resources will be used. The model acknowledges that dealing only with the immediate causes will never lead to long-term improvements, which are dependent on the societies' view as to how resources will be used and distributed in society to maximize the health and well-being of all members of society. These arguments do not apply only to developing countries; how governments prioritize the use of taxation is a function of the underlying values of the society (as expressed through the election of governments that reflect the popular view); for example, the balance of spending priorities between education, health and defense, or priorities for agricultural policies that subsidize farmers but not manufacturing industry. Policy decisions as to the priorities on spending are complex and reflect a balance of tensions and pressures that often pull in different directions. Policy will be discussed in more detail later in this chapter.

In reality, in most countries there is a recognition that a narrow (individual and immediate cause oriented) approach needs to be balanced with addressing, at least to some extent, the basic and underlying (broad) causes. Most governments acknowledge that there are differences in health outcomes in different sectors of society and that state resources should be used to try to redress these differences. The food supply is regulated in all countries, even if the regulation is restricted to issues of food safety. Many of the first efforts in public health were about developing regulations to protect the public against the adulteration of staple foods. It has always been recognized that freedom of choice does not operate in a vacuum. Many countries have regulations about the accuracy of information contained in labels. There are few countries where the government does not intervene in the food supply to some extent, either through legislation to recommend the fortification of foods or to subsidize the production of some foods, such as in the Common Agricultural Policy in Europe and farming subsidies in the USA and elsewhere.

In developing a public health perspective it is important to balance the narrow with the broad. Striking the right balance is difficult and influenced by philosophical and political considerations. As a public health nutritionist, when trying to solve a local or national problem, it is important that both the narrow and broader determinants of behavior are considered and that it is not assumed that knowledge and individual choice are all that matters.

Recently, the UK Faculty of Public Health has agreed the key concepts that underpin public health. These reiterate to some extent the debate about broad versus narrow approaches to public health (Box 1.1). The key issues are a population approach to promoting and protecting health and well-being. They also highlight the importance of information.

Epidemiology

Nutritional epidemiology underpins Public Health Nutrition. This is covered in Chapter 2. It provides a

---

[1]The preferred terminology for developed and developing countries is North and South, or low, medium and higher income groups.

Box 1.1 Concepts that underpin public health

- Surveillance and assessment of the population's health and well-being
- Promoting and protecting the population's health and well-being
- Developing quality and risk management within an evaluative culture
- Collaborative working for health
- Developing health programs and services and reducing inequalities
- Policy and strategy development and implementation
- Working with and for communities
- Strategic leadership for health
- Research and development
- Ethically managing self, people and resources

Reproduced with permission from the UK Faculty of Public Health.

scientific basis for the development of the evidence upon which public health action can be implemented. It also provides guidance on the approaches as to the best way to evaluate and monitor the effectiveness of programs designed to improve health. Epidemiology is the only setting in which it is possible to ask questions about what factors affect processes in the whole population. The questions that are asked in epidemiological studies need to emerge from metabolic and clinical research; it is important to have some sense of the underlying mechanisms and processes involved in the way the body seeks to maintain optimal function. It is also essential to understand that the biological processes that maintain functional capacity in humans do so in a wider context. As mentioned above, epidemiology is not the only source of information essential to a public health perspective.

Health promotion

Health promotion is defined as any process that enables individuals or communities to increase control over the determinants of their health. The Ottawa Charter for health promotion (www.who.int/hpr/archive/docs/Ottawa.html) outlines an internationally accepted framework for health promotion that includes five approaches:

- building healthy public policy
- creating supportive environments
- developing the personal skills of the public and the practitioners
- reorienting health services
- strengthening community action.

Figure 1.2 summarizes Beattie's model of health promotion. This model further highlights the implications of the different underlying philosophical basis of public health discussed above. The two axes of the level at which promotion operates (individual to group/society) and the approach (authoritative to negotiated) highlight the range of options available. Often a range of approaches will be used. The key point is to use the approach that is going to be most effective and sustainable. In order to be effective, it is important that the strategy to be used has been shown to be effective in the target group, and that it addresses the most important constraints or rate-limiting steps, be they knowledge, attitudes, access or intentions. Understanding what the rate-limiting step is requires an understanding of the balance of factors that affect why

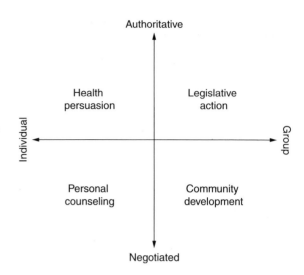

Figure 1.2 A model for health promotion. Reproduced from Beattie (1981) with permission from Thomson Publishing.

people eat what they eat (see Chapter 8). In some circumstances, a legislative approach, which requires no action at the individual level, may be the most effective way to achieve the desired health gain. A simple example is the decision to fortify flour in the USA with folic acid (see Chapter 17).

Nutbeam and Harris (1999) have summarized the theoretical models that underpin a health promotion approach. It is beyond the scope of this chapter to review all the models and theories described, and they are covered in more details in Chapters 5 and 6. The main point to emphasize here is that at whatever level one operates, there is a theoretical model that has been developed and should be considered as a basis for organizing the planning of work. A summary of models relevant for the different levels at which health promotion works is shown in Table 1.2.

A health promotion planning and evaluation cycle has been described and involves seven steps:

- problem definition
- solution generation
- resource mobilization
- implementation
- impact assessment
- immediate outcome assessment
- outcome assessment.

For all but the last step in the cycle, theories have been developed as to how to perform each step most

Table 1.2 Summary of models relevant for the different levels at which health promotion works (from Nutbeam and Harris, 1999)

Area of change	Theories or models
Theories that explain health behavior change by focusing on the individual	Health belief model Theory of reasoned action Transtheoretical (stages of change) model Social learning theory

Theories that explain change in communities and community action for health	Community mobilization:
	    Social planning
	    Social action
	Diffusion of innovation

Theories that guide the use of communication strategies for change to promote health	Communication for behavior change Social marketing
Models that explain changes in organizations and the creation of health-supportive organizational practices	Theories of organizational change Models of intersectoral action
Models that explain the development and implementation of healthy public policy	Ecological framework for policy development Determinants of policy making Indicators of health promotion policy

effectively: to identify targets for intervention; to clarify how and when change can be achieved in targets, and how to achieve organizational change and raise community awareness; to provide benchmarks against which actual can be compared with ideal programs; and to define outcomes and measurements for use in evaluation. The precede–proceed model is another way that has been used to encapsulate the steps in a health promotion cycle and this will be described in more detail in Chapter 6. These ideas have been taken and used as a basis for the development of the public health nutrition cycle, which is described in more detail later in this chapter.

1.4 What are the key public health problems?

The chapters in the latter part of this book cover in detail the public health problems that have the greatest public health impact. Here, the aim is to give a broad overview of the overall balance of global nutrition-related health problems, and to highlight, in particular, the double burden of both overnutrition and undernutrition that many transitional countries suffer (Figures 1.3–1.6, Table 1.3; http://www.who.int/whr/previous/en/). Data are presented in two ways, which are important to distinguish; Figures 1.3 and 1.4 present the proportion of deaths attributable to each major cause, whereas Figure 1.5 and Table 1.3 show the

absolute numbers of deaths or disease burden. From a public health perspective the total burden of disease gives a sense of the demands placed on the health services and infrastructure. Figure 1.3 and 1.4 show the burden of infectious diseases in developing countries compared with developed countries; Table 1.3 shows the high burden of human immunodeficiency virus (HIV) and acquired immunodeficiency syndrome (AIDS) in sub-Saharan Africa. Although cancer, as a percentage of overall deaths, is lower in developing than developed countries, in absolute terms (Figure 1.4) more people die of cancer in developing countries. In Africa and south-east Asia (Figure 1.5) the burden of communicable diseases is high, compared with Europe; in south-east Asia the burden of noncommunicable diseases is nearly as high as communicable diseases and is also higher than in Europe. The higher burden of cancer in developing countries may be a function of both a higher underlying incidence and poorer case finding and treatment (owing to limited access to health facilities). The impact of HIV on overall mortality and life expectancy is illustrated in Figure 1.6, which shows that in a number of African countries life expectancy has actually fallen since the late 1980s, after a steady rise from the 1950s to 1985.

In addition to the burden of death and disability the burden of chronic undernutrition is heavy in many developing countries. It is a stark figure, but 14 000 children die every day from malnutrition-related

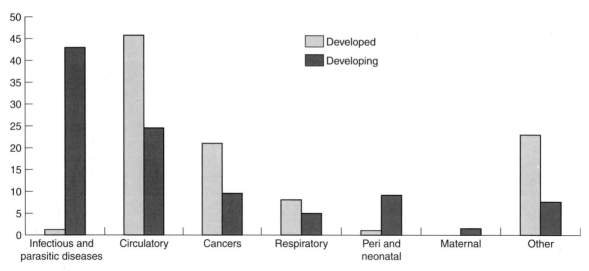

Figure 1.3 Percentage distribution of causes of death. Reproduced with permission from the WHO. (http://www.who.int/whr/previous/en/).

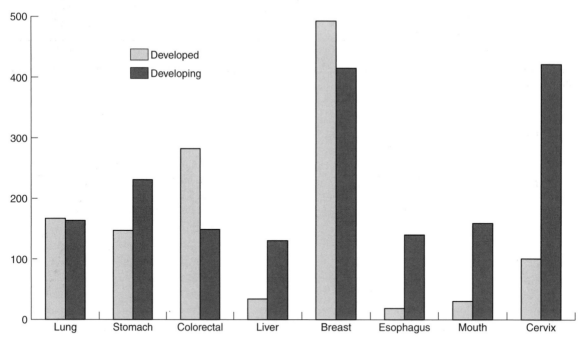

Figure 1.4 Burden (number per 1000) of cancer in developed and developing countries (women). Reproduced with permission from the WHO. (http://www.who.int/whr/previous/en/).

causes. Among those who survive, the effects on growth and development are profound and long-lasting. A quarter of all babies born in south Asia weigh less than 2500 g at birth (UNICEF, http://www.unicef.org/statis/2001). In India (44%) and Africa (29%) many children are underweight, while the proportion of the adult population becoming obese is also rising. Food insecurity continues to be a major problem for many people around the world, and not just in developing countries (see http://www.euro.who.int/ Nutrition for European data and http://www.nlm. nih.gov/pubs/cbm/nutritionsummit.html#51 for US

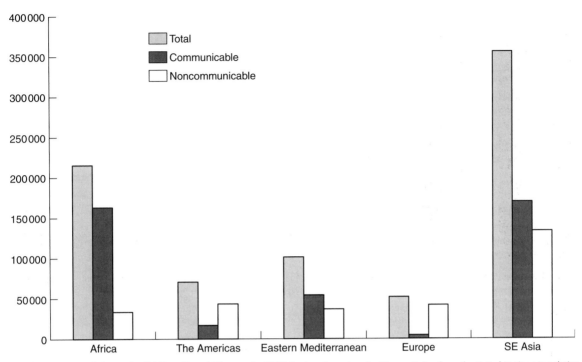

Figure 1.5 Burden of disease in diability-adjusted life-years by WHO Region. Reproduced with permission from the United Nations Population Division. (http://www.who.int/whr/previous/en/).

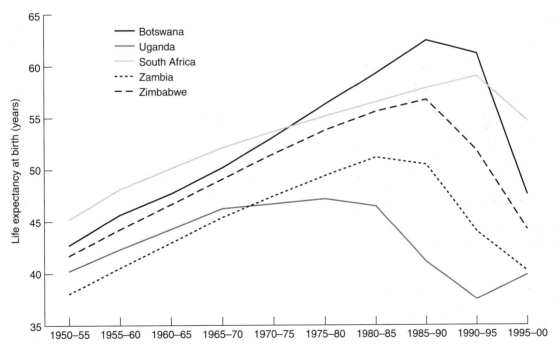

Figure 1.6 Changes in life expectancy in selected African countries with high HIV prevalence, 1950–2000. Reproduced with permission from the United Nations Population Division.

data). The Food and Agriculture Organization (FAO) provides a great deal of information about the nutrition situation in most countries (http://www.fao.org/es/esn/nutrition/profiles_en.stm). More details about the burden of undernutrition are covered in Chapter 10.

The double burden of problems of communicable and noncommunicable diseases, related to malnutrition (overnutrition and undernutrition) in the widest sense, was extensively described by Popkin (2002), who summarized the stages of the health, nutritional and

Table 1.3 Leading causes of mortality in sub-Saharan Africa, 1999

Rank	% of total
1 HIV/AIDS	20.6
2 Acute lower respiratory infections	10.3
3 Malaria	9.1
4 Diarrheal diseases	7.3
5 Perinatal conditions	5.9
6 Measles	4.9
7 Tuberculosis	3.4
8 Cerebrovascular disease	3.2
9 Ischemic heart disease	3.0
10 Maternal conditions	2.4

Reproduced with permission from the WHO.

demographic transitions (Figure 1.7). Many countries in the developing world have subpopulations in different stages of these transitions, which makes national data difficult to interpret. The complexity also places a particular burden on health services with limited resources.

1.5 Food and nutrition policy

Nutbeam and Harris (1999) highlight that a key area for achieving change is to understand where policies come from, so that they may be influenced to address a particular problem. Policies develop in a dynamic way that is influenced by many factors, one of which is the scientific evidence (Figure 1.8). Although an individual public health nutritionist may feel that it is outside the scope of his or her capacity or job to be able to influence policy, it is important to have a sense of what factors and forces influence policy. One of the aims of his chapter and book is to give a sense of where individual public health nutritionists fit into the grand scheme of things, and that there is actually a bigger picture. This does not mean becoming a lobbyist and involved in policy, but to recognize that policies are developed that influence the priorities in society that

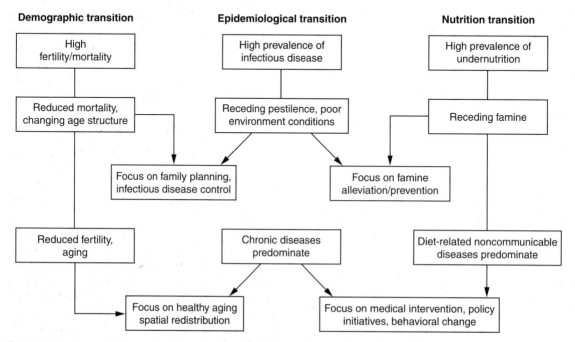

Figure 1.7 The stages of demographic epidemiological and nutrition transitions in public health nutrition. Reproduced from Popkin (2002) with permission from The Nutrition Society.

affect the work of public health nutritionists and their capacity to do their job. It is important to separate out the process and principles of gathering evidence, and the subsequent judgment that arises from that evidence as to what to do or not do about what the evidence implies for health.

There are several key players in the development of policy:

- policy holders (usually government politicians)
- policy influencers (lobby groups representing vested interests)
- the public
- the media.

The key determinants of policy development are:

- the social climate
- identifiable parties that influence policy
- what the interested parties will gain from the policy
- the ability of those interested parties to make their voices heard.

A policy about a particular issue may or may not develop because the social climate is not right, there are competing interests or priorities, or the case has not been properly organized to justify the policy. In simple terms, politicians, who make policy, need to see that if they develop a policy it will achieve what they want and in a way that will give them the credit (or that works). In public health nutrition this means that to move policy in a way that we believe is desirable for improved health requires:

- that the climate is right for action around improving nutrition

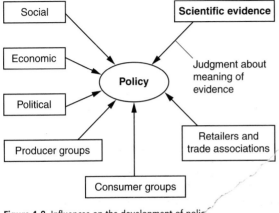

Figure 1.8 Influences on the development of policy.

- that the profession has its act together and can be effective in presenting its case
- that when asked it can deliver.

Without policy level commitment, it will be difficult to achieve change. It has been easier to gain support for policies around ensuring that the food supply is safe, and today most countries follow internationally agreed recommendations, mainly summarized in Codex Alimentaris. Policies about what to eat to maximize health are more complex than policies to ensure safety. Moreover, there is considerable debate amongst stakeholders and a wider range of vested interests that contribute to this debate, making politicians less likely to support nutrition policies related to health. Without policies that define goals and targets it is often difficult to mobilize support for action.

Food and nutrition policy

There is lack of clarity about the differences, and drivers for, food compared with nutrition policies. Food policy is concerned about how the food is grown and made available to consumers. It is mostly driven by concerns about agricultural practices and food production, manufacture and distribution. Nutrition policy is driven by a consideration of the impact of the food supply on health. A great deal more is written about food than about nutrition policy. From a public health nutrition perspective it should be clear that the primary question to be asked when considering policy issues is: "Will it make any difference to improving health, particularly in those with the greatest burden of poor health, usually the poorest in society?"

Advocacy and evidence-based policy

It is relevant to discuss briefly and to be able to distinguish between advocacy and evidence-based policy. Advocacy may be defined as the active support of an action or a cause and therefore an advocate is someone who upholds or defends that action or cause. Advocacy for a policy or action is usually based on a mix of values, beliefs and judgments that the course of action or policy is the right thing to do. The extent to which it is supported by evidence may depend on the underlying beliefs of the advocate. It is important that a clear distinction is drawn as to where the evidence stops and where judgments based on other factors start. The decisions that are made in society and from which policies and action arise do not do so in a vacuum, and even if something appears to be obvious and important, this does not mean that it will be supported and implemented.

1.6 The public health nutrition cycle

Public Health Nutrition is about solving problems. A public health nutrition (PHN) cycle has been developed to help to achieve this aim (Figure 1.9). This cycle has been designed to identify the key steps required to develop a logical approach to the best way to go about solving problems. At each step in the cycle it is important not to lose sight of the purpose of the efforts and activity. Individuals or society should not be asked to change unless there is good evidence that that change will be beneficial. Producers and retailers should not be asked to change the food supply if that change is not going to improve health and well-being. The government should not be asked to develop policies and programs of work that will not benefit the health of the population. Programs of work should certainly not be recommended that increase inequalities within a society. In other words, whatever is done needs to have the most benefit for the most people in the most efficient way possible. This may involve a combination of approaches that combine a broad and narrow approach to health. Ideology should not be allowed to hinder doing what is best.

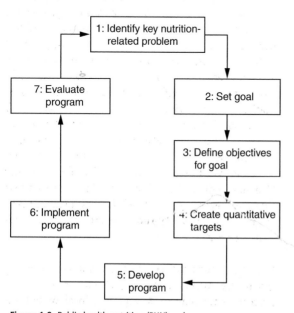

Figure 1.9 Public health nutrition (PHN) cycle.

The PHN cycle resembles a generic policy cycle. Several international organizations and governments use the "Triple A" (AAA: assessment, analysis and action) planning cycle (e.g. UNICEF and the South African Department of Health).

The Triple A cycle has a number of steps:

1. Assessment: situation analysis; identify problems and select opportunities for improvement (Where are we now?)
2. Define the problem operationally (Where do we want to go?); goals, indicators and objectives.
3. Identify who needs to work on the problem.
4. Analyze and study the problem to identify major causes.
5. Develop solutions and action for quality improvement (How will we get there?)
6. Implement and evaluate quality improvement efforts (How do we know when we arrive?)

The PHN cycle is used here to encapsulate an iterative, continuous process that starts from an identification of the public health problems in a population (be it local, national or regional level) and leads to a program of work that is designed to solve the problem. Progress through each step in the cycle should be evidence based. This includes an evidence-based approach to target setting, program development and evaluation. This cycle provides a helpful guide through the related but various aspects of public health nutrition. Sections 1.7–1.13 describe the seven steps involved in the PHN cycle.

1.7 Step 1: Identify key nutrition-related problem

The purpose of public health nutrition is to solve problems. Therefore, one should start by checking what the key nutrition-related problems are within the relevant area of work or country. The following questions should be asked before proceeding to action.

What are the big public health problems in your country/region?

Consider how to answer this question. What information is needed? Is this information available at the required level?

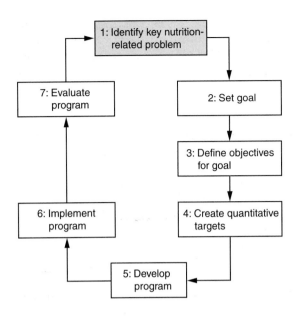

Measuring health and quality of life, mortality and morbidity, incidence and prevalence

International agencies produce a great deal of data that can be used to give some indication of the burden of poor health in a country. These data are generally freely available on the world wide web. Routine data have been most widely available for overall mortality, or broad groupings of causes of mortality, for most countries. These estimates, which are compiled centrally, are based on locally collected data and caution must be exercised in drawing conclusions from such data. Ideally, estimates of health burden should be derived using data from high-quality, purpose-specific surveys. Routine data on morbidity are much less readily available than data on mortality. If one is interested in a specific cause of illness (morbidity) or death, in some countries there will only be limited data from which to assess whether it really is a public health problem. Incidence data give an indication of new cases emerging over a particular time-frame, whereas prevalence estimates are a function of the underlying incidence and the duration of the illness. For many chronic diseases the estimates of the incidence and prevalence of mortality will be adequate. For infectious diseases with a short duration, incidence data will be required.

In some countries when a person dies a death certificate, with underlying causes of death, must be signed by medical practitioner. However, in most developing countries, particularly in remote areas, when a person

dies very often the underlying cause of death is not recorded by a medical practitioner and therefore may not be noted. It is important when comparing countries to be aware that differences may be attributed to differences in the way data are obtained. Always check the assumptions before using routinely collected data.

The WHO in its World Health report in 2002 used healthy life expectancy (HALE) as a summary measure of the level of health (www.who.int/whr/en). Although there have been several similar composite measures of health in the past, the universal use of HALE – calculated centrally by means of standard methodology using internally consistent estimates of levels of health – is a major advance. HALE is designed to be sensitive to changes over time and differences between countries in the overall health situation. Nevertheless, HALE based on self-reported health status information may not always be comparable across countries, owing to differences in survey instruments and methods, differences in expectations and norms for health, and cultural differences in reporting health.

In 2003 the WHO launched the Surveillance of Risk Factors related to noncommunicable diseases (www. int/mediacentre/factsheets/2003/fs273/en/). This lists all available data for eight risk factors: tobacco and alcohol use, patterns of physical activity, low fruit/vegetable intake, obesity (body mass index), blood pressure, cholesterol and diabetes (blood glucose), broken down by age groups and gender for all member states. The data are available on a compact disk, which includes details of the study populations and methods used to gather the data for each country. Appendix 3 of the report lists the data available by country. Of the 46 countries listed in Africa none has data on all eight risk factors: South Africa and Seychelles have information on seven risk factors, and only Nigeria and Cameroon have data on diet. In Europe data on all eight risk factors are available for 10 out of the 51 countries. In the Americas data for all eight risk factors are available for Brazil, Canada, Chile, the USA and Uruguay. India is the only country in south-east Asia that has data on all eight risk factors. Data are presented with a measure of the uncertainty of the estimates for each member state.

Specific groups affected: age, socioeconomic group, geographical region, ethnic group

National data may mask regional, local or within-household variation. If the burden of poor health falls only on a subsector of a society it is important to know because this may influence the approach to solving that problem. Data are rarely available in sufficient detail (and with power) to be certain about exactly which subgroups are most at risk.

Evidence-based review of link between nutrition and the problem

If one believes that there is a problem, the next stage is to check whether there is any evidence that links nutrition to that problem. This requires a systematic review of all available evidence and a critical appraisal of the studies. From a public health perspective the aim of this review is to identify nutrition risk factors for which the evidence is sufficiently strong and consistent to suggest a casual relationship and therefore justifies action. This review should also identify whether the risk is in all groups, or only in specific subgroups, either because of specific nutritional factors that only operate in that group, or because there are other basic or underlying differences that may confound or interact with nutrition.

It is a good idea to check whether government or some other agencies have already reviewed the evidence and made some specific recommendations about changes in diet and activity. Even if the nutritionist's review does not agree with these recommendations, it is important to know what has been recommended.

Developing critical appraisal skills is an essential part of developing a scientific approach to evidence-based public health nutrition, or any other aspect of research. The checklist in Box 1.2 may be useful to begin with.

Are the nutrition risk factors identified relevant to the target population?

Does the research identify levels of consumption that may be harmful or beneficial? Can the risk estimates be translated into consumption levels?

Often, the epidemiological study will present an estimate of the risk associated with one level of consumption compared with another. This is known as a relative risk of, for example, consumption in the highest third of intake compared with the lowest third of intake. It is not always presented in absolute terms. For example, the risk of colon cancer may be 0.5 in those in the highest third of vegetable consumption compared with those in the lowest third, but this does not

---

Box 1.2

- Are the study aims clear and precise in terms of the question being asked?
- Have they described the methods used to:
  - assess main exposure measure (e.g. weight, food intake energy intake, attitudes)
  - assess main outcome measure
  - assess other variables?
- Have they told you anything about the validity of the measures used?
  - information bias
  - social desirability bias
  - relevant time-frame.
- Have they described how they derived the sample?
  - sampling frame
  - response rate
  - selection procedure.
- Have they described interview or data collection standardization?
- Have they presented the data (tables) in a clear way?
- In their discussion have they been objective about the strengths and weaknesses of their study design?
  - Have they thought about the impact of what went wrong in the way they did their study?
  - Be very skeptical if the authors claim that they did a perfect study: no such study exists.
- Do their conclusions reflect the results presented?

---

indicate how much vegetable consumption there is in each third. What is more helpful is a measure of the population attributable risk; this gives a sense of the likely impact on health if the population changed their exposure from the lowest to the highest third of intake. The public health impact also depends on how common the health outcome is: if it is common a small reduction in risk will affect many people; if it is relatively uncommon, even a large relative risk will have only a small impact on the population burden of ill-health. Ideally, the targets for intervention should be those exposures that have the biggest effect on health, and on health problems that place the biggest burden on the target society.

What is the level of consumption in the target population?

If individual country level data are not available from either routine surveillance or specific studies, a crude estimate of average intake can be made from food balance sheet data, produced for all countries by the FAO. The FAO data are crude in that they are a measure of the gross movement of food moving into and out of a country divided by the population. Both the numerator and the denominator may be inaccurate in many countries. These data will give an estimate that may be useful, but will not give data about variation within a country or for individual levels of consumption. Where more detailed individual-level data are available, the concern will be as to whether these data are collected from a representative sample of the target population. If the epidemiology suggests that a particular group of people is at risk, are the data available relevant for that at-risk group?

Is consumption within the range that suggests possibility for beneficial change?

If the level of consumption in the target population is already above the level considered beneficial, then there is no need for a program to try to improve consumption. It may be that at a national level consumption appears adequate, or at least availability may seem adequate, but that the specific target group of interest does not achieve the national average. If the target group is below the desired level (from the epidemiological evidence) it is important to ask why. Is the supply rate limiting or is it some other aspect of the sociostructural environment?

Is it plausible that level of consumption could change from the current level to the level suggested to convey benefit?

In public health terms the estimates of risk need to be translated into levels of consumption. If, for example, the level of consumption associated with a 50% reduction in risk was 10 servings per day, and the average daily consumption in your target population was one serving per day, is it realistic to expect a 10-fold increase in consumption? It may be helpful to look at trends in intake and assess whether, and by how much, they have changed over the past 10 years. If intake has been relatively flat, and particularly if there have been many campaigns aimed at increasing intake, it is unlikely that big changes can be achieved. However, if a change of one serving a day could lead to a 5% reduction in risk, and if the risk (outcome) affects many people, then this level of change may still be very worthwhile trying to achieve. It is important to be realistic and to consider the cost–benefit of the effort required to achieve the desired change in the diet and ultimately the health outcome.

Theoretical models of relevance

At this stage it may help to begin to think about what the major constraints to change might be. The relevant theories to consider at this stage may relate to individual beliefs about the proposed intervention, social norms, or issues of institutional or societal organizational practices. If the evidence suggests fundamental changes in dietary practices in society, it is important to consider whether the social, cultural and political environment is likely to be amenable to the changes that appear to be required.

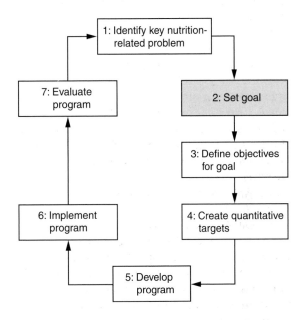

1.8 Step 2: Set goals and broad aims

Unless there are clear goals and broad aims it will not be possible to measure the impact of any programs aimed at improving health. It should be clear that the aims of public health nutrition programs are to improve nutrition-related health outcomes. The success of programs against this quantitatively defined background of work should be judged. No matter how programs may appear to be delivered, the key measure of impact is a measurable change in health outcome.

These goals inform and direct government policy at the highest level. These are the broad statements that politicians sign up to and use to argue for fiscal support and political leverage to achieve them. They need to be clear and concise and integrated into the overall health and other relevant policies of the government. They set the tone of the approach and highlight the government's priorities. The way in which these goals are achieved will vary depending on political ideology, but they are an essential first step in gaining political support.

The economic circumstances of a country play an important part in the priorities that a government places on health in general, and within the health budget on the emphasis on preventive versus curative services. In most countries preventive services only receive a small proportion of the overall health budget, even though politicians will say that prevention is important. These broad aims signal the political commitment required to leverage support for the programs aimed at improving health.

From the review of the major public health problems affecting the target population, is it possible to define a broad goal, such as reducing coronary heart disease (CHD) or cancer by 20% by 2010, or reducing the infant mortality rate from 55 to 30 in the next 10 years in rural Kenya or maternal mortality from 10 to 5% in Nigeria, or gender-specific regional variation in cancer death rates by 20% by 2010. Achieving these broad goals may only be partly determined by nutritional behaviors, and it is important to recognize what other factors may also need to be addressed to allow better nutrition to have an effect on these hard endpoints. For example, if the underlying incidence of disease is the same in two centers, differences in death rates may still occur because of differences in rates of survival associated with different health service provision.

1.9 Step 3: Define objectives

Having defined the goal, the next step is to identify the key factors that are known to be important determinants, and sources of variation in, the goal within the target population. Nutrition, or food intake, may be only one of a number of objectives that need to be defined and addressed to achieve the goal. The point of highlighting nutrition objectives is to ensure that they are not lost alongside other objectives that may have more political leverage, such as provision of services or more treatment centres. At this level the nutrition objectives may be broad, such as to encourage people to eat a healthy diet, increase physical activity or improve household food security. For example, the goal may be to reduce maternal mortality; one objective to achieve this may be by increasing household food security, while another may be to reduce the burden of infectious diseases or to control parasitic infections.

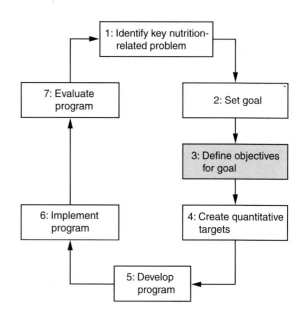

For the goal of reducing CHD or cancer mortality the objectives may be: improve access to health services, reduce serum cholesterol, reduce blood pressure, reduce obesity, increase physical activity, and increase fruit and vegetable intake. Nutritional issues may be relevant to more than one of these objectives and, if so, it will be important to ensure that a coherent and coordinated approach is adopted to address all objectives in as efficient a way as possible.

The goal must be measurable and able to be monitored over time to assess change. If the goal is subgroup specific it will be important to be sure that data are available at that subgroup level.

1.10 Step 4: Create quantitative targets

Having defined a range of objectives, the next step is to develop a specific target for each nutrition objective. There may be a number of targets that could be set for each objective. One must decide which are most likely to be achievable, and for which ones there is evidence to show that if that target is achieved it will make a difference to the objective and thereby the goal. There is a need to balance ambition with reality in setting targets. Although it is sensible to think about a wide range of targets, it may be better to be realistic about what can be achieved within the required time-frame and with the available resources. Targets need to be expressed in such a way that they can be measured with

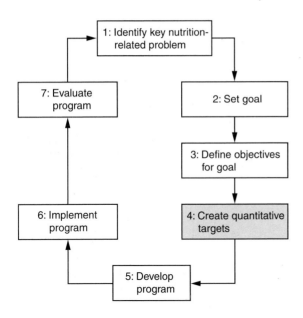

the required accuracy for the purpose of group- or population-level assessment. Without measurable targets it will not be possible to evaluate whether the target has changed. Even if the target is achieved, it may not lead to the expected change in the objective and goal, because other factors that also influence the objectives may have changed adversely. If these potential confounding factors are also assessed, it may be possible to disentangle which factors have caused which changes. It is therefore essential to be able to measure the targets at baseline and after the intervention (program) to be able to show whether the target has been achieved. It is important to consider whether the monitoring tools are available to measure change in the target population.

Targets need to be specific to facilitate evaluation, but also to make it easier to consider the program options that may adopted to achieve the target. The objective of encouraging people to eat a healthy diet needs to be reduced to the key components of what is considered a healthy diet for the target audience ("healthy" may differ in different groups at different times); for example, increase fruit and vegetable intake by 100–300 g/day or eat 15% more whole-grain cereals. The target may focus on one key aspect of a healthy diet, or even a single nutrient (such as folate, iron or vitamin A) because this may be most likely to be achievable, and also to have the greatest impact on health. The following series of questions regarding these targets needs to be addressed.

How to define these targets?

From the evidence-based review, it should be possible to identify which aspects of diet will have the greatest impact on health in a target population. From the review of dietary patterns and considering the local practical environment, it is essential to define quantitative targets. It may be unrealistic to set the international recommendation of 400 g/day of fruit and vegetables as the target, when current consumption is around 250 g/day and has not changed by more than 10% over the past 10 years. If the aim is to increase intake by 150 g/day in 5 years, but this is not achieved, the program may seem to have failed, but if the aim is to increase intake by 10% (from 250 to 275 g/day), although this is modest it may be more achievable and may still be a worthwhile improvement. It is also important to consider whether the target is to increase the average consumption by shifting the distribution in the whole population, or whether it is aimed at increasing consumption only in those with the lowest level of consumption. This distinction is rarely made and may have series implications for developing interventions. The constraints on behavior in the lowest consumers may be different from those in higher consumers. If a whole-population approach is used, there must be no risk of already high consumers exceeding upper safe limits. For many nutrients there is evidence of a U-shaped relationship between consumption and risk; too little or too much is not good for you, and there may well be a narrow optimal range. Another potentially important issue is whether the background nutritional status of the population influences the requirements for nutrients. For example, when an underweight woman becomes pregnant are her nutrient requirements different to those of a normal weight woman? Do wasted or stunted children have different nutrient needs to well-nourished children, with or without infections? Here the issue may be to make sure that things are not made worse for a subset of the population while trying to improve another section of society.

Are the targets clear and achievable?

Is it possible to be clear as to exactly which foods need to be changed? If the objective is to reduce saturated fat intake from 13% energy from fat to 11% energy from fat, what will this mean for changes in food patterns? What are the main sources of saturated fat in the diet of the target population, how feasible is it to change those foods, and what impact will these changes have on other aspects of diet? It would not be sensible to alter dietary patterns to reduce saturated fat intake, but in so doing to reduce the intake of fiber or micronutrients, which would then lead to an increased risk of other problems. If dietary patterns are being targeted, there is a need to ensure that all relevant health outcomes (good and bad) are carefully considered. The area of food-based dietary guidelines and their development is covered in Chapter 7.

If the target is to increase fruit and vegetable intake, it may be important to consider which fruits and vegetables to target; this may depend on the underlying nutrients contained in those foods that are thought to be important. It may be that the whole food is thought to be the key exposure. Which fruits are locally available or which can be imported and at what cost? Not all fruits and vegetables contain the same nutrients.

The guidance to increase olive oil consumption, if followed through by the whole population, would exceed the current capacity to grow olives. A similar problem may exist for targets set for long-chain n-3 polyunsaturated fatty acids, where fishing quotas are falling. If demand exceeds supply price tends to rise and this may limit consumption in the target group.

Over what time-frame are the targets set?

These need to be realistic. The steps involved in achieving the required change need to be carefully considered. If the aim is to increase fruit consumption by one serving a day in schoolchildren within a 1 year period, what has to be in place to produce, distribute and deliver this amount of fruit? Is there enough fruit available, is it available for those who have the worst intake and therefore are in greatest need of an increase, and what impact will this have on price (will the fruit be given away)? If fruit intake does increase, how long will it take for that increase to lead to changes in measures of health and well-being (school performance, blood pressure, etc.)?

Can the targets be monitored?

Can the required changes be monitored with sufficient accuracy to be able to measure the real underlying trend? If, for example, the aim is to increase fruit consumption by one serving a day, and the methodology used to measure fruit intake is not able to differentiate one from two servings a day, it will not be possible to measure any true underlying change.

Unless the targets are quantitatively clear and realistic within a defined period it will not be possible to assess whether the changes have been made, and ultimately whether these changes have led to improvements in health. The more clearly all of the above issues are considered in setting targets the more likely these targets will inform a program of work that can be most effective. Specific targets help to focus attention on the best ways to achieve change, discussed in step 5.

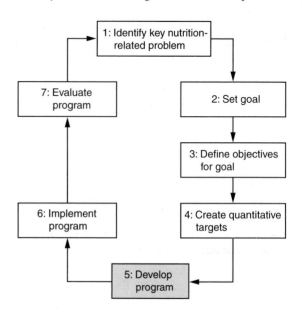

1.11 Step 5: Develop program

Once clear and quantitatively precise targets have been set, the next step is to consider the most effective approaches to achieve these targets. All potentially relevant options need to be considered, with the pros and cons of each weighed up before making the final decision on the approach(es) that will be taken. There is the temptation to try to do too many things at once; although this may seem sensible it may waste a lot of time and effort on activities that have no real benefit.

In developing a program of work, one should:

- identify determinants
- assess risk benefits or likely impact
- assess needs/constraints in society
- identify appropriate theoretical models
- identify and appraise options; decide what to do
- choose indicators for evaluation.

Each of these issues will be considered in the following section.

Identify determinants

What are the key factors that determine current patterns and where are the rate-limiting steps to success? It should not be assumed that lack of knowledge about healthy eating is the key and/or only determinant of behavior. If the target is to increase folate intake to 400 μg/day in the whole population, all the options must be considered; it should not just be assumed that the best way to achieve this is to tell people which foods are a good source of folate. The constraints on behavior that affect the target group should be considered. For example with folate, the aim would probably to increase intake in those with the lowest levels of consumption. Why, at present, does this target group eat a low-folate diet? It may be a combination of income and availability, attitudes to folate-rich foods, cooking skills for folate-rich vegetables, and so on. The constraints may change from time to time and may be dynamic depending on competing priorities. The precede–proceed model groups the factors that may constrain or influence behavior into three levels:

- predisposing
- reinforcing
- enabling.

These will be discussed more fully in Chapter 6. The point to note here is that if circumstances in the target community limit that group's ability to act on what is being put in place to achieve the target, they will not be able to achieve the target, even if they want to. The following are illustrative examples, rather than complete and exhaustive facts; one needs to think about a specific target and consider the options for that.

If the target population is not eating enough of the target food or nutrient, ways to increase consumption by changing the food supply should be investigated. The steps from the farm or producer to the consumer's plate need to be considered. The steps will differ for different people in different countries; most people living in large urban centres will not grow their own food, and so will depend on others growing and bringing the food to a place where they can buy it. Whether a person eats enough of the target food or nutrient will depend on the food being affordable and available (accessible). Government policies may subsidize certain foods for certain sectors of society. In broad terms, there is theoretically more than enough food available in most countries, provided people have the income to pay for it. If the food supply is not locally available, even if people have the money to buy it, it is usually because of dramatic external factors such as war or political unrest, which should not last. In other words, it is important to consider the chronic constraints, and not only think about acute constraints, although acute can become chronic if not addressed. War or conflict in many countries is chronic and disruptive to the poorest in those countries; sustainable solutions to nutrition-related health problems will be unlikely in a politically and economically unstable environment.

The way in which the food is processed may be a major constraint on an individual making informed choices about, for example, the fat, salt or sugar content of a food or ready-prepared/packaged meal. The majority of salt in the diet comes from processed foods, and discretionary use of salt at the table only affects about 10% of total intake. This may vary in countries where people eat meals that are prepared at home from raw ingredients.

For people who grow and eat their own food, the factors influencing consumption will be quite different from those who buy their foods. Constraints may be more about the amount and type of food that is grown, availability of land, labor, seeds, water, fertilizer and so on. All the factors that influence production and access need to be considered. If the food is grown, there may not be enough fuel or water to prepare the food properly or there may be some complex social issues within families whereby there is a hierarchy of access to food and those at the bottom of this hierarchy may not have enough food.

For people in most countries the availability of food, at least in urban areas, is left to market forces within a broad legislative framework. It is assumed that supply will equal demand, and that price will reflect this balance. However, on a global level trade is not free; many countries, usually the most affluent, have some form of tariff protection to protect within-country producers from cheaper imports from outside. The governments of most G8 (the richest and most powerful eight countries) countries distort the international markets, and this usually has a detrimental effect on producers from poor countries, which in turn affects local producers and consumers. The terms of international trade favor rich consumers and producers at the expense of poor consumers and producers (see http://www.christianaid.org.uk/g8evian/). If food supply is rate limiting it is probably more at this level, rather than in simple terms of lack of physical production worldwide. For more information about the World Trade Organization refer to http://www.wto.org/english/thewto_e/thewto_e.htm. See also the Organization for Economic Cooperation and Development (http://www.oecd.org/EN/home/). For a more critical review of subsidies and tariffs read Millstone and Lang (2003).

For some targets the way in which food is processed may have some adverse effects on consumption of specific targets in the at-risk population. For example, much of the fat removed from milk is added back into the food chain in cakes and biscuits or other products. Retailers now have enormous power in terms of the market share they control, and they can use this power to force producers to alter their production processes. A large proportion of foods sold in supermarkets are now "own brand" products made to the retailers' recipes. Recent years have seen a growing range of "healthy" products available. These products often have a price premium. Does this mean that these products lead to "healthy" changes in consumption? If a retailer approach to changing intake is to be considered, it will be important to assess whether the target population would eat the food, and if they would, whether they could afford the new foods.

With more meals being prepared and eaten away from the home in economically more affluent countries, the consumer has less control over the composition of the diet. There may be advantages and disadvantages in this from a public health point of view. The preparation of food at fewer places provides opportunities to control the nutrient supply in the diet, for better or worse. Programs aimed at reducing the salt content in the diet require that manufacturers reduce the amount of added salt, particularly in staple foods such as bread.

If the target is to increase the intake of certain foods, then at some point it is essential to ensure that the right foods are locally available. A reliable and affordable supply is necessary. Supply, however, may not be the main constraint on behavioral change.

Fortification and supplementation

When should the use of fortification or supplementation be considered? Fortification is a potentially attractive approach that requires no conscious involvement by the consumer; the consumer may not even know that they are eating a food fortified with nutrients. There are at least two important points to consider: what substances should be added, and to which foods? It cannot simply be assumed, for example, that the benefit of a diet high in fruits and vegetables is because of the vitamin C or carotenoid intake, at least without clear evidence. One of the difficulties in selecting which nutrients to add is that in most dietary patterns there is a complex mix. The other issue is which food to use as the vehicle; it must be reliably available to the target audience and an affordable price, and it must be possible to add the nutrients in a form that is both stable and biologically active when prepared and consumed in the normal way.

There is a long history of food fortification, although consumer acceptability varies greatly around the world. In some countries no foods are allowed to be fortified, whereas in others there is a liberal approach to their use. In some countries there are laws requiring some foods to be fortified. Iodized salt has had a beneficial effect on the prevalence of goiter in many countries. Problems have arisen, however, when the supply has been irregular or where iodized salt is more expensive than uniodized salt.

If the target is to increase intake substantially (e.g. of folate from 200 to 400 µg/day) it may be difficult to construct a diet that meets this level without substantially altering the whole dietary pattern, particularly if the target group is a low-income group and unlikely to achieve the changes required. It may be worth considering the possibility of fortifying key foods to achieve the desired change. If a particular sector of society requires the greatest increase in intake, it will be important to select a food widely eaten by that target group, such as bread or the staple cereal. There is no point fortifying foods that are too expensive or rarely eaten by the target group. Another factor to consider in selecting the food is whether quality control can be maintained by the producer to ensure delivery of the required amount.

If fortification is considered it is necessary to ensure that there will be no adverse effects of excess consumption in subgroups who eat a lot of the fortified foods. One of the concerns with folate fortification has been the possibility of masking vitamin B_{12} deficiency, especially amongst the elderly. With careful prior thought, however, the cost–benefit of fortification can consider and monitor these potential adverse outcomes,

---

Box 1.3

- Education (knowledge attitudes, beliefs) and an adequate flow of information
- Economic and physical access
- Knowledge, attitudes and perceptions
- Skills
- Social and environmental factors
- Training for professionals
- Regulatory measures (labeling, fortification); are new regulations required?
- Economic measures (subsidy, price and taxes, import/export policies)

---

for example by checking vitamin B_{12} status in potentially vulnerable older men and women in the population to be fortified with folate (see Chapter 17).

Some people are philosophically opposed to fortification, arguing that if people have enough resources they can buy all the food they need to supply all the nutrients they require and so do not need to eat fortified foods. However, if a government makes the decision to fortify foods as the only practical option, and this substantially reduces disease, there is a wide societal benefit from that in terms of reduced health costs and improved quality of life, with no effort at an individual level.

Before deciding to develop a program of work that includes one or more of the components listed in Box 1.3 it is important to ask whether there is any evidence that it is important in affecting behavior. This list is not exhaustive but illustrative. It includes factors that operate at the individual level and others that operate at the societal level. The balance of the emphasis between the individual and societal approach is often determined by political ideology; different governments have different approaches: Rarely, however, is the approach either totally societal or totally individual.

Assess risk benefits or likely impact

Likely benefit or harm of intervention

Before implementing the program of work, it is important to make sure that the proposed changes will not have any harmful or adverse effects on diet or health. For example, if the target is to increase fruit consumption, will there be any foods that are displaced from the diet that may affect nutrient intakes adversely? It is important to consider when a dietary change is being made that it does not lead to any undesirable

changes in overall nutrient intakes. If dietary fiber intake increases will this lead to a reduction in the bioavailability of any micronutrients; if consumption of animal products decreases, iron intake may not be adequate. It is also important to consider whether any subgroups in the population may be adversely affected by the dietary targets. In the elderly, if appetite is decreased it is important to consider the nutrient density of the diet, and to ensure that they obtain enough energy. It is also important to consider whether the target group will eat the recommended foods; this may be affected by practical, mechanical factors, or by culture or beliefs.

Target most vulnerable

If a particular target group has been identified, will the proposed intervention reach that group? It cannot be assumed that an approach aimed at shifting the whole distribution of consumption will affect those at the top and bottom of the distribution in the same way.

Expected size of effect

It is important to consider what size of effect is realistic in the target population, and not to overestimate the impact of the intervention or to set unrealistic targets.

Potential to succeed

When all things are considered, how likely is it that the target will be achieved by the proposed program of work? If it is only, say, 10%, is this worthwhile? How is this judged?

Assess needs and constraints in society

Assessing needs

Although the scientific evidence may show a clear potential benefit for changing to the target, it is important to consider whether the target population has the same concerns and priorities. If the target group does not perceive that the target is important to them, it may be difficult to motivate them to change their behavior, even if all other conditions are optimal. Needs can be defined in different ways:

- normative: defined by experts according to their own standards
- felt: perceived by an individual or a community
- expressed: felt needs that have progressed to demand
- comparative: when a community sees a lack compared with another area.

When people are asked what their needs are they may not consider longer term preventive health benefits as being as important as improving local services and access to, for example, acute care. People are most concerned when they think someone else is doing something to them over which they have no control, so people are often unsure about the safety of the food supply, or about what manufacturers are doing to their food. When asked, people often seem to know what others should do to improve their diets, but do not think that they need to change their own behavior. This is known as optimistic bias. If the target requires individuals to cooperate the perceptions of need of the target population must be considered.

Potential constraints on achieving targets

The UNICEF conceptual model shows that many basic and underlying causes may make it very difficult for an individual to meet the target. There may be many factors over which they have no control that affect their ability to implement the changes required, even if they are very positive and know what changes they should make. The factors affecting food supply have already been highlighted, and the current focus is more on whether people have enough money to buy the food, access to shops, or control of choices over the food purchases made in the family.

Identify the appropriate theoretical model

This is covered in more detail in Chapter 6. The main point to mention here is that it is important to have a conceptual framework within which to develop the approach to the intervention. Put another way, it is important to be able to predict theoretically the key constraints in the target population, and to predict how the changes proposed are likely to be translated into effective action. Of all the potential determinants of behavior, which are the most important, and what is required to change them?

The recent report of the EURODIET project contains some very useful papers (www.eurodiet.med. uoc.gr). In particular, Yngve and Sjöström (2001) develop a clear framework for action in Europe aimed at achieving the breast-feeding target. They identified five levels of determinants:

- demographic attributes
- psychosocial attributes
- health-care attributes and biomedical constraints

- community attributes
- public policy.

The precede–proceed model was used to develop an understanding of the health promotion needs in the target population. The stages of change model has been used to characterize the readiness of individuals to accept or act on health promotion.

Deciding what to do

Having considered all the options, it is now time to decide what to do. The following may help in making the decision as to the approach to be adopted.

Identify decision-making criteria

- Effectiveness (efficacy helps to define what might work, effectiveness tells you what has worked in the past)
- feasibility
- acceptability
- cost.

Consider types of intervention that may be appropriate

- Policy (strategic level)
- programs aimed at individuals or groups that address key determinants in the target group
- programs aimed at agencies that address underlying causes such as food supply, access and availability issues (producers, retailers, government)
- programs aimed at addressing the basic causes such as poverty and inequalities.

Ultimately, the approach should be the most cost-effective and have the greatest impact on nutrition-related health. If a combination of approaches is required and can be adequately supported then this should be used.

Choose the indicators for evaluation

In developing a program it is important to identify the indicators that will be used in assessing the efficacy of the intervention, whereby any change or improvement can be directly attributed to the intervention.

1.12 Step 6: Implementation

Step 5 enabled a program of work to be selected that is believed to be most likely to deliver the target established in Step 4. The next step is to implement this

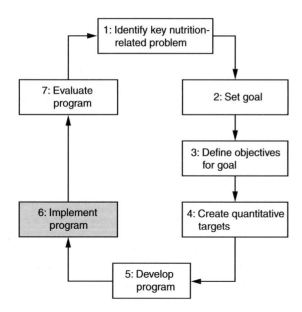

Factors that need to be considered before implementation of a program can begin

- Take account of the social and political environment and its changes.
- Define and revise specific tasks and activities (deliverables and milestones) with time-frames, priorities for action, responsibilities.
- Determine resources and reporting requirements.
- Coordinate implementation.
- Ensure accountability.
- Learn from other experiences.
- Consider efficacy and effectiveness.

Project planning

In planning a project the following need to be considered:

- what needs to be in place where and when
- who needs to be recruited and trained to do defined tasks
- what equipment and resources are required,
- timelines and management of flow of activities.

It is important to make sure that where decisions are made there is political commitment to support the role of nutrition. In the development of any policy there will potentially be winners and losers, those with a vested interest. Therefore, there is a need to consider the following questions.

- Who may be affected?
- Who has knowledge?
- Who has previous experience?
- Who may be upset?
- Who will implement?
- Who will oppose?

These groups need to be informed and as supportive as possible of the objectives. There is increasing discussion about public–private initiatives to improve diet, but care needs to be exercised to ensure that vested interests do not manipulate the balance.

1.13 Step 7: Evaluation

The objective of evaluating the program of work is to provide information that can be used to judge whether the goal was achieved, and if not why not, or if so, under what conditions or at what cost. Evaluation provides information for policy and decision makers. The policy maker may require different information to the

program of work. The practical details of how the program will be delivered must be considered; a good idea may not work because it cannot be implemented. The planning of the implementation therefore needs to consider everything that needs to be in place to deliver the program, and to consider how to remove all the constraints to effective implementation. Even if the program is very carefully developed, unexpected or unforeseen factors may hinder progress. Another, unrelated program may be implemented at the same time, the budget may be cut because of a change in government, or staff may become sick and cannot be replaced. A step that is often neglected is gathering all the stakeholders together and agreeing or exploring their views as to what will or will not work; the researcher may not agree with some of their views, but it is important to understand the drivers for all those who can influence the success of the program.

Some things cannot be planned for, but it is always a good idea to anticipate the worst things that could happen and work out how to deal with them before they happen. Some of these are summarized in Box 1.4.

Develop budget

What will the project cost? Staff, equipment infrastructure and all costs involved in setting up and delivering and evaluating the program must be considered.

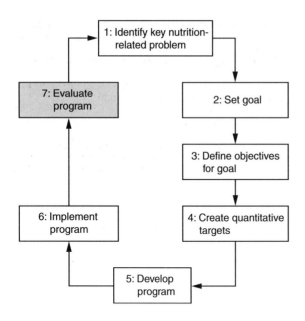

public health nutritionist. Evaluation may be broadly divided into: was the program delivered (process or formative evaluation, or may be called performance) and did it achieve the goal (outcome or impact evaluation)? Information will be required to evaluate both.

Habicht *et al.* (1999) have written a very helpful leading article that discusses how to design evaluations. Although it is well recognized that intervention programs should be evaluated, there is often too little money allocated to achieve the type of evaluation that is required; ideally, the approach to evaluating a program should be considered at the initial planning and budget development stage. One form of evaluation may be to ask the community members or leaders, or donor agencies what they think of the program.

The example in Box 1.5 is used to illustrate some key issues and from it the following lessons can be drawn.

- Goals are often easier to measure than targets; there are often systems in place to measure goals using health services or some government agencies (if they are still operating properly).
- Targets can be more difficult to measure; they may require trained staff to undertake specific field measurements.
- Process evaluation (was the program delivered?) is not the same (nor is it sufficient or acceptable to infer) as measuring outcome. Clear milestones and deliverables are required to measure whether the program is delivered.

Box 1.5

Set goal: to reduce maternal mortality from 10 to 5% in Zimbabwe in 10 years.

Define objective: to achieve this reduction in mortality by improving household food security.

Target: to increase the fruit and vegetable intake in the mothers from 160 to 240 g per day during pregnancy.

Develop program: develop a home vegetable garden.

To evaluate the program: we need to be able to measure maternal mortality with sufficient accuracy among all women to be able to see a 50% decline from 10% to 5%. This means that every time a woman gives birth someone must be able to record whether the woman died during childbirth or not, and we also need to know how many women give birth each year. Is there likely to be differential reporting and data gathering (rural bias, low-income and poor groups?) The target was to increase fruit and vegetable consumption during pregnancy: are routine data available on food intakes of women during pregnancy? Generally not, and certainly not for the whole population, so what should one measure? A number of different approaches to measuring intake should be piloted before rushing into any one method. From experience, a very important first step is to go to the community and talk to them about how they describe their diet and ways of cooking and eating. From this it may be possible to identify a number of key indicator foods that can be used to measure change in intake. Remember that the aim may not be to measure accurately individual intake, but to describe trends over time in groups of women, that is the aim is not always to be able to link intake (measures of the target) with a measure of the outcome as one might want to do in a controlled experiment. Although more detailed measures may be used in the pilot phase to check the method used in the main program, it is important to remember that the aim is to have a system that can work as part of some sort of routine activity, where there is not the same quality control that applies to a laboratory experiment. This does not mean that any old rubbish will do, but it does mean that the measure has to be simple and robust and reliable in the field.

   Did the program of work that was planned actually get delivered? In the example the question to ask is, were more home vegetable gardens developed, and did this result in the target women eating more vegetables? If the answer is no, it is important to identify where in the delivery process the program failed. Was it that there was no land set aside for the home gardens; did the women not have the skills or support to know how to grow the vegetables; did the vegetables get produced, but they were eaten by pests, or other people in the household; were they grown but sold for cash because there were other pressing needs within the household?

- If a program is not delivered, it cannot achieve the target; if a program is delivered, it still may not lead to the desired or expected change in the target or goal.
- It is essential to collect information on changes in other factors that may change during the delivery of the program that may undermine or falsely enhance the apparent effectiveness of the delivery of the program.

Further reading

Beattie A. Knowledge and control in health promotion: a test case for social policy, pp. 162–201. In: The Sociology of the Health Service, (Gabe J, Calnan M, Bury M, eds). London: Routledge, 1991.

Habicht JP, Victora CG, Vaughan JP. Evaluation designs for adequacy, plausibility and probability of public health programme performance and impact. Int J Epidemiol 1999; 28: 10–18.

Millstone E, Lang T. The Atlas of Food: Who Eats What, When and Why. London, Earthscan, 2003.

Nutbeam D, Harris E. Theory in a Nutshell: A Guide to Health Promotion Theory. Roseville: McGraw-Hill, 1999.

Popkin B. An overview on the nutrition transition and its health implications: the Bellagio meeting. Public Health Nutr 2002; 5: 93–103.

Yngve A, Sjöström M. Breastfeeding in countries of the European Union and EFTA: current and proposed recommendations, rationale, prevalence, duration and trends. Public Health Nutr 2001; 4: 631–645.

Website

Codex Alimentaris. www.codexalimentarius.net

2
Nutritional Epidemiology

Michael Nelson, Shirley AA Beresford and John M Kearney

Key messages

- Epidemiology deals with associations, analyzing strengths and seeing how specific they are. Nutritional epidemiology does not establish factual cause, but it can provide powerful circumstantial evidence of association.
- One of the aims of nutritional epidemiology is to disentangle the complex relationship between diet and disease to establish a relationship between the two.

- To optimize study design, it is essential to consult a statistician before proceeding with sample selection and recruitment.
- A key purpose of nutritional epidemiology is to inform public health nutrition, a population approach to the prevention of illness and the promotion of health through nutrition.

2.1 Introduction

Nutritional epidemiology is the application of epidemiological techniques to the understanding of disease causation in populations where exposure to one or more nutritional factors is believed to be important. Epidemiology aims to:

- describe the distribution, patterns and extent of disease in human populations
- understand why disease is more common in some groups or individuals than others (elucidate the etiology of disease)
- provide information necessary to manage and plan services for the prevention, control and treatment of disease.

Much of the focus of nutritional epidemiology has been on the elucidation of the causes of chronic disease, especially heart disease and cancer. However, the onset, development and expression of these diseases are complex, and the role of diet in the initiation of disease may be different from its role in the progression of disease. The dietary factors that contribute to the occlusion of an artery may not be the same factors that increase the acute risk of myocardial infarction. Disentangling these complex relationships is one of the aims of nutritional epidemiology.

Another important function of nutritional epidemiology is to evaluate the quality of the measures of exposure or outcome that are made. It is notoriously difficult to measure exactly how much food people eat or to determine the nutrient content of the diet. Determination of the severity of disease (e.g. the degree of blockage in the arteries of the heart) and measurements of physiological states (e.g. blood pressure) are also subject to inaccuracies. Extensive misclassification of exposure or outcome in an epidemiological study will seriously undermine the ability to determine diet–disease relationships.

A key purpose of nutritional epidemiology must be to inform public health nutrition, a population approach to the prevention of illness and the promotion of health through nutrition. Public health nutrition puts nutritional epidemiological findings into a wider social and ecological context to promote "wellness" through a healthy lifestyle, including good diet. A glossary of terms used in nutritional epidemiology is presented in Box 2.1.

Box 2.1 Glossary

Term	Definition
bias	Deviation of results or inferences from the truth, or processes leading to such deviation. Any trend in the collection, analysis, interpretation, publication or review of data that can lead to conclusions that are systematically different from the truth
case–control study	An epidemiological study that starts with the identification of persons with the outcome of interest and a suitable control group of persons without the disease. The relationship of an exposure to the outcome is examined by comparing the group with the outcome to the control group, with regard to levels of the exposure
causality	The relating of causes to the effects they produce. Causality may defined as "necessary" or "sufficient". Epidemiology cannot provide direct proof of cause, but it can provide strong circumstantial evidence
cohort study	An epidemiological study in which subsets of a defined population have been or may be in the future exposed to a factor hypothesized to be related to the outcome of interest. These subsets are followed for a sufficient number of person-years to estimate with precision, and then compare, the rates of outcome of interest
confounder or confounding variable	A variable that can cause or prevent the outcome of interest, is not an intermediate variable, and is associated with the factor under investigation
cross-sectional study	A study in a defined population at one particular period that investigates the relationship between health characteristics and other variables of interest
crude death rate	A crude rate is a simple measure for the total population. The crude death rate for a given year is the number of deaths in that year divided by the midyear count of the population in which the deaths occurred
ecological fallacy	The bias that may occur because an association observed between variables on an aggregate level does not necessarily represent the association that exists at an individual level
effect modifier	A factor that modifies the effect of a putative causal factor under study
exposure	Factor or characteristic that is a presumed determinant of the health outcome of interest
incidence	The number of new outcome events in a defined population during a specified period. The term incidence is sometimes used to denote incidence rate
incidence rate	Expresses the force of morbidity in a cohort of persons while they are free of the outcome. It is the number of new events during a defined period, divided by the total person–time units of experience over the period
misclassification	The erroneous classification of an individual, a value or an attribute into a category other than that to which it should be assigned. The *probability* of misclassification may be the same in all study groups (nondifferential misclassification) or may vary between study groups (differential misclassification)
morbidity	Any departure, subjective or objective from a state of physiological or psychological well-being
mortality	Death
odds ratio	An approximation of relative risk based on data from a case–control study
outcome	Identified change in health status
period prevalence	The total number of persons known to have had the disease or attribute (outcome) at any time during a specified period
person-years at risk	A unit of measurement combining person and time (years), used as a denominator in incidence rates. It is the sum of individual units of time (years) that the persons in the study have been exposed to the condition of interest
point prevalence	See prevalence
population	A defined set of units of measurement of exposure or outcome. The members of a population can be individuals or experimental units, e.g. schools, hospitals, doctor's surgeries, towns, countries
prevalence	The number of instances of a given outcome in a given population at a designated time (specified point in time)
quality-adjusted life-years	The product of length of life and quality of life score. A measure of the length of life or life expectancy adjusted for quality of life
quality of life	Quality of life may be used as a global term for all health status and outcomes including objective and subjective outcomes. In specific use it is an evaluation of one's position in life according to the cultural norms and personal expectations and concerns, and thus is inherently subjective

(Continued)

Box 2.1 (Continued)	
Term	**Definition**
rate	A rate is a ratio whose essential characteristic is that time is an element of the denominator. In epidemiology, the numerator of the rate is all cases or outcome events derived from the population at risk, during a given period. The denominator is the population at risk, as defined for the same period
ratio	The value obtained by dividing one quantity by another
relative risk	The incidence of disease (or other health outcome) in those exposed to the risk factor under investigation divided by the incidence of disease in those not exposed
sample	A sample is a selection of items from a population. It is normal practice to make the sample representative of the population from which it is drawn
sampling frame	A list of the items in a population from which a sample can be drawn

Based on John Last's "A Dictionary of Epidemiology".

Historical context

The history of nutrition as a science dates back just over 100 years. The history of nutritional epidemiology is even shorter. Observations of associations between diet and health date back to Greek times. In 1753 James Lind observed that British sailors who took fresh limes on long sea voyages escaped the ravages of scurvy, at that time a common cause of morbidity and mortality. This observation led to changes in practice (and the epithet "limeys" for British sailors). Systematic observation of populations did not become common until the mid-nineteenth century, and then focused more on infective than on chronic disease.

The understanding of the role of nutrients in deficiency disease gained ground early in the twentieth century with the discovery of vitamins and the acceptance that a lack of something in the diet could be a cause of ill-health. It was not until the second half of the twentieth century that an understanding of the role of exposure in chronic disease became well established, mainly through the model of smoking and lung cancer. In addition, complex multifactorial models of causation became better accepted. Statistical techniques and the advent of computers added a further boost to these disciplines by facilitating the disentanglement of complex exposures which often included causal elements that were correlated or that interacted. For example, the effects of vitamin C and other antioxidant nutrients on the risk of heart disease were difficult to disentangle from the effects of smoking, because smokers typically consume diets with lower levels of antioxidants and smoking itself increases the requirement for antioxidants.

A further boost to nutritional epidemiology was the clarification of the ways in which measures of dietary exposures were imperfect. What a person reported in an interview or wrote down about their consumption was not necessarily the truth. It had been recognized that confectionery and alcoholic beverages were regularly underreported (comparison of average consumption based on national surveys of individuals and national sales figures typically show two-fold differences). Other, more subtle misreporting of consumption took much longer to come to light. This was particularly true in the case of people who were overweight and who, on average, underreported their food consumption. This recognition of underreporting was one factor that helped to explain why the association between fat consumption and heart disease was observed internationally but not at the individual level. This issue of misclassification is discussed in detail in Section 2.4.

The most recent development in nutritional epidemiology has been the inclusion of genetic risk factors in models of causation. Genetic influences work in two ways: genes influence the ways in which nutrients are absorbed, metabolized and excreted; and nutrients influence the ways in which genes are expressed. It will be a challenge over the next 50 years to elucidate the role of nutrition-related genetics in the etiology of disease.

Measurements of exposure and outcome and how they relate

The aim of most epidemiological studies is to relate exposure to outcome. The epidemiologist must define exactly which aspects of exposure and outcome are believed to be relevant to disease causation or public health. In nutritional epidemiology, there will be a chain of events starting with the diet and ending with ill-health, disease or death. The principal tasks of the nutritional epidemiologist are to decide which aspect of dietary or nutritional exposure is relevant to the understanding of causation, and to choose a method of measurement that minimizes misclassification.

For some diet–disease relationships, this may be relatively straightforward. If there is a deficiency of a single nutrient (e.g. iodine) that is strongly and uniquely associated with an adverse outcome (cretinism in the offspring of iodine-deficient mothers), only one set of measurements will be required. Iodine intake, for example, can either be measured directly by collecting duplicate diets, or estimated indirectly by collecting 24 h urine samples (the completeness of which needs to be established). It is then possible to identify a threshold for iodine intake below which the risk of an adverse outcome increases dramatically.

Exposures relevant to the causation of heart disease or cancer, in contrast, are enormously complex. Not only is there a large number of possible dietary influences (energy intake in relation to energy expenditure, total fat intake, intake of specific fatty acids, intake of antioxidant nutrients, etc.), but different nutrients (and non-nutrients) will have different influences on disease initiation, progression and expression at different points in time. Moreover, many important non-nutritional influences (e.g. smoking, blood pressure, activity levels, family history/genetic susceptibility) will need to be taken into account when analyzing the results, and some of these factors (e.g. smoking and blood pressure) will have links to diet (e.g. high calcium intakes are associated with lower blood pressure, smoking increases the body's demand for antioxidant nutrients).

Causality

Central to the understanding of how diet and health outcomes relate to one another is the notion of causality. Epidemiology deals with associations, analyzing their strengths and how specific they are. Thus, nutritional epidemiology does not establish cause per se, but it can provide powerful circumstantial evidence of association.

Causality is often categorized as necessary or sufficient. Most communicable diseases, for example, have a single identifiable cause (a pathogenic bacterium or virus) that is responsible. Thus, it is both necessary (i.e. it must be present) and sufficient (no other factor is required). However, people do not catch a cold every time they are exposed to a cold virus. This is because other factors influence the ability of the virus to mount a successful attack. These include the state of the immune system, which in turn depends on a person's general health and (in part) their nutritional state.

A more complex example would be the risk of developing lung cancer. Smoking increases the risk, but not everyone who smokes develops lung cancer, and there are people who develop lung cancer who have never smoked. Thus, smoking may be sufficient but is not strictly necessary. There are other factors that can cause lung cancer (e.g. exposure to asbestos) and factors that may protect against the damage caused by smoking (e.g. a high intake of antioxidant nutrients).

Hill was the first to set out a systematic set of standards[1] for causality. Others have since elaborated Hill's work. The following have been considered when seeking to uphold causality.

Strength

Strong associations are more likely to be causal, while the converse is not always true (weak associations are non-causal). For example, the association between smoking and heart disease; it is more likely that weak associations exist either because of other factors that contribute to the presence of something as common as heart disease, or because there are undetected biases in the measurements that lead to the appearance of a spurious association, or because of confounding. Strong associations may also occasionally be explained by confounding. For example, low intake of fruit and vegetables is associated with short stature in children, but is explained by the effects of social class. "A strong association serves only to rule out hypotheses that the association is entirely due to one weak unmeasured confounder or other source of modest bias." (Rothman and Greenland 1998.)

Consistency

If the same association is observed in a number of different populations based on different types of epidemiological study, this lends weight to the notion of causality. Lack of consistency, however, does not rule out an association which may exist only in special circumstances.

---

[1]Rothman and Greenland note that Hill used the word "standard" and not "criteria" in order to avoid the temptation to calculate a score based on the number of criteria met as a way of determining the likely validity of the causal hypothesis.

Specificity

Hill argued that specificity was important (it certainly is in infection), but Rothman and Greenland regard the criterion as having little value in understanding diseases that may have multicausality because one exposure (such as smoking) can lead to many effects.

Temporality

It is presupposed that cause precedes effect. However, circumstances in which the suspected cause is present only after the outcome appears (e.g. markedly raised blood cholesterol levels after a myocardial infarction) do not mean that there may not be a role for the putative factor when measured in other circumstances.

Biological gradient

This is the dose–response criterion: as exposure increases, the likelihood of the outcome increases. Risk of lung cancer increases with the number of cigarettes smoked. Risk of heart disease increases with increased intake of saturated fatty acids. Not all relationship are linear across the range of exposure. Some relationships show a threshold effect: in sedentary societies such as the UK and USA, when calcium intakes exceed 800 mg/day, there is no obvious association with bone mineral density in postmenopausal women, whereas below 800 mg, there is a direct relationship. Even more complex is the J-shaped curve showing that moderate intake of alcohol (10–30 g/day) is associated with a lower risk of heart disease than either no intake or intakes above 40 g/day, where risk increases with increasing intake. Some of the explanation may be due to confounding.

Plausability

There must be a rational explanation for the observed association between exposure and outcome. Lack of a plausible explanation does not necessarily mean, however, that the association is not causal, but simply that the underlying mechanism is not understood.

Coherence

The observed association must not contradict or conflict with what is already known of the natural history and biology of the disease. It is the complement of plausability.

Experimental evidence

This refers to both human and animal experimentation in which the levels of exposure are altered and the changes in the outcome of interest are monitored. More often than not, however, the reason for undertaking an epidemiological study is that the experimental evidence is lacking. This is especially true in nutrition, where long-term exposures that may be responsible for the appearance of disease are virtually impossible to model in an experiment. Thus, the use of experimental evidence to corroborate epidemiological findings is usually limited to short steps in what may be a long and complex causal pathway.

Rothman and Greenland include "analogy" as a final criterion, but its application is obscure. Ultimately, causality is established through a careful consideration of the available evidence. If there is no temporal basis, a factor cannot be causal. Once that is established, however, the causal theory should be tested against each of the standards listed above. It should be kept in mind that confounding may be operating (e.g. children moved from inner cities to the countryside were quickly cured of rickets, supporting the bad air or miasma theories and not the notion of a missing vitamin or exposure to ultraviolet light).

Bias and confounding

Bias is defined by Last as:

> Deviation of results or inferences from the truth, or processes leading to such deviation. Any trend in the collection, analysis, interpretation, publication, or review of data that can lead to conclusions that are systematically different from the truth.

Bias can arise because of measurement error, errors in reporting, flaws in study design (especially sampling), or prejudice in the reporting of findings (the more conventional lay use of the term). Last describes 28 different types of bias that can arise. These relate to errors of ascertainment (not selecting a representative group of cases of illness or disease), interviewers (asking questions in different ways from different respondents), recall (how much respondents can remember) and so on. Most researchers work hard to identify likely sources of bias and eliminate them at every stage. Failure to do so will produce information that is misleading.

One of the most important sources of bias is confounding. Confounding bias leads to a spurious measure of the association between exposure and outcome because there is another factor that affects outcome that is also associated with the exposure. For example, there is a strong apparent association between consumption of alcohol and risk of lung cancer. However, people who drink are more likely to smoke, which in turn increases their risk of lung cancer. Thus, in a study of the effect of alcohol intake per se on risk of lung cancer, smoking is a confounding factor. Failure to take into account the effect of smoking will lead to a spurious overestimate of the effect of alcohol intake on the risk of lung cancer.

The two most common confounders are age and gender. Exposure (e.g. diet) changes with age and differs between the genders. Moreover, there are many factors such as hormones, body fatness and health behaviors that differ according to age and gender.

For any given study, the list of confounders may be very long. While it may be possible to match in study design for age and gender, matching may not be feasible for all other confounders. Modern statistical analysis facilitates the control of the effect of confounding. The important issue, therefore, is to make sure that all of the important likely confounders are measured with good precision.

A particular problem in nutritional epidemiological studies is that confounding variables are often measured with greater precision than dietary variables. As a result, there are fewer errors in classification of subjects according to the distribution of the confounding variables than the main dietary variables of interest. In sequential analyses, the apparently significant effects of a dietary factor often disappear when confounding variables are introduced. This may be due to genuine confounding of the dietary factor, or it may be that the effect of the dietary exposure is masked because of the greater precision of measurement of the confounding variable. For this reason, attention to the measurement of errors is critical in nutritional epidemiological studies.

Statistical interpretation and drawing conclusions

One reason that many students do not like epidemiology is the complexity of the statistical analyses and the difficulty of their interpretation. In the most straightforward designs, statistical analysis may be uncomplicated. Suppose that a researcher wanted to investigate the short-term benefit of using a cholesterol-lowering margarine on circulating cholesterol levels. An appropriate group of subjects (e.g. men aged 45–54 years with moderately raised serum cholesterol levels and no history of cardiovascular disease) could be defined; they could be divided into treatment and control groups and asked to consume on average 20 g of the margarine per day (giving them "treatment" margarine in one group and "control" margarine in the second group), and the change in serum cholesterol levels could be measured after 6 weeks. Anaylsis could be by unpaired t-test (if the subjects had not been matched, but the two groups were similar in composition) and a clear conclusion drawn.

Alternatively, if a researcher wanted to investigate the effects of polyunsaturated fatty acid intake on risk of heart disease in a case–control study, also in men aged 45–54 years, conditional logistic regression could be used to determine the odds ratio (the approximation of relative risk) and control for the effects of age, smoking, blood pressure, body size, adiposity, waist/hip ratio (WHR) and other aspects of diet (e.g. dietary fiber, cholesterol, saturated and monounsaturated fatty acids, antioxidant nutrients). How the outcomes are interpreted then depends on the familiarity of the researcher with the ways of expressing the results and the errors likely to arise within the measurements.

2.2 Types of study

Epidemiological studies

The science of epidemiology has taken the statistical tools of experimental design that were developed first in the area of agricultural experiments, and developed formalized systems for inference using other designs. These designs are not experimental, but mimic the principles of experimental design as closely as possible. One key principle is to compare like with like. Another principle is to set up the study so that inferences may be made back to the population from which the study subjects arose (i.e. that the samples are selected so as to make them representative of the population from which they are drawn). These key principles are often referred to as internal and external validity, respectively.

This general philosophy of avoiding bias in the interpretation of an exposure–disease association is put into practice by using appropriate techniques both at the design stage and at the analysis stage in an epidemiological investigation. Careful design can avoid many biases, and other potential biases can be adjusted for or controlled for in the statistical analysis.

The choice of study design is typically dictated by the nature of the research question and progress to date in addressing a particular question. New hypotheses or the search for a hypothesis can often be investigated initially using the ecological approach. Alternatively, a cross-sectional study carried out in a representative sample of the population can yield clues to associations. Once there is justification for a particular hypothesis, it is then appropriate to design a careful observational study that uses the principles described above. The choice will depend on the relative ease of constructing groups of people based on their exposure levels or on their disease end-points. If groups are based on exposure, the groups can then be followed forward in time until sufficient disease end-points have accrued (cohort study). If groups are based on end-points, retrospective information on prior exposures is obtained (case–control study).

Ecological studies

Ecological designs are so called because they often take the form of comparing regions of a country with other regions, or countries with other countries. This class of study also includes comparisons over time. Alternative names include indirect studies and population studies. The defining characteristic is that the average exposure for a study unit is compared with an average disease rate. If there is any variation about that average within regions or countries, there is a possibility that those exposed do not overlap with those diseased, in which instance false inferences (known as the ecological fallacy) might be drawn.

Geographical comparisons are often useful for obtaining clues as to the role of dietary factors in disease risk. For example, mortality rates from coronary heart disease and dietary fat calories using countries as data points were examined in several ecological studies. This led to cohort studies of fat and animal fat and coronary heart disease risk. In addition, studies have examined dietary fat and breast cancer mortality, and dietary fat and colon cancer mortality using the ecological method. In a careful study of fish consumption and risk of cardiovascular disease, three different periods were used to study correlations using data from 36 countries. Fish consumption data were obtained from food balance sheets collected by the World Health Organization (WHO) from 1980 to 1982 for each country. Age-standardized mortality rates per 100 000 per year, standardized to 45–74 years of age, were also obtained from the WHO, and averaged for the most recent 3 years. Considerable scatter was found about the regression line, but overall there was a significant inverse association ($p < 0.001$) between the log-transformation of fish consumption as percentage energy and the log-transformation of all-cause mortality.

Cross-sectional studies

Cross-sectional studies collect information on exposure and outcome from a common period. There is no way to state unequivocally that the exposure preceded the disease (or vice versa). The strongest design in this class is the cross-sectional design that is a census or representative sample from the population.

Cohort studies

Cohort studies are observational epidemiological studies that identify exposures in a defined population (that becomes the cohort), and then follows the cohort through time, identifying outcomes as they occur. They avoid the difficulties of recall bias that are suspected in case–control studies, but are very costly and extremely inefficient as a method for studying rare outcomes.

In a cohort study, subjects are measured at baseline for exposure to factors thought either to promote or to protect against disease (Table 2.1a). The subjects are then followed up over time. Naturally, not everyone who is exposed to the factor develops the disease. Conversely, some people who have not been exposed will get the disease. The incidence of disease in the exposed group is then compared with the incidence in the unexposed group. The comparison of the rates is known as the relative risk (RR). See Box 2.2 for an example of a cohort study.

Table 2.1 Design of (a) cohort and (b) case–control studies

		Diseased	Not diseased
(a) Cohort			
Exposed	Looking forward in time →	a	b
Unexposed		c	d
(b) Case–control		Looking backwards in time ↓	
Exposed		a	b
Unexposed		c	d

Box 2.2

In the Iowa Women's study, the cohort was defined as responders to a baseline survey that was mailed to a random sample of postmenopausal women. Dietary factors were assessed using a food frequency questionnaire, and women were followed for 11 years, recording incident cases of diabetes and other diseases.

Case–control studies

Case–control studies are unique to epidemiology, and are a clever and efficient method of comparing people with different outcomes with respect to their exposures. Some of the earliest case–control studies were those of lung cancer in relation to cigarette smoking. They are designed to use a retrospective method to mimic a prospective investigation (Table 2.1b). The principle is that people who have the disease of interest (cases) are assessed retrospectively for relevant exposures to causative factors, and compared for these same factors with people without the disease (controls).

The calculation of relative risk cannot be carried out directly based on case–control data because of uncertainties about the representativeness of the data on the unexposed group. For this reason, the relative risk is approximated by the odds ratio (OR). See Section 2.6 for more details about the calculation of the odds ratio.

The case–control study is a powerful design if conducted and analyzed carefully. Cases are identified within a defined population, in a reproducible fashion. The choice of a control or comparison group is a particular challenge, and dealing with confounding and interaction also needs to be done carefully.

This design is often used in studies of cancer, since the validity of the association measure rests on the rarity of the outcome. For example, this method was used in a study of rectal cancer and dietary factors including fat, carbohydrate, iron, fiber from vegetables, grains and some micronutrients.

Experimental studies

As was implied in the previous section, experimental studies provide the most powerful tool for making inferences concerning the relationship between exposure and outcome (dietary factor and disease). Experimental studies include those that are most rigorous, involving random allocation to one group or another, but also studies that intervene in one group and make comparisons with another group, or compare before and after the intervention.

Clinical trials

Rigorous experimental studies involving individual humans are called randomized controlled trials or clinical trials. Such studies cannot always be applied to answer a question, because the state of knowledge in

the area may not meet the accepted criteria, which include the following.

- There should be substantial evidence from observational studies that a hypothesized risk factor is associated with a disease outcome, but also that there is some indication of possible adverse effect such that a trial is necessary to sort out the balance of risks and benefits.
- The comparison group should receive no less than standard care, and the benefits to the intervention group should be expected to exceed the possible risks.
- Because of the powerful design, emphasis is placed on internal validity and the expectation that as many individuals randomized to the trial as possible will be followed to its conclusion. This leads to efforts to select individuals for the trial carefully, and run-in procedures are often used to assist in this choice.
- Consequently, participants may not be representative of a general population group in the same way as is attempted in observational studies. External validity is therefore less important.

The degree of selection of suitable individuals distinguishes what has been termed an efficacy trial (typically one in which the best possible conditions exist for detecting an effect of an intervention) from an effectiveness trial (in which conditions as close as possible to the real world are mimicked). An example of an efficacy clinical trial is given in Box 2.3.

Community trials

A natural extension of the effectiveness trial is the community randomized trial. In this design whole communities, or large groups of people, are randomized as community units. The group or community is the unit of randomization, and therefore also the unit of analysis. These trials are large and expensive to conduct. Interventions have to be sufficiently powerful to yield a measurable effect throughout the whole

---

Box 2.3

In the MRC trial of folic acid, multivitamins and neural tube defects, women who had experienced a neural tube defect-affected pregnancy who were interested in having another child were recruited. They were randomized to one of four groups and followed until they became pregnant and then throughout pregnancy. The four groups were folic acid supplement alone, multivitamin alone, both, and placebo. The rates of neural tube defects that occurred in each group were compared.

Table 2.2 Suitable dietary assessment methods to use for different types of study

Epidemiological study	Dietary assessment
Aggregate population/ecological	Food disappearance Household budget surveys Group estimates
Cross-sectional	Food records 24 h recall, FFQ Biochemical markers
Case–control	FFQ of present or past diet Diet history
Cohort	Food records 24 h recall FFQ Biochemical markers
Trial	Food records 24 h recall FFQ Diet quality indices Biochemical markers

FFQ: Food frequency questionnaire.

community for such a study to be worthwhile. Different statistical approaches are used to analyze these trials, including the use of linear mixed models which allow for the community unit and, within the community, the individual unit to be examined in the same model. An example of a community trial is shown in Box 2.4.

Nutritional measures in the context of epidemiological studies

As alluded to earlier, the assessment of dietary intake is subject to both typical and unique biases. In the context of epidemiological studies, nutritional measures need to be simple enough that they can be obtained in very large numbers of people, without imposing undue burden. For studies that are population based (the goal of all epidemiological studies), it is important that the requirement of assessing dietary intake does not in itself affect which people agree to participate in the study. Some candidate measures were designed to reflect current dietary intake (that may or may not be considered as a snapshot of usual diet), and some were designed to capture usual intake directly, sometimes even in the quite distant past. Measures commonly used in the different types of study are shown in Table 2.2.

2.3 Study design: sampling, study size and power

Once the research question has been posed and the basic design of a study appropriate to addressing that question has been decided upon, the next stage is to choose a sample. There are three basic questions that need to be answered:

- From which population is the sample to be drawn?
- How is the sample to be drawn?
- How big should the sample be?

The answers to these questions are neither obvious nor straightforward.

Choosing a sample

Populations and sampling frames
The first task is to define the population from which the sample is to be drawn. Although it is conventional to think of populations in terms of the people residing in a particular country or area, in epidemiological terms the word population means a group of experimental units with identifiable characteristics. Populations of individual people might be:

- all people resident in England and Wales
- members of inner-city families with incomes less than the 50% of the national average
- vegans
- male hospital patients aged 35–64 on general medical wards
- nuns.

Populations can also be defined in terms of groups of people. The population in an ecological study is typically a set of populations of individual countries or regions. The population in a community trial may be a set of primary schools or doctors' surgeries in a specified town or region, in which the measures of exposure may be based on catering records of food served (schools) or percentage of patients attending well-man or well-woman clinics (surgeries), and outcomes based on average linear growth (schools) or morbidity rates (surgeries). The imaginative selection of a population is often the key to a successful study outcome.

In case–control studies, two populations need to be defined. The cases need to be defined in terms of the population with the disease or condition that is being investigated. This population will have a typical profile relating to age, gender and other factors that may influence the risk of disease. The controls then need to be selected from a population that is similar in character to the cases. The key principle is that the risk of exposure to the suspected causative agent should be equal in both cases and controls. Potential confounders (e.g. age and gender) should be controlled for either in the matching stage or in analysis.

Once the population(s) have been defined, it is necessary to devise a sampling frame. This is a list of all of the elements of the population. Sampling frames may preexist as lists of people (telephone directories, lists of patients in a general practice, electoral registers, school registers) or other experimental units (countries with food balance sheet data). Some sampling frames are geographical (e.g. list of postal codes). Alternatively, they may build up over time and only be known retrospectively (e.g. patients attending an outpatient clinic over a period of 4 months), but the rules for their construction must be made clear at the outset.

Once the sampling frame has been defined, a subset of the population (the sample) must be selected. In order for the findings from the sample to be generalizable, it is important that the sample be representative of the population from which it is drawn. The underlying principle is that the sample should be randomly drawn from the sampling frame. In general, it can be argued that the larger the sample size, the more likely it is to be representative of the population. This will not be true, however, if the sampling frame is incomplete (not everyone owns a telephone and is listed in the telephone directory) or biased (older people with more stable lifestyles are more likely to appear on an electoral register or be registered with a doctor).

Once it has been established that the sampling frame contains the desired elements for sampling, a simple random sample may not necessarily yield the desired representativeness, especially if the sample is relatively small. To overcome this problem, some form of stratification or clustering may be appropriate. For

example, the sampling frame can be divided according to gender and age bands, and random samples drawn from each band or subset. This increases the likelihood that the final sample will be representative of the entire population. Moreover, if the aim is to limit the geographical spread of the sample, cluster or staged sampling is appropriate. For example, there may be four stages. At each stage, a random sample is drawn of:

- towns representative of all towns in a country or region
- postal sectors representative of all postal sectors within the chosen towns
- private addresses representative of all private addresses within the chosen postal sectors
- individuals representative of all individuals (possibly within a designated age and gender group) at those addresses.

This yields a highly clustered sample (making the logistics of visiting respondents much more simple and efficient) which in theory remains representative of the population as a whole.

In epidemiological studies generally, it is helpful to have a wide diversity of exposures to the causative agent(s) of interest. This maximizes the possibility of demonstrating a difference in risk of outcomes between those with high exposures and those with low exposures. However, if the diversity of exposure is associated with a confounding variable (e.g. gender or age), there may be too few observations in each subgroup of analysis to show a statistically significant relationship between exposure and outcome once the confounders have been taken into account. There are two ways to overcome this problem. The first is to generate a "clean" sample in which the influence of confounding is kept to a minimum. This can be achieved by having clearly defined inclusion and exclusion criteria when defining the population. For example, in a cross-sectional study of the effect of antioxidant vitamin intake on the risk of diabetic foot ulcer, it would be sensible to limit the selection of subjects to newly diagnosed patients who:

- are between the ages of 45 and 69 years
- have type 2 diabetes mellitus
- are nonsmokers
- have foot ulcers that are both neuropathic and ischemic (rather than exclusively neuropathic) in

origin, as this is more likely to include subjects in whom diet is a contributory factor.

While this selection process may limit to some degree the range of dietary exposures, it dramatically reduces the likely confounding effects of age, type 1 (versus type 2) diabetes, smoking, and nondiet-related causes of foot ulcer. It may also improve the quality of the dietary data collected by excluding subjects over the age of 70 years, whose ability to report diet accurately may on average be less good than in a younger group.

The second way to overcome the problem of too few subjects in a subgroup of interest is to choose stratified and weighted samples, as described in the next section.

Probability sampling versus weighted sampling

Subjects (experimental units) can be selected in a number of ways. In equal probability sampling (EPS), subjects are chosen in proportion to their number in the population (or, strictly speaking, in proportion to their number in the sampling frame). In staged geographical sampling schemes, the first stage (e.g. based on towns and villages) may involve making the probability of a town or village being selected proportional to the number of people who live there [probability proportional to size (PPS)]. While the aim in most studies is to generate a sample that is representative of the population from which it is derived (to improve generalizability), there may be a wish on the part of the researcher to investigate phenomena in a subgroup of the sample (e.g. investigating the relationship between diet and risk of heart disease in people of south Indian origin living in England, or examining access to health care amongst people who live in rural areas). In both EPS and PPS, however, too few observations may be collected in subgroups of special interest to facilitate analyses from which firm conclusions can be drawn.

To address this problem, it is desirable to carry out nonproportional sampling. Strata are defined according to the analyses of interest (e.g. by ethnic origin or locality). The number of subjects (or experimental units) to be selected is then determined not according to their proportion in the population, but according to the number of observations needed to have sufficient power to conduct analyses in specific subgroups. Random, representative samples of a specified size are drawn from each stratum. If the results from all of the observations in the study sample were used in analyses, the final results would not be representative of the population as a whole. Instead, they would be biased towards those groups who had been overselected (i.e. who were present in a higher proportion in the sample than in the population). To correct for this when generating results for the study overall, the results from each stratum would need to be weighted so that the results reflected the proportions of subjects in the strata in the population rather than their proportion in the sample.

Matching

The next approach to the problem of excessive diversity in the sample is to collect observations in a suitably matched control group (without the disease). This is a prerequisite of case–control studies. Cohort studies also include matching. In both case–control and cohort studies, the cases are defined according to the objectives of the study (e.g. people who develop colon cancer). The controls are then selected with matching for age and gender plus any key confounders (e.g. in the foot ulcer example above, a control group may be a group of diabetics matched for age, gender, smoking and the duration and severity of diabetes, but without foot ulcer). This allows for a broader range of cases to be included in the study. However, it introduces the problem of finding suitably matched controls. The more selection criteria there are, the longer it will take to find the controls. Thus, gains in terms of rate of recruitment of cases or diversity of exposure may be lost if the time taken to recruit controls increases substantially.

In epidemiological terms, the matching introduces bias into the sample selection. If the bias is focused exclusively on the true confounders (factors associated with both exposure and outcome, e.g. age and gender), this will improve the efficiency of the study (the ability to demonstrate exposure–outcome relationships) provided the confounders are taken into account in the analysis. The alternative approach is to allow for biases in a control group to be taken into account in analysis without having to match. This approach can be successful provided there is sufficient overlap in the characteristics between cases and controls (i.e. there are enough controls in each of the subgroups created by the stratification of the confounding variables in the cases). This is a risky strategy to follow, however. Failure to match initially may lead to situations in which (statistically speaking) there are too few controls in particular subgroups to permit adequate or statistically robust adjustment of confounders in analysis.

If the selection bias is associated with factors that are associated only with the exposure, this will lead to overmatching. Overmatching occurs when so many matching criteria are included (e.g. in the foot ulcer example, smoking and characteristics of diabetes, plus social class, religion, physical neighborhood, family doctor, marital status, etc.) that there is little scope for the controls to differ from the cases in relation to the exposure of interest. Controls are no longer representative of the population of people potentially at risk. The study then becomes focused on issues of individual (including genetic) susceptibility rather than population risk, and its value as an epidemiological study is reduced. If the selection bias is associated with factors that are associated with the likelihood of becoming a case, but not with exposure (e.g. proximity to a specialist referral center), this will have no effect on the estimates of disease risk, but may reduce the efficiency (and increase the costs) of the selection process for controls.

The efficiency of case–control and cohort studies increases substantially if between two and four controls are selected for each case. This is because the control group becomes increasingly representative of the population and true case–control differences are more likely to be revealed. The more complex the selection of the controls, the more the efficiency gains are eroded. The efficiency gains typically plateau above four controls per case.

Determining study size and number of observations

Even if issues concerning study design, sample representativeness and matching of controls have been properly addressed, a study may still fail to yield statistically significant findings for two reasons:

- there are too few experimental units
- there are too few observations within each experimental unit.

Both of these problems relate to diversity of measurement. The first is related to diversity between subjects. The second is related to diversity within subjects.

The number of items in the sample must be sufficient to estimate the true variability of the exposures in the population. If there are too few respondents, for example, the standard error of the mean ($s/\sqrt{n}$) will be large and s (the best estimate of the population variance σ) may also be an overestimate. It may thus be difficult to demonstrate that the mean of the observations in one group is statistically different from the mean in another group. A similar problem arises in relation to analysis of proportions (chi-squared analysis), and regression and correlation (showing that the coefficients are statistically significantly different from zero). Provided that the sample is not biased, increasing the number of subjects or experimental units reduces the size of the standard error and increases the likelihood of demonstrating statistically significant relationships, should they exist. It is worth noting the corollary of this premise also: if a sample is biased, increasing the sample size will not yield results that are representative of the population and the results may therefore be misinterpreted. Thus, a large biased sample size does not increase the likelihood of identifying statistically significant relationships.

The problem of within-subject variation is really a phenomenon relating to the correct classification of subjects. For example, if the aim is to classify individuals according to their iron intake, it would require approximately 10 days of valid dietary data to be confident that at least 80% of subjects had been classified in the correct extreme third of the distribution of iron intake. Fewer observations would result in an increased number of subjects being misclassified, not because the measurements were in error, but simply because the day-to-day variation in diet was not taken adequately into account when estimating each individual's intake. The more that subjects are misclassified, the less likely it is that the study will have the ability to demonstrate diet–disease relationships. This problem is independent of survey bias.

The degree of confidence of correct classification is reflected in the values given by ρ (Greek lower-case letter 'rho') (Table 2.3). The value for ρ is given by the expression

$$\rho = \frac{\sigma^2}{\sigma^2 + \tau^2}$$

where σ^2 is the true between subject variability in exposure[2] and τ^2 is the measurement error. The greater the measurement error in relation to the true

---

[2]The true between-subject variance needs to be estimated using analysis of variance to distinguish between- from within-subject variability. This is different from a calculation of the standard deviation based simply on a set of observations in a sample. The latter will include components of the within-subject variability and will therefore be far more likely to be an overestimate of σ.

Table 2.3 Correct classification by thirds of the exposure distribution

ρ	% Correctly classified
0.1	42.8
0.2	46.5
0.3	51.4
0.4	54.8
0.5	59.2
0.6	63.2
0.7	67.9
0.8	73.4
0.9	81.0

between-subject variance, the more likely the misclassification of subjects.

Measurement error can be reduced by increasing the number of observations in each subject, thereby improving the estimate of the true value of each individual's measurement of exposure. It will also have the effect of reducing the estimate of σ^2 (the less extreme the individual measurements, the smaller the value for σ^2). An approximation of the value for ρ is given by the expression

$$r = \sqrt{\frac{n^2}{n^2 + \dfrac{s_w^2}{s_b^2}}}$$

where n is the number of observations made within the individual and s_w^2 and s_b^2 are the unbiased estimates of the within- and between-subjects variances, respectively. As the day-to-day or measure-to-measure variability (s_w^2) increases in relation to the between-subject variability (s_b^2), so the value for r decreases and the number of subjects correctly classified in the extremes of the distribution goes down. This can be offset by increasing the number of observations made within each subject (e.g. days of diet record, measurements of blood pressure). Again, the expression assumes that the observations are unbiased and also normal in their distribution.

Power

When designing a study, it is essential to plan how many observations to collect. There need to be enough observations to be able to demonstrate the truth regarding the hypothesis, but not so many that time and money are wasted.

Statistical significance is usually expressed in terms of p values: $p < 0.05$ can be interpreted as saying that there is less than a 5% chance of observing what was observed if the null hypothesis is true. When p is small (i.e. <0.05), by convention the null hypothesis is rejected. Remember, also, that when rejecting the null hypothesis because p is less than 5%, there is always the chance of making a mistake, i.e. the null hypothesis really is true and it has been rejected incorrectly. This is called a type I error. The chance of making a type I error (designated by the Greek lower-case letter α) is the same as the value for p.

Power is the probability of being able to demonstrate a statistically significant finding, should one exist.[3] The underlying assumption regarding power, therefore, is that the null hypothesis is false. However, just as there was the chance of making a type I error (the incorrect rejection of a true null hypothesis), so there is the chance of making a type II error (the incorrect acceptance of a false null hypothesis). The greater the power in a study, the less likelihood of making a type II error. Power can therefore be defined as follows:

$$\text{Power} = (1 - \beta) \times 100$$

where β is the probability of making a type II error. Normally, the aim is to have not less than a four out of five chance of demonstrating a statistically significant finding, that is, power is at least 80% and β is equal to 0.2. The smaller the value chosen for β, the greater the power in the study and the smaller the probability of making a type II error. The relationships between significance level and type I error and power and type II error are summarized in Table 2.4.

It is important to remember that the null hypothesis is either true or false. It cannot be both. The two probabilities α and β are therefore independent.

Optimizing study design: power, significance level and number of observations

Power, significance level and number of observations are linked in the following expression:

$$n = \frac{2\sigma^2(Z_{\alpha/2} + Z_\beta)^2}{d^2}$$

---

[3] Collecting more and more observations does not necessarily imply an increased likelihood of finding a statistically significant finding: there may not be one.

Table 2.4 Relationships between the null hypothesis (H_0), p, power, and type I and type II errors

	The decision	
The true situation	Accept H_0	Reject H_0
H_0 is true	Correct decision: probability = $1 - \alpha$	Incorrect decision *(type I error)*: probability = α (level of significance)
H_0 is false	Incorrect decision *(type II error)*: probability = β	Correct decision: probability = $1 - \beta$ Power = $(1 - \beta) \times 100$

Table 2.5 Values for $(Z_{\alpha/2} + Z_\beta)^2$ used in the calculation of sample size according to levels of α (probability of making a type I error) and β (probability of making a type II error) and power [equal to $(1 - \beta) \times 100$]

		β	0.2	0.1	0.05
		Power	80%	90%	95%
		Z_β	0.842	1.282	1.645
α	$Z_{\alpha/2}$		$(Z_{\alpha/2} + Z_\beta)^2$		
0.05	1.96		7.85	10.51	13.00
0.01	2.576		11.68	14.88	17.82
0.001	3.291		17.08	20.91	24.36

Values for $Z_{\alpha/2}$ are two-tailed, values for Z_β are one-tailed.

where σ is the variability in the observations, d is the expected outcome (in this example, the difference between two group means), $Z_{\alpha/2}$ is the normal standard deviate relating to the chances of making a type I error (e.g. equal to 1.96 when $\alpha = 5\%$), Z_β is the normal standard deviate relating to the chances of making a type II error (e.g. equal to 0.84 when $\beta = 20\%$), n is the number of observations (taken as the integer value greater than or equal to the calculated value for n) in each group being compared (not the total number in the study).

For given levels of α and β, the number of observations required (n) will increase as the variability in the observations (σ) increases or as the predicted difference between two means (d) decreases.

Table 2.5 gives values for the expression $(Z_{\alpha/2} + Z_\beta)^2$. As the chances of making a type I or a type II error go down, so the value for the expression increases and, by implication, the number of observations in a study increases.

An example of how to determine sample size is shown in Box 2.5.

2.4 Measuring exposure

Nutritional exposures fall under a number of headings according to the influences on health outcomes being investigated. These may relate to:

- eating habits
  - consumption of food or drink (including alcoholic and nonalcoholic beverages)
  - nutrient intake
  - nonnutrient intake, including biochemical modifiers of metabolism (e.g. nonnutritive antioxidants), food additives, food contaminants and toxins
- biochemical exposures
  - levels of the nutrient and nonnutrient in circulation or in tissues
  - hormones
  - genetic modifiers of absorption or metabolism
- anthropometry
  - height, weight, body mass
  - circumferences (e.g. waist, hip, head, chest, arm) and circumference ratios (e.g. WHR)
  - skinfold thicknesses
  - growth centiles
  - wasting and stunting
- physiological characteristics and responses
  - body composition (e.g. % adipose tissue)
  - infection and infestation (acute or chronic)
  - disease states and severity (e.g. diabetes, cancer, inflammatory bowel disease)
- sociodemographic characteristics
  - household composition
  - age of householders
  - occupation
  - income
  - food and nutrition security (e.g. access to shops, car ownership)
- cultural factors
  - knowledge, attitudes and beliefs about food
  - religion
  - level of education.

Not all of these variables are direct measures of nutrients or food or the direct consequences of consumption, but many of them (e.g. hormones, infection,

---

Box 2.5

In assessing treatment of anemia in rural women working on tea plantations in the Cameroon, the mean hemoglobin (Hb) level was 10.0 g/dl, and the standard deviation (σ) was estimated to be 1.5 g/dl.[1] If the women were randomly allocated to two groups, and one group was given an iron supplement for 12 weeks and the other group was given a placebo, how many subjects would be needed to show that a Hb of 11.0 g/dl in the iron supplement group was statistically significantly different from the Hb in the placebo group (assuming it stays at 10.0 g/dl), at $p = 0.05$ and with a power of (a) 80% or (b) 90%?

The formula for the number of subjects required is:

$$n = \frac{2\sigma^2(Z_{\alpha/2} + Z_\beta)^2}{d^2}$$

If $P = 0.05$ then $Z_{\alpha/2} = 1.96$, and if power $= 0.80$ (i.e. 80%) and power $= 1 - \beta$, then $\beta = 0.2$, $Z_\beta = 0.842$ and $(Z_{\alpha/2} + Z_\beta)^2 = 7.85$. So

$$n = \frac{2 \times 1.5^2 \times 7.85}{1.0^2} = 35.3$$

The next largest integer is 36, so at least 36 subjects per group (36 in the treatment group and 36 in the placebo group) would be required to achieve 80% power.

If $p = 0.05$ but the desired power $= 90\%$, then $(Z_{\alpha/2} + Z_\beta)^2 = 10.51$ and $n = 47.295$, so at least 48 subjects would be required in each group.

If you had the resources to study only 30 subjects, then you could solve the equation above to work out the power (i.e. the chance of finding a statistically significant difference if one exists) by solving for Z_β:

$$Z_\beta = \frac{d\sqrt{n/2}}{\sigma} - Z_{\alpha/2}$$

and in this example $Z_\beta = 0.6220$. Looking this value up in the normal table[2] (use ½p because β is one-tailed), $\beta = 0.2669$ and power $1 - \beta = 0.7331$, or around 73%. At this level of power, you may decide not to do the study. Alternatively, if by extending the length of the intervention from 12 to 20 weeks you think it may be possible to show a change in Hb of 1.5 g/dl rather than 1.0 g/dl, then d in the expression above would be equal to 1.5, $Z_\beta = 1.913$, $\beta = 0.0279$ and the power $[(1 - 0.0279) \times 100]$ would be over 97%.

With intelligent application of the formulae for n, Z_β and d, it may be possible to manipulate the design of a study so as to maximize the likelihood of a fruitful outcome. Different formulae are used for other types of study design where the significant outcome desired may be a correlation, odds ratio or other statistic. Many statistical packages (such as Epi-Info, SPSS and Minitab) have a routine for estimating power, n or d, but some judicious substitution of the appropriate values given in the various formulae may be required to obtain a sensible answer for n.

[1] In most circumstances, you will need to estimate σ by looking in the literature for published values that relate to the variable of interest. There will not be published an *exact* value for σ, but instead a range of values for SD in different articles. Choose an SD value that you think is representative of σ. A very high value for σ will increase the value that you calculate for n, thereby increasing the likelihood of having a high power to your study. But the largest published value for SD is not necessarily the most representative, so use common sense. In circumstances when a good estimate for σ is not available, it will be necessary to use common sense to estimate the likely size of the different (or other measure) in percentage terms and the value for σ in terms of the coefficient of variation, CV (the standard deviation expressed as a percentage of the mean). The formula for these alternate data is then:

$$n = \frac{2CV^2(Z_{\alpha2} + Z_\beta)^2}{(\% \text{ difference})^2}$$

[2] Values in the normal table are usually given for one tail of the distribution (½p). This is appropriate for Z_β, which is a one-tailed function (i.e. you can never do worse than have a one-in-two chance of finding a statistically significant relationship, should one exist). Statistical significance, however, is two-tailed; hence the difference in the choice of values for determination of $Z_{\alpha/2}$ and Z_β.

---

income) have a direct bearing on food or nutrient availability or nutrient metabolism. They therefore gain importance as primary factors likely to affect nutrition-related health outcomes.

Some items may be regarded as both exposure variables and outcome variables. For example, rate of growth in the first year of life could be regarded as an exposure variable in studies of risk of subsequent childhood infection or adult hypertension. Rate of growth in the first year of life could be an outcome variable

in a study of breast-feeding practices and food availability during episodes of famine.

"True" exposure

"True" exposure is that factor or set of factors that is responsible for the outcome being investigated. In practice, true exposure cannot be measured directly. This problem arises for two reasons.

- *The precise factor is not known*: in a study of the effects of vitamin C intake on risk of stomach cancer, the foods in the diet, their vitamin C content and the amount of vitamin C that arrives in the stomach are all important. But of critical importance in relation to cancer will be the effects of vitamin C on stomach biochemistry, the interaction of vitamin C with putative carcinogens in relation to DNA mutations and the effects on cellular proliferation (possibly in combination with other nutrients, carcinogens and promoters).

- *The precise factor cannot be measured*: using the example above, it is likely that in the development of stomach cancer, vitamin C intake is important over a period of many years. Such long-term or cumulative exposures are virtually impossible to measure. Even short-term exposures are difficult to measure.

Relevant exposure

In most nutritional epidemiological studies, it is not the true, underlying cause of the outcome that is measured but a factor or set of factors that are related to the true exposure. In designing a nutritional epidemiological study, the first task is to define exactly what is meant by the relevant exposure and how it relates to the true (unmeasurable) exposure.

The relevant exposure is one that the study attempt is to measure. It will be defined according to a number of parameters.

Study type
Ecological, cross-sectional, analytical and experimental studies require measurements made at different levels: national, community, household or individual.

Time period
Nutritional exposures can be chronic or acute in their effects. Deciding on the time at which to assess an exposure is critical to the purpose of the study. A cohort study that characterizes nutritional status in terms of both dietary intakes and blood biochemistry may provide information relevant to the initiation of cancer, but not necessarily to its progression.

Point of measurement
Relevant exposures can be measured in terms of food consumption, nutrient intake, blood and tissue levels of nutrient, functional consequences of nutrient action (including genetic interaction) and excretion.

Type of measurement
The list of exposures given at the start of this section provides examples of exposure measures that are direct

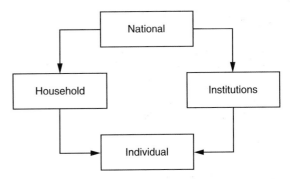

Figure 2.1 The points in the food chain where diet can be assessed.

(foods, nutrients), functional or metabolic (physiology, biochemistry), cumulative (anthropometry) and indirect (sociodemographic and cultural).

Dietary exposure

Diet can be usefully assessed at four points in the food chain (Figure 2.1).

National
Information is compiled from food producers, importers, exporters and those responsible for stocks of foods. The findings are referred to as food balance or food disappearance data and are published annually by the Food and Agriculture Organization of the United Nations. The nutrient content of the food can be estimated using food composition tables. Results are usually expressed per person, where numbers in the population are based on census data.

This method obtains national availability data only. No information is acquired on actual consumption, wastage, or variations in consumption by region, locality, household or individual.

Household
The most common form of recording is the food account method. This often forms part of a household budget survey (HBS) in which respondents record all expenditure (including that on food). Respondents keep a record of all food acquisitions (purchases, food from gardens, farms and allotments, gifts of food, etc.) typically over a period of between 1 week and 1 month. In the better HBS, respondents are asked to record amounts of food and drink acquired as well as expenditure. Such records may or may not include changes in larder stocks, foods obtained and eaten outside the

household food supply (e.g. restaurant meals), and specific items such as alcoholic beverages and confectionery. Alternative methods at the household level include the inventory method (in addition to the food account, respondents keep a record of change in larder stocks), the household record (the interviewer visits each household several times per day and records how much food has been used to feed the family) and the list-recall method (in which respondents recall how much food was acquired over the previous week or 2 weeks, with the aid of detailed questionnaires and till receipts). Collection of sociodemographic data facilitates comparisons by region, and by household characteristics such as income, occupation and education. Results are usually expressed per person rather than per household to facilitate comparisons by sociodemographic variables.

This method usually lacks information on food eaten outside the household food supply and on selected food items (alcoholic beverages and confectionery especially). No information is obtained on the distribution of consumption within households or food wastage.

Institution

Data are compiled from catering records of food acquisitions or at the point of food delivery. Total food availability or total food served is divided by the number of people for whom the food is intended. Diets available in hospital, residential institutions, schools (for school meals), and so on, may be characterized.

This method may not take account of additional food available (e.g. food bought from vending machines or brought by friends and relatives to patients in hospital). No information is obtained on actual levels of consumption by individuals.

Individual

There are two broad approaches to estimating diet at the individual level, prospective and retrospective. The prospective methods usually entail some form of record keeping, although this can be as simple as putting a tick next to the name of a food or drink on a preprinted list each time the item is consumed, or as elaborate as a 7 day food diary. Retrospective methods are sometimes regarded as more suitable for nutritional epidemiological studies, but prospective methods have been used successfully, and the retrospective methods have disadvantages regarding the identification of possible misreporting of diet and often provide no information on

day-to-day variation in diet. Questionnaires have the advantage of being able to enquire about diet in the distant past (although the validity of responses may be difficult to demonstrate). The need for assessing diet in the past arises in case–control studies of cancer, which typically has a long latent period. For such studies, the only tool available is the food frequency questionnaire (FFQ). A summary of the methods, with their advantages and disadvantages, is shown in Table 2.6.

Biomarkers

Biomarkers are substances measured in body tissues or excreta that can either act as proxy measures for nutrient (and nonnutrient) intake or provide information on the levels of exposure of body tissues to substances in circulation or in tissues, including nutrients and biochemical derivatives of nutrients or related compounds.

Biomarkers may indicate consumption over the short term (hours to days) or the longer term (weeks to years). Short-term markers relating to intake over the previous 1–2 days include:

- urinary excretion of nitrogen, potassium, iodine or vitamin C
- serum levels of vitamins B_1, B_2 and C
- breath hydrogen or methane (relating to intake of nonstarch polysaccharides).

Longer term markers include:

- adipose tissue or erythrocyte membrane fatty acid composition (specific fatty acid intakes over the previous 6–12 weeks)
- hemoglobin (iron intake over the previous 3 months)
- toenail selenium (intake over the previous 6–12 months)

Figure 2.2 gives a summary of the timescale over which various markers may usefully provide information. There is no fixed demarcation between time intervals, as indicated by the shading in the figure.

The functionality of biomarkers is dependent on a complex interplay between the amount and form of substances present in the diet, on the one hand, and the absorption, storage, metabolism and excretion, on the other. Vitamin E, for example, shows a more or less linear relationship between blood and dietary levels across a broad range of intakes. Riboflavin appears in urine only after tissues are saturated and any excess is

Table 2.6 Summary of methods for dietary assessment at the individual level

Name of method	Technique	Advantages	Disadvantages
Prospective			
Duplicate diet	Collect exact duplicates of all food consumed	Current diet Direct observation	Labor intensive for respondent and data entry
Weighed inventory	Weigh all items of food and drink at the time of consumption	Daily variation described Length of recording can be varied to suit study needs	Requires respondent skills (numeracy and literacy)
Household measures	Record all items of food and drink in household measures (including photographs of food portion size)		Underreporting likely in some population subgroups Expensive
Food checklist	Tick food or drink name in preprinted list each time item is consumed		
Retrospective			
Food frequency questionnaire	Indicate frequency of consumption of preprinted list of items of food and drink over previous month, season or year. May include portion size measures	Quick Cheap Low subject motivation Lower literacy and numeracy skills than needed for prospective methods	Reliant on memory Conceptualization skills needed to describe accurately frequency of consumption and food portion sizes Observer bias possible Reported diet may be a distortion of usual diet
Diet history	Detailed interview (1½–2 h) of usual food and drink consumption over previous month, season or year	Good cooperation Can be sent and collected by post	May lack measure of day-to-day variation in diet
24 h recall	Detailed interview (20–40 min) of usual food and drink consumption over previous 24 h. Repeat to obtain information on daily variation in diet		Requires regular eating habits Dependent on food composition tables

	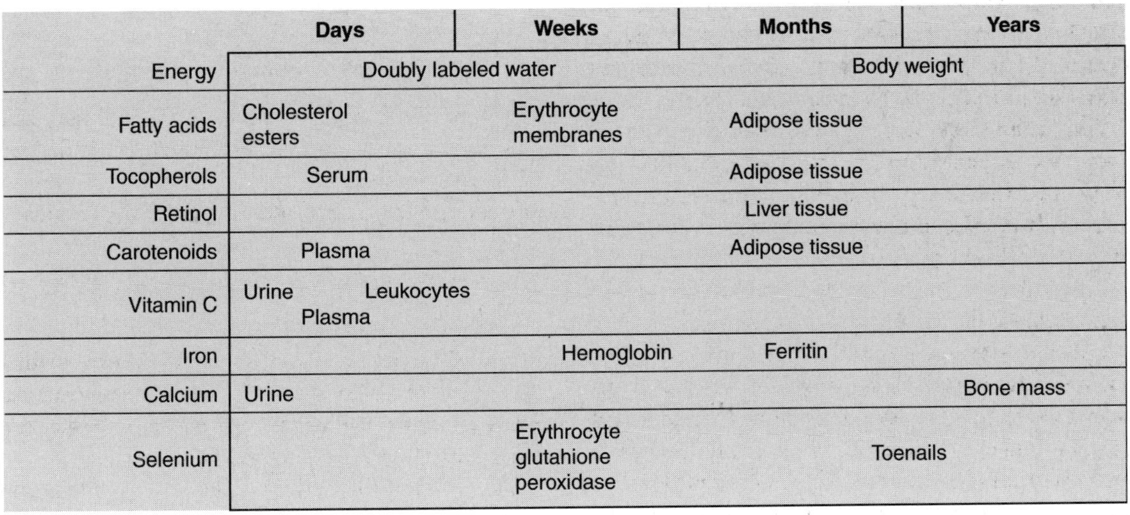 Days	Weeks	Months	Years
Energy	Doubly labeled water		Body weight	
Fatty acids	Cholesterol esters	Erythrocyte membranes	Adipose tissue	
Tocopherols	Serum		Adipose tissue	
Retinol			Liver tissue	
Carotenoids	Plasma		Adipose tissue	
Vitamin C	Urine / Plasma	Leukocytes		
Iron		Hemoglobin	Ferritin	
Calcium	Urine			Bone mass
Selenium		Erythrocyte glutahione peroxidase	Toenails	

Figure 2.2 Temporal association between biomarkers and nutrient intake.

being excreted. Vitamin C in serum or buffy coat layer is a poor marker at low levels of intake, increases in sensitivity as a marker of intake across the middle range of intakes (20–60 mg/day) and is poor once again at high levels of intake where excess vitamin is excreted in the urine. Retinol is stored in the liver and its level in blood is controlled homeostatically; it is therefore a useful marker only for low intakes.

These relationships are further complicated by issues relating to the efficiency of absorption [e.g. the creation and availability of transport proteins and their cofactors, mucosal integrity, and nutrient (and nonnutrient) interactions in the gut], storage (e.g. calcium in bone and factors affecting bone turnover), metabolism [e.g. conversion of vitamin D_3 to 25(OH)-vitamin D_3 in the liver] and excretion (e.g. kidney failure). Some markers can therefore function as markers of dietary intake (e.g. urinary potassium) and others as markers of function but not diet [e.g. circulating levels of 25(OH)-vitamin D_3, which reflect dietary intake, exposure to ultraviolet light and metabolic effects].

Biomarkers may be affected by illness, infection, infestation or disease. Measles, upper respiratory tract infection and diarrheal disease are likely to reduce circulating levels of retinol. Hookworm infestation will have a negative effect on iron status, meaning that intakes may be normal, but iron status indicators show iron deficiency. In a case–control study of diet and stomach cancer, metabolic failures relating to absorption (such as achlohydria, loss of intrinsic factor) will affect circulating levels of iron, vitamin B_{12} and other nutrients. Some types of tumor are known to be avid for thiamin and other B vitamins. Thus, using biomarkers to compare cases and controls may give a misleading impression of the relative importance of nutrients in the causation of disease because the differences have in fact arisen as a consequence of functional or metabolic failures associated with the disease process itself.

Biomarkers provide a snapshot at a single point in time. For markers that reflect medium- to long-term intake or status, a single measure may be sufficient. For markers that reflect short-term intake or status, more than one measure may be necessary. For example, the correlation between the analyzed sodium content of three 24 h duplicate diets and the sodium content of three 24 h urine collections [completeness validated with para-aminobenzoic acid (PABA)] was 0.31. Over 7 days, the correlation was 0.81. Thus, for markers that reflect short-term intake it is necessary to collect more than one sample for analysis. The number of samples will depend on the variability in both diet and tissue.

Anthropometry

Anthropometry has an important role to play in nutritional epidemiological studies. Body dimensions typically reflect a cumulative exposure to diet (especially the energy content of the diet) and illness. The measures can also be interpreted in relation to international standards for growth in children and for body size and associated risks of morbidity or mortality in adults.

The most commonly used measures are:

- height, weight, body mass
- circumferences (e.g. waist, hip, head, chest, arm) and circumference ratios (e.g. WHR)
- skinfold thicknesses.

Height (or recumbent length in children under 2 years of age) and weight appear to be relatively straightforward measurements. Nevertheless, training and monitoring of technique are essential to produce reliable results. Errors tend to be greatest in young children (who may have difficulty keeping still or standing correctly) and older subjects (whose posture may be compromised by skeletal deformity or deterioration). Body mass index (BMI) is defined by the expression

$$BMI = \frac{Weight\ (kg)}{Height\ (m)^2}$$

The values for BMI are usually taken to reflect adiposity and indeed they correlate well with other independent estimates of percentage body fat. Very muscular individuals may have a high BMI with low percentage of body fat. Although the measure is intended to be independent of height, for a given percentage of body fat, short people tend to have a higher BMI value than taller people.

Circumferences and skinfold thicknesses are generally less reliably measured than height and weight. This is partly due to a preliminary stage that requires the location of the measuring instrument on the trunk or limb. The waist is typically taken to be the halfway point between the bottom rib and the iliac crest, but in an obese subject these reference points may be difficult to locate. Fat deposits in older people tend to be more lumpy than in younger subjects, and repeat measures, especially of skinfold thicknesses, are often highly variable. Thus, a procedure for obtaining consistent repeat measures is important, and at least two measures (even of height and weight) should be routine. Forms for recording this information should be designed to facilitate at least three observations, allowing for at least one failure.

Once consistent measures have been obtained, they may be used directly as measures of exposure or outcome in nutritional epidemiological studies. In children, however, rapid changes in body size and proportion and differences between genders mean that making comparisons between groups may be problematic if groups to be compared differ in composition according to age and gender. This can be overcome by using appropriate reference standards.

Reference standards may be either internal or external. Internal reference standards are usually generated by expressing growth either as a percentage of median value or as a Z-score (number of standard deviations above or below the mean). These are typically calculated for age–gender groups at 1 year intervals. Differences between groups heterogeneous for age and gender can then be determined by comparing the mean of height or weight as a percentage of median values or the mean of the Z-scores. It is not good practice to compare groups that are too diverse in composition, as changes in rates of growth (e.g. between a preschool child and an adolescent) may make difficult a sensible interpretation of apparent differences in standardized measures of anthropometry.

External standards such as the United States Growth Charts (USGC) are available directly and through Epi-Info software. These are intended to reflect optimal rates of growth and are based on the National Health and Nutrition Examination Survey (NHANES) data on nutritional health from the USA. In addition to percentage of median and Z-scores, the USGC data allow for determination of centiles by age and gender. The centile indicates the point in the distribution for each variable. For example, a child on the 25th centile for height will be taller than 25% of their age- and gender-matched peers and shorter than 75%. International reference standards are currently available for centile distributions of height and weight, and centile distributions for BMI are available for selected populations (e.g. France and the USA).

For BMI, reference ranges in adults are commonly used to indicate overweight ($25–29.99\,kg/m^2$), obesity ($30–34.99\,kg/m^2$) and gross obesity ($>35\,kg/m^2$). These are measures of convenience for classification purposes. In the analysis of BMI data in epidemiological studies, it is likely to be more revealing to use the original values rather than to group subjects in to categories based on health risk assessments not necessarily appropriate for the outcome under consideration.

Sociodemographic and psychosocial variables

Sensible interpretation of nutrition–health relationships in the context of epidemiological studies often requires knowledge of living circumstances that may influence health behaviors and health outcomes. The important variables include ethnic origin, social class, occupation, level of education, residential area, marital status, household composition and housing tenure. Other factors relating to access to food, car use, income, proportion of income spent on food, and hunger can be used to develop a picture of food and nutrition security. There are also cultural factors concerning knowledge, attitudes and beliefs about food, religion, norms and values, role obligations, social pressures and other health behaviors that may be relevant in the interpretation of exposure–outcome relationships. These sociodemographic and psychosocial factors may be important because they confound the relationship between nutritional exposures and outcomes. For example, an older person who has a poor social network may have low vitamin D status and poor bone health because of poor access to shops (and dietary sources of vitamin D), limited activity levels and lack of exposure to ultraviolet light. The underlying cause of low bone mineral density may therefore be a social or sociomedical rather than a nutritional problem. Nutrition is in the causal pathway but is not the underlying cause of poor bone health.

Determining validity and reliability

Measuring diet is one of the most demanding tasks in nutritional epidemiological studies. There are two fundamental problems:

- Subjects tend to change their eating habits when asked to record information.
- Subjects tend to report information about consumption that is different from their actual consumption.

Failure to overcome these problems is one of the primary reasons that nutritional epidemiological studies may not show statistically significant relationships between nutritional exposures and outcomes even when such relationships exist.

It is important to define the terms that are to be used.

Reproducibility

This is the extent to which a tool is capable of producing the same result when used repeatedly in the same circumstances. The terms repeatability and reliability are often used synonymously with reproducibility, but the former implies the process of establishing reproducibility, while the latter is a quality of a measure that has reproducibility. A measurement may have good reproducibility and yet have poor validity, but a measurement which has good validity cannot have poor reproducibility.

In reality, the same circumstances can never exist in relation to biological material, because the diet, serum retinol, and so on of every individual varies on a daily, weekly and seasonal basis. Because many measures seek to assess usual intake, part of the variation in observations collected will relate to genuine variability in diet or metabolism, and part will relate to biases associated with the method. Due consideration must be given to these time-related factors when evaluating the reproducibility and validity of dietary measures, and a well-designed validation study will separate the variability associated with reproducibility from that associated with genuine biological variation.

Validity

This is an expression of the degree to which a measurement is a true and accurate measure of what it purports to measure. Establishing validity requires an external reference measure against which the test measurement (the one being used in the main survey or research activity) can be compared. In nutrition, there is no absolute reference measure of the truth.[4] Every measurement of dietary intake, for example, includes some element of bias. The best that can be managed is to assess relative or congruent validity of measurements, comparing results obtained with the test instrument with what are believed to be more accurate measures of food or nutrient intake obtained, for example, from a biological marker.

Absolute versus relative validity

There are two main problems arising from inaccurate measurements:

- incorrect positioning of a country, household, or person in relation to an external reference measure (e.g. dietary reference values)
- incorrect ranking of countries, households or people in relation to one another.

The first is a problem relating to absolute validity. In spite of the fact that in reality there are no absolute

measures of nutrient intake, it is possible to approximate the truth of the relevant exposure and to model the likely error. The likely sources of error are discussed in the following section.

The second problem is related to the correctness of classification in the ranking of observations, or relative validity. The key issue here is that even if the absolute true measures are not known, it is possible to evaluate health in relation to nutritional exposures according to whether subjects are at the top or the bottom of the distribution of exposures.

It is important to understand that no measurements will be without error. Some of the error is due to biological variation, or natural changes in values over time. Some is due to bias in the measurements. Some is due to differences in the amount of error between subjects. Each of these types of error needs to be assessed if the data are to be interpreted intelligently.

Validation studies

The problems of measurement error can be partially addressed using validation studies. These studies are designed to measure the degree to which the observed measures are likely to differ from the true measures. They compare measurements that are collected in the same way as in the main study with other, more objective or accurate measures that are likely to have less bias. An alternative approach to making inferences in the face of measurement error has been termed triangulation.

Validation studies are carried out in a sample that is similar in character to the main study sample. It should be possible to take into account the major likely confounders (e.g. age, gender, body weight) so that errors associated with the confounders can be controlled for in the analysis of the data from the main study. The exact list of confounders or effect modifiers that needs to be evaluated will vary from one study to the next. A list of common factors is given in Table 2.7. Some factors are associated with the subject; others are associated with the method of measurement.

One of the difficulties with the interpretation of findings from a validation study is that it is never possible to replicate exactly the circumstances that are likely to be encountered in the main study. This is particularly true if the aim is to understand the errors associated with a dietary measurement. This is due partly to the order of administration of the test and reference measures and partly to the type of person who is likely to participate

---

[4]The term "gold standard" was once fashionable, but it has been abandoned in favor of "reference measure", which more accurately reflects the reality that there is no wholly objective measure of the truth.

Table 2.7 Confounders and factors with potential to cause differential misclassification

Related to the subject	Related to the measuring process
Age	Portion size
Gender	Interviewer
Region	Learning effects
Social class	Recency effects[c]
Education	Lag time[d]
Language	Number of foods
Culture	Database
Social approval[a]	
Social desirability[b]	

[a] The wish to be approved of by the interviewer.
[b] The wish to be seen to be normal in relation to other people or successful in relation to one's own aspirations.
[c] The tendency to report recent events even when being asked about events in the past.
[d] The difference in time between relevant exposure and outcome (e.g. in the development of heart disease or cancer).

in a validation study, even if they are also participating in the main study.

Typically, a dietary reference measure might be a weighed record of diet collected over a given period (e.g. 7 days), validated for completeness using urinary nitrogen, the urine samples themselves validated for completeness using PABA. The test measure may be an FFQ. In the main study, the respondents will be exposed only to the FFQ. If the FFQ is administered first in the validation study, the period (e.g. dietary habits in the previous month) will not be the same as that associated with the reference measure (a prospective record of 1 week measured after the FFQ). To make the two measures coincide in time, the FFQ would have to follow the weighed inventory. Then, however, the subject will have had the benefit of thinking about their diet before the administration of the FFQ, making the circumstances different from those in the main study. In addition, the subject will have had training in dietary assessment. The people who are willing to devote the extra time and effort required in a validation study may be different from the subjects in the main study (i.e. more interested in keeping records, more willing, more numerate). They may not be representative of all people likely to take part in the main study. The validation study may therefore yield a better estimate of the level of agreement between the test measure and the truth than would be found in the main study.

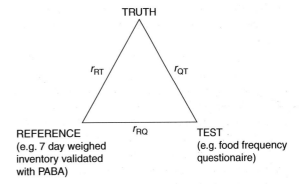

Figure 2.3 Associations between the test and reference measures and the truth. PABA: para-aminobenzoic acid.

There is no way around these problems. Elements of training and a more skilled sample are likely to make the results from a validation study an overestimate of the true relationship between the test measure and the truth. That said, not carrying out a validation study is like failing to calibrate equipment in the laboratory, thereby undermining the ability to interpret sensibly the findings from the main study. Nevertheless, the following rules should be followed in validation studies.

- The sample in the validation study must be representative of the sample in the main study. One way to achieve this is to use a nested design in which the validation study data are collected at the same time as the data in the main study.
- Everything must be measured at least twice. This will help to separate issues of validation from issues of repeatability.

Interpreting data from validation studies

The main purpose of a validation study is to understand the way in which the test measure relates to the truth. Suppose that two measures of iron intake have been collected in a validation study, one based on an FFQ (the test measure) and the other from a 7 day weighed inventory (the reference measure). Assume that there are no systematic differences in measurement between subgroups of the sample, that is, that any errors in measurement are due to noise in the system (natural biological variation) or random sources of imprecision in the measuring instruments (e.g. the scales are accurate only to 2 g). Figure 2.3 then represents the relationship between the reference measure, the test measure and the truth.

If these relationships are measured in terms of correlation coefficients (i.e. rank agreement), then they are related by the expression:

$$r_{QR} = r_{QT} \times r_{RT}$$

where r_{QR} is the correlation of the intake of the test and reference measure (FFQ and weighed inventory), r_{QT} is the correlation between the test measure and the truth, and r_{RT} is the correlation between the reference measure and the truth.

If the reference measurements are assumed to be unbiased, then r_{RT} can be estimated by the expression:

$$r_{RT} = \sqrt{\frac{n^2}{n^2 + \frac{s_w^2}{s_b^2}}}$$

where n is the number of repeat measures (e.g. 7 days of dietary data) and s_w^2 and s_b^2 are the within- and between-subject variances described previously. The relationship of the test measure to the truth (r_{QT}) is then given by the expression:

$$r_{QT} = r_{QR}/r_{RT}$$

and the likely extent of misclassification of subjects can be determined from Table 2.3. If misclassification is high (i.e. r_{QT} is small), then the lack of association between the exposure and outcome may be due to imprecision of the dietary measurement. If the level of classification is good (i.e. r_{QT} is large), then it may be reasonable to assume that any observed association between exposure and outcome (or the lack of association) is a true association (assuming that the validity of the outcome measure has also been established).

The same principles can be applied if there is a third measure available (e.g. serum ferritin). In this case, there are three expressions that can help to relate the likely association between each measure and the truth (Figure 2.4). Again, the likely (theoretical) true classification of subjects will be reflected by the various expressions for ρ which are functions of the observed correlations r between the three measures. The extent of misclassification given for (say) thirds of the distribution will be given by the values for ρ given in Table 2.3, as before. The modeling is not always perfect (the values under the square root sign are sometimes greater than unity, or negative). For most related measures, however, it provides a useful way of utilizing data from three sets of observations.

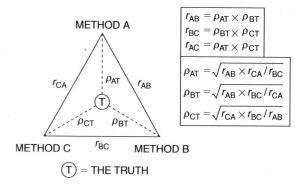

Figure 2.4 Association between three measures and the truth.

Required accuracy

It is important to know that the relevant nutritional exposure to be assessed can be measured to the desired level of accuracy with the resources available. Assuming that the measures are made without bias, the desired level of accuracy is usually achieved by ensuring that the number of measurements obtained in the sample is sufficient to achieve a standard error $SE = s/\sqrt{n}$ of a given size. The value for n is normally dictated by the power calculations.

Measurement error

The following expression defines the components of a given measurement X_i:

$$X_i = \beta T_i + \alpha + e_i + \varepsilon_i$$

where X_i = what is observed for a given measurement, T_i = the true value, β represents a proportional bias associated with the method of measurement, α represents a constant bias associated with the method of measurement, e_i is the random error associated with the noise in the variable (e.g. day-to-day variation in nutrient intake), such that for a set of individuals over a sufficient number of observations $\Sigma e_i = 0$, and ε_i is the error associated with the measurement process in a given individual. When $\Sigma \varepsilon_i \neq 0$ the method of measurement is regarded as biased, i.e. the error is systematically different in some subgroups of subjects compared with others. This is the source of differential misclassification.

One important aim in nutritional epidemiological studies is to understand the contribution made by each of these sources of error. Table 2.8 shows some possible sources of error for three different measurements. Similar examples can be constructed for most variables,

Table 2.8 Possible sources of error for three methods of measurement relating to nutritional exposures

Measurement	Method	Component of error			
		B	α	e_i	ε_i
Weight (kg)	Personal spring balances	Springs on scales are old and no longer stretch in proportion to weight; all weights underrecorded by 3%	Scales not level on hard surface. All weights underrecorded by 0.5 kg	Weight varies over the course of the day: lightest just after arising, heaviest just after evening meal	Heavier subjects may eat and drink less than normal if they know they will be weighed as part of the study
Fat intake (g/day)	Food record in household measures	Small portions overreported, large portions underreported	Use of photographs promotes average overestimation of portion size by 5%	Fat content of diet varies from day to day	Heavier subjects differentially underreport consumption of fat-containing foods
Serum ferritin (μg/l)	Elisa	Temperature on autoanalyzer too low; all reactions too slow, ferritin levels underestimated by 5%	Standard solution overdiluted; all ferritin levels overestimated by 6 μg/l	Ferritin levels vary according to timing of fluid consumption and serum dilution	Subjects with moderate to severe infections will have ferritin levels overestimated

ELISA: enzyme-linked immunosorbent assay.

often for more than one source of error. It is important when designing studies and developing strategies for analysis of data that all of the likely major sources of error are considered and that suitable quality control procedures are put in place to avoid unknown sources of error influencing the interpretation of the findings.

Misclassification

One of the primary reasons for carrying out validation studies is to understand the extent of misclassification that is likely to occur in the main study. Misclassification occurs for one of two reasons:

- There is noise (truly random error) in the system.
- There is a bias in the measurements made in particular subgroups of the sample.

The effects of these errors are shown in Figure 2.5.

Ideally, everyone in a study would be classified correctly based on the measurement used (Figure 2.5a). In this case, the influence of exposure on outcome would be clear. In practice, no measurement is perfect. If the errors are unbiased, then the noise in the system will result in an even misclassification of subjects (Figure 2.5b); any misclassification that occurs is equally likely to occur in all subgroups in the sample. This is nondifferential misclassification. This will attenuate (weaken or reduce) the ability to detect diet–disease relationships, but will not lead to bias in the interpretation. Figure 2.5(c) shows the effect of differential misclassification. In differential misclassification, the type and extent of misclassification is different in different subgroups. Figure 2.5(c), for example, might represent estimates of fat intake in subjects who are overweight. Subjects in the top third of the distribution are more likely to underreport their fat consumption than subjects who are not overweight (whose distribution could be represented by Figure 2.5b). A higher proportion of the overweight subjects are therefore likely to be classified in the bottom of the distribution of fat intake. Note that the Xs for "All observed" in (b) are the same size and correspond to the size of the Xs for "All correctly classified". In contrast, in (c), the "All observed" Xs are larger for the low-intake group than for the high-intake group, and different in size from the Xs for "All correctly classified". If the aim is to investigate the association of fat intake with risk of heart disease, the true association will be obscured because those who are at higher risk (overweight subjects) will have underreported their fat intake. Thus, the influence of fat intake appears to be far less than that of other factors (e.g. body weight, hypertension) that are measured with less misclassification.

True classification	Observed classification			
	High	Medium	Low	All correctly classified
High	X			X
Medium		X		X
Low			X	X
All observed	X	X	X	

(a) What we would like to see (no misclassification)

True classification	Observed classification			
	High	Medium	Low	All correctly classified
High	X	x	x	X
Medium	x	X	x	X
Low	x	x	X	X
All observed	X	X	X	

(b) What we often see (nondifferential misclassification)

True classification	Observed classification			
	High	Medium	Low	All correctly classified
High	X	x	x	X
Medium	x	X	x	X
Low	x	x	X	X
All observed	X	X	X	

(c) What we do not want to see (differential misclassification in one subgroup)

Figure 2.5 Classification of subjects (a) if the observed measures correspond exactly with the truth, (b) if there is noise in the system, and (c) if there is bias in measurements in one subgroup. The size of the Xs in the boxes represents the number of observations.

There is one final point to make about misclassification (and measurement error) with regard to validation studies. The assumption is that the measurements (and their associated errors) are truly independent. In practice, it is possible that the errors in the measurements are not independent in one of two ways:

- A person who tends to underreport their diet using one method may underreport their diet using another method.
- A person who tends to underreport their diet using a given method on one occasion is likely to underreport their diet on another occasion.

This leads to the concepts shown in Figure 2.6.

If the errors between methods are correlated, this will result in an overestimate of the extent to which the test measure and reference measure agree (r_{QR} is an overestimate of ρ_{QR}). If the errors within methods are correlated, this will result in an underestimate of the extent to which the test measure and reference measure agree (r_{QR} is an underestimate of ρ_{QR}).

2.5 Measuring outcomes

How do we measure health? There are many facets of health: physical, mental, social, spiritual, and so on. Although several measures have been developed to reflect these facets, the most widely accepted measures of health are really measures of ill-health, or disease. The most objective of these is mortality as a binary variable: dead or alive. Causes of death provide more information, and are relatively robust measures. Morbidity measures (measures of sickness or ill-health, short of death) include hospital discharge data and length of stay in hospital. Quality of life measures are designed to take into account the different facets of health, and are sometimes used as integrative measures of health status, including quality-adjusted life-years remaining.

Morbidity

Morbidity, the measure of sickness, may be either a general measure of ill-health or a disease-specific measure. In some countries, including the USA, there is a collaborative system or standard agreed upon by the hospitals with inpatient services. Discharge data are collected routinely, coded in a standardized fashion and reported to a central agency. In the USA, this is the National Center for Health Statistics or, for about 40% of the hospitals, the Commission on Professional and Hospital Activities. Diagnoses on discharge are coded according to the International Classification of Diseases

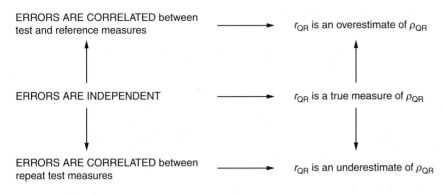

Figure 2.6 Effects of interdependence of measurement errors on the apparent agreement between methods in validation studies.

scheme, and so have parallels with the mortality data described below. Data on procedures and length of stay are also collected. From these data admissions and bed-days can be calculated. In the UK, two similar data sets are used, the Hospital In-Patient Enquiry, which reports diagnosis on admission for 10% of all patients admitted to National Health Service hospitals; and the Hospital Activity Analysis, which reports 100% of diagnoses at discharge.

Mental health can be measured in terms of symptoms with particular severity and duration, as classified in the Diagnostic and Statistical Manual of Mental Disorders (DSM-III), as well as in terms of discharges from mental hospitals, in parallel with other hospital discharge statistics.

Mortality

Measures of death are not limited to vital status. Cause of death is important information, particularly in studies of nutritional epidemiology where dietary factors are under investigation. It is important to understand where the cause of death information comes from. On the death certificate there is space for the medical recorder to complete up to three proximate causes of death and an underlying cause of death. Conventions dictate that the underlying cause of death is typically what is used in mortality data. The proximate causes are also recorded and data entered, allowing the possibility to study mortality in a different way.

The simplest measure of mortality is the crude death rate (total number of deaths in 1 year divided by the total number of people in the population). In practice, however, comparison of crude death rates between countries or regions may be misleading simply because the risk of death is so heavily dependent on age. Thus, an area that has proportionately more older people will have a higher crude death rate than an area with fewer older people, even though the age-specific death rates (e.g. number of deaths in people aged 65–74 years divided by the number of people in the population aged 65–74 years) may be lower in the former than the latter. Some form of age adjustment in the measure of mortality is essential. Adjustments may also include gender. These are known as standardized mortality rates. An alternative to standardized mortality rates is standardized mortality ratios (SMR). Typically, these compare, in percentage terms, the number of mortality events in a given area with the average for all areas being compared (e.g. regional rates compared with national mortality statistics, where the national value is set equal to 100), and take into account the variations in age and gender distribution between areas. The same types of adjustment can be applied to morbidity data as to mortality data.

The complement of mortality is survival. In expressing health status following the first diagnosis of a chronic illness such as cancer, outcome is often expressed in terms of 5 year survival rate.

Rates and ratios

It is the convention to express outcomes in reference both to the population at risk and to a defined period, usually 1 year. For example, mortality is expressed as a rate of death per population at risk per year (standardized for age).

Incidence

Incidence is the number of new cases (of the outcome of interest) in individuals who had previously not experienced the outcome (e.g. disease free with respect to the particular disease end-point in question). The new cases are applied to the numerator. The denominator is the number of people in the population who were at risk of developing the disease. Incidence is expressed in relation to a defined period, and within that period, the person-time at risk is accumulated. The measure of disease risk is the incidence rate (incidence density).

Prevalence

Prevalence (or, strictly speaking, point prevalence) is the number of existing cases of the outcome of interest at a given point in time, compared with the number of people in the population at risk at that point in time. Point prevalence is the simplest measure of prevalence. The result is expressed as a proportion or ratio.

Period prevalence extends the count of persons to those with the outcome at any point in the period of interest. This forms the numerator. The denominator is not simply the count of the population at the beginning of the period. Rather, it allows for time at risk. The period before which an outcome occurs for a person contributes, as well as the entire period for those not experiencing the outcome during the period.

Standardization of rates

It is important to be able to make comparisons between population groups in a way that takes into account potential confounders such as age and gender. This is achieved by standardization. There are three basic steps in standardization.

1. Choose a standard population. It is best to use a population that is similar in character to the population in which the original rates have been measured. The standard population provides the statistical weights (numbers of people in given age and gender categories) that are used in the calculation of the standardized values. Most countries have a standard population (usually based on the last census or some projection of the population) that can be found in the national statistics website (see Further reading section). If this is unavailable, a standard population can be made up, based on the sum of the populations of the areas being compared.
2. Calculate rates for each of the groups being compared as if they were occurring in the standard population.
3. Compare rates between standardized groups.

There are two approaches to standardization.

- *Direct standardization*: the age-specific (or age and gender-specific) rates are applied to the standard population. The total number of events (morbidity or mortality) can then be determined for the standard population at the rates that applied in each of the populations being compared. The results are then expressed per 100 000 population (or per 10 000 or per million, depending on the rate in the original populations).
- *Indirect standardization*: this looks at the rates as a ratio and is usually described as the standardized mortality ratio or the standardized morbidity ratio (SMR). For example, if the aim were to compare mortality rates for colon cancer in men between regions in the UK, the age- and gender-specific rates for the UK as a whole would be applied to the population of each region to determine the expected number of events according to the number of men in the different age groups living in each region. This would then be compared with the actual number of events in the region and multiplied by 100, i.e.

$$\frac{\text{Number of events observed}}{\text{Number of events expected}} \times 100$$

For all areas taken together (e.g. the whole of the UK) the SMR is equal to 100.

Short term and long term

The influence of nutrition on disease may be short term or long term. Typically, most deficiency disease relating to nutrition is short term. For example, dietary iron deficiency follows a cascade of events over several months:

1. reduced stores of iron (reduced levels of ferritin in serum)
2. decreased production of normal sized red blood cells with a full complement of iron (increased plasma protoporphyrin levels)
3. reduced number of erythrocytes and low hemoglobin levels in circulation.

In contrast, much nutritional epidemiology is devoted to understanding the chronic effects of diet on health. Finding the association between diet and chronic disease is difficult because there may be several periods of development of disease, each of which has a different nutritional cause, and there may be many nutritional influences on a complex etiology. In heart disease, for example, the factors linked to the initiation and development of atheromatous plaques (high levels of circulating low-density lipoprotein cholesterol, low levels of antioxidants) are different from the factors that influence risk of an acute myocardial infarction (e.g. high-fat meal, short-term dietary influences on platelet aggregation). There is a wealth of data suggesting that total fat, individual fatty acids or classes of fatty acids, various vitamins (C, E, folate), carotenoids, minerals (selenium, iron, calcium), and dietary fiber are all linked to the development of heart disease over many decades. It is important, therefore, in planning a nutritional epidemiological investigation, to ensure that the factors being measured are appropriate to the time of the influence being investigated.

Intermediate risk factors or end-points

Because of the complexity of nutritional influences on chronic disease, it is often useful to use intermediate measures as a means of assessing risk and understanding etiology. For example, increased risk of stroke is associated with high blood pressure, smoking and a high WHR. Thus, if the ultimate aim is to reduce the incidence of stroke through improvements in nutrition, it would help to understand the influences of nutrition in relation to each of the intermediate or associated factors (e.g. the effect of energy balance on blood pressure and WHR, the role of fats and calcium in hypertension and the role of antioxidants in relation to the damage caused by smoking).

Qualitative measures

Quality of life

Quality of life can be a general term for health status, but also has specific meaning that allows ranking of people according to both objective and subjective aspects of their health status, and is dependent on cultural norms and relative perceptions. Health-related quality of life (HQL) encompasses functional limitation, both physical and mental, and positive expression of well-being, physical, mental and spiritual. It can be used as an integrative measure of mortality and morbidity, and as such forms a composite index including death, morbidity, functional limitation and well-being.

Quality of life studies tend to focus on lifestyle and life choices in two groups:

- patients with disease (e.g. diabetes, stroke, head and neck cancers) with quality of life dimensions such as physical and emotional functioning, effects on speech (e.g. stroke) and social interaction and feelings of acceptance (e.g. colostomy), and coping with pain (e.g. oral cancer)
- subjects whose life circumstances are changing (e.g. older subjects and the impact of aging on dentition and disposable income).

In both of these areas, there are dimensions of quality of life that may have an influence on nutrition (e.g. depression and physical barriers to eating that affect appetite in patients with head and neck cancer) or changes in availability of food or ability to eat that may have an adverse effect on self-perceived social status, social interaction or nutrition-related state of health (e.g. immune function). For example, Hammerlid et al., describe patients with head and neck cancers each having special problems at diagnosis according to tumor location. Those with tumors in the larynx tended to have more problems with communication, those with oral tumors with pain, and those with pharyngeal tumors with nutrition and pain. The patients with hypopharyngeal cancer reported the worst HQL scores. Tumor stage appeared to have the strongest impact on HQL. Patients with a more advanced tumor stage reported significantly worse HQL scores for 24 of 32 variables reflecting functioning or problems. The females scored worse than the males for some areas, in particular emotional functioning. The older patients scored significantly better for emotional and social functioning than patients aged less than 65 years, but worse for physical functioning and various symptoms. In consideration of the nutrition-related aspects of survival in this group of patients, quality of life is a key issue.

Another example comes from the work by Sheiham et al., who assessed dental health in the National Diet and Nutrition Survey of people aged 65 years and over living in Great Britain. Seventeen per cent of the free-living edentate participants (those with no natural teeth) reported that their mouth affected their pattern of daily living on a regular basis. Oral impact levels were lowest in dentate subjects with the greatest number of teeth. For the dentate, the most common oral impacts were on eating and speaking. Impacts relating to emotional stability, sleeping, relaxing, carrying out physical activity and social contact were very infrequent, but tended to be severe when they did occur. Among those with an impact on eating, 25% said it was severe and 42% had the impact nearly every day or in a spell of 3 or more months.

2.6 Measuring diet–disease (exposure–outcome) associations

Nutritional epidemiological studies set out to explore the relationships between nutritional exposures, on the one hand, and disease or health outcomes on the other. Conventional statistical approaches for comparisons between groups (e.g. *t*-test, chi-squared analysis) will apply. However, particular features of nutritional epidemiological studies make them different, for example, from a simple intervention trial in which a simple repeat measures analysis (e.g. paired *t*-test) might be appropriate. These features are:

- evidence of the relationships between nutritional exposures and health or disease outcomes in groups of people rather than individuals
- taking into account evidence that relates changing patterns of food consumption to changes in disease that occur over time
- the need to measure the average risk of disease in segments of the population who are exposed to different levels of food or nutrients
- the need to take into account simultaneously many factors that may affect disease risk and to determine the likely contribution of nutrition and nutrition-related factors.

An additional feature of nutritional epidemiological studies is that they are often commissioned by a government to investigate specific questions of population health. The results, therefore, need to be expressed in a way that can inform policy decisions regarding PHN and nutrition health promotion. The challenge in these circumstances is to present results in a form that lay people can understand without compromising the science underlying the determination of risk. It is also necessary to address the issues of mismeasurement while not undermining the importance of the findings.

Types of measurement

Measurements of exposure and outcome in epidemiological studies can be either continuous or categorical. Continuous variables include estimates of dietary intake, blood pressure and biochemical measures in blood. Categorical measures include gender, smoker versus nonsmoker and supplement user versus nonuser. In addition, continuous measures can be made into categorical measures by defining groups according to level, such as by dividing subjects into

Box 2.6

Zatonski *et al*. (1998) examined time trends in age-standardized mortality rates for ischemic heart disease plus atherosclerosis and arterial diseases in Poland between 1970 and 1995. The data show a sharp decline in disease rates for men and women aged 45–64 years after 1991. The authors also examined trends in risk factors for heart disease, including smoking, alcohol consumption and food consumption (based on food balance sheet data).

fifths of the distribution of vitamin C intake. The nature of the analysis carried out will depend on the type of measurement. Time trend, correlation and regression analysis assume that variables are continuous. Relative risk calculations typically assume that variables are categorical (although analysis based on continuous variables is possible). Typically statistical analyses based on continuous variables are more powerful (effects are more precisely estimated) than those based on categorical variables.

Time trends

Over time, rates of disease in the population change. One of the first tasks of epidemiology is to monitor these changes in ways that are comparable between the groups being compared. If data are already classified according to age and gender, then further standardization may not be required. Parallel changes over time in potentially predisposing or protective factors may suggest causal relationships (Box 2.6).

Figure 2.7 shows the changes in heart disease rates (age standardized for men and women separately expressed as mortality ratio using 1991 = 100) together with changes in consumption of vegetable fats and oils, butter and exotic (imported) fruit. Fruit consumption is based on quarterly estimates and the jagged line reflects seasonal variations. The decline in disease rates seen after 1991 coincides with a decrease in butter consumption and an increase in margarine and fruit consumption. The authors conclude that changes in dietary fat and fruit consumption offer the best explanation for the changes in disease rates, given that other factors such as smoking and alcohol consumption changed little over the same period.

This type of analysis is relatively easy to construct. It provides the opportunity to explore apparent relationships between exposure and outcome, but there are substantial weaknesses to the approach. First, there is the ecological fallacy: it may be that the individuals whose

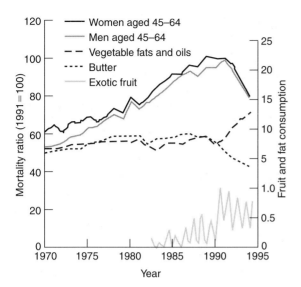

Figure 2.7 Gender-specific changes in heart disease mortality ratio versus changes in consumption of vegetable fats and oils, butter and exotic (imported) fruit in Poland, 1970–1995. Reproduced with permission from Zatonski *et al.* (1998).

reduced rate of disease is reflected in the global figures are changing their lifestyle (e.g. by smoking and drinking less) as well as participating in the general increase in margarine and fruit consumption, but it is the smoking and drinking that is changing their risk. Secondly, one would expect to see a time lag between changes in diet and changes in risk of disease. In this example, there is no time lag. This implies that the factors at work are affecting acute risks rather than chronic risks. The authors themselves cite mechanisms that could explain this association (to do with polyunsaturated fatty acid intakes and risk of clotting). The findings do not therefore address the broader issue of whether the changes in fat and fruit consumption affect chronic risk.

Correlation and regression

Variations in exposure between countries or between individuals provide the opportunity to examine how low or high levels of exposure are associated with variations in disease. For each unit of observation, exposure (x) is plotted against outcome (y). The Pearson correlation coefficient (r) is then used to describe the strength of association. It varies from $+1$

(a perfect positive correlation) to -1 (a perfect negative correlation), with a value of zero implying no association. A perfect correlation is one in which all of the variation in the dependent variable y (e.g. disease rate or index) is explained by the variation in the independent variable x (the exposure); in graphical terms, all of the x,y points would fall along a straight line. The Pearson correlation coefficient assumes that the variables are normally distributed, but there are other types of correlation analysis that do not require the assumption of normality (e.g. Spearman's correlation or Kendall's tau, based on ranks).

Regression describes the trend in association, that is, by how much the outcome changes for a given amount of change in exposure. The simplest form of regression is linear or straight line regression (often referred to as least squares linear regression analysis). The outcome is modeled mathematically as a function of exposure using the expression $Y = a + bx$ (the equation for a straight line), where Y is the predicted or average value of y for a given level of x, a is the intercept (the point at which the line crosses the y-axis) and b is the slope or gradient of the line. The derivation of the equation is based on an analysis of the x,y pairs such that the regression line shows on average how y changes as x changes. It is possible to construct more complex (multiple regression) models in which more than one predictor variable is included in the equation, for example, $Y = a + bx + cz$. Other forms of regression in epidemiology include logistic and proportional hazards models in which grouped (rather than continuous) data are used to estimate relative risk.

In statistical terms, the outcome variable is called the dependent variable in regression analysis. The relationship to be described may be written as

$$Y = a + bX + E$$

where a and b are constants and E is a random variable with mean 0, called the error, which represents that part of the variability of Y which is not explained by the relationship with X.

b is the regression coefficient. In contrast, r, the correlation coefficient, describes how close observations are (when Y is plotted against X) to a straight line. It does not describe the slope of that line (that is the job of b).

Table 2.9 Correlation and regression coefficients for the association of fruit and refined grain consumption with stomach cancer. Reproduced with permission from Jansen *et al.* (1999).

	Correlation			Regression				
	r	*p*	*r²*	*a*	*p*	*B*	*p*	*R²* (adjusted)
Mean fruit consumption (g/day)	−0.553	0.026	0.306	3.104	0.000	−0.0058	0.026	0.256
Mean refined grains consumption (g/day)	0.810	0.000	0.656	0.514	0.249	0.0067	0.000	0.632

This table shows that both correlations were statistically significant (i.e. there was less than a 5% chance of observing these values if the null hypothesis was true and there was in reality no association between the variables).

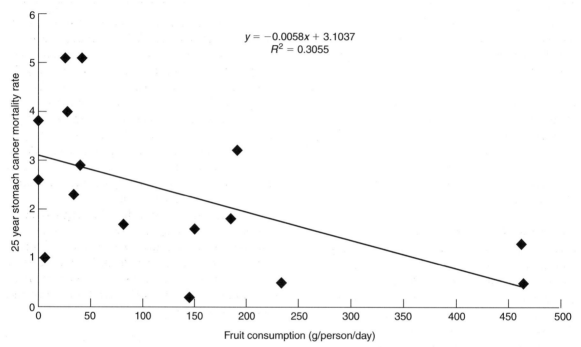

Figure 2.8   Association in 16 countries between 25 year male stomach cancer mortality rate and fruit and refined grain consumption. Reproduced with permission from Jansen *et al.* (1999).

The two are related in the following way:

$$r^2 = \frac{b^2 \times \text{Sum of squares of } X}{\text{Sum of squares of } Y}$$

(adapted from Bland, 1987).

The value r^2 (for correlation) or R^2 (for regression analysis) tells you how much of the variation in the dependent variable is explained by variation in the independent variable(s).

Jansen *et al.* (1999) describe the association in 16 countries between male stomach cancer mortality and fruit and refined grain consumption (based on food balance sheet data). The correlation between 25 year

stomach cancer rates and consumption is shown in Table 2.9. Fruit consumption was negatively correlated with stomach cancer rates, while refined grains consumption was positively associated. Figure 2.8 shows the regression line for the plotted data (together with the regression equation and unadjusted R^2 value). For each gram increase in fruit consumption, the stomach cancer rate declines by 0.006, equivalent to a decline of 0.6 for each 100 g increase in fruit consumption.

It is possible to examine the influences of fruit consumption and refined grain consumption at the same time using multiple regression analysis. This will take into account the correlation between the two independent variables ($r = -0.563, p < 0.01$) and indicate which of the two is more strongly associated with stomach cancer mortality rate. The regression equation becomes:

$$Y = 0.887 - 0.0015x + 0.006z$$

where x is fruit consumption and z is refined grain consumption. In this example, however, with both variables in the equation, the coefficient for fruit (-0.0015) is not significantly different from zero ($p = 0.477$), whereas the coefficient for refined grains is significantly different from zero ($p = 0.000$). From a statistical point of view, therefore, only refined grains are seen as a significant contributor to stomach cancer risk. The equation then becomes:

$$Y = 0.514 + 0.0067x$$

where x is refined grain consumption. This is a very simplified analysis of a potentially complex set of interactions that may involve many factors. As with the time trend data, the ecological fallacy may operate, although in fairness the authors of this particular article have argued strongly against its operation in the assessment of these data.

The concept of relative risk

Relative risk is defined as "the incidence of disease (or other health outcome) in those exposed to the risk factor under investigation divided by the incidence of disease in those not exposed". It is thus a ratio of rates and explains how the average risk in groups of people changes as their exposure changes. Although it is based on observations in individuals, relative risk does not relate to risk in any one individual.

Risk can be defined in absolute terms (e.g. lifetime risk of developing lung cancer) or in relative terms (the risk of smokers developing lung cancer compared with nonsmokers). By expressing risk in relative terms, risk in the unexposed group is equated to unity (1.0) and risk in the exposed group expressed as some multiple of the risk in the unexposed group. If the exposure is protective, then the relative risk in the exposed group will be less than 1.0. In every assessment of relative risk, therefore, there is a referent group in which the risk is arbitrarily set equal to 1.0.

Relative risk

Relative risk can be calculated directly from cohort study data because the incidence (the appearance of new cases) can be determined directly in a sample

Table 2.10 The approach to analysis in cohort and case–control studies

		Diseased	Not diseased
		Case–control study: looking backwards in time ↓	
Exposed	Cohort study: looking forward in time →	a	b
Unexposed		c	d

whose exposure has been measured at the start of the study and who can therefore be classified as exposed or unexposed. An important feature of cohort study design is that the risk of disease is theoretically the same in the exposed and unexposed groups at the start of the study. The baseline measure in a cohort study, however, is in fact likely to reflect a cumulative exposure over many years, and the early asymptomatic stages of the disease process may have already developed. Nevertheless, the cohort study provides a model that predicts over time the appearance of disease according to levels of exposure.

Table 2.1(a) and (b), regarding the design of cohort and case–control studies, is summarized in Table 2.10.

Relative risk is equal to the ratio of the incidence of disease in the exposed group divided by the incidence in the unexposed group. Using the numbers of observations indicated in the cells in Table 2.10, relative risk is defined as follows:

$$\text{RR} = \frac{\dfrac{a}{a+c}}{\dfrac{b}{b+d}}$$

where a = exposed and diseased, b = exposed and not diseased, c = unexposed and diseased, and d = unexposed and not diseased. Note that this equation is really only an approximation, which is very close to truth when the period at risk is similar for all people in Table 2.10. Incidence is more precisely defined in terms of new occurrences per person-period at risk (see Box 2.1 for a definition of incidence rate). The relative risk is still the ratio of the incidence in the exposed to the incidence in the unexposed group.

Odds ratio

The case–control study suffers from a fundamental weakness relating to the representativeness of the control group. It is not possible to equate the unexposed group in the cohort study to the sum of the numbers of unexposed cases and controls in the case–control study. One can calculate the relative odds of exposure in these studies. This is known as the odds ratio, where:

$$OR = \frac{ad}{bc}$$

The odds ratio represents the odds of being in the concordant groups (a = exposed and diseased, d = unexposed and not diseased) versus the discordant groups (b = exposed and not diseased, c = unexposed and diseased).

If the disease being investigated is relatively rare (e.g. cancer or cardiovascular disease, but not the common cold) and the controls are sampled independently of exposure, then the OR represents an approximation of the RR. This is because $a \ll c$ and $b \ll d$, such that $a + c$ can be approximated by c and $b + d$ can be approximated by d. This property of the OR is extremely useful, and is what has made the case–control study of rare outcomes such a powerful tool in epidemiology.

Exposed versus unexposed

In nutritional epidemiology, the concept of exposed or unexposed is not clear-cut. If a study is examining the risk of disease in relation to smoking, for example, people who are either smokers or nonsmokers can be identified. However, in a study investigating the effect of exposure to saturated fatty acids on risk of heart disease, there is no group of subjects who has zero exposure to saturated fatty acids. Instead, risks of subjects who have low exposure can be compared with those with high exposure.

Quartiles, quintiles and other categorical measures

Low and high can be defined as below or above the median or other cut-off point. In nutritional terms, however, it is often more interesting to compare people who are at the bottom and top ends of the distributions of intake. Instead of dividing subjects into only two groups, it is often more revealing to assess risk by comparing those in the bottom quarter or fifth of the distribution, for example, with those in the top quarter or fifth. Alternatively, there may be predefined levels of

exposure (e.g. fasting blood glucose levels to categorize subjects as nondiabetic, prediabetic and diabetic) where the numbers in the sample are not necessarily in equal thirds (see Section 2.2 for the definition of a case). It may also be appropriate to compare risks in groups defined by gender, ethnic group, and so on.

In every analysis of relative risk, it is necessary to decide which group is the referent group. Typically, this is the group with the lowest risk (so that values for RR in other groups tend to be greater than 1.0), or the most common exposure (in which case the values for RR in other groups may be greater than or less than 1.0 depending on whether the exposure is predisposing or protective), or simply an arbitrary reference group.

Confidence intervals

As with any statistical measure, the determination of relative risk and odds ratios is associated with sampling error, which needs to be reflected in a confidence interval. The null hypothesis states that exposure has no effect on outcome, so the expectation is that the values for the relative risk or odds ratio would be unity at every level of exposure. In practice, because of sampling variation, the values determined would not be exactly equal to unity, so it is necessary to compute a confidence interval around them (typically a 95% confidence interval). The confidence intervals indicates where the true population relative risk is likely to lie, based on the sample observations. If the confidence interval includes 1.0, the null hypothesis is accepted and it is assumed that the risk in the group being assessed is not different from the risk in the reference group. Because the risk in the reference group is assigned arbitrarily, there is no error associated with it, so there is no confidence interval.

Dose–response relationships and p for trend

Some diet–disease relationships conform to a threshold model and others to a dose–response model. For example, signs of nutrient deficiency appear only when intakes fall below a given level. In contrast, there is likely to be a continuous relationship between measures of overweight and risk of heart disease (the fatter a person, the greater the risk). Apparent trends in relative risk can be assessed statistically to determine whether a dose–response relationship is genuinely present or not. The findings are presented as p for trend. If $p_{trend} < 0.05$, one can reject the null hypothesis that there is no trend.

Table 2.11 Multivariate-adjusted rate ratio of postmenopausal breast cancer by anthropometric risk factors and family history of breast cancer, Iowa Women's Health Study, 1986. Source: Sellers *et al.* (2002).

Anthropometric factor	No family history					Positive family history				
	No. of cases	Total no. of women	Rate ratio	95% confidence interval	*p*-Value test for trend	No. of cases	Total no. of women	Rate ratio	95% confidence interval	*p*-Value test for trend
Weight (pounds)[a]										
≤128	206	5763	1	Reference		36	733	1	Reference	
129–140	236	5701	1.17	0.97, 1.42		59	823	1.45	0.96, 2.20	
141–155	308	6107	1.45	1.21, 1.75		67	804	1.75	1.16, 2.64	
156–174	283	5274	1.56	1.28, 1.90		52	711	1.55	1.01, 2.39	
>174	335	5754	1.83	1.49, 2.24	$p < 0.001$	68	879	1.74	1.15, 2.65	$p = 0.02$
Body mass index (kg/m²)[a]										
≤22.89	207	5700	1	Reference		47	763	1	Reference	
22.90–25.04	257	5911	1.25	1.04, 1.50		56	831	1.11	0.75, 1.64	
25.05–27.43	260	5711	1.35	1.11, 1.63		61	746	1.39	0.95, 2.05	
27.44–30.69	326	5692	1.76	1.45, 2.12		55	767	1.26	0.85, 1.87	
>30.70	318	5585	1.93	1.57, 2.36	$p < 0.001$	63	843	1.47	0.99, 2.17	$p = 0.05$
Waist/hip ratio[b]										
≤0.76	217	5156	1	Reference		35	703	1	Reference	
0.77–0.80	244	5218	1.03	0.86, 1.24		53	734	1.34	0.87, 2.06	
0.81–0.85	293	6559	0.92	0.77, 1.10		55	851	1.15	0.75, 1.76	
0.86–0.90	277	5403	1	0.83, 1.21		53	752	1.23	0.80, 1.89	
>0.90	337	6263	1.02	0.85, 1.23	$p = 0.87$	86	910	1.55	1.04, 2.32	$p = 0.06$

[a] Additional adjustment for height, waist/hip ratio, and body mass index at 18 years of age. Metric cut-off points are = 58.1 kg, 58.2–63.5 kg, 63.6–70.3 kg, 70.4–78.9 kg, and >78.9 kg.
[b] Additional adjustment for height, body mass index and body mass index at age 18 years of age. Metric cut-off points are ≤76 cm, 77–82 cm, 83–90 cm, 91–99 cm and >99 cm.

Relative risk and odds ratios: two examples

Relative risk

Sellers *et al.* used cohort data from the Iowa Women's Health Study to examine the relationship between WHR and risk of breast cancer in postmenopausal women. Because the study was prospective, they were able to use the Cox proportional hazards model to determine relative risk. Table 2.11 shows the estimates of risk of breast cancer according to weight, BMI and WHR in women with or without a family history of breast cancer.

All three variables are continuous, but for the purposes of the relative risk calculation women have been categorized into fifths of the distributions. In each case, the reference category (in which RR = 1) is the fifth at the bottom of the distribution. Assuming that weight, BMI and WHR are positively associated with breast cancer risk, the expectation is that higher levels of exposure are associated with risk significantly greater than unity.

Table 2.12 shows that among women with no family history of breast cancer, those whose weight is between 129 and 140 pounds (58 and 63 kg) have an estimated relative risk of breast cancer equal to 1.17. This value is not statistically different from the reference value, however, as the confidence interval (0.97 to 1.42) includes 1.0. Women whose weight is 141 pounds (64 kg) or greater do appear to have an elevated risk of breast cancer. This is indicated by confidence intervals that do not include unity. A similar pattern is evidence among women who do have a family history of breast cancer. The *p*-values for tests for trends for both sets of observations are less than 0.05, suggesting that there are statistically significant trends in risk, that is, as weight increases, risk increases. Note that for all of these analyses, the relationship between weight and risk has taken into account the influences of height, WHR and BMI at the age of 18 years. Other potential confounders of risk (e.g. parity, breast-feeding practices and smoking) have not been taken into account, although they were measured in the study.

Table 2.12 Effects of physical activity on breast cancer risk in premenopausal and postmenopausal Hispanic and non-Hispanic white women, adjusted odds ratios (OR)[a] and 95% confidence intervals (CI), New Mexico Women's Health Study, 1992–1994

| | Premenopausal women | | | | Postmenopausal women | | | |
| | Hispanic | | Non-Hispanic | | Hispanic | | Non-Hispanic | |
Risk factor	OR	95% CI	OR	95% CI	OR	95% CI	OR	95% CI
Total physical activity (metabolic equivalents, h/week)								
0–<25	1		1		1		1	
25–<50	1.17	0.53, 2.55	1.35	0.64, 2.85	0.74	0.40, 1.36	0.45	0.26, 0.78
50–<80	0.49	0.22, 1.07	1.44	0.67, 3.10	0.37	0.18, 0.75	0.49	0.28, 0.86
>80	0.29	0.12, 0.72	1.13	0.49, 2.61	0.38	0.18, 0.77	0.45	0.24, 0.85
Trend test	$p < 0.001$		$p = 0.741$		$p = 0.002$		$p = 0.019$	

[a] OR determined using conditional logistic regression analysis (for matched cases and controls). Analysis controls for age group, health planning district, age at first full-term birth, months of lactation, parity, years of oral contraceptive use and (in postmenopausal women) years of hormone replacement therapy use.

The findings for BMI are not as consistent as for weight. Whereas among the women with no family history of breast cancer there is an increased risk of breast cancer as BMI increases, the same is not true for women with a history, as all of the confidence intervals include unity. Paradoxically, the trend is significant in both groups. Lastly, the WHR shows no association with breast cancer risk in women with no family history, but a statistically significantly greater risk in the top compared with the bottom category in women with a family history, and a significant trend as well.

Thus, it is important to examine the confidence interval for each category of risk to ensure that it does not contain unity, as well as to look for trends in risk.

Odds ratio

In a case–control study of breast cancer risk and physical activity, Gilliland *et al.* identified contrasting influences of total activity (estimated as metabolic equivalents per person per week) on risk in Hispanic and non-Hispanic premenopausal and postmenopausal women (Table 2.12). The interpretation of the odds ratio data is similar to that of relative risk, in that at each level of exposure a confidence interval is calculated, and across categories a trend is assessed. If the confidence interval includes unity, the risk in that category is not different from the reference category. If $p_{trend} < 0.05$, a significant trend in risk exists across categories. As in the Sellers study quoted above, calculation of the odds ratio controls for potential confounders. Note in this example that as activity is deemed to be protective, risk goes down as activity levels increase. The need to analyze data

separately by categories (e.g. Hispanic versus non-Hispanic, pre- versus postmenopausal) is made clear by the differences in results shown.

2.7 Interpretation of associations

Once a study has been completed and data are in hand, with the preliminary results of statistical analysis, the investigator will examine the measure of diet–disease association. This should always be interpreted with caution. Several steps need to be followed here. The measure of association is a statistic. It has been calculated under statistical assumptions about distribution (parametric or nonparametric) and lack of bias. The first step is to compare it to a critical value (defined by the distribution and nominal significance level) if it is being used to test a hypothesis, or to take account of its confidence interval if it is being used for estimation.

Chance and bias

Could the association have arisen by chance? The comparison of the statistic with the critical value is the required step here. For example, in a study of nutritional factors and eye disease in postmenopausal women, the association of servings of whole-grain products from the dark bread group (containing phytoestrogens) with testosterone levels was examined. From the correlation of −0.20, the test statistic t was calculated:

$$t = r \sqrt{\frac{(N-2)}{(1-r^2)}}$$

for large samples, as $-0.2 \sqrt{(246-2)/(1-0.2)} = -3.19$. This is compared to the critical value of -1.96. It is a more extreme value and so is considered not likely to have arisen by chance. In fact, if there were in truth no association, such a value of r, or a more extreme value, would have arisen with a *probability* of about 0.002.

Could the association have arisen because of some bias in the data? Bias can arise in the process of selecting study subjects, in the measurement of the variables under analysis and in the configuration of other factors in the dataset. Avoiding bias is preferable to adjusting for bias. By taking care in the study design, the first source of bias can often be avoided. Measurement error is hard to avoid in diet assessment, and in some instances this actually results in bias. The role of other factors in the dataset in influencing the exposure–outcome relationship is discussed in the next section.

Confounding and effect modification

When variables are associated both with the exposure measure and with the outcome measure, such that the association between the exposure and outcome is overestimated or underestimated, the association between exposure and outcome is said to be confounded by a third factor (the confounding variable).

When the association between the exposure measure and the outcome measure depends on the level of a third factor, the third factor is said to be an effect modifier.

Correcting for measurement error: exclusion, inclusion and generalizability

Energy adjustment

There are several reasons for adjusting for energy intake in an analysis of diet and disease outcome. Each one should be considered in deciding whether and how to make such an adjustment. First, there may be instrument issues. Consider the measurement tool; for example, use of the full FFQ allows correction for systematic overreporting or underreporting by expressing nutrients in terms of percentage kilocalories or per 1000 kcal. Secondly, is calorie intake a potential confounder? Is it associated with the disease/outcome? Affirmative response calls for statistical adjustment for energy intake in the same way as any other potential confounding variable. Thirdly, mechanisms of action of the nutrient in the causal pathway to disease outcome should be considered. These mechanisms depend

both on the nutrient and on the disease, and their character may suggest the best way to adjust for energy intake in the analysis. It is important to decide, either biologically or deterministically, whether the nutrient of interest is likely to act on the outcome in question directly (perhaps because of some threshold effect), or in proportion to its dilution in the diet as a whole, or in relation to body size. In many cases the effect of the nutrient is likely to vary according to body size, since most organs have size correlated to some extent with total body size (e.g. assessed by BMI).

If the mechanism is thought to be direct, the appropriate analysis could be not to adjust for energy intake. An exception to this would be if the contribution of the nutrient of interest on outcome prediction were desired to be estimated independently of the contribution of calories. Thus, in most instances, an adjustment for energy intake is appropriate.

Adjusting for energy intake has several benefits. Adjusting for energy may reduce extraneous variation (technical and biological), allowing a more precise estimate of the diet–disease relationship. The adjustment for energy in an observational study models the intervention setting where use of an isocaloric diet is commonplace.

The choice of method depends on the reason for the adjustment. The nutrient density method is useful for correcting for underreporting or overreporting on the FFQ, but nutrient density methods do not fully remove the effect of calories. It has been demonstrated that the regression residual and the traditional regression approaches to the energy adjustment, using energy as a confounder, are equivalent in interpreting the contribution of nutrient to disease risk.

Before leaving this section on energy adjustment, a consideration that is particular to the epidemiologist's presentation of data should be discussed. For ease of interpretation, it is traditional in epidemiology to express the results of statistical association in quintiles or quartiles. Before creating these quantiles, the energy adjustment must be conducted. The results obtained if adjustment is done after the quantiles are determined are very different to those obtained in the recommended way.

Adjustment of data

Techniques for adjusting for measurement error are similar to those for adjusting for within-individual variation. Several conceptually different approaches

---

Box 2.7 Correcting the regression coefficient for measurement error (adapted from Willett, 1998)

The formula for the relationship between the "true" (i.e. removing the effects of measurement error) and observed regression coefficients is:

$$b_t = b_o \left(1 + s_w^2 / s_b^2 \, n_x\right)$$

where s_w^2 = within-subject variance, s_b^2 = between-subject variance and n_x = number of replicates of X.

X and Y are two variables. For example, Y is cholesterol intake from food frequency and X_1 is observed cholesterol from one of 4 days of diet record. Suppose X_2 is observed cholesterol from one of 28 days of diet record. The relationship between the "true" correlation (r_t) and the observed correlation (r_o), assuming no measurement error in the Y variable, is

$$r_t = r_o \sqrt{1 + s_w^2 / (s_b^2 \times n_x)}$$

where s_w^2 = within-subject variance, s_b^2 = between-subject variance and n_x = number of replicates of X, and therefore

$$r_o = r_t / \sqrt{1 + s_w^2 / (s_b^2 \times n_x)}$$

In this example, the observed correlation between X_1 and Y, say r_1, is

$$r_1 = r_t / \sqrt{1 + s_w^2 / 4 s_b^2}$$

while the observed correlation between X_2 and Y is

$$r_2 = r_t / \sqrt{1 + s_w^2 / 28 s_b^2}$$

Clearly, $r_2 > r_1$.

Box 2.8 Adjusting the odds ratio using the linear approximation method (adapted from Rosner, 1989)

Assume X is the "true" exposure, Z is the observed exposure and p is the probability of getting the disease.
  Using a validation study, we find

$$X = \alpha' + \gamma Z + \varepsilon \qquad (1)$$

The logistic model describing the relationship between disease and observed exposure can be written

$$\text{logit}\,(p) = \alpha + \beta Z + \text{error} \qquad (2)$$

while the relationship between disease and true exposure is

$$\text{logit}\,(p) = \alpha^* + \beta^* X + \text{error} \qquad (3)$$

Substituting for X in (3) using (1),

$$\begin{aligned}\text{logit}\,(p) &= \alpha^* + \beta^* (\alpha + \gamma Z + \varepsilon) \\ &= \alpha^* + \beta^* \alpha + \beta^* \gamma Z + \beta^* \varepsilon\end{aligned}$$

Comparing this with (2) yields

$$\beta = \beta^* \gamma$$

So,

$$\beta^* = \beta / \gamma$$

and the corrected OR = $\text{logit}\,(p)|_{X=1} / \text{logit}\,(p)|_{X=0} = \exp\,(\beta/\gamma)$.

---

have been suggested:

- estimating the misclassification (clinical model: sensitivity and specificity)
- using the components of variance approach (once within- and between-individual variance has been distinguished, the odds ratio can be adjusted directly or via the regression coefficient. In a similar fashion, the correlation coefficient can be adjusted)
- using a linear approximation method for adjustment.

See Boxes 2.7 and 2.8 for examples of how to do this.

Precision

The precision of an exposure–outcome relationship can be improved by incorporating the results of a validation study to estimate the within-individual variation, and then making the corresponding adjustment to the measure of association. This can be accomplished by including an internal validation study, including an external validation study or conducting a full validation study.

Triangulation

It has already been stated that all measures of nutritional assessment are subject to error. There are different schools of thought concerning whether or not all measures of nutritional assessment are also subject to bias. If one or more measures can be considered unbiased, then methods can be used in a validation study to correct estimates produced from a biased measure. Otherwise, the best approach may be to obtain three or more measures of dietary intake, with independent sources of bias and other measurement error. Consistency in the results using each of the three measures in turn lends support to the inferences made from only one of the measures. This approach is often used in studies that have dietary intake as the outcome variable, as seen in Box 2.9.

Interactions and regression analysis

Regression is a method of estimating the numerical relationship between variables. For example, a researcher would like to know the mean or expected systolic blood pressure (SBP) for individuals with a given sodium excretion, and what increase in SBP is associated with a unit increase in sodium excretion. Note that the two variables are not treated the same. One is a predictor variable (sodium excretion) and the other is the outcome variable (SBP). A regression analysis would estimate the linear association of SBP on unit change in sodium excretion. The regression coefficient estimates the slope of the regression line.

This type of analysis can be extended to multiple predictor variables or independent variables in what is known as multiple linear regression. Often the additional variables added to the regression equation beyond the original predictor variable are potential confounding variables, as discussed earlier. In some instances, it may be suspected that an interaction exists between a confounding variable and the main predictor variable. This phenomenon is also known as effect modification. It can be explored statistically by adding an interaction term, or set of interaction terms, to the regression equation. When an interaction term is in the model, the main effect terms for the predictor variable and associated confounder cannot be interpreted without acknowledging the interaction. When a hypothesized interaction is statistically significant, in epidemiological studies it is usual to subdivide the dataset by two levels of the effect-modifying variable (the confounder that has a significant interaction with the predictor on the outcome of interest). Separate regression analyses are then conducted on the two levels of effect modifier. The interaction is tested again within each subset, and if interaction remains, an additional subdivision will be necessary. If not, the analyses for the two levels of the effect modifier are presented separately.

2.8 Expressing results from nutritional epidemiological studies

In common with many epidemiological studies, it is often advantageous to present results of associations between dietary exposures and disease outcomes in terms of relative risks or relative odds by grouped categories of exposure. Common groups used are thirds, quarters or fifths. The distribution of exposure in the control or comparison group is used to define these groups. A continuous variable can then be redefined into an ordinal categorical variable with each group having a numeric code.

It is extremely important to execute any adjustments to the variable, such as adjustments for energy intake, before the cut-off points for the groups (quantiles) are defined.

The regression, logistic regression or other appropriate analysis is then conducted using dummy variables for the numeric codes for the groups (quarters, fifths, etc.) as the independent variables in the analysis. One of the groups is treated as the referent category, and relative risks of the outcome for the other quarters or fifths are estimated, with associated confidence intervals, in reference to that category. This method does not take full advantage of the powerful analyses using the dietary exposure variable as a continuous measure, but has the advantage of ease of presentation and communication of results to members of the health field. It has an additional advantage of not assuming that the relationship between diet and disease outcome is a linear one, since estimates of relative risk for contiguous fifths of exposure for example may not be monotonic.

For example, in a study of endometrial cancer and dietary fat intake, the distribution of percentage energy from fat in the control group was divided into fifths. Multiple logistic regression analysis was conducted with risk of endometrial cancer as the dependent variable, and age, county of residence, total energy intake, unopposed estrogen use and cigarette smoking as confounding variables. The results are presented in Table 2.13.

Meta-analysis

The method of critical literature review of an individual publication was formalized by epidemiologists in the 1970s, but grew into the method of information synthesis when the critical review was expanded to all available publications or unpublished articles concerning a given topic. For example, a review of dietary interventions aimed at controlling high blood pressure was based on publications identified by a MEDLINE search of published articles between 1975 and 1984 using hypertension as a keyword. The articles were rated for scientific merit and relevance to long-term behavioral change. Four articles were summarized that included random allocation to groups and at least 1 year of follow-up. The dietary components and other behaviors targeted, the types of intervention, the measures used to evaluate success, whether or not the intervention was successful and a summary of the study population were summarized.

One stage beyond the formal information synthesis is meta-analysis, which provides a quantitative summary score combining estimates of association or effect size from all studies in the information synthesis, sometimes weighting the high-quality studies higher than the lower quality studies. For example, a meta-analysis of studies of homocysteine and coronary heart disease limited the articles reviewed to those measuring fasting or basal levels of total homocysteine, and to those with population-based comparison groups.

In other applications, different estimates of the combined effect size are made within homogeneous groups of studies. For example, in an earlier meta-analysis, studies using postmethionine load homocysteine were grouped together, and studies using fasting homocysteine were also grouped together. Two combined estimates were made, one restricted to the fasting studies, and one combining all studies (Figure 2.9).

2.9 Perspectives on the future

Future nutrition research will almost certainly involve the role of the genetic link with gene–nutrient and gene–environment interactions. An increased interest in dietary patterns, rather than specific nutrients, may also be anticipated in future decades.

Nutritional epidemiology will also adopt a wider, multidisciplinary approach involving factors such as social determinants of eating patterns, food supplies and nutrient utilization on health to assist the decisions of policy makers, the food industry and consumers.

Table 2.13 Odds ratios (OR) of endometrial cancer associated with percentage energy from fat in the three-county area around Seattle, Washington, 1985–1991

% energy from fat (% kcal/day)	No. of cases	No. of controls	OR	95% confidence interval	p-Value test for trend
<30.8	107	189	1	Reference	
30.8–36.2	126	191	1.3	0.88, 1.8	
36.3–40.7	156	187	1.5	1.1, 2.2	
40.8–45.1	134	187	1.5	1.1, 2.2	
>45.1	156	191	1.8	1.3, 2.6	$p < 0.001$

OR adjusted for age in 5 year categories, county of residence (King, Pierce, Snohomish), total energy intake (continuous), unopposed estrogen use (never, <3 years, ≥3 years, missing) and cigarette smoking (ever, never).

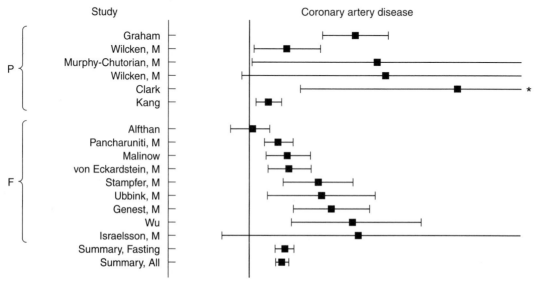

Figure 2.9 Meta-analysis of the relationship between homocysteine levels and risk of coronary heart disease (Boushey, 1995). P: postmethionine load homocysteine level studies; F: fasting homocysteine level studies. Reproduced with permission from Boushey et al. (1995).

Further reading

Bland JM. An Introduction to Medical Statistics. 3rd edition, Chapter 11. Oxford, Oxford University Press, 2000.

Boushey CJ, Beresford SAA, Omenn GS, Motullsky AG. A quantitative assessment of plasma homocysteine as a risk factor for vascular disease: probable benefits of increasing folic acid intakes. J Am Med Assoc 1995; 274(13): 1049–1057.

Cole TJ. Sampling, study size, and power. In: Margetts BM and Nelson M. Design Concepts in Nutritional Epidemiology. 2nd edition. Oxford University Press, 1997.

Frazao E (ed). America's eating habits: changes and consequences. Economic Research Service Report, Agriculture Information Bulletin 750, USDA, Beltsville, Maryland, 1999.

Gilliland FD, Li YF, Baumgartner K, Crumley D, Samet JM. Physical activity and breast cancer risk in hispanic and non-hispanic white women. Am J Epidemiol 2001 Sep 1; 154(5): 442–50.

Hammerlid E, Bjordal K, Ahlner-Elmqvist M, Boysen M, Evensen JE, Biorklund A, Jannert M, Kaasa S, Sullivan M, Westin T. A prospective study of quality of life in head and neck cancer patients. Part I: at diagnosis. Laryngoscope 2001; 111(4 Pt 1): 669–80.

Jansen MC, Bueno-de-Mesquita HB, Rasanen L et al. Consumption of plant foods and stomach cancer mortality in the seven countries study. Is grain consumption a risk factor? Seven Countries Study Research Group. Nutr Cancer 1999; 34: 49–55.

Last JM. A Dictionary of Epidemiology, 4th edn. New York: Oxford University Press, 2001.

Rosner B, Willett WC, Spiegelman D. Correction of logistic regression relative risk estimates and confidence intervals for systematic within-person measurement error. Statistics in Medicine 1989; 8(9): 1051–69.

Rothman KJ, Greenland S. Modem Epidemiology. Philadelphia, Lippincott-Raven, 1998. pp. 147–162.

Sellers TA, Davis J, Cerhan JR, Vierkant RA, Olson JE, Pankratz VS, Potter JD, Folsom AR. Interaction of waist/hip ratio and family history on the risk of hormone receptor-defined breast cancer in a prospective study of postmenopausal women. American Journal of Epidemiology 2002; 155: 225–233.

Sheiham A, Steele JG, Marcenes W, Tsakos G, Finch S, Walls AW. Prevalence of impacts of dental and oral disorders and their effects on eating among older people; a national survey in Great Britain. Community Dentistry & Oral Epidemiology 2001; 29(3): 195–203.

Willett W. Nutritional Epidemiology. 2nd edition. Oxford, Oxford University Press, 1998. Chapter 12, pp. 302–320.

Zatonski WA, McMichael AJ, Powles JW. Ecological study of reasons for sharp decline in mortality from ischaemic heart disease in Poland since 1991. British Medical Journal 1998; 316(7137): 1047–51.

Websites

http://www.cdc.gov/nchs/about/major/nhanes/growthcharts/datafiles.htm

http://www.cdc.gov/epiinfo/MANUAL/Programs.htm

United Kingdom: Population Trends (annual publication): http://www.statistics.gov.uk/themes/population/download/pt99book.pdf

United States: http://www.cdc.gov/nchs/data/IW134Pfct.pdf

World: World Population Projections to 2150 (ST/ESA/SER.A/173) (Sales No. E.98.XIII.14): http://www.un.org/popin/wdtrends.htm

3

Assessment of Nutritional Status in Individuals and Populations

Ruth E Patterson and Pirjo Pietinen

Key messages

- Accurate and detailed information on food intake and eating patterns is a critical measure for assessing nutritional status in individuals and populations, surveillance and diet–disease research.
- Choosing an appropriate nutritional status measure is a complex decision based on the objective of the data collection, whether an individual or population is being assessed, the level of accuracy sought and the amount of available resources.
- Instruments that only capture data on current intake such as food records or recalls have restricted usefulness in nutritional epidemiology research. This has prompted the development of retrospective assessment tools that assess usual intake.
- Food frequency questionnaires were developed to capture standardized, quantitative data on usual, long-term

diet and have been used to measure past diet. Their main advantages are that they have relatively low respondent burden and are simple and inexpensive to analyze because they can be self-administered and are machine scannable.
- The major limitations of height–weight measures are that they reflect variability in physical activity levels as well as dietary intake, and they are relatively insensitive to recent changes in intake or activity.
- Biomarkers are essential tools for the assessment of nutritional status because they are objective and therefore are exempt from many of the sources of error and bias in dietary self-report.
- It is recommended that large-scale studies of dietary intake should include objective biomarkers of intake for purposes of identifying and quantifying error in dietary self-report.

3.1 Introduction

Diet is one of the most important and modifiable lifestyle determinants of human health. Both undernutrition and overnutrition play a major role in morbidity and mortality, and therefore assessment of nutritional status is a cornerstone of efforts to improve the health of individuals and populations throughout the world. There are four main approaches to assessing nutritional status:

- anthropometry, which measures the dimensions and composition of the human body
- biomarkers, which reflect either nutrient intake or the impact of nutrient intake

- clinical assessment, which ascertains the clinical consequences of imbalanced nutrient intakes
- dietary assessment, which estimates food and/or nutrient intakes.

Each of these approaches has different strengths and limitations specific to their use in individuals versus populations. In addition, each varies markedly in terms of feasibility and costs associated with the data collection. Given the context of public health nutrition, this chapter will focus on anthropometry, biomarkers and dietary assessment, and largely excludes clinical assessment.

Table 3.1 Overview of issues related to assessing nutritional status in individuals and populations

Nutrition assessment purpose	Assessment data needed for	
	Individual	Population
Clinical	Determination of an individual's nutritional status for purposes of treatment or counseling	Characterization of nutritional status of a patient population by estimation of mean measures of nutritional status for the group
	Characterization of nutritional status of a patient population by determination of proportion of individuals meeting (or not meeting) some standard of nutritional status	
Public health	Nutrition monitoring and surveillance by determination of proportion of individuals in the population meeting (or not meeting) a standard of nutritional status	Nutrition monitoring and surveillance by estimation of mean measures of nutritional status for the group
Research	Research relating an individual's nutritional status to his or her nutrition-related outcome (e.g. disease status)	Comparison of mean measures of nutritional status by groups

When selecting a nutrition assessment method, an important consideration is the context in which the data will be used. The uses of assessment data can be broadly grouped as follows:

- clinical settings for determination of a person's dietary adequacy or risk and for purposes of treatment or counseling; assessment data are sometimes used clinically to characterize patient populations
- public health settings for nutrition monitoring and surveillance of populations for dietary adequacy or risk, public policy decisions related to food assistance programs, fortification, safety and labeling, and development of public health recommendations for dietary intake
- research settings for epidemiological studies on dietary intake and disease risk and for comparison of groups, such as intervention versus control groups in a randomized controlled trial.

Table 3.1 gives an overview of the differences in individual versus population assessment, depending on the context: clinical, public health or research. Although there is no rulebook with regard to selecting nutritional assessment methods, some key points for consideration are given below.

- Dietary self-report measures are the only type of nutritional status assessments that can provide detailed data on food choices, which is ultimately the behavior that must be modified to improve health

and reduce risk of disease. However, these methods tend to be costly and burdensome and are prone to significant error and bias.
- Biomarker measures are objective and can be accurate. However, many biomarkers only weakly reflect dietary intake or nutritional status because of metabolic control and other nondietary factors affecting their levels. In addition, collection and analysis of biological samples are often difficult and costly.
- Anthropometric (i.e. height and weight) measures are easy to collect and accurate. However, these measures are a function of physical activity as well as diet and only reflect long-term energy balance.

Table 3.2 provides a summary of recommendations for appropriate use of nutritional assessment measures in individuals and populations. It is clear that choosing the appropriate nutritional status measure is a complex decision based on the objective of the data collection and the target group (individual or population), with an eye towards the competing demands of accuracy and practicality. There is no right or wrong approach, but only the best measure given the objective of the assessment and the availability of resources.

3.2 Dietary assessment

Assessment of dietary intake offers considerable challenge. Over the course of a week, an individual can consume hundreds of foods, making it difficult for

Table 3.2 Recommendations for appropriate uses of major nutritional assessment measures

Assessment measure	Appropriate	Not recommended
A single, 24 h measure of dietary intake (record or recall)	For characterization of current, mean intakes of groups For international comparisons of nutrient intakes	In retrospective studies When characterization of usual diet is desired In cases where the exposure of interest (i.e. food) is rarely consumed
Replicate measures of food intake on specified days (records or recalls)	For characterization of current, usual diet in groups or individuals	In retrospective studies For studies where respondent burden must be minimized
Food frequency questionnaire	For studies of diet and health where the biologically relevant exposure is usual long-term diet In retrospective studies	If study sample size is small For surveillance and monitoring where accurate absolute intakes are required For use in a population other than that for which the questionnaire was developed, unless dietary habits are very similar in the two populations In clinical situations where precise intake estimates are needed If information on dietary patterns (e.g. meals per day or meals consumed away from home) is needed
Brief dietary assessment measures	In studies where respondent burden or cost issues prohibit comprehensive dietary assessment	Where it may become desirable to characterize entire diet When precise estimates of intake are required
Biomarkers	When an objective measure of nutritional status is needed Where an appropriate biomarker is available	Where there is lack of standardized methodology For individuals if assays are imprecise For individuals when there are no criteria for determining dietary adequacy or risk
Anthropometric assessments	For identification of long-term energy deprivation or excess	If recent changes in nutritional status are of interest For identification of specific nutrient deficiencies

respondents to report their intake accurately. Meals may be prepared by others, so that respondents may not know exactly what, or how much, they ate. Food choices typically vary with seasons and other life activities (e.g. weekends and vacations). In addition, foods themselves are often a surrogate for the variable of interest (e.g. dietary fat), which means that investigators must rely on the accuracy and completeness of food composition databases.

An additional complication with regard to studies of diet and health is that since the early 1980s research has concentrated on the identification of foods and constituents of foods (e.g. nutrients and other bioactive compounds) that cause, or protect against, the occurrence of chronic diseases. These diseases develop over many years and therefore the exposure of interest is usual dietary intake throughout the past 10–20 years. This time lag between dietary exposure and disease occurrence presents significant difficulties in the study of diet and chronic disease.

Figure 3.1 gives an overview of the options available for the measurement of food intake. The primary focus in this chapter is on the direct measurement of food intake and thus only a brief overview of indirect methods is provided.

Food balance sheets

Food balance sheets represent the "disappearance" of food, which can be a surrogate for consumption. The values are based on the difference between production of food A plus its imports, minus the export of food A plus its use in animal feed. This net value is divided by the population to calculate a disappearance value, which is measured in kilograms per capita per year. The Food and Agriculture Organization of the United Nations prepares annual food balance sheets that give, on a country-to-country basis, an indication of how the disappearance of foods has changed over time. When these foods are converted to nutrients these data can help to monitor how nutrient intakes compare with

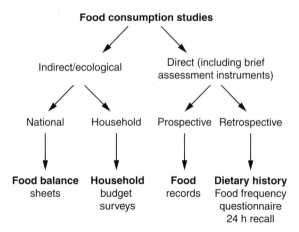

Food consumption studies

Indirect/ecological

Direct (including brief assessment instruments)

National   Household   Prospective   Retrospective

Food balance sheets   **Household** budget surveys   **Food** records   **Dietary history** Food frequency questionnaire 24 h recall

Figure 3.1 Overview of methods available for the measurement of food intake.

some reference value or how the intakes change with time. While these data are not usable for individual assessments, they have been of great benefit in international PHN. In addition, these population intakes have been correlated with disease incidence across countries in provocative hypothesis-generating studies, many of which show a strong correlation between per capita fat intake and cancer incidence. However, the use of these data requires a clear understanding of their strengths and weaknesses.

- *Strengths*: food balance sheets are an inexpensive way of routinely monitoring global food and/or nutrient intakes using a standardized methodology.
- *Weaknesses*: cross-country comparisons of food balance sheet data should be done cautiously and with an understanding of the limitations of such comparisons. First, there are problems with the denominator (i.e. the population) used in calculating these figures. Specifically, there are marked differences in the accuracy with which populations are measured. In addition, the demographic composition of populations varies widely, with a higher proportion of infants and children in less developed countries than in more developed countries. Secondly, in developed countries, there is a remarkably high level of wastage of food at domestic and catering level, which is not measured. Therefore, in developed countries, the food balance sheet estimates of energy intake exceed estimates of energy intakes using direct methods. Finally, the nutritional composition of foods may vary greatly across countries. Fat levels of meat may

vary, as will be types of meat consumed (e.g. muscle versus offal) and therefore the true nutrient compositions of a food may vary geographically.

Notwithstanding these shortcomings, such data are invaluable to those charged with the difficult task of monitoring global nutrition patterns.

Household budget surveys

Most economies conduct regular measures of household expenditure on a variety of items, including food, to calculate economic indices. If food prices are known, then household expenditure on food can be translated into household food purchase. If the composition of the household is known, then food purchase can be translated into weights of foods or nutrients per household member, which is the basis of household budget surveys. As with food balance sheets, these data have their strengths and weaknesses.

- *Strengths*: household budget survey data are relatively inexpensive to restructure for food consumption data and provide a time-trend in national food supplies.
- *Weaknesses*: one of the major limitations to these data is that in many countries, data on food purchased for consumption outside the home are not recorded. This omission can significantly distort nutrient intake given that in many developed countries as much as 30% of energy may be obtained outside the home. Household budget survey data suffer some of the same limitations of food balance sheets in that neither method records food loss during preparation or plate waste. As with food balance sheets, the denominator can be difficult to interpret in that although the food entering the home can be quantified, it is not possible to determine which members of the household consumed which foods and what proportions of them.

In summary, both food balance sheets and household budget surveys are part of a repertoire of options for measuring food intakes that national and public health nutritionists can use. They are inexpensive and widely available and therefore of great importance in countries where there is no infrastructure for the collection of dietary data.

The ensuing sections outline several dietary assessment methods:

- food records and recalls, which measure intake on specified days

- diet history and food frequency questionnaires, which measure usual intake
- brief dietary assessment instruments.

An overview of methods for assessing vitamin and mineral supplement use is also provided. Additional details on dietary assessment can be found in *Introduction to Human Nutrition*: Chapter 10: Measuring Food Intake.

Measurement of dietary intake on specified days: food records and recalls

Table 3.3 provides an overview of issues related to use of food records and recalls for assessing nutritional status in individuals and populations.

Food records

For many years, food records were considered the gold standard of dietary assessment. In brief, food records require individuals to record everything consumed over a specified period, usually 1–7 days. Respondents are typically asked to carry the record with them and to record foods as eaten. Some protocols require participants to weigh and/or measure foods before eating, while less stringent protocols use models and other aids to instruct respondents on estimating serving sizes. To ensure that sufficient detail is captured on foods and preparation methods, instruction on keeping records should be provided before the recording period and the record should be reviewed for completeness after the recording period. In theory, a food record provides a perfect snapshot of food consumed. In practice, there are considerable problems with this method for assessing food intake, including the large respondent burden of recording food intake and the impact on usual food consumption caused by record keeping. Respondents may alter their normal food choices merely to simplify record keeping or because they are sensitized to food choices. The latter reason may be more likely among women, restrained eaters, obese respondents or participants in a dietary intervention. Other sources of error by respondents include mistakes or omissions in describing foods and assessing portion sizes.

Dietary recalls

Dietary recalls are an interview in which the respondent is asked to describe all the foods and beverages consumed in the previous 24 h. Unannounced recalls are often recommended because respondents cannot change what they ate retrospectively and therefore this instrument cannot alter respondent eating patterns. The major disadvantage to dietary recalls is that they rely on the respondent's memory and ability to estimate portion sizes. In addition, it cannot be verified that social desirability does not influence self-report of the previous day's intake. A noteworthy advantage of 24 h recalls is that they are appropriate in low-literacy populations

Table 3.3 Overview of issues related to use of food records and recalls for assessing nutritional status in individuals and populations

Nutrition assessment purpose	Assessment data needed for	
	Individual	Population
Clinical	Qualitative assessment of a "usual" day's intake has a long clinical history as useful method for identifying dietary problem areas and tailoring counseling	Not typically used in patient populations because of burden to respondents, many of whom may be ill or have little control of dietary intake (e.g. hospitalized patients)
Public health	Because multiple days of intake are required to assess usual intake in an individual, these methods are less useful when the goal is to determine the proportion of individuals below some standard, such as the percentage of population consuming <30% energy from fat	A single food record or 24 h dietary recall is useful for characterizing mean intakes in a population because of the open-ended nature of assessment and relatively low burden and costs
Research	Used most frequently in small research studies where respondents are selected for willingness to record multiple days of intake or complete multiple recalls	Useful where the goal is to assess mean intakes by groups, such as dietary interventions comparing control versus intervention groups Recalls considered desirable for interventions as they are believed to be less prone to bias associated with the dietary intervention itself

for whom recording food intake is not practical. Finally, because recalls are interviewer administered, the data can be collected in a highly consistent manner from all respondents.

Use of food records and recalls for assessing nutritional status in individuals and populations

Records and recalls have proven very useful in studies of populations, particularly for purposes of nutrition monitoring. A single day's intake can provide reliable estimates of the mean intake of large groups. Because these methods are open-ended, they are appropriate for assessing intake among population groups with markedly different eating patterns. Records and recalls are often used for evaluating dietary interventions where the goal is to compare mean intakes in the intervention versus the control group.

An important limitation to these methods is that a single day's intake cannot be used to study distributions of dietary intake because on any one day, an individual's diet can be unusually high (e.g. a celebratory meal) or unusually low (e.g. a sick day). These days are not representative of an individual's usual intake even though they may be perfectly recorded. This day-to-day variation in intake is a type of random variation that does not bias the estimation of mean intake for a group. However, this variability does result in an increased distribution of observed intake (i.e. a wide standard deviation), as shown in Figure 3.2. These issues need to be considered whenever data from a single day's intake are presented. For example, when looking at the distribution of energy intake in Figure 3.2(a), it is important to remember that the unit of observation is days, not individuals. Therefore, it is correct to conclude that on 2.3% of days, individuals consumed less than 1000 kcal. However, it is incorrect to conclude that 2.3% of individuals usually consume less than 1000 kcal. As shown in Figure 3.2(b), when a mean of 6 days of intake is used to estimate dietary intake, there are no observations below 1000 kcal.

Because of the day-to-day variability in intake, several days of records are required to estimate an individual's usual food and nutrient intake. Using food record data from 194 participants in the Nurses Health Study, investigators calculated that the number of days needed to estimate the mean nutrient intakes for individuals within 10% of "true" means is: 57 days for fat, 149 days for cholesterol and 424 for vitamin A (Willett,

1998). For estimating food consumption for individuals, variability can be even greater. The number of days needed to estimate the following foods within 10% of "true" means is: 115 days for hamburgers, 152 days for cabbage/cauliflower and 206 days for hard cheese. Unfortunately, research has shown that reported energy intake, nutrient intake and recorded numbers of foods decrease with as few as 4 days of recording dietary intake. These changes may reflect reduced accuracy and completeness of recording intake or actual changes in dietary intake to reduce the burden of recording intake. In either case, it is clear that there are limitations on the usefulness of short-term dietary recording methods when the objective is to characterize usual intake in individuals.

It is worth noting that the amount of variability in dietary intake differs by individuals within a cultural context. For example, within a population, dietary patterns of individuals with routine diets may be well

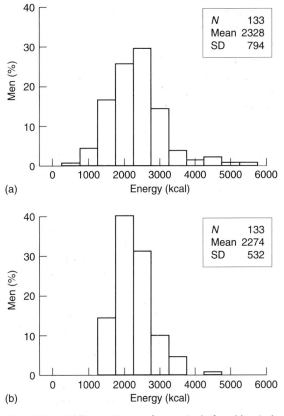

(a)

(b)

Figure 3.2 Variability in estimates of energy intake from (a) a single 24 h recall compared with (b) the mean of 6 days of 24 h recalls per person in the same population (n = 133 adult males).

characterized by 4 days of records, whereas for other respondents even 28 days may not capture usual intake. Individuals in developed countries typically have access to an extensive food supply and tend to have highly variable diets. Conversely, in less developed countries where individuals rely heavily on locally grown foods or stock, diets may not vary on a day-to-day basis, although there may be wide seasonal shifts in dietary patterns dependent on local harvests. Much of the published literature on variability in dietary intake has used data from food records or recalls collected in developed countries as part of national nutrition monitoring efforts or large research studies. Less is known about the variability in nutrient and food intake in undeveloped countries.

Measures of usual food intake: diet history and food frequency questionnaires

As noted above, much of the nutrition research since the early 1980s has focused on the associations of diet with chronic disease. Because these diseases develop over time, the biologically relevant exposure is long-term diet consumed many years before disease diagnosis. Therefore, instruments that only capture data on current intake (e.g. food records or recalls) have restricted usefulness in nutritional epidemiology research, which has motivated the development of retrospective assessment tools that assess usual intake.

The dietary history method

The dietary history method has been used in many European countries to ascertain nutrient intake in their national dietary surveys. Although the methods vary, the basic objective is to use a face-to-face interview to reconstruct a pattern of food intake typical of a recent week. Thus, one approach has been to begin by outlining meal patterns in a typical week (e.g. breakfast 4 days per week), followed by a general description of likely food components (e.g. coffee, fruit juice, cereal and toast for breakfast) and, finally, details of each food (type of juice, milk, etc.). As with all approaches, quantification can rely on a number of approaches such as assigning average values using models, household measures or food photographs.

Food frequency questionnaires

Table 3.4 gives an overview of issues related to use of food frequency questionnaires (FFQs) for assessing nutritional status in individuals and populations. FFQs were developed to capture standardized, quantitative data on usual, long-term diet and have been used to measure past diet. Although the design of FFQs can vary, they typically contain the following three sections:

- adjustment questions that permit more refined analyses of nutrient intake by asking about food preparation practices (e.g. removing fat from red

Table 3.4 Overview of issues related to use of food frequency questionnaires for assessing nutritional status in individuals and populations

Nutrition assessment purpose	Assessment data needed for	
	Individual	Population
Clinical	Seldom used because of the need for specialized hardware (scanners) and software (analysis programs) Also avoided because close-ended food list and/or inaccurate respondent responses can produce improbable nutrient estimates	Rarely used in this application (see individual assessment)
Public health	Rarely used because close-ended food lists may not be appropriate for individuals with different eating patterns Not appropriate for individuals with low literacy levels unless interviewer administered, which is costly and burdensome	Rarely used in public health settings (see individual assessment)
Research	Used frequently in epidemiological studies to rank individuals by dietary intake for comparison to an individual outcome (i.e. disease) Useful in situations where an absolute estimation of individual intake is not important	Especially useful in large studies because of low costs and respondent burden, where the goal is to compare dietary intake between two groups

meat) and the nutrient content of specific food items; for example, respondents mark what type of milk they usually drink (whole, skim, soy), which saves space and reduces participant burden compared with asking for the frequency of consumption and usual portion sizes of many different types of milk

- a food list with questions on usual frequency of intake and portion size: typical food lists range from 80 to 120 items and may include food groups, such as "Oranges, grapefruit, and tangerines"
- summary questions that ask about usual daily, total intake of fruits and vegetables; the long lists of these foods that are needed to capture micronutrient intake can lead to overreporting of intake.

The main section of an FFQ consists of the food (or food group) list. The foods are selected to capture data on:

- major sources of energy and nutrients for most people
- between-person variability in food intake
- specific objectives or hypotheses of the investigation.

The choice of a food list is part data driven and part scientific judgment. One data-based approach uses recall/record data to determine which foods are the major sources of nutrients in the diet of a specific population. However, a food item is only informative if intake varies from person to person such that it discriminates between respondents. Therefore, another data-based approach to choosing the food list is to start with a long list of foods that is completed by a representative sample of the larger population. Stepwise regression analysis is performed, where the dependent variable is the nutrient and the independent variable is frequency of consumption of foods. In this process the computer algorithm ranks foods by the degree to which they explain the most between-person variance in nutrient intake, which is reflected in change in cumulative R^2. In addition to these two data-driven methods, items may be included in a questionnaire because of specific diet–disease hypotheses (e.g. soy foods and breast cancer risk).

A particularly challenging issue in FFQ food lists has to do with assessing intake of mixed dishes. For example, many FFQs ask about frequency of pizza consumption. However, from a nutrient perspective, there is no accurate way to define "pizza". Depending on whether it is meat or vegetarian, thick or thin crust,

extra cheese, and so forth, pizza may be low or high calorie, low or high fat, and so on. Nonetheless, it is unreasonable to expect respondents to report their consumption of pizza as servings of (1) breads, (2) vegetables, (3) meats, (4) cheese and (5) added fats. Therefore, FFQs typically strike an uneasy compromise between asking about some mixed dishes such as pizza or tacos, while also asking the respondent to provide information on foods contained in their mixed dishes: "Cheese, including cheese added to foods and in cooking". Unfortunately, asking about both "Pizza" and "Cheese in cooking" presents the threat of double counting. There are little or no data to guide an investigator in making these judgments.

Finally, to save space and reduce respondent burden, foods are often grouped into a single-line item (e.g. orange and grapefruit juice). When grouping foods, important considerations include whether they are nutritionally similar enough to be grouped and whether the group will make cognitive sense to the respondent. For example, a food group composed of maple syrup, hard candy and sugar may be nutritionally sensible. However, this question could be difficult to answer because it requires summing across multiple types of food consumption occasions: breakfast (the syrup), desserts and snacks (hard candy) and a beverage consumed throughout the day (sugar in coffee).

To allow for machine scanning of these forms, frequency responses for the food list are typically categorized from "never or less than once per month" to "2+ per day" for foods and "6+ per day" for beverages. Portion sizes are often assessed by asking respondents to mark "small", "medium" or "large" in comparison to a given medium portion size. However, some questionnaires only ask about the frequency of intake of a "usual" portion size (e.g. 1 cup of milk).

Advantages of FFQs are that they have relatively low respondent burden and are simple and inexpensive to analyze because they can be self-administered and are machine scannable. A disadvantage of these questionnaires is that they require respondents to perform a fairly high-level cognitive task, estimating the usual frequency of consumption and portion sizes. These types of question can be difficult for many respondents, as evidenced by the fact that energy estimates from FFQs can be outside of the realm of what is biologically plausible. For example, it is not unusual for respondents to report usual energy intakes that are less than 500 kcal/day or greater than 5000 kcal/day. Extreme estimates of energy intake from FFQs provide one of the strongest motivations for adjusting nutrient estimates by energy intake as a way of adjusting for instrument error. For example, if a respondent underestimates both energy intake and fat intake by 50%, the estimate of the percentage of total energy derived from fat is still valid.

Use of food frequency questionnaires for assessing nutritional status in individuals and populations

The major advantage of an FFQ is that it attempts to assess the exposure of interest in many applications: usual dietary intake in an individual. A limitation of these questionnaires is that they are close-ended forms with a limited food list. Because the food list varies from questionnaire to questionnaire, every FFQ will have somewhat different measurement characteristics. In addition, a questionnaire with appropriate foods and portion sizes for one group (e.g. postmenopausal Caucasian women) could be wholly inappropriate for another group (e.g. teenage Hispanic males). Finally, if there are changes in the food supply, such as an increase in specially manufactured low-fat foods, questionnaires can become obsolete over time. FFQs have proven very useful in many nutritional epidemiological studies assessing individual intake, but when the goal is to assess mean intakes in groups with distinctly different dietary patterns the FFQ is typically not the instrument of first choice.

Brief dietary assessment instruments

In a variety of settings comprehensive dietary assessments are not necessary or practical, leading to the development of diverse brief assessment instruments.

Table 3.5 gives an overview of issues related to use of brief assessment instruments for assessing nutritional status in individuals and populations. Examples of targeted and behavioral instruments are given below.

Targeted instruments

Dietary assessment instruments that measure a limited number of foods and/or nutrients are most useful when the target food/nutrient is not distributed throughout the food supply. For example, dietary fat is widely distributed in dairy foods, meats, added fats, desserts and prepared foods. Therefore, short assessment instruments that attempt to estimate fat intake tend to be biased and imprecise. Alternatively, short questionnaires for assessing fruit and vegetable intake have been extensively used in surveillance and intervention research. The typical approach uses two summary questions to capture consumption of most fruits and vegetables ["How often did you eat a serving of fruit (not including juices)?" and "How often did you eat a serving of vegetables (not including salad and potatoes)?"], to which are added usual consumption of juice, salad and potatoes.

Behavioral instruments

The development of brief, dietary behavioral instruments was motivated by problems in assessing intervention effectiveness, particularly low-fat interventions. Traditional comprehensive instruments such as records and FFQs yield fairly imprecise estimates of fat intake that may not be sensitive to an intervention focused on changing participants' dietary behavior. One of the best known instruments of this type is the fat-related diet habits questionnaire developed by Kristal et al. (1990). This instrument was based on an

Table 3.5 Overview of issues related to use of brief assessment instruments for assessing nutritional status in individuals and populations

Nutrition assessment purpose	Assessment data needed for	
	Individual	Population
Clinical	Rarely used because intake estimates tend to be imprecise and underestimated	Not generally useful in patient populations, where energy undernutrition is typically the major concern
Public health	Limited use, although short fruit and vegetable instruments have been used for determining the proportion of the population meeting a dietary recommendation	Short fruit and vegetable instruments have been used for determining mean intakes in populations
Research	Used in large-scale studies where individual assessments must be brief and can be highly focused	Used for determination of mean intakes of targeted foods or nutrients by groups

anthropological model describing four types of low-fat dietary change:

- avoiding high-fat foods (exclusion)
- altering available foods to make them lower in fat (modification)
- using processed lower fat foods instead of their higher fat forms (substitution)
- using preparation techniques or ingredients that replace the common higher fat alternative (replacement).

An example of these behavioral questions asks whether the respondent removes the skin from chicken, where the response options are "always, sometimes, occasionally, never". These instruments typically yield a score rather than an absolute estimate of nutrient or food intake.

Use of brief dietary instruments in assessing nutritional status in individuals and populations

Because brief assessments include such diverse instruments, it is difficult to generalize regarding their use in individuals and populations. However, a few points apply. First, because they are brief, these instruments tend to produce dietary intake estimates that are imprecise and therefore have limited usefulness for assessment of an individual's nutritional status. Secondly, the accuracy of several of these instruments is particularly sensitive to differences in dietary patterns across population groups. For example, the validity of the diet habits questionnaire (see above) depends entirely on knowledge of the dietary behavior that influences fat intake in a particular culture. In populations with different dietary patterns, the instrument would provide a poor assessment of fat intake.

The biggest consideration when choosing a brief instrument is that it is often impossible to anticipate all the questions regarding diet that may appear important at the end of a study. Unfortunately, the use of an instrument targeted to only a few foods or nutrients will limit the future questions that can be addressed. Nonetheless, epidemiological research is a compromise between what is ideal and what is practical, and a comprehensive dietary assessment may not always be possible.

Overall, it is useful to remember that brief dietary assessment instruments are developed for specific objectives and care needs to be taken when applying them to other populations or using them for other purposes.

Vitamin supplement assessment

Compared with food intake, less attention has been paid to measuring vitamin supplement use. In countries where supplement use is common, assessment is important because supplement use per se is an exposure of interest for the risk of several chronic diseases. For many nutrients (e.g. vitamin E), the dose available from supplements (typically 200–1000 mg) is many times larger than can be obtained from foods (about 8–10 mg). Therefore, supplements can contribute a large proportion of total (diet plus supplement) micronutrient intake, which is another important exposure.

The most accurate approach to assessing supplement use is to conduct an inventory, record brand names, and link these data to a supplement register that provides the exact nutrient contents and doses contained in the supplements. This approach has been used in clinical settings, some nutritional monitoring applications and small-scale research studies. However, in large-scale applications where supplement use is common, the number of supplements is extensive and the types of supplements are rapidly changing, this method may not be feasible because of the practical difficulties and costs of collecting data, and entering data on the supplement information and maintaining an updated register.

Epidemiological research studies often use relatively brief questionnaires to obtain information on three to five general classes of multiple vitamins, single supplements, the dose of single supplements, and sometimes frequency and/or duration of use. In a validity study comparing this self-administered assessment method to label transcription among 104 supplement users, accuracy of the brief questionnaire varied from poor to good, depending on the micronutrient being assessed (Patterson *et al.*, 1998). The principal sources of error were investigator error in assigning the micronutrient composition of multiple vitamins, and respondent confusion regarding the distinction between multiple vitamins and single supplements. These results suggest that commonly used epidemiological methods of assessing supplement use may incorporate significant error in the estimates of some nutrients.

3.3 Biomarkers as measures for the assessment of nutritional status

Biomarkers are essential tools for the assessment of nutritional status because they are objective and therefore are exempt from many of the sources of error and bias in dietary self-report. Table 3.6 gives an overview of issues related to use of biomarkers for assessing nutritional status in individuals and populations. Major uses of these data are:

- provision of information about the accuracy of measures of dietary intake: identification and understanding the sources of error in self-reported dietary intake can aid in the interpretation of studies of diet and disease, and biomarkers can also serve as a study outcome (e.g. changes in serum carotenoid concentrations can confirm whether an intervention to increase fruit and vegetable intake was effective)
- as a direct measure of tissue exposure to nutrients or phytochemicals: because metabolic differences may influence absorption and excretion of nutrients, dietary intake may only weakly reflect tissue concentrations, which may be the true determinant of disease risk
- as measures of nutritional status for determination of dietary adequacy or risk (e.g. iron deficiency)
- to improve our understanding of disease causation: to the extent that biomarkers are part of the causal link between diet and disease, they provide mechanistic information about the pathogenesis of disease.

There are hundreds of biomarkers that can serve one or more or the above functions. This section is not intended to be a comprehensive review of biomarkers themselves, but instead presents the basic concepts and key issues around their use for assessing nutritional status.

Many biomarkers have been used in clinical, public health and research settings to investigate both individual and population dietary adequacy or overall status for a nutrient. Typical examples of useful biomakers include serum albumin to indicate visceral protein status and serum ferritin as a indicator of iron stores in the body. The usefulness of a biomarker is based on the physiological and other determinants of the measure. The concentrations of many micronutrients and other biochemical markers in the circulating pool are homeostatically regulated (e.g. serum calcium) or may be only loosely related to intake (e.g. serum cholesterol) because of endogenous production. Biochemical measures with tight metabolic regulation will not vary with dietary intake or nutritional status and therefore are not useful biomarkers. For example, although vitamin C is provided predominantly by fruits and vegetables, this measure is minimally useful as a dietary biomarker because the relationship between vitamin C intake and plasma concentration is linear only up to a certain threshold. The use of vitamin supplements often increases the intake level beyond the range in which linearity between intake and plasma concentration occurs and obscures the relationship between diet and tissue concentrations.

An understanding of the nondietary factors influencing nutrient concentrations in the tissue is necessary for interpreting biomarker concentrations. For instance, tocopherols and carotenoids are transported in the circulations by lipoproteins. Therefore, higher concentrations of these lipoproteins result in higher concentrations of these associated micronutrients in

Table 3.6 Overview of issues related to use of biomarkers for assessing nutritional status in individuals and populations

Nutrition assessment purpose	Assessment data needed for	
	Individual	Population
Clinical	Widespread use among patients, especially in assessment of protein–energy malnutrition and iron and other micronutrient deficiencies	Can characterize patient populations by provision of mean measures
Public health	Widespread use (especially of measures of iron status) in assessing individual status in public health settings and national nutrition monitoring	Widespread use when assessing mean nutritional status of groups, particularly useful when identifying at-risk subgroups for targeting of public health efforts
Research	Commonly used as an individual measure of dietary exposure, response to an intervention, intermediate marker or outcome of interest	Used to compare mean nutritional status by groups

the circulation, independent of dietary intake or total body pool. Smoking has been shown to decrease serum levels of several micronutrients, including vitamin C, tocopherols, carotenoids and folate. If nondietary determinants of biomarker concentrations are known, adjusted measures can be calculated (e.g. serum carotenoids adjusted for cholesterol levels), the other factors can be controlled for in multivariate models or reporting of the measure can be stratified (e.g. serum C concentrations for smokers versus nonsmokers).

Sensitivity of a biomarker to dietary intake is also a function of turnover rate and the relative amount of total body reserves. For instance, serum α-tocopherol represents a relatively large body pool and tissue turnover is slow compared with many other micronutrients, whereas other biomarkers (e.g. serum vitamin K) represent a small body pool and serum concentrations are labile and dependent on very recent dietary intake.

Finally, all biomarkers have a certain amount of biological variability (e.g. diurnal variation), reflecting the inherent fluctuation that is normal in the biological system. Knowledge of factors affecting such variation is important and therefore it may be desirable to obtain replicate measures to quantify this type of random error. In addition, using the average of two or more measures can be an effective method of decreasing measurement error.

Dietary biomarkers have proven especially important to the advancement of nutritional epidemiology. Recent studies using doubly labeled water to estimate energy expenditure have found significant underreporting and person-specific biases in nutrient estimates, such as the tendency for obese women to underestimate dietary intake. Identification and understanding of the effect of these biases are some of the major challenges facing nutrition research. However, progress in this field has been hampered by the lack of biomarkers. There is no known biomarker for total fat intake, and many biomarkers (e.g. serum β-carotene for total fruits and vegetables) are not on the same metric as the food or nutrient being assessed and therefore are of limited usefulness in assessing bias in self-report. Other biomarkers are simply not practical for large-scale epidemiological studies. For example, 24 h urinary sodium excretion is a reliable measure of sodium intake. However, in addition to the practical difficulties of obtaining 24 h urine samples from free-living study subjects, a single 24 h collection has all the limitations of a 24 h dietary recall with regard to being

a poor estimate of usual intake. In spite of these difficulties, there is a growing awareness of the importance of biomarker substudies for the interpretation of results of diet–disease studies that rely on dietary self-report.

Use of biomarkers for assessing nutritional status in individuals and populations

As noted above, the chief advantage of biomarkers is that they are objective and not subject to the biases of dietary self-report. However, the use of biomarkers in individuals or populations is dependent upon issues of practicality and cost. Considerations include the ability to access easily the body compartment for measurement (e.g. blood, urine, adipose tissue); the procedures necessary to collect, process and store the sample; and the resources and technology needed for laboratory analyses.

3.4 Anthropometric and other clinical measures

Intake of a diet sufficient to meet or exceed the needs of an individual will keep the composition and function of a healthy individual within normal clinical ranges. Therefore, many clinical and physical measures are most useful in populations where malnutrition is prevalent. Clinical measures include (but are not limited to) physical examinations of muscle mass, edema, hair and skin. Limitations of these measures include nonspecificity of the physical signs, examiner inconsistency and variation in patterns of physical signs.

Anthropometric measurements are typically a part of a clinical examination, and can include weight, height, skinfolds and circumferences. Height and weight are usually combined in some manner to obtain a single measure of relative weight for height, which is an indicator of long-term energy undernutrition or overnutrition. There are more precise methods for assessing body composition using underwater weighing, bioelectrical impedance, isotope dilution and a variety of other laboratory methods. However, these methods are expensive and burdensome and typically used only in clinical research settings. Therefore, this section concentrates on measures of height and weight, as these are probably the most commonly used public health measures of nutritional status because of their ease of collection and accuracy. Table 3.7 gives an overview of issues related to the use of clinical and anthropological

Table 3.7 Overview of issues related to use of anthropological measures for assessing nutritional status in individuals and populations

Nutrition assessment Purpose	Assessment data needed for	
	Individual	Population
Clinical	Widely used to determine individual overnutrition or undernutrition in patients	Used to characterize patient populations by provision of means for the group
Public health	Widely used in nutrition surveillance efforts to determine the proportion of individuals who are underweight or overweight/obese	Used to determine mean weight-for-height of populations and subgroups within populations
Research	Used as an exposure measure of individual risk Also used as an outcome to determine individual responses to dietary or physical activity interventions	Used as an exposure or outcome measure when the goal is to characterize mean weight-for-height status of groups

measures for assessing nutritional status in individuals and populations.

There is no universally accepted classification system for defining weight-for-height in terms of energy undernutrition and overnutrition, although many have been proposed. A survey of heights and weights can be used to produce population standards against which an individual can be compared using percentiles and/or standard deviation scores. However, the use of population-based height–weight data presumes that the population norms are desirable. In countries where malnutrition is common or obesity is prevalent, use of these norms to assess individual risk can be inappropriate. Ideally, cut-off points for risk or desirable standards should be linked to morbidity or mortality.

In the USA, life insurance industry statistics have been used to develop tables of "normality". These tables give weight ranges for height and frame size, which are associated with longevity in individuals who were healthy at the time of the initial examination. These data were predominantly from upper middle-class Caucasians (thereby limiting generalizability) and provide data on the basis of longevity of young people weighed in their early twenties and followed to their death. However, it is not clear whether weight changes with age are desirable or undesirable, and therefore the appropriateness of these standards is in question.

Recently there has been considerable emphasis on the use of the body mass index (BMI: weight (kg)/height (m)^2). The World Health Organization (2000) has provided BMI criteria for international use: a BMI of 18.5–24.9 is considered normal, 25.0–29.9 is overweight, and 30 and above is obese. The US National Heart, Lung, and Blood Institute issued guidelines that divided adults into six BMI categories that were based on health risks (Expert Panel on the Identification, Evaluation, and Treatment of Overweight in Adults, 1998). This classification system identified 55% of US adults as being overweight or obese. However, there is controversy about this system because it fails to account for gender, race/ethnicity, age and other differences; it stigmatizes too many people as overweight; and it ignores the risks associated with low weights and efforts to maintain an unrealistically lean body mass.

Use of height–weight measures for assessing nutritional status

The main advantages of height and weight measures are that they are quite accurate, noninvasive and inexpensive, can be performed by relatively unskilled personnel and provide information on long-term nutritional history. In addition, in developed countries, individuals generally know their height and weight and thus self-reported height and weight are useful when direct measurement is not possible or practical. However, self-report data must be treated cautiously because studies have shown that overestimation and underestimation of self-reported heights and weights can vary by gender, degree of obesity and culture. The major limitation of height–weight measures is that they reflect variability in physical activity levels as well as dietary intake and they are relatively insensitive to recent changes in intake (or activity).

3.5 Error in methods of assessment of nutritional status

Error in nutritional assessments can invalidate inferences about the nutritional status of individuals and

Table 3.8 Examples of error associated with assessment of nutritional status

Measure	Random error	Group-specific error	Person-specific error
Food and nutrient intake	Respondent skips a question Coding errors in records Day-to-day variability in intake	Instrument underestimates energy intake by 20% on food frequency questionnaire	Self-report of intake varies with psychological characteristics of the respondent (e.g. social desirability)
Biomarkers	Improper handling or storage of a sample Physiological variability in serum levels	Entire lot of samples is mishandled (exposed to heat) such that the serum level is consistently underestimated	Not applicable
Anthropometrics	Misreading a tape Transposing numbers when recording weight	Scale is not calibrated so that all subjects' weights are overestimated by 5 kg	Not applicable

populations. This section discusses this important topic and cover types of measurement error, studies of error (reliability and validity studies) and the consequences of such error.

Types of error in methods for assessing nutritional status

There are many sources and types of measurement error in measures of nutritional status, each of which will have markedly different consequences. Table 3.8 gives the major types of error and examples for each of the methods for assessing nutritional status. Random error occurs by chance. Group-specific error refers to underestimation or overestimations of a nutritional status measure across an entire population. Person-specific error occurs when characteristics of an individual bias their nutritional status measure (i.e. the measure is subjective). Because biomarker and clinical measures are objective, they are not vulnerable to this type of person-specific error.

Identifying and quantifying error: reliability and validity studies

Reliability and validity studies of methods for assessing nutritional status are an important part of understanding the type, and consequence, of variability and error associated with measures in specific populations. Reliability generally refers to test–retest reproducibility, or whether an instrument or assay will give the same finding twice in the same subjects. Therefore, a reliability study simply compares repeat measures from two administrations of an instrument or assay in the same group of subjects. Validity, which refers to the accuracy of an instrument, is a higher standard. A validity study compares a practical assessment method with a more accurate but more burdensome method in the same subjects. An example of a validity study may involve comparing a simple, instant assay of serum cholesterol levels used in health fair screenings with serum cholesterol levels determined by a specially certified laboratory.

Illustration of the importance of validity studies

Many nutrition surveillance surveys and research studies collect dietary intake data and height and weight measures. Analyses of these data have led to the observation that, against all expectations, energy intake and obesity were not related or were even inversely correlated. These observations generated hypotheses that obese individuals had lower metabolism or other biological differences from normal weight individuals. Some researchers suggested that obese individuals had low levels of physical activity. An alternative explanation was that obese individuals were consciously trying to reduce their energy intake (e.g. dieting) and therefore this type of cross-sectional analysis could not distinguish between cause and effect.

The development and use of accurate biomarkers of energy intake (whole body calorimetry and doubly labeled water) have resolved this paradox by demonstrating that in most published research, self-reported energy intakes (from any assessment instrument) were biologically implausible. There is also evidence that certain people are more likely to underestimate intake, in particular women, unmotivated respondents, weight-conscious and/or obese adults, and individuals

Table 3.9 Methods for assessing nutritional status in individuals and populations: a summary of the major advantages, disadvantages, errors and usefulness of these measures

For each method of assessing nutritional status, summary of the major or most important

Method	Advantage(s)	Disadvantage(s)	Error	Usefulness in individual or population assessment
Food record	Open-ended format appropriate for all eating patterns Provides highly detailed information on eating patterns	Requires literate, motivated respondent Needs multiple days to estimate usual intake in an individual Recording intake affects food choices	Systematic underreporting of intake Person-specific biases associated with gender, obesity, etc. Even multiple days are weak surrogate for usual intake	Multiple days (per person) of data can be used to estimate usual intake in an individual To estimate mean intakes in groups/populations
24 h dietary recall	Open-ended format appropriate for all eating patterns Provides highly detailed information on eating patterns Method cannot affect food choices	Needs multiple days to estimate usual intake in an individual Relies on respondent's memory and ability to estimate portion sizes	Systematic underreporting of intake Person-specific biases associated with gender, obesity, etc Even multiple days are weak surrogate for usual intake	Multiple days (per person) of data can be used to estimate usual intake in an individual To estimate mean intakes in groups/populations
Food frequency questionnaire	Captures data on usual intake Machine scannable and therefore appropriate for large studies Can be used for retrospective data collection	Limited food list will not be appropriate for all respondents Requires literate respondent	Respondent may be unable to report accurately on usual intake because of cognitive difficulties or an inappropriate food list Person-specific biases associated with gender, obesity, etc.	To rank individuals by intake for studies of association with disease risk
Brief assessment	Typically inexpensive with low respondent burden	Noncomprehensive assessment limits future questions that can be addressed	Intake generally underestimated and imprecise	To rank individuals by intake of targeted foods or nutrients to address specific hypotheses
Biomarkers	Objective measures are not subject to biases of selfreported data	Require biological samples, which can be expensive or impractical Lack of available biomarkers	Metabolic regulation and nondietary factors influence concentrations Laboratory error	To rank individuals by a measure of dietary adequacy/risk For comparison to measures of self-reported intake
Anthropometric measures	Easy to collect Accurate	A function of physical activity as well as dietary intake Reflect long-term energy balance only	Error in self-report of height and weight measures	Assess individual risk Population surveillance and monitoring

with higher levels of social desirability. Finally, investigators have suggested that some dietary components (e.g. fat or desserts) may be underestimated more than other components.

This finding regarding widespread energy underestimation has resulted in considerable controversy regarding the validity of dietary self-report. Nonetheless, it is clear that nutritional health cannot be studied in isolation from food consumption. From an analytical/perspective, it is possible to eliminate dietary intake estimates that fall below a certain cut-off point of plausibility. For example, investigators typically delete FFQ results above or below a certain point (e.g. <1000 kcal or >5000 kcal) under the assumption that such FFQs were not completed in a reliable manner. Measurements of height and weight permit calculation of basal metabolic rate for comparison with reported energy intake, thereby allowing a more fine-tuned identification of implausible intakes that could be used to delete questionable FFQs or records/recalls. However, without a clear understanding of participant characteristics associated with dietary underestimating or overestimating, this procedure has the potential to introduce some unknown selection bias that could lead to erroneous findings or inferences. Many investigators are now recommending that large-scale studies of dietary intake include objective biomarkers of intake for the purposes of identifying and quantifying error in dietary self-report.

Effect of measurement error in measures of nutritional status

Random error will introduce noise into nutrient estimates, such that the ability to find the "signal" (e.g. an association between dietary fat and breast cancer) is masked or attenuated (biased towards no association). Systematic error across an entire population will not affect measures of diet–disease relationships. However, person-specific biases may result in either null associations or spurious associations between nutritional status and outcomes, depending on whether the error differs according to the outcome (i.e. disease) being studied.

Prentice et al. (1996) used data from FFQs collected in a low-fat dietary intervention trial to simulate the effects of random and systematic error on an association of dietary fat and breast cancer. In this simulation, the investigators assumed that the true relative risk (RR) of a high-fat diet on breast cancer risk was 4.0. Assuming that only random error exists in the estimate of fat intake, the projected (i.e. observed) risk for fat and breast cancer would be attenuated to an RR of 1.4. However, assuming that both random error and systematic error exists, the projected RR would be 1.1. This simulation clearly indicates that nutritional status measures that are prone to random and/or systematic error (such as self-reported dietary intake) may not be adequate to detect many associations of diet with disease, even when a strong relationship exists.

3.6 Perspectives on the future

As noted above, choosing a nutritional status measure is a complex decision based on the objective of the data collection, whether an individual or population is being assessed, and the available resources. Table 3.9 provides a useful overview of the chapter by giving the principal advantages, disadvantages, sources of error and uses of methods for assessing nutritional status.

Accurate and detailed information on food intake and eating patterns is a critical measure for assessing nutritional status in individuals and populations, surveillance and diet–disease research. Advances in computer software, web-based applications and palm computers hold considerable promise for reducing the costs and respondent burden associated with methods of assessing dietary intake. However, these technological improvements do not address the striking problems of random error and bias in self-report that have recently been elucidated by dietary biomarker studies and other objective measures (e.g. height and weight). The use of dietary biomarkers can allow for the identification of respondent characteristics associated with reporting error and lay the groundwork for the development of statistical methods equipped to adjust for error in dietary self-report. This interface of dietary self-report data, objective measures (biomarkers and anthropometrics) and statistical methods is likely to offer the greatest opportunity for identification of dietary strategies for promoting health and increasing longevity in individuals and populations.

Further reading

Beaton GH, Milner J, Corey P et al. Sources of variance in 24-hour dietary recall data: implications for nutrition study design and interpretation. Am J Clin Nutr 1979; 32: 2546–2549.
Campbell DR, Gross MD, Martini MC et al. Plasma carotenoids as biomarkers of vegetable and fruit intake. Cancer Epidemiol Biomarkers Prev 1994; 3: 493–500.

Expert Panel on the Identification, Evaluation, and Treatment of Overweight in Adults. Clinical guidelines on the identifications, evaluation, and treatment of overweight and obesity in adults: executive summary. Am J Clin Nutr 1998; 68: 899–917.

Kristal AR, Shattuck AL, Henry HJ, Fowler AS. Rapid assessment of dietary intake of fat, fiber, and saturated fat: Validity of an instrument suitable for community intervention research and nutritional surveillance. Am J Health Promotion 1990; 4: 288–295.

Patterson RE, Kristal AR, Levy L *et al*. Validity of methods used to assess vitamin and mineral supplement use. Am J Epidemiol 1998; 148: 643–649.

Prentice RL. Measurement error and results from analytic epidemiology: dietary fat and breast cancer. J Natl Cancer Inst 1996; 88: 1738–47.

Rock CL, Lampe JW. Biomarkers in nutrition research. In: Research: Successful Approaches, 2nd edn (Monson E, ed.). Chicago, IL: American Dietetic Association, 2003.

Strawbridge WJ, Wallhagen MI, Shema SJ. New NHLBI clinical guidelines for obesity and overweight: will they promote health? Am J Public Health 2000; 90: 340–343.

WHO. Obesity: preventing and managing the global epidemic. Report of WHO Consultation. Geneva, World Health Organization, 2000 (WHO Technical Report Series, No 894).

Willet W. Nutritional Epidemiology. 2nd edn. New York: Oxford University Press, 1998.

4
Assessment of Physical Activity

Michael Sjöström, Ulf Ekelund and Agneta Yngve

Key messages

- For the majority of European adults, who neither smoke nor drink excessively, the most significant controllable risk factors affecting their health are what they eat and how physically active they are.
- Nutrition and physical activity are usually considered as two different specialties, but this is hardly optimally suited to today's needs in health promotion and disease prevention. The links between diet and physical activity and their combined impact on health is a central issue in public health nutrition.
- There is strong epidemiological evidence indicating that physical activity is highly beneficial for health. Higher levels of physical activity are associated with lower overall mortality rates, and lower risks of cardiovascular disease and mortality, type 2 diabetes and cancer.

- Physical activity is a complex behavior. To understand the relationship between physical activity and health accurate methods are needed for assessing the total amount and the patterns of physical activity at individual level and energy expenditure related to physical activity.
- Such methods are currently emerging; however, no single physical activity assessment method can assess simultaneously all different dimensions and aspects of physical activity.
- The amount and patterns of physical activity in the general population are more or less unknown. Accurate assessment methods are needed to assess physical activity and identify risk groups in the population. Such methods are under development.

4.1 Introduction

Nutrition, physical activity and public health nutrition

Historically, the science of medicine has differentiated into various specialties based on disease categories, organs in the human body, age, gender, special techniques or medical setting. Current health-care systems, international organizations, medical education, research and patient organizations are still deeply embedded in this structure and are served reasonably well by it.

However, this organizational structure, which may convey the impression of territorialism, also represents a major barrier to collaborative efforts between the different disciplines. Yet it is an interdisciplinary approach that may be critical for the success of research and developmental work, as well as for securing funding, especially in health promotion and disease prevention.

Primary prevention directed at risk factors for cardiovascular disease, for example, often depends on experts from diverse areas such as behavioral medicine, nutrition, physical activity and epidemiology.

That today's structure still considers (clinical) nutrition and physical activity (exercise physiology/orthopedy) as two different medical specialties is a result of history rather than of logic. It is hardly optimally suited for today's needs in health promotion and disease prevention. For the majority of adults, the most significant controllable risk factors are what they eat and how physically active they are. Preventive research and the development of public health work will not reach its full potential until a more holistic view is adopted.

Collaboration between experts has certainly increased. Public health exemplifies such a multidisciplinary approach to promotion and prevention research, capitalizing on the variety of available expertise, but there is still much room for improvement. This book focuses on public health nutrition, a relatively new specialty, which embraces the promotion of good health through nutrition and physical activity and the prevention of related illness in the population. The links between diet and physical activity and their combined impact on health is a central issue for this rapidly growing multidisciplinary specialty.

This chapter describes some fundamental aspects of physical activity and defines the modern terminology used. It focuses on methodology for the assessment of the amount and character of physical activity at individual as well as at population levels. It is essential for public health work that information is available about the current level of physical activity in the population, and that risk groups are better identified, to make health promotion and disease prevention, and evaluation of the outcome, more meaningful and efficient.

The different instruments available for measuring physical activity and energy expenditure in individuals, groups and populations will be surveyed, with the main focus on methods that can be used in free-living people. The principles, feasibility, advantages and disadvantages associated with the different methods will be discussed, as well as the choice of method for a particular study. In addition, the precision (validity and reliability) of the different methods will be commented upon.

Evolution

The genetic constitution of humans has developed through billions of years of evolution. In the same way as all other living organisms, our ancestors evolved specific characteristics through a process of natural selection. Up to the time of the agricultural revolution, approximately 10 000 years ago, our ancestors were hunters and gatherers, a lifestyle characterized by physical activity. It has been estimated that such a lifestyle would involve daily movement ranges of 10–15 km, mainly through brisk walking.

In contrast to the enormous societal changes associated with the agricultural and industrial revolutions, our genetic pool has remained relatively unaltered during the past 40 000 years. Thus, the biological constitution of modern people remains similar to that originally developed for stone age life. In modern society, motorized transportation, labor-saving devices and sedentary leisure activities, such as watching television and using computers, have reduced the amount of physical activity to levels much lower than those for which our genome was selected.

Thus, from an evolutionary perspective it comes as no surprise that physical inactivity is recognized as a major health problem.

Physical activity and health

There is strong epidemiological evidence indicating that physical activity is highly beneficial to health.

- Higher levels of daily physical activity, or regular exercise, are associated with lower overall mortality rates and a lower risk of cardiovascular disease and mortality.
- The decrease in the risk of coronary heart disease attributable to regular physical exercise is of a similar magnitude to that achieved by refraining from cigarette smoking.
- Regular physical exercise prevents or delays the onset of high blood pressure and lowers the blood pressure in hypertensive people.
- Regular physical exercise, and maybe also a high level of daily activity, is associated with protection from some types of cancer.
- Regular physical exercise reduces the risk of developing type 2 diabetes.
- Physical activity helps to maintain energy balance and thereby prevent obesity.
- Weight-bearing physical activity is essential for the development of the skeleton during childhood and adolescence and for achieving the peak bone mass in young adults.

To gain an even better understanding of the relationship between physical activity and health there is a need for more accurate methods for determining patterns of physical activity and energy expenditure associated with physical activity. Further, the actual amount and patterns of physical activity in the general population are more or less unknown. Thus, to be able to monitor physical activity and identify risk groups in the population, accurate methods for the assessment of physical activity are required. The appropriate design of public health interventions requires the availability of accurate epidemiological data. These data, in turn, depend on valid methods for assessing physical activity.

4.2 Definition of commonly used terms

The terms physical activity, exercise and fitness are often used interchangeably and incorrectly, and therefore they need to be defined.

Physical activity

Physical activity is a complex multidimensional form of human behavior, or rather, a class of behaviors, that theoretically includes all bodily movement from fidgeting to participating in marathon running. Although physical activity is behavioral, it has biological consequences. Usually, physical activity refers to the movement of large muscle groups, as when moving the arms and legs. Physical activity is generally defined as any bodily movement produced by skeletal muscles that results in energy expenditure.

Physical activity and energy expenditure are not synonymous. Physical activity is a form of behavior, whereas energy expenditure is an outcome of that behavior. The relationships between body movement, physical activity and energy expenditure, and examples of different assessment methods are shown in Figure. 4.1.

Characterization of habitual physical activity is often of interest, since this reflects the long-term patterns of physical activity, and most of the health benefits derived from physical activity are a result of regular physical activity performed over extended periods (months and years). However, in many people the physical activity patterns differ between weekdays and weekends, between winter and summer, and from year to year.

To quantify habitual physical activity, different aspects of daily life (domains) in which physical

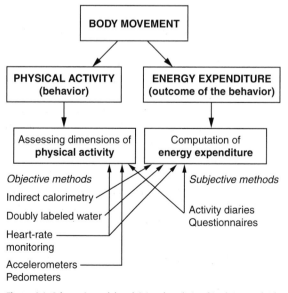

Figure 4.1 Schematic model explaining the relationships between body movement, physical activity and energy expenditure. Examples of objective and subjective assessment methods are included.

activity takes place need to be recognized. These domains usually include occupational physical activity, transport or moving from place to place, household chores, gardening, and leisure time and recreational physical activity.

Exercise

Exercise is defined as a subset of physical activity that is planned, structured, and repetitive bodily movement done to improve or maintain one or more components of physical fitness. Thus, exercise is a minor part of the total volume of physical activity and is performed with a specific purpose. Both exercise and physical activity can be performed at a wide range of intensities (see below). It is generally believed that the exercise intensity has to be vigorous to improve fitness or health. Although this may be true for improving aerobic fitness, many other health benefits can be obtained from moderately intense physical activity.

In fact, the latest physical activity recommendations for public health purposes in adults emphasize the accumulation of 30 min of moderate physical activity every, or nearly every day. This recommendation is similar, with regard to intensity, to the recently published recommendations for young people, according to which all young people (5–18 years of age) should be physically active for at least 60 min every day. In addition, some of these activities should help to enhance flexibility and muscular strength. A detailed description of the evolution of physical activity guidelines, from exercise prescription to public health promotion, is given in Physical Activity and Public Health: A Report from the Surgeon General (http://www.cdc.gov/nccdphp/sgr/sgr.htm).

Physical fitness

Physical fitness is defined as a set of attributes that people have or achieve that relates to the ability to perform physical activity. Physical fitness is an attribute or a physiological state and is therefore clearly distinguished from physical activity and exercise, which are different types of behavior. It is generally considered that physical fitness can be classified as health-related fitness and performance-related fitness. Although these terms seem to overlap to some extent, there is a clear distinction (Figure 4.2). Health-related fitness refers to those components that are specifically related to health and in some instances related to performance, whereas performance-related fitness components relate

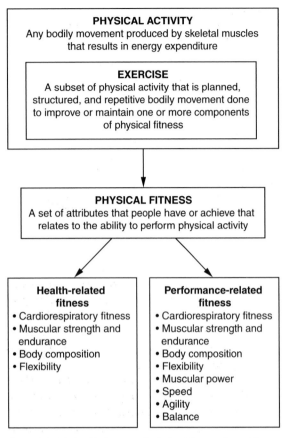

PHYSICAL ACTIVITY
Any bodily movement produced by skeletal muscles that results in energy expenditure

EXERCISE
A subset of physical activity that is planned, structured, and repetitive bodily movement done to improve or maintain one or more components of physical fitness

PHYSICAL FITNESS
A set of attributes that people have or achieve that relates to the ability to perform physical activity

Health-related fitness
• Cardiorespiratory fitness
• Muscular strength and endurance
• Body composition
• Flexibility

Performance-related fitness
• Cardiorespiratory fitness
• Muscular strength and endurance
• Body composition
• Flexibility
• Muscular power
• Speed
• Agility
• Balance

Figure 4.2 Relationship between physical activity, exercise and fitness.

only to athletic performance. Health-related fitness has been said to include cardiorespiratory (aerobic) fitness, muscular strength and endurance, body composition and flexibility.

Cardiorespiratory fitness relates to the ability of the respiratory and circulatory systems to provide the muscles with oxygen during physical activity. Maximum oxygen uptake ($V_{O_2\,max}$) is often used as an indicator of an individual's cardiorespiratory fitness. $V_{O_2\,max}$ is usually measured by indirect calorimetry during a graded exercise test to exhaustion and is considered the best marker of aerobic fitness. However, various submaximal exercise tests, for example ergometer bicycle tests and walking tests, have been developed for the assessment of cardiorespiratory fitness.

Muscular strength is the ability of the muscle to exert force, whereas muscular endurance is its ability to continue with physical activity without fatigue. The body composition is generally considered to be a part of

health-related fitness and may be defined as the relative amounts of body fat, muscles, bones and other parts of the body (fat-free mass). The assessment of body composition and its relation to health and disease has been extensively discussed (see *Introduction to Human Nutrition*, Chapter 2). Flexibility is the potential range of motion of a specific joint.

Specific components of performance-related fitness are muscular power, speed, agility and balance. These components are almost entirely related to athletic performance. Muscular power is the rate at which the muscle can perform work. Agility is the ability rapidly to change the position of the body in space and speed is the ability to perform a movement of the whole body within a short period. Finally, balance is the ability to maintain equilibrium while stationary or moving.

4.3 Dimensions of physical activity

There is no assessment method available today that is able to capture all the different dimensions of physical activity. Researchers have to choose which dimensions of activity they are interested in measuring and then decide upon an appropriate method. Further, there seems to be a relationship between cost, time and effort, on the one hand, and the precision of the method, on the other. The methods that yield data with the highest precision are those that are the most sophisticated and the most time and labor consuming. Thus, when choosing a particular instrument the scientist has to strike a balance between precision, cost, the characteristics of the subjects, time, the number of subjects, feasibility and the overall objectives of the study.

When assessing physical activity, there are at least four main dimensions that are of interest, namely the type, the frequency, the duration and the intensity of physical activity, all of which are important for both descriptive and analytical purposes. The type or mode of physical activity refers to the different specific activities in which the subjects are engaged. This could be of importance for different specific research questions. It is well known, for example, that weight-bearing activities and strength-conditioning exercises are related to bone health.

Most people spend the vast majority (approximately 85–90%) of their awake time in sitting, standing and walking activities, and the relative contribution of each is of importance. Perhaps even more important is the

Table 4.1 Relative and absolute classification of physical activity intensity

	Relative intensity		Absolute intensity (METs) in different age groups[a]			
	$V_{O_2 max}$ (%)	HR_{max} (%)	Young (20–39 years)	Middle-aged (40–64 years)	Old (65–79 years)	Very old (>80 years)
Light	25–44	30–49	3.0–4.7	2.5–4.4	2.0–3.5	1.26–2.2
Moderate	45–59	50–69	4.8–7.1	4.5–5.9	3.6–4.7	2.3–2.95
Hard	60–84	70–89	7.2–10.1	6.0–8.4	4.8–6.7	3.0–4.25
Very hard	≥85	≥90	≥10.2	≥8.5	≥6.8	≥4.25
Maximum[b]	100	100	12.0	10.0	8.0	5

Adapted from: Physical Activity and Health: A Report from the Surgeon General (1996).

[a] Absolute intensity values are approximate mean values for healthy men and usually 1–2 metabolic energy turnover units (METs) lower in women.

[b] Maximum values are approximate values achieved during maximum exercise.

$V_{O_2 max}$: maximum oxygen uptake; HR_{max}: maximum heart rate.

type of activities in the remaining part of the day, since this time may include activities of higher intensity and thereby contribute significantly to the total daily energy expenditure.

The frequency of physical activity refers to the number of sessions of physical activity per unit of time. The duration of physical activity is the length in time spent in this activity. In theory, the frequency and duration of physical activity seem easy to assess, since most subjects who are exercising on a regular basis remember the length and number of exercise sessions. It is much more complicated to recall the frequency and duration of less frequently performed activities or activities of lower intensity. Furthermore, in children and adolescents the assessment is even more complicated. First, the activity pattern of young people is much more complex and multidimensional than that of adults. Secondly, the cognitive ability of children to recall physical activity is not normally as well developed as in adults. These problems can at least partly be solved by using objective measures of physical activity.

The intensity of physical activity is commonly described as low or light, mild or moderate, hard or vigorous, and very hard or strenuous (Table 4.1). These intensity categories can be defined in absolute and relative terms. A frequently used absolute categorization of the intensity of physical activity is the metabolic energy turnover (MET) classification. One MET corresponds to the energy expenditure during rest, about 3.5 ml O_2/kg per minute. The MET classification is a useful tool when calculating energy expenditure from subjective assessment instruments such as activity diaries and questionnaires. A wide range of specific activities has been classified according to their respective MET values. Table 4.2 summarizes the average MET values for a number of physical activities. However, the use of an absolute intensity categorization is to some extent limited (see Box 4.1).

Another limitation of the use of MET values relates to differences in the energy cost of movement between subjects with different body compositions. The absolute MET value for a weight-bearing activity (e.g. walking), calculated as the oxygen cost of the activity divided by the resting metabolic rate (RMR), is significantly elevated in obese subjects. Thus, the energy expenditure in obese subjects may be underestimated when calculated from self-report methods using standard MET values (Table 4.2).

Physical activity can also be assessed in terms of the total volume of, or energy expenditure associated with physical activity. Some of the available assessment instruments are able to capture the frequency, duration and intensity, as well as the total volume of physical activity. When assessing physical activity for public health purposes the total volume of physical activity may be of importance, as it seems that this dimension has a significant impact on the health status. If the researcher is interested in a more detailed picture of the activity behavior, an instrument that is able to measure the frequency, duration and intensity may be preferable.

The total volume of physical activity can be quantified in MET-hours per day or week. That is, the intensity of all different activities performed during the assessment period expressed in MET equivalents multiplied

Table 4.2 Average metabolic energy turnover (MET) values from a selected range of commonly performed physical activities[a]

Activity	MET value	Activity	MET value
Occupational		Driving motorcycle	2.5
Construction, general outside	5.5	Bicycling, general, to and from work (<16 km/h)	4.0
Carpentry, general	3.5	Bicycling (16–22 km/h)	6.5
Carrying heavy loads	8.0	Bicycling (>22 km/h)	>10.0
Forestry, general	8.0	Walking, strolling, slow (<3.2 km/h)	2.0
Sitting, light office work, meetings, light assembly/repair	1.5	Walking, moderate (4.8 km/h)	3.5
		Walking, brisk (6.4 km/h)	4.0
Standing, light (store clerk, hairdressing, etc.)	2.5		
Standing, moderate (lifting light goods)	3.5	*Sport and leisure*	
		Basketball, general	6.0
Home and garden activities		Basketball, game	8.0
General cleaning	3.5	Bowling	3.0
Washing dishes (standing)	2.3	Golf, general	4.5
Cooking (standing)	2.5	Ice hockey, general	8.0
Ironing	2.3	Horseback riding, general	4.5
Scrubbing floors	5.5	Skateboarding	5.0
Multiple household tasks	3.5	In-line skating	7.0
Playing music, general	2.5	Soccer, game	10.0
Child-care	3.5	Soccer, general	7.0
Lying or sitting quietly (watching TV, listening to music)	1.0	Squash	>10.0
		Table tennis	4.0
Home repair, automobile repair	3.0	Volleyball, game	8.0
Home repair, painting	4.5	Volleyball, beach	8.0
Home repair, washing and waxing car	4.5	Running (8–10 km/h)	8.0–10.5
Mowing lawn, power motor	4.5	Running (11–13 km/h)	11.5–14.0
Mowing lawn, hand mower	6.0	Running (14–16 km/h)	14.5–17.0
Picking fruit off trees	3.0	Skiing, general	7.0
Gardening, general	5.0	Skiing, cross-country, uphill, vigorous	16.0
Planting	4.0	Skiing, downhill, general	6.0
Shoveling snow, by hand	6.0	Swimming, general	4.0
Transportation			
Driving car	2.0		
Riding bus, train	1.5		

Reproduced from Ainsworth *et al.* (1993) with permission from Lippincott Williams & Wilkins.
[a] Intensity levels in METs are approximate mean values. The individual variation could be high as a result of body composition, aerobic fitness and economy of movement.

Box 4.1

For example, a specific activity such as walking at 6 km/h is approximately equal to 4 METs. This intensity (absolute) requires a greater percentage of the maximal aerobic capacity in an old individual than in a young subject since the maximal aerobic capacity is decreased with increasing age. For an older subject this intensity may be equal to approximately 75% of his or her maximal aerobic capacity. Walking at 6 km/h can therefore be classified as light exercise for a 20-year-old-individual, whereas the same activity can be regarded as vigorous for a 60-year-old.

by time spent in all activities. This is a common way to express the total volume of physical activity when using questionnaires. When activity monitors are used, the total volume of physical activity is expressed in terms of total counts or the ratio of total counts to registered time. The key dimensions of physical activity and energy expenditure are summarized in Figure 4.3.

If an instrument is designed to quantify the total energy expenditure over a specific period, it is possible to calculate the average daily energy expenditure (ADEE) or total energy expenditure (TEE). The TEE comprises RMR, diet-induced thermogenesis (DIT) and energy expenditure in physical activity (see *Introduction to Human Nutrition*, Chapter 3). The basal or resting energy expenditure consists of 60–70% of the ADEE, and the DIT constitutes about 10% of the total energy expended per day.

Energy expenditure from physical activity is by far the most variable component of the ADEE. In

PHYSICAL ACTIVITY
• Intensity (e.g. METs, kcal/min)
• Frequency (e.g. no. of sessions)
• Duration (time)
• Total volume (e.g. MET-h, counts)
• Type

ENERGY EXPENDITURE
• Resting metabolic rate (RMR)
• Activity energy expenditure (AEE)
• Total energy expenditure (TEE)
• Diet-induced thermogenesis (DIT)

Figure 4.3 Key dimensions of physical activity and energy expenditure. MET: metabolic energy turnover.

extreme cases, the energy expended in physical activity is more than four times the resting energy expenditure. Such extremely high values have been reported in endurance elite athletes, for example cyclists racing in the Tour de France. By subtracting estimated or measured RMR from ADEE, the activity energy expenditure (AEE) can be calculated. The AEE is a useful measure, since it quantifies the total amount of energy associated with physical activity. The calculation of AEE usually takes into account DIT, assuming that 10% of TEE is due to DIT.

$$AEE = TEE - (RMR + TEE \times 0.1)$$

Although the calculation of AEE provides an estimate of energy expenditure devoted to physical activity, it may not differentiate between subjects or groups of subjects with different levels of physical activity. Comparisons of activity levels between individuals require correction of energy expenditure for body size. If two subjects with different body weight do the same weight-bearing activity (e.g. walking or jogging), the gross energy expenditure is higher in the heavier subject even if their movement economy is the same. In contrast, if the subjects do exactly the same amount of work in a nonweight-bearing activity (e.g. bicycling) their gross energy expenditure is almost the same. In attempts to adjust for differences in body size several options are available. TEE or AEE can, for example, be divided by body weight, although the use of ratios (TEE/kg or AEE/kg) to express energy expenditure data has been questioned on the grounds of the variability of the nonzero intercepts between the numerator and denominator, which are necessary if a ratio is to remove the confounding effect of the denominator. Unfortunately, there is no simple approach to adjusting AEE for differences in body size.

Thus, other adjustments for body size differences may be more appropriate. One such approach is to quantify the total amount of physical activity by expressing TEE as a multiple of the resting or basal metabolic rate. The physical activity level (PAL) is

Table 4.3 (a) Physical activity level (PAL) values for different lifestyles and activity levels in adults, and (b) suggested PAL values corresponding to different intensities of habitual physical activity in children and adolescents

(a) Adults (>18 years)	PAL
Chair-bound or bed-bound	1.2
Seated work with little or no option to move and little or no vigorous leisure activity	1.4–1.5
Seated work with requirement to move around move and little or no vigorous leisure activity	1.6–1.7
Standing work	1.8
Significant amounts of vigorous leisure physical activity (≥3 times per week)	+0.3
Hard manual work or highly active leisure activity	2.0–2.4

(b) Children and adolescents

Age (years)	Gender	Habitual physical activity		
		Light	Moderate	Vigorous
1–5	M, F	1.45	1.60	–
6–13	M	1.55	1.75	1.95
14–18	M	1.60	1.80	2.05
6–13	F	1.50	1.70	1.90
14–18	F	1.45	1.65	1.85

Adapted from Shetty et al. (1996) and Torun et al. (1996). Reproduced with permission of Nature Publishing Group.

calculated as the ratio of ADEE over RMR. PAL can be a useful indicator of the overall physical activity, although it assumes that the variation in ADEE is dependent on body size and physical activity. Nevertheless, PAL is frequently used for interindividual comparisons of physical activity, since it provides a way to adjust for differences in age, gender, body weight and body composition.

PAL values have been estimated for different lifestyles and activity levels in adults, and for low, moderate and vigorous intensities of physical activity in children and adolescents. A summary of these values is given in Table 4.3. In general, PAL values vary between 1.2 and 2.4. It has been suggested that a PAL value of 1.2 is the lowest "survival" level in a free-living individual. However, lower values for PAL have been reported from wheelchair-dependent individuals.

At the other extreme, there is a distinction between the physical activity that is maximally achievable in short period (weeks) and the maximally sustainable long-term physical activity (years). It has been proposed that a PAL value of 2.5 is the maximal value for longer periods. Such PAL values have been reported, for example, for athletes in regular training and for women during the harvest season in developing countries. Although referring to a limited period (1–3 weeks), even higher PAL values (>4.0) have been obtained for athletes during intense training or competition.

Each dimension of physical activity differs from the others. This fact contributes to the difficulties for the researcher in choosing an appropriate method and comparing results between studies. Furthermore, each dimension may demand its own assessment method. A combination of methods could be an alternative and this possibility should be considered when designing a new research project.

4.4 Reliability and validity of physical activity assessment instruments

All measurements are associated to some extent with measurement errors. Reliability and validity are important issues in connection with all measurements, not least when measuring physical activity.

Reliability

Reliability may be defined as the consistency of measurements or the absence of measurement error. When assessing physical activity, reliability can be considered as the amount of error deemed acceptable for the use of a particular assessment instrument. When testing or developing a new instrument, the test of reliability is the first step, since an instrument cannot be valid if it is not reliable, that is, consistent over time.

Several terms have been used interchangeably with reliability, such as repeatability, reproducibility, stability and agreement. In physical activity assessment, reliability most often refers to repeatability or test–retest repeatability.

Repeatability is the extent to which an instrument produces the same result on different occasions, assuming that the respondents do not alter their behavior between administrations. When assessing physical

activity using subjective instruments, such as questionnaires, it is important to ensure that the instrument provides the same result over time. That is to say, when developing a new questionnaire, or applying an old instrument in a new population, a repeatability study is not only recommended but also warranted. For other types of instrument (i.e. objective methods), such as heart-rate monitors and activity monitors, the interinstrument reliability is critically important; that is, a high degree of agreement between two (or more) instruments of the same type.

A relatively high intraindividual day-to-day variability is expected in physical activity assessment. Therefore, when using some types of objective instruments it is of importance to estimate the critical minimum number of days that can be assumed to reflect the overall or long-term pattern of physical activity. Researchers have attempted to define the minimum number of days of assessment required to reflect usual physical activity. It has been clearly demonstrated that both weekdays and weekend days should be included. The minimum number of days that need to be assessed is dependent on the intraindividual and interindividual variability in physical activity and the variability of the assessment method. Thus, different assessment methods require measurement of different lengths of time.

This type of reliability is referred to as stability. Stability has been defined as the day-to-day variability in measurements. It has recently been suggested that 4–5 days of monitoring is necessary to achieve a stability coefficient of 0.8 in children, and that a 7 day monitoring period, including both weekday and weekend days, will provide reliable estimates of habitual physical activity behavior in children and adolescents when an activity monitor is used as the assessment instrument.

Similar data have been reported for other objective assessment methods, such as heart-rate monitoring. Since the activity patterns of young people in general are more variable than those of adults, a 7 day monitoring period also seems to be appropriate in adults. However, a 7 day monitoring period does not take into account seasonal variations. Repeated measurements throughout the year may therefore reflect the habitual physical activity behavior more closely.

Validity

Validity may be defined as *the extent to which an instrument assesses the true exposure of interest*, in this case physical activity. More precisely, this definition of validity is frequently referred to as internal validity. This implies that there is an absolute measure of the variable of interest against which the alternative assessment instrument is compared. Since physical activity is a multidimensional exposure, an accurate definition of physical activity is fundamental to the design of a subjective assessment instrument (e.g. a questionnaire) and its validation. The above-cited definition of physical activity includes all physical activity and refers to energy expenditure as the outcome variable. The selection of a comparison instrument is fundamental to the design of a validation study. The perfect validation instrument would measure physical activity objectively with uncorrelated error from the method being validated.

Indirect calorimetry is one option when choosing a criterion instrument for validating a specific instrument (e.g. activity monitors) during specific physical activities over a limited period. However, although portable, lightweight indirect calorimetry systems have been developed, they are not suitable for measuring energy expenditure over longer periods.

The doubly labeled water (DLW) method (see below) is considered a gold standard method for measuring TEE over longer periods, such as weeks. This method is therefore probably the best criterion method for validation of an instrument aimed at assessing the total amount of physical activity or energy expenditure. Often it is not possible to use a gold standard method. If a more practical instrument is chosen, it should be highly correlated to a gold standard method. When an assessment instrument that is considered from previous research to be accurate is used as a criterion for validation, the validity studied is referred to as relative validity or concurrent validity.

In some studies, a subjective instrument (e.g. a questionnaire) for assessment of physical activity has been validated against another subjective instrument (e.g. an activity diary) or compared with other questionnaires. Although a high correlation between two subjective instruments suggests validity, the instruments are not of a different type and may be subject to correlated error. A study aiming to validate a subjective assessment instrument should therefore include a comparison with an objective instrument. A suggested validation schema is shown in Figure 4.4. Criterion methods should preferably be used when validating objective assessment techniques, and self-report methods should at least be validated against an objective method that has previously been shown to be precise.

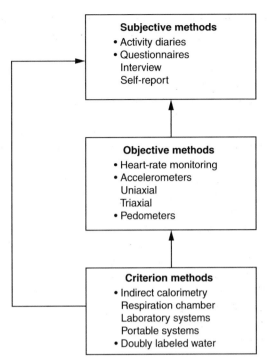

Figure 4.4 A study aimed at validating a subjective assessment instrument should include a comparison with an objective instrument. A suggested validation schema is shown.

4.5 Physical activity assessment methods

Laboratory-measured energy expenditure

Laboratory methods are not generally applicable to the assessment of physical activity in field situations. The methods include direct measurement of energy expenditure (heat production) and indirect measurement of oxygen uptake (V_{O_2}) and carbon dioxide production (indirect calorimetry). The oxygen uptake and carbon dioxide production are measured either in a respiration chamber or through an open-circuit system. Although these laboratory methods do not apply directly to the assessment of physical activity in the field, it is important to understand the basis of indirect calorimetry for several reasons.

- Field methods are often validated against indirect calorimetry in the laboratory.
- Indirect calorimetry is frequently used to determine the energy costs of specific activities.
- The development of portable indirect calorimetry systems has made it possible to measure energy expenditure in the field.

These methods are covered in detail in *Introduction to Human Nutrition*, Chapters 2 and 3.

The latest approach in indirect calorimetry is the development of portable systems. A portable system was introduced as early as in 1909 by Zuntz and Leowy, but the microelectronic advances have contributed to lightweight (600–1200 g) systems with reasonable accuracy. Thus, today it is possible to measure energy expenditure during specific activities in the field with a high degree of accuracy.

There are at least two important applications in the field of physical activity assessment where these systems can be used. First, other assessment instruments, such as activity monitors and heart-rate monitors, can be validated under field conditions. Secondly, energy expenditure during specific activities can be accurately measured. The latter approach will further improve the calculation of energy expenditure from subjective assessment instruments, such as questionnaires and activity diaries. The suggested MET values in Table 4.2 apply reasonably well when energy expenditure is calculated in adult groups. However, in specific groups, such as children, and elderly and obese subjects the corresponding MET values may be different. Thus, there is a need to obtain appropriate MET values for a variety of activities in these groups.

Objective assessment methods

The most commonly used methods for objective assessment are the DLW method, minute-by-minute heart-rate monitoring and motion sensors (activity monitors). The use of objective methods may be limited with regard to sample size, although some of the methods are well suited to large-scale epidemiological studies. When physical activity is assessed in children and adolescents the use of objective methods is highly recommended in view of the sporadic and intermittent nature of the physical activity in these groups. Furthermore, the reliability and validity of children's self-reported physical activity may be limited by their inability to recall such activity with accuracy.

The doubly labeled water method

The DLW ($^2H_2{}^{18}O$) method is considered the most accurate technique for measurement of energy expenditure during free-living situations. This method measures the carbon dioxide production, from which, combined with an estimate of the respiratory quotient, energy expenditure can be calculated. The respiratory quotient can be obtained through dietary assessment or an assumed value can be used. The DLW method is an important development in the assessment of energy expenditure, as it is both precise and usable over relatively long periods. It can be applied in free-living subjects with minimal interference with daily living.

The accuracy of the DLW method has been extensively validated. Energy expenditure measured by this method has been compared with energy expenditure measured by indirect calorimetry in metabolic chambers. The accuracy of the DLW method is high, generally within 5%.

Development of the doubly labeled water method

The use of the DLW method for measuring energy expenditure in small animals was first described in 1955 by Lifson and colleagues, who demonstrated that carbon dioxide production estimates obtained by this method were similar to those provided by standard respiratory measurements. However, the theory underlying the method was dated a few years earlier. In 1949, Lifson and colleagues showed that the oxygen in body water was in complete isotopic equilibrium with the oxygen in expired carbon dioxide. Thus, if an isotopic label of oxygen were eliminated from the body by both water and carbon dioxide, an isotopic label of hydrogen would be eliminated by water only. Thus, the difference in elimination of the two isotopes would provide a measure of the carbon dioxide production and indirectly of the energy expenditure. Because of the extremely high cost of the ^{18}O isotope, the method was limited to small animals until the 1980s. By that time, improvements in the precision of isotope-ratio mass spectrometers had made the method 100 times more precise than it was in the 1950s. The high dose of isotopes needed earlier was no longer required and the cost was reduced. The first validation study using the DLW method in human subjects was published in 1982 by Schoeller *et al.*

Principle of the doubly labeled water method

The DLW method assesses the carbon dioxide production rate by measuring the differential disappearance of the stable isotopes ^2H (deuterium) and ^{18}O (oxygen-18) from the body. The isotopes are stable, that is nonradioactive. Stable isotopes occur naturally and are present in everything we eat or drink. To determine the individual isotope enrichment a baseline sample of blood, urine or saliva is taken immediately before administration of the DLW dose. The background levels differ between subjects and over time, even within the same population using the same tap water.

At time zero the subject is given an individually weighted oral dose of water labeled with deuterium and oxygen-18. This dose increases the baseline level of deuterium by approximately 150 part per million (ppm) and of oxygen-18 by approximately 300 ppm. The volume given is about 80–160 ml in adults. Carbon anhydrase causes a rapid exchange of oxygen-18 between water and carbon dioxide within the body, leading to an isotopic equilibrium of oxygen-18 in carbon dioxide and body water. The disappearance rates of the isotopes can be calculated in two ways: by the multipoint method or by the two-point method.

In the multipoint method serial samples of body water are used and exponential disappearance is assumed. The two-point method requires only two samples, one at the beginning of the measurements and one at the end. Samples from body water, usually through urine, are taken over a period covering one to three biological half-lives of the isotopes, which is from 3 days in extremely active subjects to 30 days in sedentary elderly people. A 14 day measurement period is frequently used in normally active adult subjects. Oxygen-18 is eliminated from the body water pool as carbon dioxide ($CO_2{}^{18}O$) and water ($H_2{}^{18}O$), whereas deuterium is eliminated only as water ($H_2{}^{18}O$). The calculation of the carbon dioxide production rate is based on the difference in turnover rates between the oxygen and hydrogen labels. For measurement of the deuterium and oxygen-18 contents in biological fluids, gas-isotope-ratio mass spectrometry is used. Oxygen-18 is measured in water vapor produced from the samples by vacuum distillation. Deuterium is measured in hydrogen gas, produced from the samples either by the hot uranium technique or by the hot zinc reagent technique.

The calculation of energy expenditure demands an assumption of the dilution spaces for deuterium (Nh) and oxygen-18 (No). The ratio of Nh to No has been estimated to be approximately 1.03 to 1.04 as a population-based average. The use of a fixed ratio based on the population mean of a study group seems to be preferable to individual ratios. The use of different Nh/No ratios affects the calculated energy expenditure.

In order to calculate TEE from the carbon dioxide production, information about the subject's respiratory quotient (RQ) is needed. The imprecision of the RQ may increase the error in the estimated energy expenditure by 3%. Under most circumstances the use of an assumed RQ value of 0.85 does not introduce significant error. Nevertheless, it has been suggested that the use of food quotients (FQs) calculated from food records will reduce this potential error. The FQ, calculated from the dietary intakes of fat, carbohydrates, protein and alcohol, is assumed to be equal to RQ provided that the subjects are in energy balance. A measured or predicted FQ can be used in place of RQ, since energy balance is usually maintained over the DLW measurement period.

The DLW method is no doubt the most useful method for measuring energy expenditure in free-living subjects. It is ideal for field studies, since it is noninvasive and nonradioactive, requires minimal subject compliance and does not interfere with normal living. The method has many advantages, but like all other methods for physical activity assessment it also has drawbacks. The advantages and disadvantages are summarized in Table 4.4. The main limitation of the method is the cost and the limited supply of the stable isotope, oxygen-18, which together with the complicated and expensive analytical procedures rule out its use in epidemiological studies.

However, the DLW method is the best available technique today for validating other physical activity assessment methods aimed at assessing the total amount of physical activity, that is the TEE. Together with the measured RMR, the method provides accurate information regarding the energy expenditure due to physical activity (AEE) as well as the physical activity level (PAL). The method has significantly added to our knowledge of the validity of other assessment techniques.

Minute-by-minute heart-rate monitoring

Heart-rate monitoring is an objective and frequently used method for assessing habitual physical activity. It does not measure of physical activity directly, but rather is a marker of the relative stress upon the cardiopulmonary system resulting in increased oxygen uptake. Nevertheless, it is generally accepted as a reliable and valid field method.

The method is not new and originates from work by Berggren and Christensen. It is based on the principle that there is a close linear relationship between heart rate and oxygen consumption (energy expenditure) throughout a large proportion of the aerobic work range. When this relationship is known, the oxygen uptake can be estimated and energy expenditure calculated from heart-rate data. In earlier studies using

Table 4.4 Summary of the advantages and disadvantages associated with different physical activity assessment methods

Method	Advantages	Disadvantages
Doubly labeled water	Provides an accurate measure of the average daily energy expenditure Provides an accurate measure of the energy cost of physical activity (computed as ADEE − RMR) Simple and noninvasive for subjects Can be used over the entire age span (from premature to elderly) Causes minimal interference with normal daily living	Technically complex (requires expertise and the use of advanced analytical instruments) Analyses are time consuming Cost (one single dose costs US$200 to >1000, depending on body size)
Heart-rate monitoring	Provides a measure of both TEE and the intensity, frequency and duration of physical activity Applicable to children and adults Causes minimal interference with normal daily living Can be used during water activities Large amount of data can be stored before downloading	Indirect measure of physical activity Heartrate is affected by other factors beside physical activity (emotional and environmental factors, body position, type of activity) Time and labor consuming as it requires individual calibration of subjects
Motion sensors	Provide a measure of the total amount of physical activity Provide a measure of the intensity, frequency and duration of physical activity Direct measure of physical activity Applicable to children and adults Cause minimal interference with normal daily living Large amount of data can be stored before downloading	Do not capture all types of movements (uniaxial accelerometers) Unable to detect energy expenditure due to static work Need algorithms for computing energy expenditure from activity counts
Activity diaries	Provide a measure of both TEE and the intensity, frequency and duration of physical activity Low cost Large number of subjects can be assessed simultaneously	Subjective method High effort for subjects under investigation Require the use of tabulated values for energy expenditure calculations May interfere with normal daily living Probably less valid in children
Questionnaires	Low cost Large number of subjects can be assessed simultaneously Different types of physical activities can be assessed Do not interfere with normal daily living	Subjective method Rely on subjects memory Absolute amount of time spent in physical activity may be overestimated Require the use of tabulated values for energy expenditure calculations Less valid in children

ADEE: average daily energy expenditure; RMR: resting metabolic rate; TEE: total energy expenditure.

heart-rate monitoring, energy expenditure was estimated from the average of the heart rate over 1 or more days.

The use of an averaged heart rate may introduce an error in the calculation of energy expenditure, since the heart rate is not a good predictor of energy output at rest and at low levels of activity. The development of light-weight heart-rate recorders that are able to store data on a minute-by-minute basis for up to approximately 10 days has contributed to overcoming the drawbacks of relying on the heart rate as an index of sedentary energy expenditure. Heart-rate data can be analyzed minute by minute and energy expenditure can be calculated separately for sedentary and exercising activities. Various, commercially available heart-rate monitors have been shown to provide reliable heart-rate values compared to with electrocardiogram recordings.

The minute-by-minute heart-rate monitoring method has been extensively validated against indirect calorimetry in a metabolic chamber, as well as during free-living conditions against the DLW method in different groups with various levels of physical activity. In general, the method provides relatively close agreement for TEE on a group level, whereas the individual variation is high.

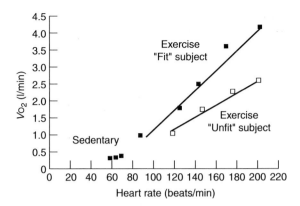

Figure 4.5 Relationship between oxygen uptake (V_{O_2}) and heart rate during sedentary activities and during exercise. Note the differences in slopes between sedentary and exercise and between the "fit" and "unfit" subjects for the exercise activities.

Principle of the minute-by-minute heart-rate monitoring method

During aerobic exercises, there is a close linear relationship between heart rate and oxygen uptake (Figure 4.5). The between-subject variation in the slope of the regression line is high, mainly as a result of interindividual differences in aerobic fitness. That is, a fit subject can perform a specific workload with a lower heart rate than a less fit subject, even though the oxygen consumption is the same. This implies a need to establish individual regression equations for heart rate (HR) versus oxygen uptake (V_{O_2}) at several levels and intensities of activity. In practice, the heart rate and oxygen uptake are measured simultaneously by means of indirect calorimetry during exercise, usually walking and running, at different intensities on a treadmill. The exercises are performed for at least 5 minutes each so that a true steady state is achieved at each stage. Heart rate and oxygen uptake data are generally averaged over the last 2–3 min at each stage. Some researchers have used other types of exercise such as stationary cycling and bench stepping. Opinions vary as to the type and number of activities necessary to calibrate heart rate versus oxygen uptake, but it is unlikely that the HR–V_{O_2} relationship established in the laboratory can capture in detail the cardiovascular response associated with free-living energy expenditure. This is one of the key factors influencing the precision of the method.

In addition to the individually established HR–V_{O_2} regression during exercise, heart rate and oxygen uptake are measured during sedentary activities, usually supine, sitting and standing. The slope of the regression line for the sedentary activities is significantly different from the slope for exercise (see Figure 4.5). An individually determined heart rate, the HR FLEX, defined as the average of the highest heart rate during sedentary activity (usually standing) and the lowest heart rate during exercise, is used to discriminate between resting and physical activity during the monitoring period.

The definition of the transition point (HR FLEX) is the second key factor that influences the precision of the method. Different researchers have used different definitions of HR FLEX. Some have used the "true" average between resting and exercising heart rates, whereas others have defined HR FLEX as the average of the highest heart rate during sedentary activities and the lowest exercising heart rate + 10 beats/min. Still others have defined HR FLEX as the average of heart rate from all sedentary activities and the lowest exercising heart rate. Thus, there is no consensus on how to define HR FLEX, probably because little is known about the extent of its variation within and between subjects. The intraindividual repeatability of HR FLEX over time is critical, especially when examining total daily energy expenditure in largely sedentary subjects, since in these subjects a large proportion of the heart rate will lie daily around the HR FLEX, where the predictive power of the method is poorest. It is likely that HR FLEX is group specific. That is, in aerobically fit subjects (e.g. athletes and children) the lower HR FLEX seems appropriate, whereas in unfit or sedentary subjects HR FLEX + 10 may be the most appropriate definition. This is due to the fact that in aerobically fit subjects the resting heart rate during standing can be as high as, or even higher than the lowest exercising heart rate.

In fit subjects, the elevated resting heart rate during standing is at least partly due to the orthostatic reaction (pooling of blood in the lower extremities, which decreases venous return and consequently stroke volume). In unfit subjects, the orthostatic reaction again occurs, but the exercising heart rate during walking is normally increased beyond the "standing" heart rate.

The calculation of total daily energy expenditure from the minute-by-minute FLEX heart-rate monitoring method includes:

- energy expenditure in physical activity calculated minute by minute for all time when HR > HR FLEX, using the individually established relationship between heart rate and energy expenditure

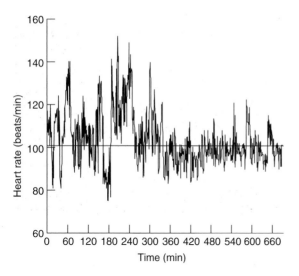

Figure 4.6 Typical heart-rate registration during 1 day in a free-living subject. The individually identified HR FLEX is 104 beats/min.

- energy expenditure in sedentary activities, calculated minute by minute for all time when HR ≤ HR FLEX, using the average energy expenditure while supine, sitting and standing
- energy expenditure during sleep, using the measured or estimated RMR:

$$\text{TEE} = \text{EE}_{act} + \text{EE}_{rest} + \text{EE}_{sleep}$$

The continuous monitoring of heart rate during free-living conditions should be performed within a few weeks after the HR–V_{O_2} calibration procedure, preventing intraindividual changes in the HR–V_{O_2} relationship. Heart rate is usually monitored during awake time for a minimum of 3 days, including one weekend day. A typical heart-rate recording is shown in Figure 4.6.

Alternative procedures used for the conversion of heart-rate data into energy expenditure estimates include the use of linear regression and second order polynomial regression. These methods do not rely on a FLEX heart rate, since all data points are fitted into one line.

Advantages and disadvantages of the minute-by-minute heart-rate monitoring method

Field monitoring of heart rate should, at least theoretically, present few problems. The available heart-rate monitors are robust and designed to function under many field conditions, including water activities. The data storage capacity is good, allowing heart-rate data to be collected on a minute-by-minute basis for more than 2 weeks without downloading. The method is generally well accepted by the subjects under investigation and is applicable to both children and adults.

The assessment of children's physical activity by heart-rate monitoring merits some further recognition. A number of unexpected problems may be encountered, including lost transmission due to fiddling with the receiver unit, loss of contact due to poorly fitting transmitter belts because of small ribcages, and the loss of entire monitoring units.

Heart-rate monitoring meets many of the criteria for evaluating free-living physical activity. One of the major advantages of the method is its ability to capture different dimensions of physical activity. TEE and its derivatives can be accurately assessed on a group level. If maximum aerobic fitness ($V_{O_2 max}$) is measured during the calibration procedure, this will provide a measure of patterns of physical activity, that is, time spent in physical activity of different intensities during the monitoring period.

However, the minute-by-minute heart-rate monitoring method does not measure activity per se, only an individual's physiological response to activity. Other factors besides physical activity affect the heart rate. These include emotional factors, the ambient temperature, body position, food intake, the nature of the muscular work (isometric or dynamic contractions) and whether the activity is continuous or intermittent. The extent to which these factors affect the total daily energy expenditure calculated by this method is unknown. The advantages and disadvantages are summarized in Table 4.4.

It should be noted that many researchers using heart-rate monitoring, especially in children and adolescents, did not calibrate their subjects in terms of their unique HR–V_{O_2} relationship. In such studies, a cut-off point of 140 beats/min is commonly used as an indicator of physical activity of moderate intensity. Although this approach is time and labor saving, the use of an arbitrary heart-rate threshold detracts from the validity of heart-rate data.

When a fixed heart-rate threshold is used, individual differences in aerobic fitness, body fatness, age and gender are not taken into account, factors that undoubtedly affect the HR–V_{O_2} relationship. In view of the inherent errors in such an approach, it is strongly recommended that individual calibration is used if heart-rate monitoring is chosen as the assessment method. The minute-by-minute heart-rate monitoring method has been used to assess the total daily energy expenditure and associated patterns of physical activity in a few relatively large-scale studies, comprising up to 800 subjects.

Motion sensors

Motion sensors or activity monitors have been developed to reflect human body movement, that is, physical activity. In contrast to heart-rate monitoring, motion sensors provide a direct measure of physical activity. The pedometer is a mechanical device for counting steps taken or estimating distance walked. It was probably the first motion sensor to be developed. One of the first pedometers was designed and constructed by Leonardo da Vinci approximately 500 years ago.

The principle of mechanical pedometers is that steps are counted in response to vertical accelerations of the body, which cause a balance arm to move vertically and a gear to rotate. Studies on mechanical pedometers have generally led to the conclusion that they are inaccurate at counting steps or measuring distance walked. The new generation of commercially available electronic pedometers provides a reasonably accurate estimate of these variables; however, the number of steps may not be equivalent to energy expenditure.

For example, the energy expenditure per unit of time during running may be three times as high as that during walking, even though the number of steps taken during walking is larger. The principle of electronic pedometers is similar to that of the mechanical ones, except for the gear. In the electronic version, each movement of the lever arm makes an electric contact and one event (one step) is marked, providing a total count of the accumulated number of steps taken. In one study an electronic pedometer (Digiwalker DW-200, www.digiwalker.com) was validated against indirect calorimetry during various activities performed by children in a laboratory environment.

The validity of electronic pedometers for use in free-living situations remains to be elucidated. Although they do not provide an accurate estimate of TEE or capture the intensity, frequency or duration of physical activity, electronic pedometers may be an alternative for assessing the total amount of physical activity (i.e. the number of steps taken) in large-scale population studies.

Further development of human body movement sensors has led to accelerometers, in which transducers

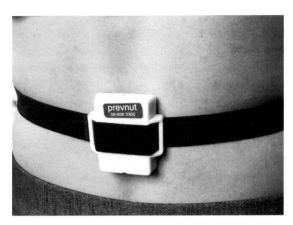

Figure 4.7 Activity monitor on the lower back.

are used to measure the acceleration and deceleration of the body in one or more directions. Accelerometers have the potential to reflect not only body movement, but also its intensity, duration and frequency.

Currently there are several commercially available accelerometers, including uniaxial types [e.g. Caltrac, www.muscledynamics.net; Manufacturing Technology Inc. (MTI) activity monitor, WAM 7164, www.mtifwb.com; Mini Motionlogger Actigraph, www.ambulatory-monitoring.com; Kenz, Select 2 model, Nagoya, Japan; and Biotrainer, www.biotrainer.com] and triaxial models (e.g. Tritrac-R3 D, www.stayhealthy.com). In addition, triaxial accelerometers have been produced for noncommercial use (e.g. Tracmor).

Accelerometers

Accelerometers and pedometers are generally worn in a belt around the waist (Figure 4.7). In this position, a uniaxial accelerometer measures the acceleration of the body in the vertical plane, whereas the triaxial accelerometer measures not only the vertical acceleration but also the mediolateral and anteroposterior dimensions of acceleration. Thus, in theory, triaxial accelerometers should be able to detect a greater amount of movement than any separate dimension on its own.

All of the accelerometers mentioned above have been validated against indirect calorimetry during short-term protocols of standardized activities. In general, accelerometers seem to be valid for the assessment of walking and running, as well as for discriminating between different intensities of walking and running. Additional validation studies of accelerometers have included comparisons with energy expenditure measurements made in metabolic chambers and with the DLW method.

Drawing general conclusions about the validity of the different accelerometers is complicated, despite the choice of energy expenditure measurements as a validation standard. The Caltrac accelerometer has been found to underestimate energy expenditure in adults, to overestimate energy expenditure in children and to show a close agreement in obese women. It routinely displays TEE calculated from body acceleration and the subject's characteristics (weight, height, age and gender).

Thus, the primary evaluation consists more or less of conversion of the subject's characteristics into energy expenditure estimates, since the RMR accounts for approximately 60–70% of the variation in TEE. The explicit built-in equations for the calculation of TEE from Caltrac data have not been published. The Caltrac accelerometer can be programmed to monitor raw movement counts in a similar way to that of the Tritrac, the MTI activity monitor and the Tracmor accelerometer. The results from the validation studies of the latter accelerometers are similar, and the MTI activity monitor and the Tracmor seem to provide reasonably valid data on the total amount of physical activity under free-living conditions in children and adults.

The Tritrac three-dimensional accelerometer has been compared with energy expenditure measured in a whole room calorimeter. Tritrac-estimated energy expenditure was based on predicted RMR and on AEE predicted from body acceleration (with the Tritrac), with a correlation of 0.91.

Activity monitors are usually worn around the waist (hips or lower back), although they may also be attached at the wrist or ankle. The addition of an activity monitor attached at the wrist increased the explained variation in estimated energy expenditure by no more than 2.6% compared with a single monitor placed at the hip. The placement around the waist is chosen since it is close to the center of gravity, and therefore represents whole body movements. The effect of different positions has not been extensively studied, although there may be differences between monitors. Placement around the waist is recommended when assessing free-living physical activity. Furthermore, the monitor should be tightly strapped to the body to prevent registrations due to nonhuman movements.

Calculation of time spent in physical activity of different intensity levels

One of the features of activity monitors is their ability to assess the intensity and duration of physical activity.

Thus, time spent in physical activity of different intensity levels can be calculated. Cut-off values corresponding to different intensity levels have been published for at least one of the available activity monitors (MTI). The cut-off values differ significantly between different studies as a result of different calibration procedures.

Calculated cut-off points for moderate, vigorous and very vigorous intensities of physical activity during treadmill walking and running have been found to be significantly different to those calculated from a variety of activities, including overground walking and different recreational and household activities of moderate intensity. The cut-off values for moderate physical activity varied by a factor of 10, from 190 counts/min when calculated for a combination of activities to 1952 counts/min for treadmill walking and running.

Thus, the time spent at a specific intensity level as calculated on the basis of an activity monitor depends on the cut-off points applied. Even if multiple types of activity are included when cut-off points are established, it is not known whether this will improve the accuracy of the calculated time spent at different intensity levels when assessing physical activity in free-living subjects. Future studies, perhaps including a combination of methods (e.g. heart-rate monitoring and activity monitors) for assessing physical activity in free-living subjects may help to establish optimal cut-off points for activity monitors.

Until optimal cut-off points that are known to reflect normal daily life have been established, the main application of activity monitors may be in the assessment of the total amount of physical activity. An activity monitor recording from one subject is presented in Figure 4.8. Figure 4.8(a) shows the activity pattern during a day when the subject spent most of the time in sedentary activity, and Figure 4.8(b) shows a recording including an exercise session (jogging) for about 80 min.

Principle of motion sensors

The basic principle of accelerometers lies in the mechanical laws of Newton. The second law of Newton states that "the rate of change of momentum is equal to the externally applied force". Thus, force can be defined as any influence that acts to change the state of rest or motion of the body, as measured by the rate of change in momentum. The unit of force is the newton (N), which is the force producing an acceleration of

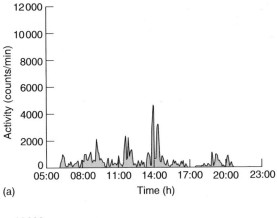

(a)

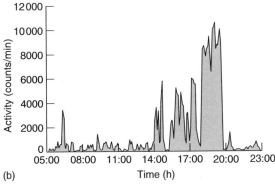

(b)

Figure 4.8 Physical activity assessed with an activity monitor (a) during a day with predominantly sedentary activities and (b) during a day including an 80 min exercise session.

1 m per second every second (1 m/s^{-2}). When a subject moves the body it is accelerated in proportion to the muscular forces responsible for the accelerations.

According to the definition of physical activity, all physical activity is due to muscular contractions, which will lead to energy transformation, resulting in heat loss and external work (i.e. energy expenditure). Muscular work has dynamic dimensions, as in walking, and static dimensions, as in weight bearing. All dynamic work will have its concurrent accelerations and decelerations. Since there is a strong linear relationship between the integral of body acceleration and oxygen uptake (energy expenditure), a measure of the integral of the absolute value of body acceleration can be used as an estimate of physical activity.

Static work and muscular work against external forces are not detected by changes in body accelerations. This has to be considered when interpreting accelerometer data, and researchers have to assume that these types of muscular work will only be a small part of the daily habitual physical activity.

Most available accelerometers are equipped with filters, which are used to discriminate human movement from vibrations. Therefore, nonhuman movements such as traveling by train or by car will not be recorded as physical activity.

Advantages and disadvantages of motion sensors

This section focuses on the advantages and disadvantages of motion sensors based on accelerometry. The main reason for this is the limited reliability and validity of pedometers. However, the latest versions of electronic pedometers have been found to give an accurate assessment of the number of steps taken, at least for a walking speed greater than about 4.8 km/h. At lower walking speeds the number of steps taken seems to be underestimated.

Some electronic pedometers have built-in device for energy expenditure calculation based on body weight and number of steps taken, although the validity of this option has not been tested during free-living situations. Thus, if pedometers are chosen as an instrument, it is recommended that raw data be used, that is the number of steps taken, keeping in mind that this number may be underestimated at lower walking speeds. Pedometers are inexpensive and cause minimal discomfort to the subjects under investigation. Furthermore, pedometers may be particularly useful in intervention studies if, for example, the subjects are encouraged to walk a certain number of steps every day. When used in this way, these instruments provide excellent feedback for the subjects.

Modern activity monitors are robust and lightweight, and thus ideal for use in both children and adults. They are equipped with computer microchips, which allow vast amounts of data to be stored and later recalled for analysis. Start and stop times can be specified, and a detailed analysis of patterns of physical activity in real time can be produced. They are also socially acceptable and can be worn under the clothes.

The main limitation of uniaxial motion sensors is their inability to capture nonvertical movements (e.g. climbing and crawling), typical activities performed by children. This suggests that a triaxial activity monitor may be more appropriate for the assessment of children's physical activity. Older commercially available triaxial activity monitors are somewhat larger than uniaxial accelerometers and may interfere with children's normal activity; however, the latest generation of commercially available triaxial accelerometers is significantly smaller.

Another limitation of activity monitors is their inability to detect increased energy expenditure due to static work, for example carrying loads or lifting weights. Although the proportion of the TEE due to static work is assumed to be negligible in normal living, it may be substantial during specific activities. Nevertheless, activity monitors seem to be among the best available objective instruments for the assessment of the total amount of physical activity in large-scale studies, not at least in children.

Subjective assessment methods

Subjective methods for assessment of physical activity include activity diaries and physical activity questionnaires. Activity diaries are self-administered, whereas questionnaires can be either self-administered or interview administered through personal or telephone contact. These methods are generally the only choice for use in large-scale surveys.

Activity diaries

The activity diary is a subjective instrument, which demands cooperation from the subjects under investigation. When using such a diary, the subjects are asked to record their activities over a specific period. The length of this period is critical both in terms of accuracy of the data recorded and regarding the burden on the subjects. A long period (e.g. >1 h) may result in inaccurate data, since physical activity can vary tremendously over the period, whereas a very short period (e.g. <5 min) may interfere with the subject's normal physical activity.

Normally, subjects choose activities from a prepared list of physical activities with different intensities. One example of an activity diary is the one developed by Claude Bouchard. This diary is divided into 96 blocks of 15 min and the subjects are asked to record their main activity within each block. Activities are ranked on a scale from 1 to 9 according to their intensity. As with objective instruments, the number of days recorded is critical. It is generally assumed that at least 3 days, including one weekend day, and preferably 7 days of recording are needed to provide reliable data.

The activity diary method seems to yield a good estimate of the TEE of groups, with an error of about 3–6%, whereas the individual error is relatively large.

The method may underestimate TEE in specific groups. It has been reported that the method underestimated TEE in athletes by approximately 25% compared with that calculated from the HR FLEX method. The discrepancy between these two methods is probably due to the values used for categorizing hard and very hard intensity in the diary. Thus, the physical activity status of the subjects may be needed to be investigated when activity diaries are used.

Principle of activity diaries

When using activity diaries, the subjects are asked to log their main physical activity in the diary for a specific period. For accuracy, it is important that the subjects record the activities on a regular basis, for example every 15 min or every time the activity changes. The dominant activity for each period should be logged. The logging of figures corresponding to specific intensity levels is thereafter summarized over the measurement period. TEE can be computed by multiplying the amount of time spent in each category by the intensity (MET values) of that category and by the estimated or measured basal metabolic rate (BMR). TEE can be computed in two ways. One option is the use of tables of energy costs (i.e. MET values) for specific activities (see Table 4.2). Another way is to measure the oxygen consumption by indirect calorimetry during activities, which represent common activities recorded in the diary. The latter option is often called the factorial method and may be more accurate, although much more time and labor consuming.

TEE is calculated from activity diaries as follows.

1. BMR is measured or calculated from predictive equations.
2. The time spent in different activity categories is calculated.
3. The time spent in each activity category is multiplied by an appropriate intensity (MET value) and by the BMR.
4. The energy expenditure in the different activity categories is summed = total daily energy expenditure (TEE).

Advantages and disadvantages of activity diaries

Activity diaries are well suited for large-scale epidemiological studies of physical activity. The method is inexpensive and data can be collected from a large number of subjects simultaneously. In addition, the method provides an estimate of TEE as well as information on the length of time spent in physical activity of different intensities. Thus, data on the major dimensions of physical activity can be obtained.

The activity diary is a self-administered assessment method. Much effort is devoted to the subjects and complete cooperation is of critical importance if accurate data are to be obtained. Even so, the researcher is not able to check for wrong data entry or to find out whether subjects forget to record all activities performed. Furthermore, owing to the boring process of recording all data, the longer the data collection the less accurate the data may be. Having regular personal contact with the subjects during the data collection period may prevent this, at least to some extent. As with other subjective methods (e.g. questionnaires), activity diaries are considered less accurate in children, at least below the age of 10 years. However, the method has been shown to be valid for group estimation of TEE in adolescents.

Another disadvantage associated with the activity diary method is the computation of TEE based on tabulated values. The intensity or energy cost of each activity or activity category has to be estimated. Although the energy costs of a wide range of activities have been published in the literature, the use of published values may introduce a source of error. It has been suggested that the accuracy of the method may be improved if the RMR is measured in each subject and combined with intensity values, based on MET values for each activity.

When the diary method is used in specific groups, such as athletes with a known high maximal oxygen uptake, the intensity values for physical training and intense exercise have to be adjusted. The commonly used MET value (approximately 8 MET) for high-intensity activities seems to be far too low to be used in aerobically well-trained subjects. A further limitation of the method is the risk that the subjects may alter their activity behavior knowing that they are under investigation.

Physical activity questionnaires

The development of objective instruments for physical activity assessment since the 1980s has added to the knowledge on the amount and patterns of physical activity in the general population, as well as the relationship between physical activity and health-related outcomes. However, these methods may not be appropriate for all kinds of physical activity research.

In large-scale epidemiological studies, the number of subjects is of critical importance in order to reach statistical power. In these studies, questionnaires are the

Box 4.2

For example, if women's physical activity were of interest, questions about household chores and care-taking activities have to be included. For a study interested in bone health, questions about strength-conditioning exercises and weight-bearing activities seem to be appropriate. For surveillance systems, a few questions about time spent in moderate and vigorous intensities of physical activity may be sufficient. The latter allows ranking of subjects as well as an estimate of the number of subjects considered physically active according to existing physical activity guidelines.

most practical and widely used technique. Another situation in which questionnaires are the only feasible alternative is in surveillance systems for monitoring health risks and states of health conditions. Surveillance systems include systematic collection, analysis and interpretation of specific health data, integrated with dissemination of these data to those responsible for preventing and controlling disease and injury.

Physical activity questionnaires vary considerably in their complexity, from single-item questions ("Do you exercise"? Yes or No) to multiple-item questions about lifetime physical activity behavior. It might be assumed that the accuracy of the instrument will increase with the number of questions asked. However, increasing the number of questions will also entail a risk of overreporting. The number and details of questions asked depend on the specific purpose of the survey (Box 4.2).

Factors to consider when using questionnaires

Questionnaires are administered in two main ways. Self-administered questionnaires are usually sent or delivered to respondents with written instructions, and completed without further assistance. Interview-administered questionnaires can be conducted by telephone or personal contact. An advantage of the latter questionnaires is that the interviewer can ask additional questions and can clarify things for the respondents. However, if more than one interviewer is responsible, they have to be trained in the same way to give the same information to the respondents. Interview-based questionnaires are both time and labor consuming and differences in interpretation between interviewers may introduce a source of error.

When using a self-administered questionnaire the investigator must take the respondents' age and educational level into consideration. It has been considered that self-reports of physical activity should not be used in children until they are about 13–14 years old, because of the inability of younger children to recall physical activity accurately. Furthermore, the patterns of physical activity found in children are much more sporadic in both duration and intensity compared with those in adults, which makes recall even more difficult.

Questionnaires may also vary according to their reference period or time-frame. In an activity questionnaire the subject may be asked either about physical activity during a usual week or about activity during a specific period, such as the previous day, previous 7 days or previous year. A short time-frame (previous day or last week) has the advantages of being less vulnerable to recall bias and is easier to validate against an objective criterion instrument. However, since physical activity behavior may change substantially from one week to another, a short time-frame is not likely to reflect usual behavior. Thus, each investigator needs to decide what time-frame of a physical activity questionnaire will most adequately answer the research question. For some purposes, it may be appropriate to attempt to assess the lifetime physical activity, as some chronic diseases, such as osteoporosis and cancer, tend to have a long developmental period.

Most questionnaires do not cover all domains of physical activity. Earlier studies in physical activity epidemiology focused mostly on physical activity performed at work. Thus, the type of occupation (blue-collar or white-collar) was considered to determine the activity level. Later, questions regarding the intensity, frequency and duration of physical activity at work were included. However, since occupational physical activity has declined in most Western societies, leisure-time physical activity has been the assumed to be the domain that reflects most closely the activity level of a population.

Several physical activity questionnaires have been developed, and frequently used to assess leisure-time physical activity (including sports participation) or leisure-time and occupational physical activity. Surprisingly few questionnaires have been designed to reflect all domains (occupational, transportation, leisure time and household chores) of physical activity.

Reliability and validity of physical activity questionnaires

When designing a new questionnaire or using an existing one in a new population, there is a need for reliability and validity testing. Reliability is usually assessed in terms of agreement between different occasions of measurement (repeatability or test–retest reliability).

An implicit assumption underlying most repeatability studies is that the behavior is stable over time. In the case of a questionnaire with a short reference period (e.g. the previous week), there would seem reason to doubt that this assumption holds. People may change their behavior substantially over a short period. Thus, low reliability can be due either to true variation in the activities reported or to poor measurement characteristics, or both. It is therefore recommended that the questionnaire be administered on two occasions approximately 3 days apart, with reference to exactly the same period.

This approach ensures that the reliability is not influenced by differences in physical activity in different reference periods. If a questionnaire is designed to assess the usual physical activity behavior, it is recommended that the questionnaire be administered on two occasions 2–3 weeks apart. It is important that the instructions to the respondents on how to fill in the questionnaire are standardized and presented in exactly the same way on both occasions. Another inherent problem with reliability testing is that some respondents report no involvement in physical activity on both the test and retest occasions. These identical values reported (usually zero) on both measurement occasions will inflate the reliability coefficient.

To test the internal validity of a physical activity questionnaire the use of an objective criterion instrument aimed at measuring physical activity directly (motion sensors) or of a physiological marker of physical activity (DLW, heart-rate monitoring) is highly recommended. The internal validity of a questionnaire cannot be measured by comparing two questionnaires with each other, since they may be subject to correlated error.

The choice of validity test of the questionnaire is dependent on the selected reference period. For example, if the questionnaire is designed for use with a short reference period (previous week), the criterion instrument chosen may be of a different type to that chosen for a longer reference period (previous year). In practice, physical activity will be measured by the criterion instrument for 1 week and the questionnaire will be administered in connection with this. If a longer reference period (previous year) is chosen, the validation requires the use of a repeated design.

Physical activity should be assessed by the criterion instrument at least three or four times during the reference period. If the questionnaire is designed to enquire about lifetime physical activity, the validation should include indirect measures of physical activity, such as aerobic fitness, body composition, muscular strength and endurance, and lipid profiles. In addition, if a questionnaire is intended to assess TEE, then the criterion instrument should measure this variable. Conversely, if the questionnaire is designed to assess the length of time spent in physical activity of different intensity levels then the criterion instrument should be able to measure this variable accurately.

A checklist has been developed, which can be used to judge the quality of methods of validation of physical activity questionnaires. The checklist includes the following issues (adapted from Rennie and Wareham, 1998).

- Has the dimension of physical activity that the instrument is purported to measure been clearly defined?
- Does the validation method chosen measure the true exposure of interest?
- Has the validation method been applied in the same reference period as the questionnaire?
- Has correlated error between the validation method and the questionnaire been avoided as far as possible?
- Is the sample chosen representative of the population to which the questionnaire will be administered?
- Have appropriate statistical methods been employed to assess the validity of the questionnaire?

A comprehensive review of physical activity questionnaires used in the general population, questionnaires for older adults and questionnaires used in major population-based surveys has been compiled by Kriska and Caspersen (1997). The publication includes a description on the use of the questionnaires, data on reliability and validity testing, instructions for administration and details on how to calculate summary estimates from each questionnaire.

In general, reliability scores are higher for vigorous or hard intensities of physical activity and lower for moderate and light intensity. People seem more able to recall their participation in physical activity of vigorous intensity (i.e. exercise and sports) that in moderate and light physical activity. It is not known whether the higher scores for vigorous physical activity are affected by a large number of zero respondents, as discussed above. There seems to be an inverse relationship between test–retest reliability scores and the length of time between administrations. That is, the longer the

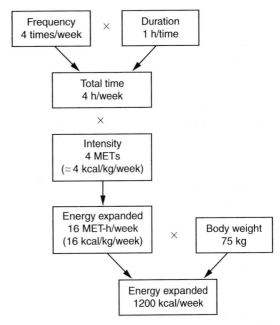

Figure 4.9 Principle of the computation of energy expenditure from questionnaire data. MET: metabolic energy turnover.

time between the first and second administrations the lower the reliability score.

A large number of frequently used physical activity questionnaires, not least those used in large population surveys, has not been rigorously tested for their validity. Most questionnaires do not provide accurate estimates of the absolute amount of physical activity, and young people and adults tend to overestimate their physical activity, particularly high-intensity activity, when answering questionnaires. The principle of calculating energy expenditure from questionnaire data is shown in Figure 4.9. In this example a subject with a body weight of 75 kg is walking at a brisk pace (4 MET) for 1 h four times per week. The computed energy expenditure for this activity is approximately 1200 kcal/week.

Advantages and disadvantages of questionnaires
Questionnaires have the following advantages.

- They are low cost and relatively convenient to administer.
- They are the only feasible method for assessing physical activity in large population surveys.
- They can be used to rank or classify respondents into different groups.

- Depending on the design of the questionnaire, information on different dimensions of physical activity as well as the type of physical activity is identifiable.
- A questionnaire is unlikely to affect the physical activity behavior of the subjects under investigation.

Questionnaires have several limitations.

- They rely on the subject's capability to recall previous physical activity accurately.
- People tend to overestimate either time spent in physical activity or the intensity of physical activity, or both.
- If the questionnaire is designed to assess the intensity of physical activity, different intensity levels have to be described and clarified for the respondents. For example, moderate intensity is described as "something that makes you breathe harder than normal" and vigorous intensity is described as "something that makes you breathe much harder than normal". An aerobically fit individual will probably judge a specific activity differently to an unfit subject if the judgment is based on breathing patterns.
- If the questionnaire data are to be converted to TEE or energy expenditure associated with physical activity, the calculation relies on tabulated values of energy expenditure for different activities, which may introduce a source of error.
- As with activity diaries, questionnaires may provide less accurate information when used in children.

4.6 Perspectives on the future

Physical activity is a complex, multidimensional form of human behavior. Despite considerable advances in the development of physical activity assessment techniques no single method can be used to assess all different dimensions and aspects of physical activity simultaneously.

More sophisticated and therefore more expensive methods provide more accurate information, although these methods may be limited to smaller samples. The DLW method is considered the gold standard method for measuring TEE in free-living subjects. Minute-by-minute heart-rate monitoring does not measure physical activity per se, but has been shown to give results in close agreement with those of the DLW method in groups. This method also provides information about the intensity, frequency and duration of physical activity.

Activity monitors, particularly accelerometers, assess body movement in one or more directions. They can describe the intensity, frequency and duration of physical activity, and at least some of the commercially available accelerometers seem to provide valid data on the total amount of physical activity. Subjective methods, including activity diaries and questionnaires, may be the only feasible instruments in large-scale surveys because of their relatively low cost.

Activity diaries seem to be valid for group estimation of TEE. Only a limited number of questionnaires has been rigorously validated against objective criterion measurements, and even fewer have been designed to include all domains of physical activity. Each investigator needs to decide whether the method chosen is accurate enough to answer the research question adequately.

A further development of physical activity assessment techniques includes the use of a combination of methods, such as DLW or heart-rate monitoring in combination with activity monitors and perhaps the global positioning system. The latter, however, is currently limited to specific environmental conditions ("open sky"). In the near future, wearable computers using tiny programmable microprocessors, which can be incorporated in clothing and embedded into accessories, will make it possible to collect a large amount of data. Heart rate, muscle activity, respiration and skin conductivity will be measured noninvasively and correlated to a microdigital camera worn by the subject. Thus, the development of objective assessment methods has just started, and in the near future, techniques will be in use which today can only be imagined.

Although enormous development is taking place in computer technology for the application in assessment of physical activity, for surveillance systems and for global monitoring of trends of physical activity, there is a current need for a universal, internationally standardized questionnaire that has been thoroughly tested for reliability and validity. The International Physical Activity Questionnaire (IPAQ, www.ipaq.ki.se) may have the potential to fill this gap (Craig *et al.*, 2003).

Further reading

Ainsworth BE, Haskell WL, Leon AS *et al.* Compendium of physical activities: classification of energy costs of human physical activities. Med Sci Sports Exerc 1993; 25: 71–80.
Berggren G, Hohwu Christensen E. Heart rate and body temperature as indices of metabolic rate during work. Arbeitsphysiologie 1950; 14(3): 255–60.

Craig C, Marshall A, Sjöström M *et al.* IPAQ Consensus Group, IPAQ Reliability and Validity Study Group. International Physical Activity Questionnaire (IPAQ): a comprehensive reliability and validity study in twelve countries. Med Sci Sports Exerc 2003; 35: 1381–1395.

Kriska AM, Caspersen C, eds. A collection of physical activity questionnaires for health-related research. Med Sci Sports Exerc, 1997; 29 (Suppl).

Mahar K, Ainsworth B, eds. Measurement of Physical Activity (Special Issue). Res Q Exerc Sport 2000; 71 (Suppl): 1–158.

Montoye HM, Kemper HCG, Saris WHM, Washburn RA. Measuring Physical Activity and Energy Expenditure. Champaign, IL: Human Kinetics, 1996.

Murgatroyd P, Shetty P, Prentice A. Techniques for the measurement of human energy expenditure: a practical guide. Int J Obes 1993; 17: 549–568.

Rennie KL, Wareham NJ. The validation of physical activity instruments for measuring energy expenditure: problems and pitfalls. Public Health Nutr 1998 Dec; 1(4): 265–71.

Sallis J, Owen N. Physical Activity and Behavioral Medicine. Behavioral Medicine and Health Psychology 3. Thousand Oaks, CA: Sage, 1999.

Schoeller DA, van Santen E. Measurement of energy expenditure in humans by doubly labeled water method. J Appl Physiol 1982 Oct; 53(4): 955–9.

Shetty PS, Henry CJ, Black AE, Prentice AM. Energy requirements of adults: an update on basal metabolic rates (BMRs) and physical activity levels (PALs). Eur J Clin Nutr 1996 Feb; 50 Suppl 1: S11–23.

Sirard J, Pate R. Physical activity assessment in children and adolescents. Sports Med 2001; 31: 439–454.

Speakman J. Doubly Labelled Water: Theory and Practice. London: Chapman and Hall, 1997.

Torun B, Davies PS, Livingstone MB, Paolisso M, Sackett R, Spurr GB. Energy requirements and dietary energy recommendations for children and adolescents 1 to 18 years old. Eur J Clin Nutr 1996 Feb; 50 Suppl 1: S37–80; discussion S80–1.

Welk G, ed. Physical Activity Assessments for Health-Related Research. Champagne, IL: Human Kinetics, 2002.

Website

Physical Activity and Health. A Report from the Surgeon General, 1996. http://www.cdc.gov/nccdphp/sgr/sgr.htm

5
Public Health Nutrition Strategies for Intervention at the Ecological Level

Kim D Reynolds, Knut-Inge Klepp and Amy L Yaroch

Key messages

- The ecological approach was developed by social scientists and adapted by researchers and practitioners in health promotion to help understand and influence health behaviors.
- In the ecological approach, health behavior is believed to be determined by multiple levels of influence, including intrapersonal factors and environmental factors.
- The ecological approach recognizes the importance of individual factors in determining nutrition behavior, but is also concerned with factors outside the individual and with the interaction between the individual and the environment.
- Interventions designed using the ecological approach move beyond individual one-on-one encounters with a nutrition educator, and can occur in a number of settings including schools, churches, grocery stores and state legislatures, to name just a few.
- When an intervention is developed using the ecological approach, it is important to define the level of the organization that will be targeted by that intervention. Some interventions will target factors at the intrapersonal level, some will target the social and cultural level, and others will attempt to influence the physical environment.
- Different aspects of the ecological model can be used to change eating habits across diverse cultures and geographical areas.

5.1 Introduction

The actions that people take are determined by a wide range of factors. Individual beliefs, friends and family, laws and regulations, and the physical environment are all factors that help to determine how people live their lives. The ecological approach was developed by social scientists to help to understand this complex web of influences on behavior. This approach has been adapted by researchers and practitioners in health promotion to help to understand and influence health behaviors. This chapter will describe the ecological approach and its use in understanding nutrition behavior. In addition, the chapter will explain how this approach can be used to develop effective interventions to change people's eating patterns.

5.2 Definition of the ecological approach

It is helpful to begin our exploration of the ecological approach by defining some of its key elements. Green and colleagues stated "The ecological model of health promotion presents health as a product of the interdependence between the individual and subsystems of the ecosystem (e.g., family, community, culture, physical and social environment)." That is, health is not determined solely by an individual and his or her personal actions and characteristics. Rather, health is determined by:

- individual actions and characteristics
- factors outside the individual
- an interaction between the two.

For example, the incidence of overweight and obesity has been increasing around the world and has reached epidemic proportions, according to many health authorities. Overweight and obesity result from positive energy imbalance. That is, when people burn too few calories through physical activity, relative to their intake of calories from eating, they gain weight. Eating and physical activity patterns are individual characteristics. Individuals decide how much physical activity to take and which foods to consume. However, according to the ecological approach, these personal decisions about exercise and eating patterns are only part of the story. The amount and type of food a person eats, and the amount of physical activity they take are also determined by factors outside the individual. These environmental factors include the availability of different types of foods and the demands for physical activity placed on a person by their social and physical environment. According to many researchers, the current epidemic of obesity may be due to long-term changes in the availability of energy-dense foods, to societal changes that support consumption of these foods, to reduced demands for physical activity, and to reduced opportunities and support for physical activity in our societies. There is evidence, for example, that the portion size of foods people consume outside the home has been increasing for many years. As a result, the number of calories consumed by people may have increased. Thus, portion size is a factor in the ecosystem that exists outside the individual, which can influence the number of calories a person consumes and which can have an influence on weight and health status.

In the ecological approach, health behavior is also believed to be determined by multiple levels of influence, including intrapersonal factors and environmental factors. For example, a preference for low-fat foods (intrapersonal factor) will partially determine whether a person eats low-fat snacks. However, the availability (environmental factor) of low-fat snacks in the home, restaurants and cafeteria where a person works also determine whether that person will eat low-fat snacks. A person's friends and colleagues also influence how he or she eats through social pressure, social norms and modeling (environmental–interpersonal factor). Thus, a person's ability to eat low-fat snacks may be limited or facilitated by their physical and social environments.

Defining characteristics of the ecological approach are summarized in Box 5.1.

> **Box 5.1** Defining characteristics of the ecological approach
>
> - Behavior is determined by multiple levels of influence, including intrapersonal factors and environmental factors.
> - Health is a product of the interdependence between the individual and subsystems of the ecosystem (e.g. family, community, culture, physical and social environment).

5.3 Individual versus ecological approaches

It is important to understand the distinction between individual-level approaches and ecological approaches to explaining nutrition behavior. Individual-level approaches focus solely on factors within the individual, or on the individual's perceptions of their environment to explain nutrition behavior. Factors within the individual such as knowledge, positive or negative attitudes, and personal beliefs about social norms are used in the individual approach to explain nutrition behavior. For example, if an individual holds positive attitudes towards low-fat eating, they are more likely to limit consumption of high-fat snacks, to prepare foods with less fat and to select lower fat meals when eating out in restaurants or cafeterias. The ecological approach recognizes the importance of individual factors in determining nutrition behavior, but is also concerned with factors outside the individual (i.e. environmental factors), and with the interaction between the individual and the environment. The interaction between individual influences and environmental influences, in particular, is what sets the ecological approach apart from the individual approach. The interaction means that various individuals may be influenced by different environmental factors or in different ways by the same environmental factors. For example, a person at a high income level may not be influenced by fluctuations in the price of produce and may purchase the same amount of fruit and vegetables regardless of these fluctuations. However, lower income individuals may be readily influenced by price fluctuations and may be less likely to purchase and consume fruit and vegetables when prices are high.

Individual versus environmental factors in the ecological approach are summarized in Box 5.2.

The use of the ecological approach does not minimize the importance of changes in knowledge and psychosocial factors within the individual. Rather, this approach seeks to identify additional levels of influence

> **Box 5.2** Individual versus environmental factors in the ecological approach
>
> - Individual causes of nutrition behavior are recognized in the ecological approach.
> - Environmental causes of nutrition behavior are also seen as important.
> - The interaction between individual and environmental causes of behavior is important in the ecological model.

> **Box 5.3** Examples of factors included in the intrapersonal level of the environment
>
> - Perceived barriers to dietary change
> - Perceived benefits of dietary change
> - Perceived social norms for eating different foods
> - Perceived self-efficacy for dietary change
> - Knowledge related to nutrition
> - Intention to eat specific foods
> - Taste preferences
> - Skills for food preparation.

on behavior, and incorporate these to help in the understanding of human behavior. The nutrition educator can take advantage of these additional levels of influence to produce stronger changes in nutrition behavior by intervening directly on environmental factors. Interventions designed using the ecological approach move beyond individual one-on-one encounters with a nutrition educator, and can occur in a number of settings including schools, churches, grocery stores and state legislatures, to name just a few.

5.4 Key principles in the ecological approach

Various models have been proposed to describe the ecological approach. These models share several common elements that are described below.

Levels of organization in the ecological approach

The ecosystem is very complex. Models of the ecological approach attempt to characterize the ecosystem by dividing it into various levels. This chapter uses one of the simpler formulations that includes three main levels of the ecosystem. These include the intrapersonal, social and cultural, and physical levels. The ecological approach suggests that each of these levels is important in determining behavior. Thus, it is important to understand each level as a means of understanding nutrition behavior and designing interventions to change that behavior.

Intrapersonal level

These are attitudes, beliefs and perceptions that individuals hold towards dietary behavior. Many of these variables have been examined in research projects and are related to nutrition behavior. These attitudes, beliefs and perceptions exist within the individual and may or may not be shared with other people. For example, perceived self-efficacy is an individual's

belief in their ability to change a specific behavior such as increasing fruit and vegetable consumption or reducing fat consumption. Higher self-efficacy leads to greater change in behavior. If a woman believes that she is able to prepare more vegetarian meals, she is more likely to do so than a woman who does not believe that she is capable of preparing these meals. Another example of an intrapersonal factor is perceived barriers to changing one's diet. People differ in their perceptions of the barriers encountered in changing their nutrition behavior. Some people perceive a high number of barriers, while others perceive a low number of barriers. If perceptions of barriers are high, this may inhibit a person from changing the way they eat. For example, a man may believe that fruit and vegetables are expensive, that they spoil quickly and that they will make his meals less enjoyable. These could be seen as perceived barriers to eating more fruit and vegetables. If he believes that a large number of barriers exist, he is less likely to purchase fruit and vegetables. Numerous theories exist to describe the effects that these intrapersonal factors have on nutrition behavior, including social cognitive theory, the Health Belief Model and the Theory of Planned Behavior. In addition, these factors have often been used to design nutrition education programs.

Examples of factors included in the intrapersonal level of the environment are listed in Box 5.3.

Social and cultural environments

This level of the ecological approach includes the interactions that people have with family, friends, institutions (e.g. churches, schools, worksites) and government policies or laws. Broad cultural influences are also often considered a part of the social and cultural environment.

In the ecological approach, these different factors (e.g. family, worksite, government) can influence one another. Thus, a complete understanding of nutrition behavior requires an analysis of the diverse relationships between these factors, and their ultimate linkage to the behavior of individuals. For example, changes in national dietary guidelines by the federal government are typically covered by the media, which in turn produces increases in awareness by individuals. These individuals may then make different food purchasing decisions that affect the price and availability of food items in stores. Thus, the modification of a dietary guideline can trigger changes in individuals, and in the social and cultural, and physical environmental levels of the ecosystem.

A plausible target for intervention using an ecological approach is to change organizations, rather than individuals within organizations. For example, a nutrition intervention based on the ecological approach may change the types of foods offered in a worksite cafeteria. The elimination of high-fat foods and high-fat preparation methods from the cafeteria is a legitimate target of an ecological intervention. These changes in offerings may lead directly to reduced fat consumption among the employees of the worksite. This intervention does not aim to change intrapersonal factors, but can produce a change in eating patterns by intervening directly in the social and cultural environment. The intervention may also reduce fat consumption indirectly by exposing workers to new low-fat food options and changing their preference for these foods. This modification in taste preferences may then carry over into other environments, influencing the foods consumed at home and in restaurants.

A large number of avenues for nutrition intervention can be identified within the social and cultural level of the environment. Examples are a mass media campaign mounted to alter the cultural norms for healthy eating, and a church-based intervention in which members support one another in preparing low-fat, high-fiber foods for church events, and where the pastor models and supports healthy eating.

Physical environment

The presence of different types of food, and other characteristics of the physical infrastructure that help to determine what we eat, define this level of the ecosystem. The most obvious example of the physical environment is the availability of different types of food. Foods that are more available are more likely to be consumed. Conversely, foods that are not available will not be consumed. Thus, efforts to make more fruit and

vegetables present in restaurants, cafeterias and homes may well lead to increases in consumption. Similarly, the removal of high-fat and high-salt food items from vending machines in schools, worksites or other locations may lead to reduced consumption of these food items. The physical environment may also extend beyond the simple availability of certain food items. For example, if a family does not have a refrigerator, some food items may not be kept at home because of problems with spoilage. Such a family may be forced to consume large quantities of canned foods or fast foods, which may be higher in sugar, fat and salt than alternatives that must be kept refrigerated. As noted earlier in this chapter, portion size is an environmental factor that has received increasing attention among nutrition researchers and which may contribute to increased energy intake and the epidemic of obesity being experienced in many countries around the world. The increasing tendency for families to eat meals that are prepared outside the home, and the typically higher energy density and fat content of these foods, can greatly impact the quality of the diet. The labeling of food items is another form of physical environmental change that can impact dietary habits. The presence of food labels that are easy to understand, and that provide appropriate information for people to make decisions about the foods they purchase and eat, could impact eating habits.

Finally, the seasonal availability of foods, and the impact that this availability could have on prices, is another example of an environmental factor that may influence eating habits. If foods are less available in the winter, or prices are higher owing to lower supply and higher import costs, people are less likely to purchase these foods. The influence of seasonal factors may have been diminished in recent years in many countries because of the greater availability of low-cost imported fruits and vegetables.

Levels of organization in the ecological approach are shown in Box 5.4.

Box 5.4 Levels of organization in the ecological approach

- Intrapersonal: including knowledge, attitudes and beliefs.
- Social and cultural: including friends and coworkers, settings such as schools and churches, organizations such as local governments, and laws and policy.
- Physical environment: including climate, geography, and availability of foods in the home and neighborhoods.

5.5 Intervention

Targets of intervention

When an intervention is developed using the ecological approach, it is important to define the level of the organization that will be targeted by that intervention. Some interventions will target factors at the intrapersonal level, some will target the social and cultural level, and others will attempt to influence the physical environment. Although each of these interventions is attempting to improve the diet of individuals, their influence may be produced through change in social and cultural or physical levels of the environment. Targets of the intervention are usually considered more important than the settings in which the interventions occur. Targets receive intervention in the hope of making changes that will ultimately benefit the individual clients.

Settings for intervention

The setting is a particular organization, community or society through which clients for an intervention are identified. The setting for an intervention and the targets of the intervention are not the same thing. Individuals may be selected as a target for an intervention, with those individuals being reached through churches, which provide the setting for the intervention. Alternatively, one may be interested in changing the policies of the churches themselves, making churches the target of the intervention, and the setting is both the church and the community from which the church is drawn.

Intervention strategy

To develop an intervention based on the ecological approach, it is important to define an intervention strategy that describes how the intervention targets interact within a given setting to produce change in individuals. An intervention may be designed first to produce changes in an organization, which then lead to changes in the individual clients. For example, nutrition educators may work directly with fast food restaurants to offer a low-fat alternative to their usual high-fat meals. This is a change in the policy of the fast food organization (social and cultural level), which will lead to increased availability of low-fat menu items (physical environmental level), increased consumption of low-fat foods by customers (intrapersonal level) and

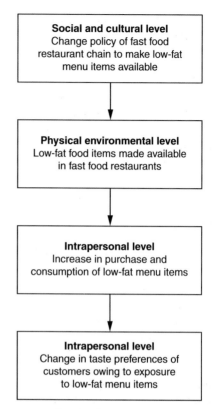

Figure 5.1 Strategy for a fast food intervention using the ecological approach.

perhaps a change in the customers' preferences for low-fat foods (intrapersonal level) (Figure 5.1). Another example can be drawn from the 5-a-Day for Better Health program conducted in the USA. In this program, the National Cancer Institute, a federal government agency, collaborated with wholesaler producers of fruit and vegetables to increase the consumption of fruit and vegetables in ways consistent with national guidelines. This collaboration led to the use of several major intervention activities at the social and cultural level of the environment. These activities included a national media campaign, the licensing of fruit and vegetables retailers to promote fruit and vegetables in their stores, the formation of state coalitions to promote fruit and vegetables in their states, and the completion of carefully evaluated community intervention studies. The combination of these activities at the social and cultural level of the environment led to additional changes in individuals' knowledge, attitudes and preferences about fruit and vegetables (intrapersonal level), to changes in the availability of fruit and vegetables (physical environmental level), and eventually to changes in the consumption of fruit and vegetables by individuals (intrapersonal level).

The examples above illustrate the importance of defining the strategy to be used for the intervention when an ecological approach is used. Since three levels and many factors within each level can be used to mount an intervention, a planning process is crucial to maximize the efficiency and the effectiveness of the intervention.

5.6 Advantages and disadvantages of this approach

Importance of the ecological approach

The ecological approach is important for several reasons. First, interventions that consider multiple levels of influence on nutrition behavior may be more effective. For example, a program that increases preferences for fruit and vegetables, but does nothing to increase the availability of those foods, is probably going to produce smaller increases in consumption than a program that addresses both preferences and availability. Secondly, ecological interventions can also improve nutrition behavior without the need to change individual's knowledge, attitudes, beliefs or skills directly. For example, reducing the amount of fat present in foods served in school cafeterias can reduce overall fat consumption without altering children's beliefs or attitudes about low-fat foods. This type of program is often referred to as a passive intervention program. Passive interventions, once established, can be maintained more readily at a lower cost than active interventions. Such interventions can also last longer, since they require less support and are often built into schools, worksites or other community settings as a policy that remains in force until changed, or as a physical environmental change that lasts until modified. Nutrition behavior can be altered through passive interventions that do not require ongoing educational interventions.

Limitations of the ecological approach

Although it has many advantages, the ecological approach also has its limitations. Understanding the levels, and factors within levels, of the ecosystem that can influence nutrition behavior is a very complex undertaking. For example, the foods that are available in supermarkets and restaurants, the dietary preferences

> **Box 5.5** Limitations of the ecological approach
>
> - It is difficult to understand all levels of ecological influence on eating patterns.
> - Levels of ecological influence interact, making the model even more complex.
> - Intervening at more than one level of the ecosystem can be difficult and costly.

of family members, individuals' beliefs about the types of food that will make them healthy and attractive, and the policies of the government about food labels, may all influence the food that a person eats. The ecological approach suggests that the levels of the ecosystem and the factors within levels interact with one another. For example, the types of food available in the grocery store are influenced by government import policy, and the government import policies may be influenced by the demand exerted by the public for certain types of food. To simplify our understanding of the diverse ecological influences on nutrition behavior, it is often necessary to consider a limited set of ecological influences and how they interact with one another at a given time. Intervening at more than one level in the ecosystem can be difficult and costly. For example, a comprehensive effort to reduce the amount of fat used for cooking by families may require lobbying efforts with local supermarkets to remove lard from the store shelves, community education efforts to alter the perceptions of food preparers about what constitutes healthy cooking practices and efforts to change the taste preferences of individuals. Limitations of the ecological approach are summarized in Box 5.5.

5.7 Guidelines for using the ecological approach to design nutrition interventions

Several guidelines have been put forward by researchers to aid in the development of interventions using the ecological approach. These guidelines are briefly described in the paragraphs below and summarized in Box 5.6.

It is important to examine the many ways in which the intrapersonal, social and cultural, and physical levels of the ecosystem can influence people's nutrition behavior. This requires thoughtful consideration of each level, and the impact that each level may make in determining the foods that people eat.

> **Box 5.6** Guidelines for intervention using the ecological approach
>
> - Examine ways in which the physical and social environment influence health.
> - Consider the relationship between individual and environmental factors.
> - Intervention should enhance the fit between people and their surroundings and give people greater control over their environment.
> - Focus intervention on leverage points.
> - Multiple levels of the environment must be considered when designing interventions.
> - Interventions that include more than one level of the ecosystem will be more effective.

It is important to consider the relationship between intrapersonal factors and the social and cultural, and physical levels of the environment in designing nutrition interventions. For example, individuals with a strong family history of heart disease may be given priority for the receipt of nutrition intervention to reduce levels of serum cholesterol.

Nutrition intervention programs should enhance the fit between people and their surroundings and give people greater control over changes in their environment. For example, people should be given the opportunity to dictate the types of low-fat snacks made available in vending machines where they work. Perceived control over environments can promote healthy behavior.

Interventions should be focused on high-impact leverage points. A large number of factors can be addressed within an ecological nutrition intervention. However, some factors may have a greater and wider impact than others. These are referred to as leverage points. For example, many factors may influence the consumption of fast foods that are high in fat and sodium. Inappropriate perceptions of the health value of these foods, taste preferences, and the speed with which foods can be purchased and consumed may all influence the amount of fast food eaten. However, the most appropriate intervention may target time management, allowing the individual to make greater time available for healthy food preparation, as well as exercise and enhanced family relationships.

The multiple levels of the ecosystem must be considered when determining the causes of a behavior and designing interventions to modify the behavior. The ways in which physical and social environments interact are particularly important to consider in this regard. Physical and social environments can serve to moderate or to mediate effects on health. For example, an extremely busy working environment can lead to great stress and to strained interpersonal relationships among the workers. As a result of this stress it is possible that workers may eat more high-fat "coping" foods and also do not receive support to eat more low-fat options. In this case, stress mediates the effects of the physical environment on dietary consumption. As an example of a moderator, the busy working environment mentioned above may lead directly to workers selecting more high-fat coping foods in the cafeteria, unless they have a supportive social group that values low-fat eating. In the latter case, workers will be encouraged by one another to eat more low-fat items, limiting (i.e. moderating) the negative effects of the busy work environment.

Since levels of the ecosystem interact, interventions that include more than one level are more likely to be effective. For example, an intervention to increase the number of fruit and vegetables consumed by parents is more likely to be effective if it includes both intrapersonal components, designed to increase skills for food preparation, and a component designed to label recommended fruit, vegetables and juices in the local grocery stores. Unintended side-effects can also occur because levels of the ecosystem interact. For example, convincing a primary food preparer to use less fat in cooking (intrapersonal level) can lead to complaints from the family (social and cultural level) about changes in the way that foods taste. It remains possible that this could lead to other members of the family purchasing more fast food with even higher levels of fat. Thus, possible unintended effects should be considered and interventions designed to avoid them.

5.8 Ethical issues to consider

The ecological approach includes both intrapersonal aspects of behavior and environmental aspects that are beyond the control of individuals. Because of this, nutritionists, nutrition educators and other public health professionals who wish to explain health behavior are less likely to place all responsibility for unhealthy behavior solely on the individual. This is considered a strength of the ecological approach. The tendency to place sole responsibility on the individual for unhealthy behavior is sometimes referred to as "blaming the victim" or "victim blaming."

Because the ecological approach includes causes of behavior that fall outside the control of the individual, it may guide program designers towards intervention strategies that take control away from individuals. For example, various nutrition guidelines call for the consumption of prudent amounts of fat in the diet, and at levels lower than are currently consumed by the general population. Education directed at individuals is one way to reduce the amount of fat consumed. However, the ecological approach calls for the use of broader strategies, such as raising beef with lower fat content in the meat and restricting the availability of high-fat foods in some settings (e.g. school lunches, fast food restaurants). These strategies may be highly effective in reducing fat consumption; however, they also restrict the number of options available to individuals in selecting their meals, and may reduce the enjoyment that some people derive from their meals.

The appropriate balance between nutrition education approaches that maximize individual choice, and approaches that involve changing the social or physical environment, which may limit individual choice, will vary depending on the nutrition behavior that is being changed and the types of people who are targeted by the intervention. In general, many more individual educational approaches have been used, provoking more past concern about the blaming of individuals when change in nutrition behavior did not occur. In the future, as ecological approaches become more common, nutrition educators will more frequently face the need to balance individual choice against environmental control. Nutrition educators should consider these ethical issues when designing interventions, perhaps striving to maximize the impact possible through environmental change, while maintaining sufficient elements of individual choice. Ethical considerations in using the ecological approach are summarized in Box 5.7.

Box 5.7 Ethical considerations

- Individual education approaches can foster "victim blaming".
- The ecological approach reduces victim blaming by highlighting other causes of dietary behavior.
- The ecological approach can reduce individual control.
- Nutrition educators must consider these issues and identify the correct balance between nutrition education approaches that emphasize individual choice, and ecological approaches that produce change outside the control of the individual.

5.9 Ecological interventions to change eating habits

The following sections describe interventions that have been designed in Africa, Europe and the USA using an ecological approach. The programs vary, but they all share the use of an ecological approach as a guiding principle to their design. The use of programs from three different continents will help to demonstrate the adaptability of the ecological model to the explanation and modification of nutrition behavior across diverse cultures and geographical areas. This will also illustrate the way in which different cultural, geographical and political climates lead to an emphasis on different aspects of the ecological model in developing intervention programs.

Example 1: Black Churches United for Better Health

The Black Churches United for Better Health Project was conducted among 2519 rural African–American adult church members in eastern North Carolina, USA. The researchers cite using churches as the setting to conduct the study because of the high percentage of African–Americans attending church in the southern USA and also because of the importance of churches within the African–American community. The aim of the intervention was to increase fruit and vegetable consumption in this population. The study was conducted throughout 10 counties and 50 churches. The results of this study showed an increase in fruit and vegetable consumption among the intervention group. Specifically, subjects in the intervention group consumed 0.85 servings more than subjects in the delayed intervention group at follow-up. This increase in fruit and vegetable servings is considered substantial.

In this section, the various levels of the ecological model (intrapersonal, social and cultural, and physical environments) will be described and examples provided within each of these categories. This will be followed by a description of how the researchers applied the guidelines for using the ecological approach in designing the intervention. In conclusion, Black Churches United for Better Health is summarized within the ecological framework.

Ecological approach used by Black Churches United for Better Health

This intervention used all three levels of the ecological model in program design. Although primarily targeting the intrapersonal level, researchers also influenced the social and cultural, and physical environments. Therefore, multiple variables within each of the three levels were targets of this intervention.

Intrapersonal level

The intrapersonal level variables targeted for change in this intervention included stages of change related to fruit and vegetable consumption (what stage a person is at in their willingness to change a particular behavior), knowledge, self-efficacy for eating five servings of fruit and vegetables per day, and perceived availability of fruits and vegetables at church functions. One activity designed to facilitate these changes and ultimately to increase fruit and vegetable consumption included tailored bulletins, where each participant received personalized messages related to their own fruit and vegetable consumption, stages of change, barriers to eating fruits and vegetables, beliefs and social support, based on information obtained from their baseline surveys. Another activity involved the creation of a cookbook, where modifications were made to participants' favorite recipes to meet guidelines set by 5-a-Day and recipes were included in a cookbook given to members. The intrapersonal factors related to this activity included increasing self-efficacy and preferences related to fruits and vegetables.

Social and cultural environment

The social and cultural environment for this intervention was the community setting of churches. Churches provided the social network to the community and African–American participants of this program. By choosing to conduct this intervention in churches, the researchers set up a system where the tenets of the program (i.e. eating at least five portions of fruit and vegetables per day) could potentially be maintained and continued through this setting (i.e. if the pastors and church community adopted and continued various activities originally initiated in the study). At the end of the study, church coordinators (members who helped to arrange, manage and implement intervention activities) were interviewed and all but one of the 22 contacted stated that they would continue at least some parts of the study through the churches. Specific activities reported by coordinators as being sustained were printed materials and serving fruit and vegetables at church functions. Furthermore, some churches had incorporated intervention activities into their budgets and were still receiving reduced prices on fruit and vegetables from local grocers. An activity specifically targeted towards the social and cultural environment included pastor support, where pastors were encouraged to support the project in sermons from the pulpit in each intervention church. In addition, pastors received educational material, such as newsletters and a manual designed for the pastors to help them to convey aspects of the program to church members. Another example included church-initiated activities, where other activities besides those developed by the researchers were specifically created and conducted through the church, such as "5-a-Day Sundays".

Physical environment

The researchers of this intervention manipulated the physical environment to help to increase fruit and vegetable consumption among participants. Activities developed specifically designed to change the physical environment and increase the availability of fruit and vegetables included gardening (having victory gardens and fruit trees planted by members at church sites), serving more fruit and vegetables at church functions such as vacation bible school, and grocer–vendor involvement (promoting locally grown produce by the distribution of coupons, recipes and posters to church members and neighboring markets).

Guidelines applied in the development of this intervention

The researchers clearly applied many of the guidelines for using the ecological approach in designing their intervention. The first guideline was used in understanding that multiple levels of the ecological environment affect behavior change. Specifically, the researchers targeted all levels in their intervention, including intrapersonal, social and cultural, and physical environments. Each of these levels was recognized for its importance and incorporated into the design of the intervention.

The researchers addressed the second guideline by considering the relationship between the individual and the environment in targeting a traditionally underserved, at-risk population. The population in this case comprised rural African–Americans, who are especially in need of nutrition interventions, owing to higher rates of cancer and other chronic diseases in comparison with other ethnic and racial groups.

The third guideline was incorporated by the researchers in that participants in this intervention were given greater control over changes in their environment by including their input in various activities (e.g. inclusion of their favorite recipes to be modified and used in the cookbook, and including church members as lay health advisors).

The next guideline to be addressed by the researchers was the sixth guideline, since this intervention included more than one level of the ecosystem by using a "kitchen sink" approach. The drawback to conducting an intervention impacting many levels is that it is problematic to separate out the different effects and determine exactly which aspects of the intervention are actually impacting behavior.

Summary

The Black Churches United for Better Health intervention was successful in increasing fruit and vegetable consumption in a rural adult African–American population in the southern USA. In addition, improvements were also seen in intrapersonal factors (psychosocial variables) such as stages of change, self-efficacy, knowledge, and perceived availability of fruit and vegetables at church. This intervention successfully applied the ecological model, incorporating the various levels to a population in need of this type of intervention. Churches were used as the setting to deliver the intervention, with the notion that the church is important in the African–American community and that this venue would aid in promoting and hopefully maintaining behavioral change in this population.

Example 2: A fruit and vegetable subscription program in Norwegian schools

The fruit and vegetable consumption in Norway is lower than that seen in most other European countries, and lower than the current Norwegian recommendation of "Five-a-Day". Thus, a major objective of the Norwegian Food and Nutrition Policy is, and has been since it was first formulated in 1975, to increase the consumption of fruits and vegetables in the Norwegian diet. Schoolchildren constitute an important target group in this effort to promote fruits and vegetables. A national survey conducted in 1993 found that the average consumption among 13-year-olds was only about two portions a day, and that only 4 and 9% of boys and girls, respectively, met the recommendation of "Five-a-day".

In Norway, school lunch for most children consists of open sandwiches brought from home. Until recently most schools did not provide any food for the children, and few students bring fruit or vegetables as part of their lunchpacks. Milk, however, has for many years been provided at school as part of a subscription program. Parents pay a fee at the beginning of each school semester, and each student is handed a carton (250 ml) of milk at school each school day. The dairy industry provides transportation to schools, and also offers the schools refrigerators to store the milk.

In 1996, a similar concept for distributing fruit and vegetables to schoolchildren was pilot tested. The goal was to increase fruit and vegetable consumption among schoolchildren (grades 1–10) by providing each child with one portion of fresh fruit or vegetables at school on every school day.

Ecological approach used by the fruit and vegetable subscription program

This intervention is primarily aimed at changing the physical environment by making fruit and vegetables available at school. However, it also includes a promotional component targeting parents and students with the aim of persuading them to sign up for the program (intrapersonal level), and it will influence the social environment by providing student role models for fruit and vegetable consumption (social and cultural level).

Intrapersonal level

Students are initially recruited into the program by means of a brochure sent home to all parents. This brochure provides information regarding the health benefits of eating more fruit and vegetables, how the program is operating in the schools, and detailed information regarding cost and payment by parents. A webpage provides more information for those interested (www.skolefrukt.no). Thus, in addition to recruiting students to the subscription program, this information fosters increased parental awareness regarding the importance of fruit and vegetable consumption among schoolchildren. This, in turn, could potentially lead to more parents making fruits and vegetables readily available at home, or those parents who decide not to sign their children up for the subscription program choosing instead to include fruits or vegetables as part of the children's lunchpack.

Social and cultural environment

The social and cultural environment for this intervention is the public, mandatory school system (grades 1–10). Making fruit and vegetables available is a very direct way of stating the importance placed on fruit and vegetables as a critical component of a healthy diet. As the children eat the fruit and vegetables during the school day, they model this behavior for each other. Peer modeling has been found to be an important influence on a number of health-related behaviors among schoolchildren. When children eat fruit and vegetables together at school this may help to create more positive attitudes towards fruit and vegetables and thus contribute to increased consumption outside the school setting. Finally, the children are involved in the distribution of the fruit and vegetables within their own class (on a rotation system), and this involvement may further help to foster positive attitudes among participating students.

Physical environment

Increased availability at school is seen as an important measure to increase the total intake of fruit and vegetables among children. Most children and young people seem to like fruit and vegetables and tend to eat them when they are served fresh.

The fruit and vegetable subscription program is a public–private partnership, and it is being implemented in cooperation between the National Council on Nutrition and Physical Activity (responsible for the Norwegian "Five-a-Day" recommendation), the Norwegian Fruit and Vegetables Marketing Board, the county health authorities and private, local wholesale distributors. For NOK 2.50 (€0.30/US $0.35) a day the participating students receive an apple, a pear, a carrot, a banana or an orange at lunchtime. Parents are invited by the school to subscribe for 6 months or a year at a time. Wholesalers ordinarily deliver the fruit and vegetables twice a week directly to each school. The schools are responsible for administering the program. In 2001–02 the program was granted NOK 10 million (€1.25 million/US $1.46 million) in subsidies through the collective agricultural agreement between Norway's farmers and the agricultural authorities to reduce the cost to the parents.

Experience to date

The program, which began as a pilot project in a single county in 1996, has now been introduced in 17 of Norway's 19 counties. About 56 000 students in more than 1100 schools took part in the program during the 2001–02 school year. The goal is for all primary schools (grades 1–10) in Norway to offer the program to their students.

No formal evaluation of the impact of the program is yet available from Norway. Process evaluation data indicate that 90% of the participating schools report that the arrangement functions well or very well. The main concerns in order to ensure further dissemination and sustainability of the program are that the quality of the produce delivered remains high, and that the local wholesale distributors are able to make a profit. It is also of concern that some parents and children are not participating because of the cost. Thus, the program could potentially serve to increase, rather than reduce, the social inequality seen with respect to fruit and vegetable consumption. As a result, the National Council on Nutrition and Physical Activity is working to ensure that the program is paid for by the government and offered to all students for free.

Similar efforts to provide fruit and vegetables for schoolchildren have been initiated in a number of European countries, including Denmark, the Netherlands and the UK, and outcome evaluation studies are underway.

In conclusion, the Norwegian fruit and vegetable subscription program demonstrates how an ecological intervention is aimed at changing the physical environment by making health-promoting food items available in a specific setting (schools). Such an intervention also contributes by influencing factors at the intrapersonal level and in the social environment.

Example 3: The Baby-Friendly Hospital Initiative

Breast-feeding has universally been regarded as the ideal form of infant feeding, especially in the first 6 months of life, during which no other foods are necessary for optimal growth. In resource-poor settings in Africa, breast milk is an important source of energy and protein for the first 2 years of life. It reduces the incidence and severity of infectious disease, thereby lowering infant morbidity and mortality. Breast-feeding also helps to establish a strong emotional bond between mother and infant. Furthermore, breast-feeding protects the mother's health by decreasing postpartum bleeding, and reducing the risk of breast and ovarian cancers. Finally, in many resource-poor settings the infertility associated with breast-feeding is a major factor preventing birth rates from rising, and it provides women with a way of controlling their own fertility.

In sub-Saharan Africa, breast-feeding rates have traditionally, and still largely are, high. However, urban

---

Box 5.8 Breast-feeding objectives

- To enable mothers to make an informed choice about how to feed their newborns.
- To support early initiation of breast-feeding.
- To promote exclusive breast-feeding for the first 6 months.
- To ensure the cessation of free and low-cost infant formula supply to hospitals.

Box 5.9 WHO/UNICEF Baby-Friendly Hospital Initiative: 10 steps to successful breast-feeding

To became a Baby-Friendly Hospital, every facility providing maternity services and care for newborn infants should:

1. Have a written breast-feeding policy that is routinely communicated to all health care staff
2. Train all health-care staff in skills necessary to implement this policy
3. Inform all pregnant women about the benefits and management of breast-feeding
4. Help mothers initiate breast-feeding within half an hour of birth
5. Show mothers how to breast-feed, and how to maintain lactation even if they are separated from their infants
6. Give newborn infants no food or drink other than breast milk, unless medically indicated
7. Practice rooming-in: allow mothers and infants to remain together 24 hours a day
8. Encourage breast-feeding on demand
9. Give no artificial teats or pacifiers (dummies or soothers) to breast-feeding infants
10. Foster the establishment of breast-feeding support groups and refer mothers to them on discharge from the hospital clinics.

Reproduced with permission from the WHO.

---

residence and modernization have contributed to a decline in breast-feeding. During the past few decades a trend towards decreased breast-feeding and increased use of breast-milk substitutes for infant feeding in several developing countries has been observed. Aggressive marketing and easy availability of breast-milk substitutes are important influences that affect the choice of infant feeding practices. Unsupportive health-care practices and negative attitudes among health personnel towards breast-feeding have further been identified as reasons for the decline in breast-feeding.

Although overall breast-feeding rates largely remain high in sub-Saharan African countries, exclusive breast-feeding is rarely practiced, as it is common to introduce water and other weaning foods early. Furthermore, in many societies it is not common to use the colostrum and the initiation of breast-feeding is often delayed.

To reverse a trend of declining breast-feeding, the Baby-Friendly Hospital Initiative (BFHI) was launched in 1991 by the World Health Organization (WHO) and the United Nations Children's Fund (UNICEF). It is a global initiative that seeks to improve breast-feeding early in life, when it should be exclusive. Breast-feeding objectives are summarized in Box 5.8.

Health-care facilities providing maternity services and care for newborn infants are eligible to become part of the BFHI network. To obtain status as a Baby-Friendly Hospital, the facility has to fulfill the 10 criteria listed in Box 5.9.

Ecological approach used by the Baby-Friendly Hospital Initiative

The BFHI is a policy intervention aimed at changing the social and cultural environment of health-care facilities providing maternity services and care for newborn infants to promote early and exclusive breast-feeding. As mothers are given information and skills to breast-feed their infants more effectively, the intrapersonal level is also being addressed. The physical environment of the facilities is also changed to allow mothers and infants to remain together 24 hours a day, and by the removal of artificial teats and pacifiers, and food and drinks other than breast milk.

Intrapersonal level

As can be seen in the criteria above, providing the women with information about the benefits and management of breast-feeding, as well as skills related to breastfeeding initiation and continuation, are three of the 10 steps of the BFHI. Thus, explicit goals of this objective are to increase the knowledge of the women regarding the health benefits associated with breast-feeding, to foster positive attitudes supporting breast-feeding, and to help the women to overcome barriers that might otherwise limit both the initiation and duration of breast-feeding.

Social and cultural environment

The social and cultural environment for this intervention is the health-care facilities providing maternity services and care for newborn infants. Having a written breast-feeding policy and providing relevant training for all health-care staff (steps 1 and 2) are very direct ways of communicating with the staff and securing a climate supportive of breast-feeding. Furthermore, encouraging breast-feeding on demand and fostering the establishment of breast-feeding support groups (steps 8 and 10) clearly have the potential to provide a supportive, but noncoercive social environment regarding breast-feeding. Increased breast-feeding rates at the hospitals, clinics and support groups will serve to provide more breast-feeding role models for the women, and will further help to provide a supportive social and cultural environment.

Physical environment

The BFHI changes the physical environment within the hospitals and clinics by making sure that infants are not given food or drink other than breast milk (unless medically indicated) and by banning artificial teats and pacifiers (steps 6 and 9). Furthermore, allowing mothers and infants to remain together 24 hours a day may require a physical restructuring of the hospital wards or clinics. Allowing mothers to be with their children constantly will greatly increase the availability of breast milk for the infant. At the same time, constant mother and infant interaction also impact the social environment within the health-care facility.

Experiences from Nigeria

BFHI is a global initiative, and evaluation studies of its implementation and effects have been conducted in a number of countries. Nigeria is one of the African countries where a drastic decline in the duration of breast-feeding was observed during the 1970s and 1980s. Mothers' misconceptions as to the insufficiency of breast milk to support the growth of the child for the first 6 months of life were seen to be one of the major factors for early introduction of breast-milk substitutes and the decline of longer durations of breast-feeding. Thus, the BFHI was introduced in Nigeria in 1991 by the Committee of Chief Medical Directors of Teaching Hospitals. A formal evaluation was undertaken to investigate the impact of the BFHI at the Obafemi Awolowo University Teaching Hospital Complex in Ile-Ife in 1997. Nursing mothers attending an urban health centre designated a BFHI centre were compared with nursing mothers attending a rural maternity centre not designated as a BFHI centre. The two groups did not differ with respect to age, educational level or occupational status. Women attending the BFHI centre were significantly more likely to initiate breastfeeding within 30 min after delivery (61 vs 39%), to practice exclusive breastfeeding (75 vs 35%) and to position their children correctly on the breast (66 vs 18%) compared with the women attending the reference site.

It is not clear from this study exactly how the health-care staff were trained and how they practiced the steps of BFHI. There seems, however, to be compelling evidence that the initiative had a profound impact on the breast-feeding practices within the Ife township. This indicates that this global initiative has been translated and implemented in such a way that it has been seen as highly relevant and feasible in the context of local Nigerian health workers and nursing mothers.

Breast-feeding in the era of HIV and AIDS

As the acquired immunodeficiency syndrome (AIDS) epidemic has unfolded in sub-Saharan Africa, increasing numbers of children are born to human immunodeficiency virus (HIV)-positive mothers. It has been estimated that the risk of mother-to-child transmission of HIV in sub-Saharan Africa could be as high as 21–45%, with breast-feeding accounting for at least one-third of that risk. Guidelines on breast-feeding and HIV prepared jointly by UNAIDS, WHO and UNICEF in 1998 recommend that breast-feeding should continue to be protected, promoted and supported among HIV-negative mothers and among mothers of unknown infection status. These guidelines further promote fully informed, free choice of infant feeding method for HIV-infected mothers, but introduce artificial feeding as a viable alternative to breast-feeding for HIV-positive mothers. This has led to a heated debate regarding the best feeding method in resource-poor settings for infants whose mothers are infected with HIV (see Chapter 16).

In resource-poor settings with high HIV rates and strong social stigma associated with HIV, exclusive breast-feeding as promoted by the BFHI still seems to be the most viable option for mothers. However, as HIV testing and counseling become more readily available, along with antiviral drug treatment before and during delivery, mothers are being confronted with contradictory messages: breast milk as the best form of infant feeding and breast milk as a source of a deadly virus. To ensure that a poor, often illiterate mother is able to make a fully informed, free choice of infant feeding method, when she may have just learned that she is HIV positive, requires an extremely skilled counselor.

Thus, from a practical and a theoretical point of view, there is an enormous challenge to design interventions at the ecological level that minimize the risk of HIV infection, as well as that of intestinal infections and malnutrition among infants, and at the same time to support and promote the health and the dignity of the mothers.

5.10 Perspectives on the future

As seen by the ecological approach, an individual's health status and his or her health behavior are controlled by multiple levels of influence. These include the intrapersonal, social and cultural, and physical environmental levels of the ecosystem. To improve the eating habits of people, it is important to understand how these three levels of the ecosystem operate to determine nutrition behavior. Guidelines have been established by researchers to assist in the development of interventions using the ecological approach. These guidelines start by emphasizing the need to understand diverse ecological influences on nutrition behavior, including interactions between the different levels of the ecosystem (intrapersonal, social and cultural, physical environmental). They emphasize the need to maximize the fit between people and their surroundings to give people greater control over their environment. These guidelines also highlight the need to target multiple levels of the ecosystem in a nutrition intervention and to focus on high-impact leverage points that are likely to produce the most change in behavior. Finally, health professionals developing intervention programs using the ecological approach need to be mindful of the trade-off between individual choice and environmental control in designing these intervention programs. While the ecological approach provides a powerful framework for understanding nutrition behavior and for designing intervention programs that will modify that behavior, further research needs to determine the means for identifying the high-impact leverage points that will result in the greatest behavioral change.

Research is also needed to determine how much the target of intervention varies depending on the particular public health issue being tackled.

Further reading

Breslow L. Social ecological strategies for promoting healthy lifestyles. American Journal of Health Promotion 1996; 10: 253–257.

Green L, Richard L, Potvin L. Ecological foundations of health promotion. American Journal of Health Promotion 1996; 10: 270–281.

Richard L, Potvin L, Kishchuk N et al. Assessment of the integration of the ecological approach in health promotion programs. American Journal of Health Promotion 1996; 10: 318–328.

Sallis J, Owen N. Ecological models. In Health Behavior and Health Education. Theory, Research, and Practice, 2nd edn. (Glanz K, Lewis F, Rimer B, eds), pp. 403–424. San Francisco, CA: Jossey-Bass, 1997.

Stokols D. Establishing and maintaining healthy environments: toward a social ecology of health promotion. Am Psychol 1992; 47: 6–22.

Stokols D. Translating social ecological theory into guidelines for community health promotion. American Journal of Health Promotion 1996; 10: 282–298.

Stokols D, Allen J, Bellingham R. The social ecology of health promotion: implications for research and practice. American Journal of Health Promotion 1996; 10: 247–251.

6
Public Health Nutrition Strategies for Intervention at the Individual Level

Barrie M Margetts

Key messages

- Intervention programs should be developed to address specific goals and targets.
- Interventions are aimed at directly changing intake, or indirectly influencing factors that affect behavior (knowledge, attitudes, perceptions).
- Programs aimed at directly changing dietary intake need to consider factors that affect the translation of efficacy to effectiveness.

- Programs aimed at influencing factors affecting behavior should consider both the theoretical models that underpin behavior and the practical constraints that limit intentions being put into action.
- Guidelines to maximize the effectiveness of intervention programs should be followed.
- Programs should be evaluated for their ability to achieve their targets and goals.

6.1 Introduction

This chapter focuses on the best approaches to developing effective interventions at the individual level. Chapter 5 covered ecological level interventions. The distinction between an ecological (groups, communities or whole population) and an individual-level intervention is the level at which the intervention is targeted, and thus also the level at which the impact is evaluated. To some extent, the desire to use an ecological rather than an individual approach arises out of a broader perspective of health, with a desire to address the basic and underlying causes of problems. The ecological approach accepts that health is determined not solely by an individual's behavior, but by an interaction between an individual and the wider environment. Even if an individual wants to change their behavior they may be constrained by wider socioeconomic factors. An individual approach fits more comfortably with a narrower view of public health that seeks to address risk factors at an individual level and focuses on removing illness.

In this chapter the focus is on interventions at the individual level. These interventions are likely to be more effective if supported by a consideration of the wider social, economic and political context in which the individuals live their lives. Interventions can vary from the simple provision of information to intense individual support. The choice of the intervention most likely to be effective will depend on the target group. Several interventions may be used to reinforce the message that is trying to be communicated. However, if people cannot afford to do what is being asked, or they do not have the skills required, it will be unlikely that the intervention will be effective or sustainable.

Possible approaches to intervention

Having identified what the problem is, and defined a goal and targets (as outlined in Chapter 1), the aim should be to develop a program of work that will be most effective in achieving the required change. Before starting work the aim should be to weigh up the pros and cons of all the different potential programs of work, and then select the most effective approach or approaches. It is somewhat artificial to separate out the individual and ecological approaches as it is likely that a mixture of both may be most effective. For example, if a program is aimed at improving the quality (nutrient density) of a diet the options for the program may include education to improve knowledge, attitudes and perceptions, skills to allow previously uneaten foods to be consumed, food-based intervention, supplementation, food fortification, income to reduce economic constraints, and improved physical access to foods (price and availability). Food fortification, income and price policies may be considered as ecological interventions, because they do not directly target each individual, but aim to change the whole population. Interventions to improve knowledge and skills, or food-based interventions or supplementation may be seen as individual-level interventions because they target the individual. It is always helpful to review previous research to identify which approaches have been shown to work.

Some problems may be conducive to an ecological or population approach. Perhaps the best example internationally is the fortification of salt with iodine, and more recently bread or flour with folate or other micronutrients. Another population approach that is gaining support is for food manufacturers to reduce the salt or sugar or fat content of foods; none of the changes requires any effort, or even awareness, on the part of individuals. There is a philosophical divide as to whether the food supply should be manipulated by producers (either under regulation or not) to change levels of consumption. As highlighted in Chapter 5, programs aimed at increasing the desire by individuals to eat more fruits and vegetables will not be effective unless the desire can be translated into action by the foods being available (physical and economic access).

It should not be assumed that the only approach to achieving change is by attempting to change knowledge or attitudes in an individual. Nor can it be assumed that these are the major constraints to individuals making changes to their diet or level of physical activity without evidence. Caution should always be exercised in generalizing from one population or subgroup to another, and the interplay of factors may be quite different. It may also be important to consider where the push for change comes from: is it bottom–up or top–down. Is it addressing a perceived need, or is it motivated by cost (promoted by a government to save money) or an ideological perspective?

It is essential to consider all of the stakeholders that may need to be involved or who could have an influence on the effectiveness of the intervention (Table 6.1).

The rest of this chapter will focus on past experience and summarize what is known about the most effective approaches to achieving change at the individual level, within a public health rather than a clinical context. Examples will be taken from three important reviews (Roe *et al.*, 1997; Allen and Gillespie, 2001;

Table 6.1 Factors influencing effectiveness of intervention

Question	Stakeholder	Type of involvement	Desired outcome
1. Who may be affected by:			
(a) the health issue	Government, nongovernmental organizations	Identification and policy, planning and implementation	Consistency of recommendations
(b) determinants	Producers, retailers, consumer groups	Identify supply and consumption issues	Identification of and commitment to objectives
(c) intervention	Transport, settings, target groups	Review regulations, etc. that affect supply	Identification of and commitment to objectives
2. Who has knowledge?	Researchers, food companies	Analyze determinants	Evidence-based approach
3. Who has previous experience?	Government, campaign groups	Analyze determinants	Identification of best practice options
4. Who may be upset?	Organizations	Identify level of participation required	Support for strategy
5. Who will implement the intervention?	Health sector, industry	Agree goals	Identification of roles and responsibilities
6. Who will oppose the intervention?	Groups that may have to change	Identify issues	Resolution of concerns and support for the strategy

Table 6.2 Key steps involved in planning, implementing and evaluating an intervention

A. Planning the program (PHN cycle steps 1–5)
Identify the problem: epidemiological evidence
  I. Identify the determinants:
      (a) food supply (economic and physical access)
      (b) knowledge, attitudes and perceptions
      (c) skills
      (d) social and environmental factors

 II. Assess risks and benefits for possible or likely impact of the program:
      (a) likelihood of health risk or benefit (relative and absolute risk, population attributable risk, risk difference, number needed to treat)
      (b) vulnerable and target groups at greatest risk:
            (i) population and/or targeted approach
      (c) assess expected health benefit of intervention (change in risk estimates)
      (d) potential to succeed
      (e) nature and strength of evidence
      (f) other sources or causes of the same risk; interaction and overlap in population
      (g) impacts on other factors

III. Assess needs and constraints in the population, including any subgroups:
      (a) structural, social and other determinants of behavior
      (b) barriers to change
      (c) environmental influences
      (d) educational and organizational (predisposing, enabling, reinforcing) factors
      (e) administrative and policy factors

IV. Identify appropriate theoretical models upon which to base strategy (see Chapter 1, 5 and 8 for more details)

 V. Identify and appraise intervention options:
      (a) identify decision-making criteria:
            (i)   effectiveness
            (ii) feasibility
            (iii) acceptability
            (iv) cost
      (b) consider types of interventions that may be appropriate:
            (i)   policy
            (ii) programs
            (iii) infrastructure support
      c)   consider settings and approaches for options under (b):
            (i) define best practice within each setting (social marketing, point of sale, schools, worksites, food service, community, health sector, food supply)

VI. Decide on the intervention portfolio

VII. Choose indicators for evaluation

VIII. Develop a budget for program

IX. Establish partnerships and stakeholders:
      (a) engage stakeholders and put the problem in context
      (b) establish key players and who will own activity
      (c) consider those who may be adversely affected by program (companies, lobby groups)
 X. Project planning (develop written study protocol, built-in quality control and standards)

B. Implementation of the program (PHN cycle step 6)
  I. Building the team, developing the protocol:
      (a) training and networking
 II. Implementation of the protocol:
      (a) piloting and feasibility, revision and refinement
      (b) monitoring and feedback, with sufficient flexibility to adapt project plans

C. Evaluation (PHN cycle step 7)
  I. Formative evaluation
 II. Attainment of objectives
III. Effects (e.g. behavior, risk factors, morbidity/mortality, structural or policy changes)
IV. Costs
 V. Process
VI. Other consequences
VII. Feasibility for other subgroups, regions or countries (generalizability)

PHN: public health nutrition.

Eurodiet Project, 2002). The aim is to draw out the general principles on the best way to solve problems, be they problems of overnutrition or undernutrition, and irrespective of locality.

Interventions may be broadly grouped into the following types:

- growth monitoring and promotion
- promotion of breast-feeding and appropriate complementary feeding
- communications of behavioral change
- supplementary feeding
- health-related services.

The distinction is whether the intervention includes supplementary feeding or not. The rest of this chapter will first consider interventions aimed at supplementing or changing food intake, and secondly interventions aimed at changing behavior without adding food or nutrients. The detail of identifying public health priorities, developing goals and targets and how to consider program options was covered in more detail in Chapter 1 and will not be repeated in this chapter. Table 6.2 modifies the public health nutrition (PHN) cycle to highlight the key steps involved in planning, implementing and evaluating an intervention. This is a modification of the precede–proceed model and was described in more detail in Chapter 1.

6.2 Interventions of supplementary feeding, foods or nutrients

A vast literature has been summarized by systematic reviews that explore the effects of changing diet on nutritional or health status, such as studies aimed at improving birth outcomes, childhood growth and micronutrient status. In addition, there are many reviews of the effects of changing diet on chronic disease risk factors, particularly blood pressure and blood lipids. The main findings of these reviews are summarized in the relevant chapters in this book. The aim of this chapter is to draw some conclusions and lessons about the process of undertaking these studies. Two types of question are asked: does it work in theory (efficacy), and does it work in practice (effectiveness)? In public health terms the interest is primarily in terms of effectiveness; often a program appears to work in theory, but when it comes to putting it into routine practice there are various practical (skills, resources, environment in general) factors that reduce its

effectiveness. It is therefore important to be able to identify what these practical constraints are, and how to overcome them.

Some of the reasons why programs work in theory, but not in practice, are summarized in Box 6.1.

The principles of interventions using nutrients (aimed at assessing efficacy) in a controlled trial are exactly the same as those that apply to experiments in the laboratory: they must ensure blinding, randomization, and measures of compliance and loss to follow-up, and the sample size needs to be large enough to measure the expected and biologically relevant change (see Chapter 2).

There are many examples of randomized controlled trials of nutrients that can be shown to have improved the nutritional status of women and children. The impact on health is more difficult to assess, as there is often a complex interaction of factors that alter the demands for nutrients and therefore lead to apparently different effects of changing supply, at the same level of intake. It may also be difficult to measure intermediary markers of early change in functional state or health, such as cognitive performance or fetal health. Most obvious is the impact of infection, and perhaps for pregnant women, workload and or smoking. Previous malnutrition may have longer term effects on metabolic competence that alters the effect of current intake. During pregnancy it is critical to think about when to increase consumption: before conception, during the first, second or third trimester, or throughout pregnancy? The impact of supplementation may also differ depending on the age and parity of the woman, and the effects of changing the quantity of diet may be quite different depending on the overall quality

---

Box 6.1 Some of the reasons why programs work in theory but not in practice

- Problems with the reliability of supply, delivery and distribution of foods or nutrients
- Inadequacies in institutional capacity (training, supervision, monitoring, evaluation, community involvement)
- Poor targeting and control (leakage) over who receives nutrients
- Inadequate quantity, quality or density of foods, so that target audience does not receive enough
- Culturally unacceptable foods used
- Lack of understanding of beliefs and perceptions about intra-household food distribution practices
- Lack of counseling about needs for supplementary foods
- Failure to address other important causes of undernutrition

Box 6.2 Key points required in developing an individual intervention program

- Assess behavior (diet and activity levels, breast-feeding, etc.) before the intervention and identify sources of variation within the population: identify the problem and develop goals and targets (as outlined in Chapter 1) for the at-risk or target group
- Assess options as to the most effective way to achieve the target: when, what, how, when, cost
- Assess what support and infrastructure is required, whether it available, and if not how it will be developed
- Build in an evaluation strategy early on in the development of the intervention

of the diet. It may be that increased birth weight can be achieved not only with modest changes in energy intake, but also by improving the quality (increased nutrient density) of the diet.

Key points required in developing an individual intervention program are summarized in Box 6.2.

Evaluating effectiveness

Randomized double-blind controlled trials are not possible for food-based interventions and are very difficult for assessing effectiveness. In particular, there are ethical and practical issues about a control group that does not receive the intervention. Before and after studies may be the only options for assessing the impact of community-wide interventions.

It is common to evaluate the effectiveness of fortification programs using an individual level of data collection, even though the intervention applies at a community level. For example, blood or urine samples may be taken from random samples of children both before and after fortified foods have been introduced into an area or country to assess mean changes in levels. It is not possible to link actual intake with levels because intake is not measured. It is assumed that any change in blood levels is due to changes in intake; this may be a reasonable assumption where areas with and without fortification are compared and are comparable in terms of background health status. It may be possible to randomize communities either to receive or not to receive fortified foods, but in general fortification is introduced to the whole community at once and it is therefore not possible to have a proper control group.

Factors influencing effectiveness

Lessons from anemia prevention trials can be used to illustrate the factors that influence effectiveness.

Under carefully controlled circumstances (efficacy), giving more iron increases hemoglobin levels. However, effectiveness is affected by:

- lack of supplements on a reliable basis
- lack of information
- education and communication campaigns
- skills of health workers.

Factors that enhance the effectiveness of food-based interventions aimed at promoting growth include:

- level of participation: active involvement of mothers in the program
- guidelines for decision making based on children's progress: clear guidelines used at all levels of the program
- targeting and integration of program components: close coordination, good targeting and follow-up
- community awareness and decision making: community actively involved and proud of improving results
- individual nutrition counseling: counseling intensity related to the problem, targeted materials, negotiated approach
- workers and workload: workers given help, percentage of children gaining weight, part of job performance
- training of workers: appropriate training, negotiation skills, community motivation, self-assessment
- supervision of nutrition workers and activities: feedback, visits to mothers, ongoing training
- detailed operational planning: full set of operational guidelines with options, budget for innovations, responding to local needs
- program level monitoring: data on growth used for program decisions
- commitment to sustain program: goals and targets at national level, with local resource allocation.

6.3 Changing behavior without giving foods

Roe *et al.* (1997) and Eurodiet (2002) provide good summaries of the experience of programs that work, mainly in terms of those aimed at improving diet by changing knowledge, attitudes, perceptions, skills, and so on, in the USA and Europe. Few data exist on the effectiveness of such programmes in Africa or India.

Before developing a program of work it is important to have a good idea of what is believed to be the best theoretical model to use to develop the work. An understanding is required of the key factors that constrain behaviorial change in the target population, along with how the factors that operate at an individual and society level interact to make it more or less difficult to make changes. Various models have been described that are appropriate for considering the forces that affect change at the individual level: the Health Belief model, the Theory of Reasoned Action, the Transtheoretical model and social learning theory. Irrespective of the label given, the aim should be to understand the key constraints that operate at the individual level within the target population, so that the optimal intervention can be developed to address these constraints.

Theoretical models

Health Belief model (addresses attitudes and beliefs: a psychosocial model)

The likelihood of an individual taking action is based on the interaction between:

- their perceived susceptibility to the problem
- the seriousness of the consequences of the problem
- the perceived benefits of a specified action
- the perceived barriers to taking action.

If people feel that they are at risk of a problem and that they can do something about it (self-efficacy), they will do so, provided the benefits outweigh the costs, and the social circumstances are supportive. It has been shown that advice to change diet is more effective in those who have recently been told that they have high blood pressure, or if a member of their family has recently been diagnosed with cancer or some other illness, and if there have been media campaigns that highlight the benefits of change (and that make it seem feasible).

Theory of Reasoned Action (or planned behavior)

Behavioral intentions are influenced by attitudes or belief that if a particular action is taken a desired outcome will occur. The motivation to comply with the wishes of others (normative beliefs) interacts with attitudes to influence intentions to act. Thus, a person will act if they believe their behavior will benefit their health and is socially desirable, and they feel the social pressures (from their respected peers, the media, etc.) to behave in that way. The theory also suggests that a person's intentions will be strengthened if they feel that they have some control over their behavior (self-efficacy).

Transtheoretical (Stages of Change) model

This model has been widely used in dietary-based intervention in various settings. In the UK it has been used in a number of interventions in primary care. The model was developed from experience in smoking and drug behavior programs. It looks at change as a process, and acknowledges that people have different levels of readiness or motivation to change. This model proposes six separate stages through which people may progress towards long-term positive health behaviors (Figure 6.1):

1. precontemplation (not contemplating or not ready for change)
2. contemplation (considers making a change)
3. preparation (serious commitment to change)
4. action (change is initiated)
5. maintenance (sustaining the change)
6. relapse.

The model further proposes that subjects in different stages of change benefit most from interventions tailored specifically to that stage. Subjects in precontemplation need feedback to make them aware of a need to change and attitude information to convince them of the benefits of such a change. Subjects in the contemplation and preparation stages need skills training, observational learning techniques and environmental

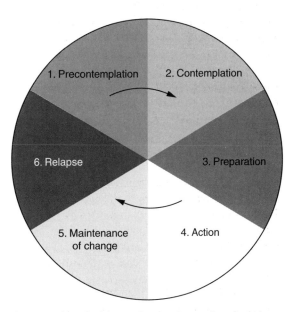

Figure 6.1 The cycle of change: six separate stages through which people may progress towards long-term positive health behaviors.

change to convince them of the possibilities and their abilities to change. The triggers and factors that support action and maintenance may also be different to those that inhibit people from moving to action.

Social learning theory

This model addresses the underlying determinants of health and methods of promoting change (subtle and complex interaction between an individual and their wider environment). The interaction between individuals and their environment is affected by the capacity to learn from others, the value they place on the outcome of different behaviors, and a belief in a personal ability to perform the behaviour successfully (self-efficacy).

Attitude, Social Influence, and Self-efficacy model

A more holistic model has been developed, the Attitude, Social influence, and Self-efficacy (ASE) model, which is derived from a number of psychosocial theories, including social learning theories and cognitive expectancy theories. The model proposes that behavior is primarily a function of motivation or intentions. Three main psychosocial factors have been identified that predict intentions: attitudes, social influences and self-efficacy. A person's attitude towards, for example, fruit and vegetables is a result of the consequences that are expected from consumption. Social influences are a result of subjective norms, examples of important others, and direct social support and pressure related to fruit and vegetable intake. Self-efficacy is a result of a subjective assessment of abilities and possibilities related to fruit and vegetable intake. The model proposes that by introducing or clarifying more positive consequences of fruit and vegetable intake, by creating or encouraging a positive social environment, and by making fruit and vegetables as easily available as possible, higher consumption of fruit and vegetables can be achieved. When applying the ASE model to nutrition behaviors, lack of awareness of personal intake levels has been identified as an important barrier to dietary change.

Another approach that is often used may appear more mechanistic, but it attempts to capture the entirety of the task being undertaken (including social, structural, community, environmental and individual aspects). This framework builds on the concept of target groups, approaches and settings.

Target groups are groups of people within the population who are linked by common characteristics, for example age, gender, physiological state, ethnicity or socioeconomic group. Examples include young people, pregnant women, school-aged children, older people, ethnic groups, people living on a low income, refugees, homeless people, professional groups and politicians.

Approaches (sometimes called channels) are ways of working to bring about change in target groups or settings, or for use by settings in influencing others. Examples include mass media, written materials, skills training, counseling, partnership working, local projects, community development and advocacy.

Settings are identifiable institutions in society that contain large numbers of people in a common environment and/or that have significant influence. They have a dual role: as a group that can be encouraged to change using individual, environmental and structural means, and as a tool to bring about changes in society outside the immediate setting. Examples include schools, workplaces, the commercial sector, primary health care, hospitals, communities, residential homes for older people and nurseries.

Examples of approaches

Mass media

Television and newspaper and magazine advertisements and articles may be useful to raise awareness about a general issue, but most people will have difficulty relating a broad general message to their own particular circumstances. Television adverts are expensive and may not be cost-effective, unless they are part of an integrated program where the advert reinforces messages taken up by other more individually tailored approaches.

Leaflets

Provision of information alone, for example, in the form of a leaflet, is a poor way of encouraging change in behavior. A leaflet may raise awareness of a general issue, but it may not lead to change because the person reading it cannot relate the message to their own personal circumstances. Leaflets are not an effective communication tool, and may exacerbate inequalities in health because it is often the better off with better health who will have access to the leaflet and who will be most likely to benefit further from the information contained within the leaflet. If a leaflet is to be used, the style and content need to be appropriate for the target audience. In a community with a variety of linguistic and cultural groups these differences need to be taken into account. It is not sufficient simply to translate the leaflet into different languages, as different cultural sensitivities need to be considered. This means that it is worthwhile ensuring that the publication is a high-quality one which meets all of its objectives. Guidelines that may be helpful in preparing a simple publication for the general public are listed in Box 6.3.

Skills training

In some circumstances, the intervention that is most appropriate may be developing an individual's skills, such as cooking, planning meals or managing a budget. Skills development must take account of the context in which the skills will be used. Several skills development programs have failed to achieve the desired changes because the new skills developed could not be put into practice owing to resource or other constraints. One example was a program to ensure that women soaked and cooked cassava for long enough to destroy the toxins in the cassava. It was found that women were not soaking and cooking the cassava for longer because of a lack of skills, but because of a lack of water and fuel.

In the past, home economics was a part of many school curricula and children (mainly girls) were taught basic cooking skills. As pressure on the curriculum has increased these lessons have often been cut, and with less cooking being done at home there are fewer learning opportunities for young people to see how to prepare food.

The development of shopping skills may also facilitate dietary changes; these may be targeted towards how to select foods to eat a low-fat diet, or to plan meals for diabetics, or simply to help shoppers to read labels and decide whether the food they are buying really is "low in fat" or "low in sugar".

Counseling

Individual counseling, usually in a primary care or health center setting, is likely to be more effective if it is seen to be addressing a problem, such as obesity, high blood pressure or high blood lipids. Dietary advice tailored to the individual is more likely to be successful than advice given to the general population; this implies that the individual's diet can be assessed and modified in an appropriate way. It also implies that changes in the diet can be assessed to monitor whether the agreed changes have occurred. Some research has suggested that if the individual signs a contract whereby they agree to make the changes recommended, it helps them to stick to the program. Prompt-sheets with agreed weekly or monthly targets have been shown to help some people to achieve and maintain dietary change.

The attitude of the health worker may also be crucial, as may the way in which the individual is recruited into the activity. The concept of helping people to take some control of their life (diet and health) has been shown to be helpful in some circumstances, at least where the individual has the resources to act. In other circumstances the individual passes responsibility for their health to the doctor; if this is the case then the counseling required will be to help to change this relationship.

Examples of settings

Schools

The school setting provides a valuable opportunity to influence health through policy measures, education and food provision. Schools provide the most effective and efficient way to reach a large proportion of the population, including young people, school staff, families and community members. Young people, in particular, can be reached at an influential stage in their lives and over a long period. For example, attitudes towards issues such as breast-feeding are often developed in adolescence, and the attitudes of both girls and boys can have a significant impact on whether breast-feeding is started and then maintained.

The most comprehensive review of nutrition education research published to date concluded that the following elements are critical with respect to effectiveness of nutrition education for schoolchildren.

- Nutrition education interventions are more likely to be effective when they use educational strategies that are directly relevant to a particular behavior (e.g. diet or physical activity) and are derived from appropriate theory and research.
- Interventions need adequate time and intensity to be effective.
- Family involvement enhances the effectiveness of programs for younger children.
- Incorporation of self-evaluation or self-assessment and feedback is effective in interventions for older children.
- Effective nutrition education includes consideration of the school environment.
- Interventions in the larger community can enhance school nutrition education.

Although, on the whole, young people are more active than adults, many have a sedentary lifestyle. There is a particularly sharp decline in activity during the teenage years. The Centers for Disease Control recently reviewed evidence for the promotion of physical activity among children and adolescents, and produced guidelines to promote lifelong physical activity. Their conclusions broadly supported previous ones, and reinforced the need for physical activity among students to be part of a coordinated, comprehensive school health program. In particular, programs should involve families and be supported by the local community. A multidisciplinary approach is important, including health education, health services, social welfare and other school support services.

Much of this thinking has been incorporated into what is becoming known as the whole school approach, which is the basis for the World Health Organization (WHO) Health-Promoting Schools initiative. This is an integrated approach to promoting health, including teaching, facilities, service provision, culture and attitudes, and draws upon the views and needs of the children.

There is a wide range of approaches to health education and to nutrition education in the different European Union (EU) member states. In some countries nutrition education is part of the school curriculum. However, a survey carried out in all 15 current (2002) EU member states, as well as Iceland, Norway and Switzerland, during the testing process of a Nutrition Education Guide for Health-Promoting Schools found no official policy or overall national policy.

Even in those countries where nutrition education is included in the school curriculum, it is not considered as a separate subject. There is also a variety of professionals (teachers, educators, nutritionists, school health workers, public health workers, physicians, etc.) with a responsibility for delivering nutrition education programs. Although teachers are often involved in nutrition education projects, teacher training in nutrition is often absent or poor.

Health-care setting

The pan-European survey examined sources of nutrition information for consumers and the trust that consumers place in these different sources. Although the main source of information is the mass media, the most trusted source of information is the health professional. In many countries a significant proportion of the population is registered with a doctor. This means that health professionals and the health-care setting are in a unique position to promote healthy nutrition and physical activity. This need not be confined to patients. In many cases doctors are in a position to influence the wider community, and medical professional organizations often form very powerful lobbies at a national level.

In 1997 Brunner *et al.* specifically assessed the effectiveness of dietary advice in the primary prevention of chronic disease. The subjects were well motivated and most studies were in either a health-care or an institutional setting. Dietary advice to reduce fat or sodium and increase fiber was included. The authors concluded that primary prevention dietary interventions could achieve modest improvements in diet and cardiovascular disease risk. They reported a 3.7% proportional reduction in serum cholesterol and a 1.4% proportional reduction in diastolic blood pressure. When these figures were applied to previous theoretical predictions, it was calculated that dietary intervention could realistically reduce coronary heart disease by 14% and stroke by 9%.

A similar metaanalysis was reported by Yu-Poth (1999). The purpose was to evaluate the effects of the two stages of dietary intervention recommended by the National Cholesterol Education Program in the USA. A 10% reduction in plasma total cholesterol was reported with the low-intensity intervention and a 13% reduction with the high-intensity intervention. Tang *et al.* (1998) focused specifically on randomized controlled trials where the intervention was individualized dietary advice to modify fat intake. Nineteen trials met the inclusion criteria. Reduction in blood total cholesterol attributable to dietary advice was 8.5% at 3 months and 5.5% at 12 months.

The systematic review of health promotion interventions by Roe *et al.* (1997) included interventions in the primary health-care setting. The authors identified four good-quality studies in this setting, which had been carried out in the previous 10 years. Although there were relatively few studies, their results were remarkably consistent, showing modest and sustained effects on both blood cholesterol and dietary fat intake. This was true whether the intervention focused on diet alone or was a multifactorial intervention. The most effective interventions had the following characteristics.

- They were intensive and often targeted those with increased risk factors.
- They were tailored to the personal characteristics of individuals, e.g. readiness to change and current eating patterns.
- They were client centered and used educational and behavioral frameworks, with the Stages of Change model being particularly useful.

The problem with these types of high-intensity intervention is that they are costly. Encouragingly, the review also reported that low-intensity interventions, such as mailed, computer-generated, personalized nutrition education material, could be effective in well-motivated groups.

The promotion of healthy weights in a population is complex and the evidence indicates that an integrated approach is essential. As part of that integrated approach, the health-care setting has a role to play, not only in promoting healthy nutrition and physical activity, but also in treating those who are already overweight or obese. The National Institutes of Health in the USA systematically reviewed the literature on the identification, evaluation and treatment of overweight and obesity in adults. They concluded that there is strong and consistent evidence that patients in well-designed programs can achieve a weight loss of as much as 10% of baseline weight. Physical activity alone results in modest weight loss, and cardiorespiratory fitness is increased, independent of weight loss; there is strong evidence that the combination of dietary change and increased physical activity produces greater weight loss than diet alone or physical activity alone. There are strong indications that behavioral strategies to reinforce changes in diet and physical activity in obese adults

produce weight loss in the range of 10% over 4 months to 1 year. Weight that is lost is usually regained unless a weight maintenance program consisting of dietary therapy, physical activity and behavior therapy is continued indefinitely. One major barrier to health professionals playing a positive role in promoting nutrition is their own lack of basic training, both in the topic and in the skills necessary to bring about change.

Workplace

The workplace has enormous potential as a setting for improving the health of the adult population because of:

- ease of access to a large number of people
- a relatively stable population
- a working community, which can offer benefits such as positive peer support
- established channels of communication, which can be used to publicize programs, encourage participation and provide feedback.

The workplace is therefore seen as a medium through which the working population's health status can be improved both directly, through supporting and allowing the individual to take action on their health, and indirectly, through the development of an overall health culture.

It also has an important role to play in enabling breast-feeding women to return to work. Some studies indicate that if women return to work, they are nearly half as likely to be breast-feeding at 4 months as women who are not working. The converse of this is that women who do not have supportive workplaces are less likely to return. Employers thus benefit from creating a supportive environment by having higher rates of return from maternity leave and lower absenteeism (breast-fed babies are less likely to suffer from illnesses than those who are formula fed). The type of support provided could include explicit policies supporting the breast-feeding woman, provision of child-care facilities, and the cultivation of a sensitive and supportive attitude amongst other staff.

The general principles for effective workplace health promotion are summarized in Box 6.4. Examples of successful nutrition and physical activity activities in the workplace are:

- healthier eating achieved through point-of-purchase labeling of healthy food choices in workplace cafeterias, and computer-generated personalized nutrition advice

- prompts at decision points, e.g. posters at stair/escalator intersections have doubled stair usage
- workplace schemes to increase cycling and walking to work, and the provision of shower facilities, safe bike storage, etc.

Commercial sector

The commercial sector has a critical role to play in shaping the food consumption of the population. It includes food manufacturers, retailers and many caterers. The data on the effectiveness of interventions in these settings are of poorer quality than in many other settings. Although the commercial sector routinely collects data to inform its decision making, this information is not in the public domain. The studies in the public domain are often not of particularly good quality, and in the most relevant systematic review the inclusion criteria had to be relaxed for this setting. The main conclusions of the review were that interventions in supermarkets, for example point-of-choice signs, advertising, supermarket tours and educational videos, could be effective, although there was very little evidence about the sustainability of any effect. The results were similar for changes to catering provision, although passive manipulation of the nutrient content of menus appeared to be promising.

Local and community food projects

There is an enormous range of local food projects. Broadly speaking, they are projects that either operate in a given community or have arisen from a local group within a community. The almost infinite variety of projects can be grouped into three main categories:

- projects that have a very specific health focus, and are often part of a larger health-related initiative
- projects that attempt to address the needs of low-income groups, these sometimes identify themselves as projects concerned with poverty or with sustainable communities
- projects that arise from food-related environmental concerns, including the way in which food is grown, distributed and sold; these are often referred to as projects concerned with a sustainable environment.

These categories are very crude and many projects have objectives that fall into all three categories. There is a very obvious link, for example, between sustainable communities and a sustainable environment.

6.4 Evaluation of programs and interventions

Table 6.2 shows seven aspects to evaluation (also see Chapter 1). Once clear goals and targets have been articulated in the planning phase, the attainment of these targets should be considered as the primary test of the effectiveness of the intervention. The program should be designed in such a way as to enable an objective assessment of whether the objectives have been achieved. It is important to ensure that delivery of the intervention is effective, and this goes beyond a description of the process used to deliver the intervention. Three types of evaluation have been described: formative, process and outcome. Formative justifies the need for the intervention, process describes the delivery, and outcome describes the impact on behavior; a program can only be said to be effective if it achieves the desired change in behavior (outcome). A final element of the evaluation may be to consider whether the approach used to achieve the change in behavior is the most time and cost-effective, or to assess the cost–benefit of the intervention. This may be described in person-years of life saved per unit of economic expenditure, or in number needed to treat to save each life.

Since the early 1990s there has been a growing understanding of which public health approaches are more likely to result in changes in attitudes, behavior, risk factors, and morbidity and mortality outcomes. However, for policy makers it is critical to distinguish between health impact effectiveness and cost-effectiveness. A recent systematic review of interventions to promote healthy eating in the general population identified the characteristics of those interventions that had the most health impact. These are summarized in Box 6.5.

For the promotion of physical activity a similar review concluded that interventions that encouraged home-based activities such as walking, and did not require attendance at a facility, were more likely to increase and sustain overall physical activity. Frequent professional contact was stressed as important in increasing adherence. Face-to-face contact appears to be important in increasing and maintaining physical activity levels. Mass media approaches have a short-term impact, but are useful in supporting professionals working at a community level.

6.5 Perspectives on the future

Increasingly, the effectiveness of intervention programs is being judged in terms of cost–benefit, that is, the health gain per unit of expenditure. The decision as to what level of expenditure is considered acceptable for what health gain is dynamic and influenced by the current social and political perceptions of the risks and benefits to society of the health problem. It also relates to the effort required by individuals and society to

achieve the change. The perception of the public of the size of the risk, and the size of the expected benefit, is likely to vary from that which is assessed by the academic community. Individuals (in rich countries in particular, where imperatives of survival are less immediate) are very concerned about safety and worried by things over which they have little direct control, such as the amount of pesticides on apples. They are less concerned about things over which they have direct influence, such as eating five portions of fruit and vegetables and their weight. This imbalance between perceived and actual risk is likely to continue to be an issue for those involved in trying to achieve change. Behavior that appears irrational is not irrational to the individual and needs to be understood; it cannot be assumed that those factors that the public health nutritionist thinks are important and will motivate change, will be perceived in the same way by the target group.

A great deal has been written elsewhere about the importance of genetics. In the context of public health, it is unlikely that the level of knowledge about the links between genes and health will be sufficiently clear and precise to help population strategies to improve public health. The main causes are already known, and are environmental. At a clinical level, it may be possible in affluent societies to identify people at increased risk because of an identifiable gene defect, and treat them accordingly. The cost of developing the technology to screen and identify such people will be vast and only affordable by the most affluent individuals in a country and only in a few such countries. For the majority of the population of the world there will not be sufficient resources to do this. Scarce resources should not be diverted away from major public health initiatives such as providing clean water, education, food security and primary health care, and the elimination of poverty and related micronutrient deficiencies.

To improve public health globally requires greater joined up and collaborative efforts internationally to address the basic and underlying causes of food insecurity in the poorest people in rich countries, and in the poorest people in poor countries. Assuming a reductionist individual/health behavior change model as the only way to address these major global problems will not succeed. Strategies need to be organized and integrated from the individual, to the group, to the community, to the country and regional level to ensure that the fundamental causes are addressed, and to enable individuals and families to have real options to control their own lives. Only when all of these constraints have been addressed should the focus shift to those factors operating at an individual level that enable people to make choices about healthy food and a healthy way of life, such as knowledge, attitudes, perceptions and skills.

Further reading

Allen LH, Gillespie SR. What works? A review of the efficacy and effectiveness of nutrition interventions. United Nations Sub-committee on Nutrition and Asian Development Bank (ADB), Manila (www.adb.org) September 2001.

Arnhold W, Dixey R, Heindl I *et al*. Healthy Eating for Young People in Europe. Nutrition Education in Health Promoting Schools. Copenhagen: European Network of Health Promotion in Schools, 1999.

Brunner E, White I, Thorogood M, Bristow A, Curle D, Marmot M. Can dietary interventions change diet and cardiovascular risk factors? A meta-analysis of randomized controlled trials. Am J Public Health 1997; 87: 1415–22.

Centers for Disease Control. Guidelines for School and Community Programs to promote lifelong physical activity among young people. MMWR Morb Mortal Wkly Rep 1997; 46(RR-6): 1–36.

Eurodiet project. Nutrition and diet for healthy lifestyles in Europe: The Eurodiet Project. Public Health Nutrition 2001; 4(2): 265–739.

Grilli R, Freemantle N, Minozzi S *et al*. Mass media interventions: effects on health services utilization. Cochrane Review of Effectiveness, 1997.

Puska P, Tuoomilehto J, Nissinen A, Vartiainen E. The North Karelia Project. Finland: National Public Health Institute, 1995.

Riddoch C, Puig-Ribera A, Cooper A. Effectiveness of Physical Activity Promotion in Primary Care: A Review. London: Health Education Authority, 1998.

Roe L, Hunt P, Bradshaw H, Rayner M. Health Promotion Interventions to Promote Healthy Eating in the General Population: A Review. London: Health Education Authority, 1997.

Tang JL, Armitage JM, Lancaster T, Silagy CA, Fowler GH, Neil HA. Systematic review of dietary intervention trials to lower blood total cholesterol in free-living subjects. BMJ 1998; 316: 1213–20.

Yu-Poth S. Effects of the National Cholesterol Education Program's Step I and Step II dietary intervention programs on cardiovascular risk factors: a meta analysis. Am J Clin Nutr 1999; 69: 632–346.

7

Dietary Guidelines

Michael J Gibney and Petro Wolmarans

Key messages

- Dietary guidelines can be expressed in quantitative or qualitative terms and can be applied at the level of the nutrient or at the level of the food as food-based dietary guidelines.
- Nutrient-based quantitative dietary guidelines can be population based, where the guideline is the target for the population mean, or individual based, where the guideline applies to all.
- Food-based dietary guidelines should reflect a public health nutrition problem and not simply a difference between population intake and some quantitative dietary guideline. They should be based on prevailing patterns of food intake and should be culturally acceptable.
- Options for food-based dietary guidelines include changing the percentage of the population who eat the target food, changing the frequency with which consumers of the food eat that food, changing the portion size when the food is consumed and switching people to a comparable alternative food.

7.1 Introduction

Dietary advice is both ancient and anecdotal, from Hippocrates' advice on the value of vinegar for "feminine disorders" to the anecdotal expectation that "an apple a day keeps the doctor away". Quantitative advice on population targets for nutrient intake emerged only during the twentieth century, when the essential nature of most nutrients had been established. This quantitative advice came in the form of recommended dietary allowances (RDAs) and covered micronutrients, energy and protein. RDA were intended to direct population nutrient intake to a level where the probability of nutrient deficiency would be low. They were not directed at the noncommunicable chronic diseases. Macronutrient balance was not deemed important until the 1950s and 1960s, when evidence emerged that coronary heart disease was linked to plasma cholesterol and that plasma cholesterol was linked to the balance of dietary fats. The first all-embracing set of dietary guidelines was issued in the USA in the early 1970s.

Since then, hundreds of committees have met across the globe to review and rereview the evidence linking nutrient intake patterns and the risk of noncommunicable chronic disease. The purpose of this chapter is to introduce students to the broad principles of dietary guidelines without engaging in detailed discussions as to the pros and cons of the deliberations of the many committees that have developed dietary guidelines.

7.2 Overview of dietary recommendations

Three main types of dietary recommendations may be produced by public health agencies.

Dietary allowances

Recommended nutrient intakes (RNI) are also called RDA, recommended dietary intakes (RDI), dietary reference values (DRV) or population reference intakes in different countries. Quantitative guidelines

---

for different population subgroups for the essential micronutrients, energy and protein primarily to prevent nutritional deficiencies are generally known as RDA. These dietary guidelines are the subject of Chapter 7 in the *Introduction to Human Nutrition* in this series, to which the reader is referred. In brief, the approach generally used is to identify the average requirement (AR) and its variance in the form of the standard deviation (SD). Some 95% of values will lie between the AR − 2SD and the AR + 2SD, leaving 2.5% beneath the first of these values and a further 2.5% above the second of these values. The RDA is defined as the AR + 2SD and covers the requirements of all the population except those 2.5% of the population above this value. RDA arose out of a need to assess whether populations or subpopulation groups were receiving enough nutrients in the food supply to meet nutritional needs. They have been compiled for whole populations and for different subgroups within the population based on gender, age, physiological status and activity level. The concept of RDA is often mistakenly misused, being interpreted as a minimum or an average amount of a nutrient required by an individual to maintain health.

Dietary goals

Dietary goals are quantified national targets for selected macronutrients and certain micronutrients aimed at preventing long-term chronic diseases such as coronary heart disease, stroke and cancer. They are generally used for planning at the national level rather than as advice for individuals and are usually expressed in terms of national average intakes in grams/day or as a percentage of energy contribution.

Dietary guidelines

Dietary guidelines are targeted at individuals. These sets of advisory statements give dietary advice for the population to promote overall nutritional well-being and relate to all diet-related conditions. Dietary guidelines are broad targets for which people can aim, whereas RDAs or RNIs indicate what should be consumed on average every day. Adopting RNI and dietary goals for a population may form part of the process for the development of dietary guidelines, which are the recommended strategies for the population to achieve nutritional well-being.

Quantitative guidelines for the macronutrients in particular, but increasingly also for the micronutrients,

aimed at reducing the incidence of noncommunicable chronic disease, are generally referred to as dietary guidelines and these will form a major part of this chapter. These guidelines can also be issued in qualitative form. Food-based dietary guidelines (FBDG) translate quantitative dietary guidelines into target foods, meals or eating habits. These will also be a major focus of this chapter.

In addition to FBDG in any country, a set of dietary guidelines expressed in scientific terms may exist, with quantitative recommendations on nutrients and food components, available for use and reference by policy makers and health-care professionals.

7.3 Quantitative dietary guidelines

Since the 1950s, when the links between diet and chronic disease began to emerge, public health nutritionists have begun to compare some ideal pattern of nutrient intakes with those prevailing in the target population. Today, students become rapidly familiar with the national dietary guidelines for their country and these play a significant part in shaping their interpretation of public health nutrition issues. To use these guidelines properly, it is necessary first to understand the principles that underlie their derivation and then to understand clearly the difference between population-based dietary guidelines and individual dietary guidelines.

Deriving quantitative dietary guidelines

The derivation of dietary guidelines is not a precise science. Rather, it is based on expert judgment following extensive review of the relevant literature. Ideally, two separate sets of quantitative data need to be linked.

Disease–risk factor associations
Nutrition epidemiology has provided quantitative data on the relationship between specific chronic diseases and risk factors for these diseases. An example of this is shown in Figure 7.1(a), which plots the age-adjusted incidence of colon cancer (cases/10^5 persons per year) against fecal output as measured in 23 populations in 12 countries. Clearly, the lower the fecal output, the higher the risk of colon cancer. This is the first set of data needed to determine a dietary guideline for fiber.

Risk factor–nutrient associations
Increasing dietary fiber intake is associated with increasing fecal output. Figure 7.1(b) summarizes this relationship from 11 different studies with 206 subjects

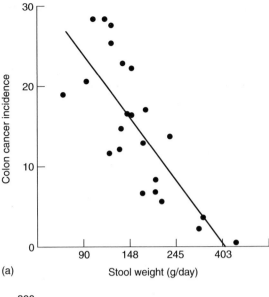

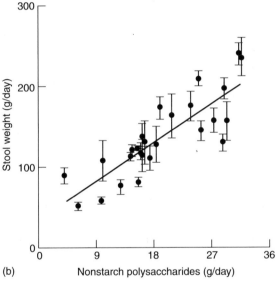

(a)

(b)

Table 7.1 Dietary guidelines to reduce the incidence of chronic disease where there is or is not an intermediate risk factor

Dietary guideline	Risk factors	Disease
Physical activity	Blood pressure	HT
	Insulin resistance	Diabetes
SFA	Plasma cholesterol	CHD
MUFA	Plasma cholesterol	CHD
n-6 PUFA	Plasma cholesterol	CHD
trans-PUFA	Plasma cholesterol	CHD
n-3 PUFA	Platelet aggregation	CHD
Cholesterol	Plasma cholesterol	CHD
Sodium	Blood pressure	CHD/CVD
Fiber	Fecal output	Colon cancer
Fruit and vegetables	Nil	Cancer
Fermentable carbohydrates	Nil	Caries
Total fat	Nil	Obesity

SFA: saturated fatty acids; MUFA: monounsaturated fatty acids; PUFA: polyunsaturated fatty acids; HT: hypertension; CHD: coronary heart disease; CVD: cardiovascular disease.

Figure 7.1 (a) Age-adjusted incidence of colon cancer (cases/10^5 persons per year) against fecal output as measured in 23 populations in 12 countries. (b) Relationship between dietary fiber (nonstarch polysaccharide) intake and fecal output as measured in 206 subjects involving 28 dietary studies. Reprinted from Cummings *et al.* (1992) with permission from the American Gastroenterological Association.

involving 28 dietary periods. In this instance, dietary fiber is defined as nonstarch polysaccharides (NSP). The relationship between fecal output (F) and NSP is F = 5.3NSP + 38.

Taking these two sets of data together, it is now possible to address the question: "What level of fiber (NSP) intake is needed to attain a level of fecal output to reduce colon cancer by 50%?" Thus, the linking of quantitative data on the link between the incidence of a disease and risk factors for the disease, on the one hand, and between risk factors for the disease and nutrient intake, on the other hand, allows a reasonably good estimate to underlie dietary guidelines.

Such elegant extrapolations are not always possible, however. For example, in the case of fruit and vegetables and their protective effect against certain cancers, there are no biological risk factors that can link epidemiological data on disease–risk factor relationships with experimental diet–risk factor relationships. This is also true for the link between fermentable carbohydrate intake and dental caries and the link between dietary fat and obesity. Table 7.1 lists nutrients for which dietary guidelines can be quantitatively established on the basis of disease–risk factor data combined with risk factor–nutrient data and those which cannot be so based. In the case of the latter, the quantitative dietary guideline is made by expert judgment of the direct link between the food or nutrient and the disease in question. In other instances, a quantitative dietary guideline can be derived by default, that is, the logical amount that arises when all other issues are considered. For example, if a guideline of 30% energy from fat is combined with an expectation of 15% energy from protein, then all carbohydrate must provide 55% of energy. If a figure of 25% is assigned for all monosaccharides and disaccharides (as in the case, for example, in the Netherlands), then by default 30% of energy should be derived from starch, assuming that dietary guidelines exclude alcohol from the calculations.

The target audience

Dietary recommendations can be issued at the level of the population (goals) or of the individual (guidelines). The difference is profound and thus must always be clear before applying dietary guidelines. Consider a population target of 10% energy from saturated fatty acids (SFA). If the SD is 2.5%, then 95% of the population will be between 5 and 15%, that is, between +2SD and −2SD above and below the mean (10% of energy) (Figure 7.2a). If 10% energy from SFA were to be a target for individuals and the goal was for, 97.5% of the population to meet this target, then 10% would have to be equal to the mean +2SD (Figure 7.2b). Thus, there is a fundamental difference between "population" and "individual" dietary recommendations,

and users should always be clear in their mind as to the target audience. For example, the guideline of 400 µg/day of folic acid for the prevention of neural tube defects in pregnancy is an individual-based dietary guideline, applying to all women of reproductive age.

Monitoring the attainment of quantitative dietary guidelines

Dietary guidelines can be expressed either in quantitative terms (five servings of fruit and vegetables/day) or in qualitative terms (eat more fruit and vegetables). The two are not necessarily exclusive and can exist side by side, with the qualitative guideline primarily aimed at the public and the quantitative guidelines used by public health nutrition professionals to monitor progress in attaining dietary guidelines. In terms of this monitory process, two approaches are possible. One is to search a nutrient intake database to determine the percentage of the sample that meet the guidelines. Although this is a widely used approach, it is probably only appropriate when the guideline in question is aimed at individuals and not populations. If the guideline is a population target, then the best approach to monitoring success or otherwise is to rank the data for the intake from the lowest value to the highest value. If the target is 11% food energy from saturates, then individuals are selected from the lowest upwards, until such time as the target of 11% food energy from saturates becomes the mean of the sample. The data in Box 7.1 illustrate how the two approaches provide

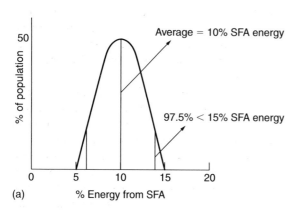

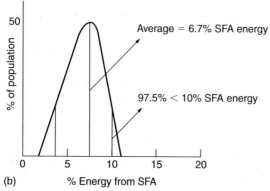

(a)

(b)

Figure 7.2 Pattern of distribution of saturated fatty acid (SFA) intake for (a) a population goal of 10% energy, and (b) an individual goal of 10% energy.

> **Box 7.1** Approaches to evaluating attainment of population dietary guidelines for total fat and saturated fatty acids in a sample of adult males using (a) an inappropriate individual approach and (b) a more correct population approach
>
> (a) Percentage of food energy from total fat (dietary guideline: 35% of food energy)
> - Of the 662 males in the sample, 32% of *individuals* ($n = 211$) have intakes below the dietary guideline.
> - For this *group* of individuals, the mean intake is 31% of food energy.
> - The largest *group*, the mean value of which meets the targets exactly, is 516, which is 78% of the population.
> (b) Percentage of food energy from saturated fatty acids (dietary guideline: 11% of food energy)
> - Of the 662 males in the sample 11% of *individuals* ($n = 74$) have intakes below the dietary guideline.
> - For this *group* of individuals the mean intake is 9.1% of food energy.
> - The largest *group*, the mean value of which meets the target exactly, is 217, which is 33% of the population.

quite different interpretations, using data from Ireland to explore targets of 35% food energy from fat and 11% food energy from SFA.

7.4 Qualitative dietary guidelines

"Eat more fiber-rich foods" is a qualitative dietary guideline. It does not specify the level of increase required and, in general, this is the type of message transmitted to the consumer. Such qualitative messages are not always popular with planners of public health nutrition, since they do not provide for an analysis of the scope of the problem or an analysis of progress in solving the problem. Nonetheless, qualitative dietary guidelines may be the best compromise when hard data on prevailing nutrient intakes are limited.

Food-based dietary guidelines

Although there is extensive international experience in the derivation of population nutrient goals, the translation of these into FBDG has received much less attention. FBDG represent the practical way to reach the nutritional goals for a population. They take into account the customary dietary pattern and indicate what aspects should be modified. They consider the ecological setting, socioeconomic and cultural factors, as well as the biological and physical environment in which the population lives. FBDG should be developed in each country and different guidelines may also be required for different geographical regions or socioeconomic groups within the same country. Whatever FBDG are developed they must be subject to critical appraisal, monitoring and review, especially in regard to unintended consequences and to ecological considerations.

The Food and Agriculture Organization and the World Health Organization have issued a report, which outlines strategies for the development of FBDG. The report outlines a number of key principles.

Food-based dietary guidelines should be based on a recognized public health issue

Quite often, local nutrient intake data show a deficit relative to various international standards for intake, be they reference nutrient intakes (RDA) for protein, energy and micronutrients or dietary guidelines for the composition of macronutrient intakes, fiber, n-3 polyunsaturates, and so forth. The existence of such a

deficit may indicate a probability that a particular public health problem exists. However, the deficit in nutrient intake alone is not proof that a public health problem does exist. The human body has a remarkable capacity to adapt to different patterns of nutrient intake and the ability to make these adaptations can be influenced by related dietary factors, physical activity, reproductive patterns, climate and many other factors. Thus, the existence of a nutrient deficit may mean a high prevalence of a public health disease or condition in a sedentary population with a given pattern of nutrient intake, but in another population which is very physically active and with a different pattern of nutrient intake, such a deficit may not have comparable public health implications. An example of this is calcium intake in Chinese women. A large study of women in Beijing showed a mean calcium intake of about 400 mg/day. This is well below every national and international standard for calcium intake. In the USA, calcium intakes (800 mg/day) are below the ideal population mean intake (1200 mg/day) that would minimize osteoporosis, a disease associated in part with low calcium intakes. On the basis of the very low calcium intakes among Beijing women, one might expect a high incidence of osteoporosis. This possibility was investigated in a comprehensive epidemiological study of osteoporosis in Beijing women. The prevalence of osteoporosis in Beijing was found to be one-sixth of that in the USA. Quite why Chinese women can adapt to such a low calcium intake is difficult to explain. They have a very high intake of phytoestrogen rich in soy protein, which may help bone homeostasis. They spend a considerable amount of time in a squatting position, which may strengthen muscles around the hips. Elderly Chinese are held in very high social regard and are never socially isolated. Their protein and sodium intakes may be lower, which would reduce calcium excretion. Whatever the reason, the calcium deficit does not at present constitute a public health problem. Thus, FBDG should not be devised simply because of a gap that may exist between prevailing nutrient intake and a numerical recommended intake for a nutrient. However, once the public health issue has been identified, the first step should be to ascertain the extent to which it may be attributable to nonnutritional factors. Specifically, infection, safe food and water, physical activity and smoking may have to be addressed for nutrition strategies to be fully successful.

Food-based dietary guidelines should be based on prevailing patterns of food consumption

It might seem anomalous to propose that a food intake pattern that fails to meet a target nutrient intake to minimize the risk of a given disease or condition should be the basis of establishing FBDG. However, unless FBDG are rooted in a food intake pattern that is socially acceptable, success is unlikely to be achieved. In this context, some level of common sense needs to be applied. If for example, a food supply simply cannot provide sufficient iodine, then FBDG rooted in this iodine-deficient food supply will be doomed to fail. However, FBDG in most instances can be used to identify optimal food intake patterns based on prevailing food intake. If prevailing food intake patterns are not used, the ensuing FBDG will be theoretically derived, that is, based on what some expert group thinks should be eaten.

Food-based dietary guidelines should always take account of the cultural context of the population to which they are addressed

The phrase "cultural context" needs to be interpreted with common sense, applying different criteria to different situations. The cultural context of the poor of a city in Asia differs from that of peasant farming communities in the mountainous regions of South America or the affluent suburbs of the West Coast of the USA. Cultural context must take account of many issues: religious beliefs, local taboos, food security, income, price, food availability, fuel availability, social norms and many more as appropriate. In applying this principle, the public health nutritionist must address the simple question: "Is my advice on food intake patterns likely to be culturally and socially acceptable?"

Options for the development of food-based dietary guidelines

A general principle for the development of FBDG is that although guidelines for their development exist, they need not be slavishly followed, but when used, some basic principles of common sense should be applied. In very many instances across the globe, FBDG will have to be developed in the absence of significant dietary survey data and with limited food composition data. Under such circumstances, the following points will need to be borne in mind.

Paucity of data

In the absence of a large nutrient database for a country, nutrition scientists have to depend on scattered dietary information obtained during cross-sectional studies on specific study groups, information from experimental studies, qualitative information on dietary intake and a good general knowledge of the dietary habits in a country. A metaanalysis of the dietary data available from different studies undertaken in a country should be undertaken to obtain an idea of national food consumption patterns. It may be difficult to conduct a metaanalysis, especially if the methods used for the collection of the data differ and the quality of the data is questionable. If this is the case, a summary of the literature on dietary intake studies in a particular country should be undertaken to provide information on food and nutrient intakes of the population. This information could then serve as a guideline for the formulation of FBDG. It is then up to the nutritionists of that country to interpret the data from this literature survey and metaanalysis against the background of a good degree of knowledge of prevailing local food customs and practices.

There are several limitations when national food consumption information is not available and assumptions have to be made based on existing data. Information from large epidemiological studies may be area specific and may not represent the dietary habits of all the inhabitants of a country. In this case, dietary data collected during studies on small sample sizes, such as the baseline of an experimental study, could be used to supplement the findings from epidemiological studies, provided the information is collected on people known to have similar dietary habits. The dietary patterns of those living in cities may differ vastly from those who live in rural areas and have a limited access to shops. For example, people living in the cities may follow a Western-type diet linked to hypercholesterolemia, while those in rural areas may still follow a low-fat diet and have a low prevalence of hypercholesterolemia. For the latter, an FBDG to use low-fat milk instead of full-cream milk may not be of paramount importance, while the former, because of their high fat intake, need to cut down on their intake of fat from animal products.

Impact of changes in food production

Data from epidemiological studies may be old and not necessarily applicable any more, since food production has changed and different products are available on the market. Because of advances in the food industry, products lower in fat and saturated fatty acids may have become available, but at the same time products high in *trans* fatty acids came onto the market. The main issue may not be to advise people to use margarine instead of butter to cut down on their SFA intake, but to stress that they should use polyunsaturated instead of hydrogenated brick margarine to limit the intake of *trans* fatty acids. In the absence of recent survey data, nutritionists need to familiarize themselves with changes in food production and the availability of new products on the market. Information from market research organizations could make an important contribution in adding to the knowledge about the food practices in a country.

Lack of food composition data

Inadequate information on food composition may also be a limiting factor, especially when there is a lack of information on the food composition of traditional foods. These foods may make an important contribution to specific nutrients, and the lack of information on the nutrient composition of these traditional foods may prevent the inclusion of these foods as part of the FBDG. It is therefore important that either nutritionists or community members who are familiar with the dietary habits of people who include traditional foods in their diet are part of the team that formulates FBDG for a country.

Within-country diversity

In a country with different ethnic and cultural groups whose dietary habits differ, one set of FBDG may not be enough to address the nutrition needs of all groups. One group may consume a typical Western diet high in fat and cholesterol, while the other may follow a prudent diet as far as fat and cholesterol intakes are concerned. The latter diet may be deficient in micronutrients. The only solution is to formulate FBDG guidelines based on available information on food and nutrient intakes and then to test these FBDG in the target population. Focus group discussions with the target population may shed some light on areas where there are gaps that need to be addressed.

7.5 Steps involved in devising food-based dietary guidelines

The ensuing sections assume that some level of knowledge of food and nutrient intakes exists and that the practitioner has these organized in some form of electronic database.

Step 1: The public health problem and its dietary and nondietary dimensions

Before using an electronic database, the practitioner must reflect on the problem to be solved. One needs to establish the public health nutrition issue to be tackled and to ascertain whether nondiet-related factors might contribute to the problem. For example, if iron-deficiency anemia is the public health issue at stake, parasitic infestation of the gut could be a complicating issue and FBDG programs would have to be conducted in association with programs to eliminate or minimize the parasitic contribution to iron-deficiency anemia.

Step 2: Consideration of target and related nutrients before intervention

Once the public health issue at stake has been identified as one not likely to be confounded by nondietary factors, the relevant nutrients need to be considered. This is not simply a case of a single nutrient related to a problem, for example, iron and anemia. A slightly wider view needs to be taken. In the case of iron, dietary factors that promote or inhibit iron absorption may need to be considered; for example, vitamin C and phytates. In the case of calcium, a related factor may be vitamin D. Table 7.2 illustrates some examples of public health nutrition problems, their nondietary confounding problems, and the target nutrients and associated nutrients.

Table 7.2 Interrelationships between nondietary factors, target nutrients and related nutrients for the management of anemia, osteoporosis and dental caries

Public health nutrition disorder	Nondietary-related factors	Target nutrient	Related nutrients
Anemia	Parasitic infestation	Iron	Phytate Vitamin C
Osteoporosis	Sedentary lifestyle Smoking Hormone replacement therapy	Calcium	Vitamin D Phosphorus
Dental caries	Oral hygiene	Fermentable carbohydrates	Fluoride

Step 3: Candidate foods for food-based dietary guidelines

This is the most important element of FBDG. Several approaches may be used depending on available data. If no food intake database is available, then local expert knowledge combined with some food composition data must be used. The following section assumes the availability of an electronic food and nutrient intake database.

Identifying major sources of the target nutrient

The percentage contribution of different foods or food categories to the intake of the target nutrient can be a useful indicator of the relative importance of different foods. However, some element of caution needs to be applied in using this approach. Its strength lies in situations where the intake of the target nutrient is predominantly met by a narrow range of foods. For example, in Western countries, milk and milk products are the main sources of calcium, to the point where patterns of intake of milk and milk products, by and large, determine calcium intake, and this is likely to apply to all segments of society excluding the lactose intolerant, those allergic to milk proteins and vegans. However, when many foods contribute significantly to the intake of the target nutrient, simply ranking their relative contributions to intake will not necessarily be useful in identifying food intake patterns that truly discriminate between high and low consumers of the target nutrient. This is illustrated in Table 7.3 for sources of dietary fat in groups with high and low intakes of fat in several European countries. More or less the same foods contribute equally well to fat intake irrespective of whether one examines high fat-consuming or low fat-consuming segments of society. This, in turn, indicates that the composition of dietary fatty acids is not influenced by fat intake level. Those with low fat intakes simply eat less of the same sources of fat. Thus, the percentage contribution of foods or food groups to intakes of the target nutrient is valuable, but needs to be used cautiously and is best applied to situations where one or two foods or food groups predominate the target nutrient intake.

Quantile analysis

Where food and nutrient intake data are available, it is possible to develop FBDG based on the food consumption patterns of population subgroups that achieve a particular nutritional goal. This allows one to discriminate between subgroups with high and low intakes of a target food or nutrient. Such foods or nutrients are often not those that would be predicted on the basis of their contribution to actual average intake of the target nutrient. Thus, it is important to determine patterns of food intake not only on the basis of the population average, but also for subgroups or even individual consumers. It is possible for two subpopulations to have equal average intakes, but to differ in terms of the proportion of consumers and their different intake levels. The intakes of a target nutrient can be divided into quantiles (tertiles, quartiles or quintiles depending on the size of the sample available), and the patterns of food consumption in each quantile can be examined in an attempt to identify patterns that distinguish between acceptable, nearly acceptable and unacceptable nutrient intakes. A major shortcoming of many such analyses, and indeed of analyses of food intake data in general, is the

Table 7.3 Sources of dietary fat (%) in groups consuming high or low levels of dietary fat in four European countries

Fat intake group	Denmark		Ireland		UK		Netherlands	
	Low	High	Low	High	Low	High	Low	High
Meat	22	21	18	23	21	21	20	19
Spreadable fats	56	48	32	25	20	17	28	33
Milk	7	9	14	9	12	10	12	11
Biscuits and cakes	NA	NA	10	12	11	15	5	4
Cheese	8	9	NA	NA	8	6	8	9
Eggs	3	4	5	5	5	5	2	2
French fries	NA	NA	NA	NA	5	4	NA	NA

NA: data not available.

failure to distinguish between consumers of a food and nonconsumers of a food. Table 7.4 presents mock data for the intake of three foods. For each food, the data are presented for those 10 subjects in the upper and lower quartiles. Since the total mock sample is 40, there are 10 subjects in each quartile.

- *Food A*: on the basis of the population average (all subjects included, even nonconsumers), those with the higher nutrient intake (higher quartile) have the highest intake of food A (45 vs 25 g/day). If one were to stop there, the conclusion would be that higher intakes of food A will increase the target nutrient intake. However, looking at the percentage of consumers, within the higher quartile, 80% of people are consumers of food A while only 50% of people in the lower quartile are consumers. Looking solely at consumers, intakes are very similar (50 vs 56 g/day) across the lower and higher quartiles. In order to alter the intake of the target nutrient, in this instance there needs to be a focus on changing the percentage of consumers rather than or perhaps in addition to the amount consumed.
- *Food B*: the average population intake of food B is higher in the higher quartile of the target nutrient intake (26 vs 14 g/day). There are no differences in percentage consumers, so the same higher intake is found among consumers only in the higher quartile of the target nutrient intake (18 vs 33 g/day).

- *Food C*: Whether one looks at the higher or lower quartile of the target nutrient intake, the mean population intake of food C is the same (35 vs 35 g/day). Because there is a large difference in percentage consumers (50 vs 20%), in the low quartile of nutrient intake consumers eat twice as much of food C as consumers in the higher quartile of the intake of the target nutrient (70 vs 35 g/day).

This mock analysis highlights the need to distinguish between the total population mean intake, which can be dramatically influenced by the presence of non-consumers, and the intake among consumers only. In effect, the use of this analytical approach should lead to decisions as to which of the following public health nutrition strategies is most relevant:

- changing the percentage of the population who eat the target food
- changing the frequency with which consumers of the target food eat the target food
- changing the portion size whenever a consumer eats the target food
- switching people to a comparable alternative food.

If a full database were used rather than this mock analysis, eating occasions could be converted from grams/occasion to portions per occasion and the occasions per week or day on which the food is consumed could be recorded. These data, together with data on the percentage of consumers and consumer-only intakes will greatly assist in making choices.

Simple modeling of the impact of changes in food choice

Table 7.5 presents data on the pattern of fiber intake in a given population. In this instance, the first column shows which foods contribute to fiber intake. Using just those data, bread would be a top priority to increase the fiber intake of this group; or would it? The third column shows that the percentage of consumers cannot be increased much more and the final column shows that attempts to increase the number of slices of bread per day will probably be unsuccessful. However, bread consumption should not be ignored. The intake of bread and its contribution to fiber intake can be used to calculate that, on average, the level of fiber in the bread consumed by this group is 4.4 g/100 g. Food composition tables give a value of 3.8 g of fiber/100 g of white bread and 7.4 g of fiber/100 g of wholemeal bread. The target now is to encourage more people to

Table 7.4 Mock data for the intake of three *foods* (A, B, C) in the lower and upper quartiles of a target *nutrient* intake (see text for explanation)

Quartile of target nutrient intake	Food A		Food B		Food C	
	Low	High	Low	High	Low	High
Target *food* intake (g/day)	0	50	12	26	60	45
	40	75	0	30	80	25
	60	0	28	42	70	35
	0	35	14	0	40	30
	0	65	0	28	0	40
	50	65	22	32	100	60
	75	85	14	0	0	10
	25	50	26	28	0	40
	0	0	18	36	0	30
	0	25	10	40	0	35
Average intake (g/day)	25	45	14	26	35	35
% Consumers	50	80	80	80	50	20
Consumer only intake (g/day)	50	56	18	33	70	35

Table 7.5 Sources of dietary fiber and contribution to fiber intake, with percentage of consumers of each source and intakes of each fiber source

	Contribution to dietary fiber intake (%)	Fiber (g/day)	Consumers (%)	Intake	
				(g/day)	(Portions/day)
Bread	33	5.5	98	125	4.5
Breakfast cereals	9	1.5	38	66	1
Pulses	9	1.5	77	66	1
Vegetables	17	2.8	100	105	2
Potatoes	11	1.8	90	140	1
Fruit	11	1.8	88	123	1

eat wholemeal bread. A quick search of the database shows that 80% of people consume white bread and 20% wholemeal bread. It is quite simple to calculate what the impact would be on dietary fiber intake of changing the existing 80:20 ratio to 60:40 or 40:60. Taking a comparable approach to all of these foods, the strategies summarized in Box 7.2 can be identified and the impact of different strategies calculated or modeled, however roughly.

The advantage of crudely calculating impact analysis is that it helps to create a reality-based prioritization within a range of public health nutrition options. It also helps to focus attention on two other key issues in the development and implementation of FBDG.

Step 4: Displacement of foods or nutrients

Previously, four strategies for developing FBDG to alter the intake of a target food were identified, of which one was encouraging people to switch to a comparable alternative (from whole-milk to low-fat milk, from lower fiber to higher fiber cereals, from soft drinks to fruit juices, etc.). In this instance there is substitution. But what if a decision was made that, to increase fiber intake, more people should consume pulses, more frequently and in larger serving sizes than at present? What food at what meal would give way for pulses? If the database allows, it may be possible to find out at which meals pulses are served and with which other foods. This may help to uncover foods that could be displaced. Displacement of vegetables would not be acceptable, but displacement of meat may be acceptable. However, displacement of red meat may cause a problem regarding iron intake. There are no guidelines to indicate which foods are likely to be displaced but the more help the consumer is given in this regard, the

Box 7.2	
Bread	Encourage more people to switch from white to wholemeal bread
Breakfast cereals	Increase the percentage of consumers
	Encourage more of these consumers to eat cereals with a higher fiber content than at present
Pulses	Encourage more people to eat pulses, more frequently and with a larger serving size
Vegetables	Leave things as they are
Potatoes	Leave things as they are
Fruit	Increase the number of portions/day

more likely the program is to succeed. However, this assumes that the program of public health nutrition knows its consumer.

Step 5: Consumer attitudinal research

The launch of a new food brand on the market is not the beginning of a project. It may be the first public release of the product, but it will have been preceded by an awesome amount of research, from the demand for such a product, by which sector of society, to its formulation, its name, its packaging and its associated advertising campaign. The manufacturer will know quite a lot about the intended buyer and their general social, educational, residential and economic profile. In general, there is little such research done for public health nutrition programs. Selling a new nutritional message is not all that different from selling a new detergent. In both instances, the campaign wants to attract consumers and then to convince them of the value of the product. The more the public health nutritionist understands the consumer, the more likely the message is to be listened to and acted upon. For example, a survey of the attitudes of 15 000

European Union (EU) adults to food, nutrition and health revealed the following key findings.

- In all 15 countries studied, "Trying to eat a healthy diet" was ranked in the top five factors influencing food choice, from a list of 15 possible factors.
- When asked, in their own words, to define "healthy eating", these consumers by and large answered correctly, i.e. the first choice was "more fruit and vegetables" and the second choice was "less fat".
- These consumers identified two broad categories of barriers to healthy eating: "internal", such as lack of willpower or not being able to give up favorite foods, and "external", such as a busy lifestyle or the constraints of job, work or studies.
- When asked as to their opinion on the following statement: "I do not need to make changes to my diet as my diet is already healthy enough", overall some 70% either "agreed strongly" or "agreed".

The conclusions are simple. These 15 000 consumers, representative of the population of 15 EU countries,

- believe that healthy eating is important
- know what healthy eating is
- want healthy eating to fit in with their lifestyle
- have already achieved a healthy diet.

The last statement is clearly wrong since dietary surveys show a significant shortfall between average nutrient intakes and the population goals for those intakes. The key message to get across is: "You may think your diet is healthy but it is more than likely that it needs considerable improvement". Packaging that message is difficult and challenging. This type of research helps to identify not only the broad issues that need to be addressed, but also where in society the biggest problem lies: by age, by gender, by social class, by place of residence, by income, and so on.

7.6 Visual presentations of food guides related to dietary guidelines

Several visual presentations of food guides related to dietary guidelines are used. The principal objective of these visual presentations of food guides is to help consumers to implement the dietary guidelines by suggesting types and amounts of foods to be consumed.

Culturally appropriate modes of presentation of the main messages should be sought, pretested and disseminated. Some commonly used examples include a two-dimensional pyramid or triangle in which food groups that should be eaten least are found at the top and staple foods that should be eaten most are across the broad base of the triangle (e.g. USDA Food Guide Pyramid 1993, Mediterranean Diet Pyramid 1994, Asian Diet Pyramid 1995).The major difference between these three pyramids is in their distinction between plant and animal proteins. Other increasingly used visual presentations are the food circle, with sectors of equal size (Sweden) or of different sizes (Finland, the Netherlands), and the health food plate, which consists of a plate with a knife on one side and a fork on the other, with sectors of different sizes, each illustrating major foods of the group (UK: Food Guide; US: AIRC New American Plate).

7.7 Perspectives on the future

At present, our understanding of food consumption patterns and indeed nutrient intakes is highly aggregated into a single value for nutrient intake and a single value for food intake. In reality, the pattern is one of multiple eating occasions, each of which has the potential to deliver a different metabolic response. In the future, much more attention will have to be paid to understanding the nature of temporal distribution of food and nutrient intake, the associations between foods as meals and the impact of particular patterns of meal consumption on metabolism. More effective FBDG may be developed taking into account this greater understanding and knowledge.

Further reading

Cummings JH *et al*. Fecal weight, colon cancer risk and dietary intake of non-starch polysaccharides (dietary fiber). Gastroenterology 1992; 103: 1783–1789

Websites

http://eurodiet.med.uoc.gr/WP2/wp2_home.html
http://www.dga2000training.usda.gov/welcome.htm
http://www.fao.org/DOCREP/x0243e/x0243e00.htm
http://www.fao.org/es/esn/fbdg/httoc.htm
http://www.sahealthinfo.org/nutrition/safoodbased.htm

8
Food Choice

David N Cox and Annie S Anderson

Key messages

- The measurement of food choice relies on a range of methodologies, including observational approaches, interview, questionnaire and diary studies, controlled intervention trials, the use of animal models to understand basic mechanisms, and sensory preference trials in the laboratory and home.
- Popular models of food choice include those that investigate perception of sensory attributes of the food (e.g. taste and texture), psychological factors (e.g. mood and attitudinal factors) and the social environment (e.g. cultural norms, advertising, economic factors and food availability).

- Access to a "healthy" diet for all requires an adequate variety of "good" food at affordable prices. Access can be influenced by area of residence, car ownership, public transport, shopping and storage facilities.
- Food choices are socially patterned, notably with respect to sociodemographic variables of age, gender and social class, as well as by ethnicity, marital status and household composition, and a range of psychosocial and intervening variables.
- Personality traits, beliefs, attitudes, mood and expectations all influence food choice.

8.1 Introduction

The study of food choice in humans involves many complex interactions, incorporating areas ranging from the biological mechanisms of appetite control, through the psychology of eating behavior, social and cultural values, to public health and commercial attempts to alter the food intake of particular populations. Food choice is apparent as both an outcome (an end) of a decision process and a mechanism or process (a means to that end). For nutritionists there is an increasing awareness that there are consequences with regard to both the end-point and the process. Understanding the factors that influence the development and changes in food selection are considered fundamental to aiding the successful translation of nutritional goals into consumer behavior. Many public health campaigns now recognize that biomedical research alone cannot address the major challenges of chronic disease prevention. Increasingly, government agencies seek to incorporate behavioral and social intervention strategies into public health interventions.

The overall aim of this chapter is to demonstrate to the nutrition student the relevance of applying the behavioral and social sciences to nutritional problems and to gain an insight to the complex interactions with nutrition in the process of food choice. This chapter will focus first on the population issues and then on the individual issues associated with food choice.

It is important to remember that the literature on food choice focuses predominantly, but not exclusively, on consumers in industrialized countries and therefore predominantly in Western cultures. As this chapter reviews the existing and established approaches to the subject much of the discussion will apply to such societies and cultures. It does not follow that such approaches are always valid in other cultures. A glossary of the terms used in the study of food choice can be found in Box 8.1.

- Acculturation: the process of cultural change from contact between cultural groups
- Attitude: a tendency, comprising affective, cognitive and conative aspects, which can be long or short-term, volatile and possibly amenable to change
- Behavioral traits: long-term dispositions for behaviors
- Commensality: eating food together
- Cultural flavor principals: the combinations of basic foods, herbs, spices and cooking methods that give foods characteristic sensory properties associated with particular cultures or regions
- Ecological validity: a quality of empirical evidence that reflects what is also observed in the real world
- Food deserts: areas of residence with few or no shopping facilities
- Food neophobia: a reluctance to eat and/or avoidance of novel foods (opposite of food neophilia: liking for new foods)
- Forced commensality: foods palatable to all participants at a shared meal, minimizing waste (adapted from commensality: eating food together)
- Hedonics: liking or disliking, the degree of pleasantness derived from stimuli such as food
- Perceived control: perceived ability to make dietary changes
- Psychohedonics: perceptions and preferences determined by pleasantness or *hedonics* (liking or disliking)
- Psychophysical perceptions (and possibly preferences) determined by the sensitivity of the physical senses
- Self-efficacy: perceived ability to make dietary changes
- Sensory-specific satiety or food-specific satiety: reduction in the perceived pleasantness of foods after a certain quantity has been consumed
- Shared cognitions: common ways of thinking about a food or meals, which may include attitudes and beliefs; one part (of three) of a definition of culture
- Standard operating procedures: agreed protocols for acquiring, preparing, cooking, eating and disposal of foods; one part (of three) of a definition of culture ·
- Subjective norm: the influence of important others (social influence)
- Unexamined assumptions: an attitude that *shared cognitions* and *standard operating procedures* are not generally questioned; one part (of three) of a definition of culture

8.2 The study of food choice

Often consumers' initial response to a question asking why they choose a particular food is "because I like the taste". Many people can rapidly give broad reasons for choosing foods. For example, a large European study focusing on influences on food choice highlighted quality and freshness, price, taste, trying to eat healthily and family preferences as the five most important factors influencing consumers' choices. This is confounded,

however, by how different consumers interpret terms such as "trying to eat healthily".

Part of the problem with trying to understand the underlying reasons why consumers choose particular foods is that they are not always conscious of their reasons for choice. Marketing researchers often describe common foods as "low-involvement" products. Involvement in a product means that consumers find it very important and invest considerable time in acquiring knowledge of the product, facilitating more informed choices and the ability to express themselves. Such involvement may vary with the particular food or beverage. Wine could be considered to be a high-involvement beverage because of its intrinsic complexity (e.g. hundreds of volatile odors) and its social status at the meal table. These facilitate a large vocabulary (but not always with common definitions) allowing expression of opinions about wine qualities and preferences. The same cannot be said for, say, cooking oil, which could be considered a low-involvement food. Compared with other consumer products, such as cars, most foods would rate as low-involvement products. Nevertheless, particular groups of consumers, for example people who are very concerned about their body weight, may have a greater involvement with foods than others or with certain foods (e.g. energy-dense foods such as chocolate). Women, largely because of historical gender roles that persist in modern society (e.g. shopping, cooking and caring for their families), tend to be more involved with food than men. There are suggestions that some cultures are more involved with food than others; for example, within southern European cultures food is considered more important than among many sections of the UK population. What does this mean when trying to understand food choice? Simply, many people find it difficult to express the underlying reasons why they choose particular foods because of their lack of involvement. Confounding this is that there is no common vocabulary for expressing the attributes of foods. People were found to be confused between different tastes (sweet, sour, bitter, salt) and used other sensory descriptors (e.g. acidic) when asked to label tastants. Therefore, the term taste, when used colloquially, can mean many aspects of the sensory attributes of foods (Table 8.1) and different things to different people. Without a common definition it is difficult to compare across people or across foods. The challenge for investigators of food choice is to seek out the underlying reasons for choice when so many

Table 8.1 Comparison of scientific and lay consumers' definitions of "taste" (variations and aspects of taste or tastes further indicate the complexity of the term)

Scientific definition of taste	Some lay understanding or use of the qualitative attribute taste	Some quantitative aspects (and scale anchors) that can interact with the attribute taste
Gustation, the five basic[a] tastes (sweet, sour, bitter, salt, umami[b]) detected by taste receptors in the oral cavity	Tasty, salty, sweet, bitter, sour, acidic, mouthfeel, texture, smell, odor, pungency, flavor[c]	Strength (weak–strong) Duration (short–long) Quality (good–bad) Hedonics (liking–disliking) Ideal point (too little–just right–too much) Time intensity (peak perception over time) Aftertaste Off-taste

[a] Not all scientists agree that there are five basic tastes.
[b] The fifth basic taste, umami, has no satisfactory English equivalent word; however, the closest could be "savory". It is rarely reported by Western consumers.
[c] The term flavor is often used to describe a combination of odor, taste and pungency.

affective (e.g. sensory–hedonic), cognitive (e.g. attitudes, traits, beliefs) and external (e.g. availability, price, other people's influence) factors are involved.

By definition, the term food choice implies a degree of volition, of control over the foods that people eat. However, it is often gauging how much choice and what influences choice that becomes the central focus. Measuring food choice relies on a range of methodologies, including observational approaches, interview, questionnaire and diary studies, controlled intervention trials, the use of animal models to understand basic mechanisms, and sensory preference trials in the laboratory and home.

Like nutrition, food choice is a complex area involving many different disciplines. Past studies have taken a transdisciplinary approach, which has sought to apply various disciplines to the food provisioning process: the acquisition, preparation, cooking, eating and disposal of food. Essentially, different disciplines have been applied to a process or problem. Such an approach has drawn upon the knowledge of social and economic scientists (from sociology, economics, marketing and anthropology) and therefore has tended to emphasize external or social factors in food choice.

Other literature has been described as cross-disciplinary. This literature has been written by investigators from the behavioral (psychology, psychiatry and sensory science) and life (physiology, pharmacology, neurology and nutrition) sciences, but has also included marketing approaches. Such an approach has

emphasized internal or individual factors associated with food choice. The areas of study tend to sit within models that locate those internal or individual factors within a culture, an economic system and a society (external factors). Different scientific backgrounds and differing collaborations have provided differing emphases on the understanding of food choice. It is therefore important to look carefully at the background of the investigators to see from which perspective they approach problems of food choice. This chapter emphasizes socioeconomic and psychological approaches to food choice, with some reference to physiology. Reference should be made to the chapter on sensory systems in *Nutrition and Metabolism*. Personal attributes will also have a major modifying effect on physiological reactions. These include perception of sensory attributes (e.g. taste, texture), psychological factors (e.g. mood, cognitive factors such as attitudes) and the social environment (e.g. cultural norms, advertising, economic factors and food availability). Various schematic models have been devised which attempt to show how factors influencing food preferences and choice interact. A popular model of food choice is shown in Figure 8.1.

Understanding the processes of food choice at an individual level is complex. It has been observed that people's life course experiences affected major influences on food choice that included ideals, personal factors, resources, social contexts and the food context. These influences, in turn, informed the development of per-

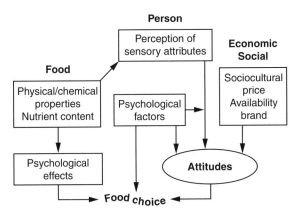

Figure 8.1 Shepherd's model. From Shepherd and Sparks (1999). Reproduced with permission from Kluwer Academic/Plenum Publishers.

sonal systems for making food choices that incorporated value negotiations and behavioral strategies.

8.3 Population issues affecting food choice

Behavior (such as eating), social and economic factors, and people's beliefs and attitudes when applied to a population or ethnic group collectively can be labeled as cultural factors influencing food choice. This section explores cultural factors and the sociology of food choice.

Cultural factors

It is thought that culture is a major determinant of human food choice. Indeed, there is evidence that traditions, beliefs and values are among the main factors influencing preference, mode of food preparation, serving and nutritional status.

The psychologist Triandis provided a useful review of many different definitions of culture and concluded that most people agreed that culture was reflected in shared cognitions, standard operating procedures and unexamined assumptions. A common theme in most definitions is that of sharing. By whatever definition (and culture is a difficult phenomenon to define), food is almost always generally considered to be major part of culture, and culture is considered to be the major influence upon food choice, specifically, a culture shares certain food choices.

Genetics or cultural influences?

Explanations for cultural food choices and preferences for particular varieties of foods have been sought in terms of differences in the perceptions of the sensory characteristics of foods. Early cross-cultural studies focused on comparison of sensory perception such as threshold, sensitivity or discrimination. Most studies looking at perception of tastes in solutions found no differences between cultures. No difference was recorded in the four basic taste (salt, sweet, bitter, sour) thresholds between Nigerian, Korean and American subjects. There is some emerging preliminary evidence that odor perception may differ between Japanese and Europeans; however, this requires more substantiation. Despite the lack of research into cultural differences in perception of sensory properties other than tastes such as flavor or texture, chemosensory abilities appear generally similar between cultures. It is well accepted that there is evidence of variation between cultures in preference for food. Research has looked at cultural patterns for liking of specific sensory properties. Taste intensity liking has been found to vary between cultures depending on the context or food. Overall, cultural variation in taste level preference seems to be product specific, with no consistency in direction or magnitude across products. These product-dependent differences appear to be related to consumer familiarity and exposure. Therefore, cross-cultural variation in food preferences appears to arise from experience, dietary habits and attitudes to food, rather than a strong genetic influence. Nevertheless, within cultures emerging evidence suggests that there is a genetic component to various food behaviors at an individual level, including stomach filling, dietary restraint, eating companions, susceptibility to social facilitation and possibly palatability of highly palatable foods.

Cultural flavor principles

Flavor principles have been suggested to characterize particular cultures food preferences. For example, tomato, olive oil, garlic and herbs are characteristic of certain cuisines of Mediterranean countries or regions. Cuisine can be structured as:

- basic foodstuffs
- manipulative techniques (particulation, incorporation, separation or extraction, marination, fermentation and the various applications of heat)
- cultural (or regional) flavor principles.

The historical perspective given to these shared processes and cultural favors introduces the concept of exposure and familiarity, which has been demonstrated to be a significant predictor of food acceptance.

Biology, culture and individual behavior

Chili, corn, manioc and sugar have been used as examples to illustrate the way in which culture and individual behavior influence and modify biology. A biological aversion to chili peppers (which contain a hot irritant) may be overridden by culture (culinary behavior) and individual psychological processes. The manioc (cassava) example sought to show how biological problems (the toxicity of manioc, perceived by the bitterness of the tuber) were overcome by processing (individual behavior) and how such processing became integrated into culture (the detoxification technology), leading to individuals using the technology and accepting the food. A nutritional example was that of corn (maize). The poor niacin, amino acid and calcium content of such a staple food (biological problem), the discovery of processing with added lime and the making of tortillas (individual), and the acceptance of such technology and cuisine (culture) led to the acceptance of corn tortillas as a staple food. However, the biological component (nutrient deficiencies) may have been overcome through the enhanced sensory acceptability route, as the addition of lime softens the corn, creating perceptions of greater palatability. In these ways culture, biology and individual behavior interact with respect to food choice.

Cuisines are rarely static; indeed, the traditional food itself is not unchanging. Tradition has been defined as "a sequence or variations on received and transmitted themes" and several scenarios of how traditional cultural cuisines change, resist change or move across national boundaries have been documented.

Cultural food choices and potential benefits to other populations

The landmark studies of Keys in the 1950s of the "cultural" Mediterranean diet led to attempts at changing trends in food choice in the latter half of the twentieth century in many industrialized countries. There has been consensus for some time on increasing fruit, vegetable and grains in the diets of Western industrialized populations, and similarly in reducing fat or, more recently, consuming different fats (e.g. less saturated and more poly unsaturated or monounsaturated fats).

These can be perceived as an attempt to use one food culture in other cultures. For example, people of Anglo-Celtic origin appear to have low intakes of fruit, vegetables and grain foods compared with southern Europeans (Italians and Greeks). Data on the eating habits of Italians and Italian migrants supports a resilience of the desirable features of the Mediterranean diet. Retaining aspects of the Mediterranean diet and encouraging its consumption in other cultures may be a useful public health nutrition strategy. An understanding of food choice is crucial in this respect.

Cultural influences and the rise of the global marketplace

In the early 1980s it was asserted that, with a global marketplace, products, including foods, were becoming standardized worldwide (or at least in the developed world) and that consumers would develop homogeneous preferences. However, this view has subsequently been modified and there is increasing consensus that certain marketing parameters may only be standardized to varying degrees, depending on the market, the product, the company and the environment.

In some respects, homogeneous preferences for "fast foods" have increased enormously since the early 1980s. Such foods may be part of a global culture of increasing perceived time poverty or choices to allocate time to other activities. These changes may have important consequences for nutritional status and deserve considerable investigation.

Cultural integrity

Evidence from some of the rapidly industrializing countries of Asia provides examples of resistance to homogeneous food preferences. For example, the food choices of Koreans and Chinese Malaysians have resisted changes and remain culturally intact. It is notable in that the South Korean economy has industrialized rapidly since the 1950s, yet the traditional foods and cuisines associated with Korean diets have been retained. As a consequence, nutrient intakes have, in comparison to other rapidly industrialized Asian countries, changed little. Contact with people of one's own culture has been shown to help maintain cultural behaviors, including food habits. In contrast, the Malay Malaysian community appears to be developing more Westernized diets with associated recent increases in chronic diseases such as heart disease and certain cancers found in Western industrialized nations. It is largely unknown which factors are most important: social, self-identity or even sensory attributes of the foods. Nevertheless, certain cultural cuisines appear to resist changes while others, even in the same country, appear to be more open to modification.

Acculturation

Acculturation is defined as "the process of cultural change from contact between cultural groups". The process of migration and immigration demonstrates how food choices can resist or be influenced by cultural change, and several cross-sectional studies of acculturation have assessed migrants to Western cultures. For example, Korean migrants living in the USA consumed more "American" foods if their acculturation was greater. In a sociological study of South Asian females living in Scotland, it was found that, in contrast to Italian migrants, fat intakes had increased markedly with migration, with an associated increase in body mass index (BMI), and incidence of heart disease and type 2 diabetes. Various possible mechanisms were described, such as body image, gender/cultural roles and the value of certain foods. British-born South Asians were more marked in this respect than Asian-born South Asians. However, South Asians placed much more emphasis on traditional foods for formal meals than their Italian counterparts, who appeared to be more flexible in their culinary choices, choosing Anglo-Celtic foods more often.

Australia presents an intriguing case as 98% of its population is migrant. The country has been dominated by white Anglo-Celtic culture, but, especially during the latter half of the twentieth century, has witnessed large migration from southern Europe (bringing a Mediterranean diet) and, since the 1990s, from Asia. Since the 1970s, Australian food choice appears to have become increasingly diverse, nevertheless, there is some evidence that distinct cultural preferences and beliefs about foods have been retained in the populations of Anglo-Celtic and Mediterranean origin. Evidence of Asian migrants' distinct food preferences is illustrated by a study of Vietnamese women resident in Australia who were found to have retained distinct food preferences and dietary profiles, particularly with regard to staple or core foods. Changes in food intakes occurred most among those who had migrated at an earlier age, which is consistent with considerable research on the development of children's eating habits.

In contrast, North American studies including data on Chinese migrants to the USA and Canada, and Korean migrants to the USA provide evidence for increasing similarity between migrants and the host cultures in terms of nutritional status as a function of greater acculturation. A Canadian study notes changes in perceived flavor, health and prestige value of foods among young boys suggesting, again, that age of migration, with consequent impression and early exposure, is important. It is possible that food choices remain culturally specific, while the relative quantities of foods move towards those of the host nation's culture, with consequent changes in macronutrient intakes. The resilience of the Korean diet in Korea, in contrast to Korean migrants to the USA, suggests that US cultural effects are stronger than mere changes in economic circumstances.

Acculturation is a complex phenomenon requiring multidimensional measures, and the evidence suggests that the end result of acculturation is not simple assimilation by the dominant host culture. Whereas cultural food choices appear to remain resilient, especially for core staple foods, changes in macronutrient intakes appear, in some cases, to move towards the host culture. Age and generation appear to be key factors and fit with the principles of early exposure and availability. However, as all studies cited are cross-sectional, relying on length of residency as a marker for changes over time, there is a need for longitudinal studies.

Media and advertising

The media, especially television, may be one of the most important sources of information about food. Government data suggest that in the UK, children aged 4–15 years spend between 17 and 18 h/week watching television, via which most food and drink images are conveyed through advertising. By the time children in the UK leave school, the time devoted to watching television will exceed the hours spent in school. Within Europe, the UK has the highest level of advertising targeted at children, while Sweden and Norway have no child-directed advertising. Most studies of the content of television food advertising highlight that a significant proportion of food adverts is for high-fat or high-sugar foods, and concern has been expressed that overweight children may be particularly sensitive to these. However, the issue remains controversial; there is no evidence to suggest that advertising is the principal influence on children's eating behavior, and it is likely to be just one influence among many factors.

The impact of advertising on children's dietary knowledge, attitudes and behavior is unclear. Food advertising is known to increase children's knowledge of brand names, to foster positive attitudes to the food and to change beliefs, but few long-term studies have monitored and quantified these effects. Children exposed to a cartoon program containing food advertisements made more bids for the advertised foods than children in a control condition. Research has demonstrated that if children enjoy a commercial and are interested in its content, their requests to have a particular food increase. Public health messages delivered to young children with adult reinforcement of the positive value of more "healthy" foods have been shown to decrease consumption of less healthy snacks by young children. It has been demonstrated, in a naturalistic setting, that the more television advertising a child sees for a particular product marketed specifically for children, the more likely it was that the product would be found in the child's household. Thus, media messages can be influential in determining requests for food items and in food selection, at least in the short term.

Food access and availability

The concept of food availability stretches from local retail provisioning to availability within the home and catering settings (notably school food provision). Food retailing is major business and a source of consumer pleasure and concern. Throughout Europe, the number of retail outlets has diminished as larger supermarkets have developed. For example, in France retail outlets have declined from 200 000 in 1986 to 150 000 in 1990, and in Italy the number of retail outlets dropped by 15% between 1985 and 1993. In the UK the number of independent food stores declined by almost 40% between 1986 and 1997. Although providing the benefits of lower costs through economy of scale to both retailers and consumers, such a concentration of retail outlets requires that consumers have access to transport, most often the private car.

Adequate food at affordable prices is necessary if people are to have access to a healthy, balanced diet. Such access can be influenced by area of residence, car ownership, public transport, and shopping and storage facilities. Access is generally considered a major factor in compliance with dietary recommendations.

In the UK, concern has been expressed over the problem of areas of residence with few or no shopping facilities, known as "food deserts", as a contributor to health inequalities. Several studies have reported higher shopping costs for "healthy" than for "less healthy" shopping baskets, and variation in costs in different urban areas of residence. A UK independent inquiry has recommended the development of policies to ensure adequate retail provision of foods to those who are socially disadvantaged. Studies in a deprived urban area in London demonstrated a four-fold difference in price between the cheapest and most expensive food prices in the area. Less than one-third of the foods that would contribute to a basic basket for a healthy diet were stocked in most outlets. However, this observation is not universal.

Within catering settings, changes in food accessibility and pricing have been shown to lead to increases in fruit and salad purchases, and decreases in the selection of confectionery and crisps. Availability of quality and variety almost certainly also influence consumption.

Social influences on food choice

Food habits are generally developed and maintained because they are effective, practical and meaningful behaviors in a particular culture. However, society refers to the people who participate in the culture, and the characteristics of those people will, in turn, affect dietary intake.

Sociodemographic factors

Food choices are socially patterned with the key sociodemographic variables of age, gender and social class, but also with ethnicity, marital status and household composition, and a range of psychosocial and intervening variables (Figure 8.1). Age will affect dietary intake through a range of biological processes (e.g. growth), current contexts and fashions, social factors and psychological factors. Even during adult life there are marked differences in food consumption (Table 8.2).

From birth it is clear that nutritional wisdom will be modified by social pressures, normative behaviors and practical constraints. Breast-feeding is a good example of this (see Chapter 16). Throughout the lifespan biological needs will interact with social factors in the formation, development and maintenance of eating behaviors. Thus, in early childhood the social construction of meanings about food by teachers and

Table 8.2 Frequency of food consumption by age of adults in the Scottish Health Survey, 1993

	Age (years)				
	16–24 years (%)	25–34 years (%)	35–44 years (%)	45–54 years (%)	55–64 years (%)
Eats crisps once a day	39	29	18	11	5
Eats root vegetables five or more times per week	16	20	23	26	32
Eats sweets or chocolate once a day or more	39	33	24	17	14
Drinks soft drinks once a day or more	46	32	19	19	16

Data from Scottish Office (1995).

pupils intersects with the policy and provisioning within schools. Likewise, in adolescence, emotions such as resentment, anger and frustration may find expression through eating habits by spitting, throwing and mashing, or through physiological responses of nausea, gagging or vomiting. In older years some authors suggest that access to food and the cost and quality of food impact upon food habits, resulting in a contrast between stated food beliefs and actual consumption patterns.

Even from early childhood it is recognized that food intake varies by gender. Dietary surveys in Europe have highlighted differences in food consumption between men and women, with men having higher intakes of meat products, alcohol and sugar, and lower intakes of fruit, vegetables and low-fat products than women. In some respects these choices make women's diets more consistent with current recommendations than men's; however, women's intakes of micronutrients, for example, iron, zinc, vitamin B_{12} and folate, are often deficient, particularly when biological requirements are greater.

Biological, social, psychological and behavioral factors associated with gender appear to interact to influence the intake of different foods and nutrients. In general, women have lower energy requirements than men owing to lower body mass. Socially, it may be considered less acceptable for women to be seen to eat large quantities of food in a culture where excess body weight is considered undesirable. Women seem to be more knowledgeable about food and nutrition and indicate higher levels of concern over food safety, health and weight reduction. Men appear to have stronger beliefs and values associating certain foods items with qualities such as strength, power and virility, and consumption may be used as a symbol of masculinity. It has also been argued that specific foods and types of meal function as symbolic markers of gender and of gender status within the nuclear family.

Social class or socioeconomic variations in food consumption are of particular concern with respect to health inequalities. Various measures have been used to access socioeconomic position, including occupation, income and education. Class is assumed to have an economic base, is measured by income or occupation, and implies some control over resources.

People belonging to higher social class groups and with a higher educational level tend to have healthier diets. For example, they have higher intakes of fruit, fruit juices, lean meat, oily fish, wholemeal products and raw vegetables compared with manual workers, who have higher intakes of energy (presumably to match energy requirements) and lower intakes of polyunsaturated fatty acids, fruits and vegetables. It is also assumed that groups with higher socioeconomic status have healthier diets because they are more health conscious and have a healthier lifestyle. Higher educational levels may also help to conceptualize the relationship between diet and health.

Disposable income and the amount of money to spend on food are also crucial factors in food choice, especially for meat, fruit and vegetables. The evidence on the relationship between diet and poverty in Europe suggests that people in low-income households are not ignorant of food issues, but are in fact highly skilled at budgeting, especially where food is often the only flexible item in the household. In the UK, households in the lowest decile of income spend the highest proportion of money on food. Data from the UK National Food Survey show that poorer households are the most efficient purchasers of nutrients per unit cost. There is also some evidence that foods that are currently recommended for a healthier diet not only cost more than cheap, filling, energy-dense foods, but are also more expensive to purchase in areas of rural and urban deprivation.

Social factors at the household level

Eating behaviors are also strongly linked to social groupings. For example, households may struggle to attain current dietary recommendations if different family members eat different things at different times. Specific influences from the social environment, which impact on eating behavior, include social pressure from friends and family, modeling behavior and social facilitation. The nuclear family has been demonstrated to play an important role in the development of food patterns. Social influences appear to be embedded in family food rules and often interact with other determinants of food intake. Mothers are generally considered to be more influential than other family members because of their nurturing role, control over food activities in the home and presence at mealtimes. Family eating habits are also influenced by cultural patterns in preference and consumption, availability of foods in the home and genetic factors. Competing factors that influence family eating include food eaten out of the home, which is more likely to be influenced by others.

The role of social facilitation in energy intake has been well described, with a positive association between the number of people present on meal and snack occasions and higher energy intakes. For example, meals eaten with other people present were on average 44% larger than meals eaten alone, and included larger amounts of carbohydrate, fat, protein and alcohol. It is assumed that this relationship is causal, reflecting a combination of increased food availability, relaxed social atmosphere, distraction, more tempting food and longer meal duration. Other influences include the gender and familiarity of the diners. Even inheritance has been found to influence meal size and frequency.

Religious, moral and ethical influences

The rituals of eating behavior are prescribed not only socially, but also by religious beliefs. Religious beliefs are dynamic and subject to change, including generational and individual modification, and so can be considered as social constructs. Six general functional categories of religious food practices have been described (Box 8.2 and Table 8.3).

In more recent years moral and ethical issues rather than strict religious issues may have become more important in exerting an influence on food selection.

Box 8.2 Functions of religious food practices

Communication with God
Demonstration of faith
Rejection of worldliness
Identification and belonging
Expression of separateness
Reinforcement of ecological pragmatism

Modified from Fieldhouse (1995) with kind permission of Kluwer Academic Publishers.

Table 8.3 The function of religious food practices

Eating behavior	Example
Food restrictions	Avoidance of beef by Sikhs
Fasting	The Islamic fast of Ramadan
Feasting	Christmas day for Christians
Respect for special days	No food preparation on the Sabbath by Jews
Respect for time of day	Buddhist monks do not eat after midday
Preparation of food	Kosher food preparation by Jews

Such issues range from boycotting the products of certain manufacturers deemed to engage in politically incorrect activities (e.g. breaking advertising codes on breast-milk substitutes), avoiding foods that may contain genetically modified materials, and vegetarianism. For many vegetarians, food concerns will extend to modes of food production, ecological issues and global sustainability.

8.4 Individual issues affecting food choice

An application of food choice to public health nutrition requires an understanding of how different groups perceive and choose foods. However, the scientific knowledge obtained depends on measuring the behaviors of individuals. It is therefore important to understand how individuals perceive and choose foods. As in all research, the phrasing of questions has a large influence on the responses. Similarly, modeling food choice through experimental designs strongly influences the outcomes. It is therefore worth noting that the science of understanding individual food choice uses a range of different measures that require definition.

Outcome measures

Individual perceptions and senses have a fundamental role in human existence. Perception and sensation must be viewed as an integrated whole if the complex interactions that occur among human sensory processes, perceptions, cognitions and behavior in everyday eating situations are to be understood. Investigators seek to understand both psychophysical and psychohedonic responses to foods.

Psychophysical measures are the relationship between sensory (affective) responses and physiology. Such differences may be particularly pertinent with the aging process, when atrophy of the sensory organs alters the perception of foods because of loss of sensitivity. There is little evidence for physiological differences determining preferences for foods across other groups, for example, cultures. However, genetically determined individual differences may play a role.

Psychohedonics is the pleasantness of a food and is influenced by cognitive (cultural, belief and attitudinal) factors expressed as subjective liking or disliking. Evidence suggests that psychohedonic responses play a major role in food choice. In this respect, investigators of food choice have claimed that the brain is the most important physical organ influencing human food choice.

At an individual level, outcome measures of food choice can be taken as:

- consumption
- hedonic response (liking or disliking)
- preference
- acceptance.

Understanding consumption as a behavior is an important end-point measure. This is because there is often poor agreement with measures of preference and reported consumption. As detailed elsewhere (*Introduction to Human Nutrition,* Chapter 10), measuring food intake in free-living individuals is not easy in terms of actual measurement, the measurement effects and the behaviors of the individual undertaking the measurement or being measured. The tendency is for investigations to concentrate on tasting particular foods, and it is rare that liking and consumption are investigated together.

Liking is often used synonymously with preference; however, distinct differences exist between the two. Preference is influenced by affective, external and cognitive factors. For a food preference to be expressed, choices must be available. The interactions of affective aspects with cognitive factors that influence preference are numerous. Several scales have been developed that

attempt to measure both the affective and the cognitive aspects of food acceptance. Care must be taken to choose the appropriate response scale for the purpose and to resist the temptation to modify those that have a sound theoretical basis.

Genetics and taste sensitivity

It would seem reasonable that genetically moderated differences in physiology may account for individual differences in taste. However, it was not until an accidental discovery by Fox (in 1931) that a marker was found that might explain such differences. After an accidental spill, Fox's colleagues could taste, as extremely bitter, the compound phenylthiocarbamide (PTC), whereas Fox could not perceive the bitterness at all. Subsequent work revealed a genetic basis for such differences. Tasters had a dominant allele (T) or a dominant allele paired with a recessive allele (Tt), whereas nontasters had two recessive allelles (tt). Subsequent work describes how distributions for tasters and nontasters were found to be bimodal. Tasters have more fungiform papillae and therefore more numerous taste buds. Using the related (safer) compound 6-*n*-propylthiouracil (PROP), sensitivity has been found to be associated with perception of some bitter compounds (e.g. quinine, naringin), and sometimes associated with sweetness perception (e.g. sucrose and some, but not all, sweeteners). Through the trigeminal nerve system, greater sensitivity to capsaicin (the hot ingredient in chilies) was found among those with greater taste sensitivities. Individuals sensitive to PROP could more easily identify the creaminess of fat and cheese and the fat content of manipulated foods, and there is some evidence that such people have lower BMI and lower dietary energy intakes. Females, and people of African and Asian origin are more likely to be more sensitive to PROP. Further work has identified a third group of medium tasters who can only just perceive the bitterness of PROP. However, the methodology is not without problems and it is now thought that the psychophysical scales used to measure people's perceptions of intensity need to be carefully anchored using, for example, a label such as "strongest sensation ever experienced" to account for differences across groups. Alternatively, using taste sensitivity as a continuous variable (rather than cut-offs of supertasters, medium tasters and nontasters) may prove more useful and may explain inconsistent results. Similarly, despite some early work on low preferences for brassica vegetables by supertasters, the evidence for the specific effects upon actual food choice is weak and this has been poorly studied. This may be explained by the lack of associations between PROP sensitivity and other bitter compounds; for example, a vegetable may contain hundreds of potentially interactive bitter compounds that may or may not be perceived. PROP sensitivity, which is more prevalent among some Asian people, is associated with capsaicin sensitivity, yet chili is an important part of many Asian cuisines. Perhaps more important, but as yet unknown, social and cognitive factors and learning processes override individual physiological differences.

Innate versus learned preferences

There is no doubt that the capacity to express hunger is innate; however, with particular preferences for tastes of foods there is debate as to whether preferences are truly innate or as a result of learning. Innate preferences mean preferences at birth; however, this does not mean that such preferences are genetic as they are likely to be learnt *in utero* or through exposure to breast milk. Essentially innate preferences could be characterized as "very early learning".

Taste

Facial expressions of infants support evidence that there is possibly an innate (or very early) dislike of bitter and sour foods and a preference for sweetened foods. The dislike of bitter foods may be related to toxic substances such as certain alkaloids present in some bitter-tasting plants and may therefore have a genetic component. There is compelling evidence for early preferences for sweet foods and almost any food becomes acceptable if it is sweet. However, the preference for sweetness may be a learnt response due to early exposure to breast milk or milk formula. Salt perception does not appear to occur in humans until 4–6 months of age. However, most experimentation undertaken with basic tastants may be a flawed methodology, as young children's salt preferences differ depending whether the salt is in a soup or a simple solution (as a tastant), suggesting that context and the particular food are important, even at a very early age.

Flavors

There is some evidence that preferences for flavors can be acquired *in utero* or through maternal milk. Repeated exposure to vegetables has been shown to increase acceptability in children who had been breast-fed, compared with children who had been formula fed, which has been explained by some evidence that flavors from maternal diets pass into breast milk.

Texture

Animal studies suggest that there may be some innate (unlearned) component to positive hedonic responses to fatty textures, particularly when deprived of food. Similarly, there may be a role for odor volatiles and specific free fatty acids in enhancing palatability. However, there is also evidence for preferences for other energy-dense foods. Given that many people live in a world of highly palatable foods and can make choices, the evidence reviewed strongly supports interactions with early experiences and learning.

Early food selection

Longitudinal data exist on French nursery children's dietary selections that suggest strong variability amongst choices, avoidance of bitter foods and control of energy density with a constant selection of starchy foods. These data suggest that selection differed according to the sociodemographic backgrounds of the children, gender and weight status. However, although offered a wide range of foods, these children made selections from a socially determined "healthy" range of foods. The self-selection of individual food choice does not appear to be separated from the social context and value judgments of others.

Energy intake and meal size

Much work has been done in the area of self-selection of energy intake and how learning through association can regulate energy intake through satiety. Manipulations of foods have shown that very young children regulate and anticipate their energy intakes as a result of the experience of familiar foods. Although meal sizes vary considerably over 24 h, energy intakes remain relatively constant. Given these skilled compensatory mechanisms, how is it that the energy imbalance seen in underweight, overweight and obesity can occur? Part of the answer seems to lie in the parent–child interactions and the child's ability to regulate energy intake. Authoritarian parenting was found to be negatively associated with self-regulation; similarly, there are strong relationships between parental mealtime behaviors and overweight in children. Peer pressure and emulation of adults' choices shape children's food choices. It has been suggested that reward systems in children's environments favor sweet products and therefore, perhaps unconsciously, reinforce preferences for sweet foods at the expense of, for example, vegetables (see Chapter 15 in *Nutrition and Metabolism*).

Both peer pressure and the degree of control are important in adolescent children's individual food choices. In contrast, there is evidence that parents, cajoling, persuading, threatening or bribing their children to eat certain socially determined healthy or appropriate foods is rarely successful. Despite initial success, bribery is rarely successful in the long term and, although some parents rationally reject such strategies, in practice they find them difficult to resist.

Exposure and conditioning mechanisms

At an individual level a cyclical process would seem to occur, involving repeated exposure, a feedback of consequences such as satiety, and reinforcing factors such as pleasant associations (Figure 8.2).

Numerous experiments in children and adults, and in other animals have demonstrated how food preference is an increasing function of exposure frequency. In other words, the more frequently a food has been tasted, the better it is liked and the more frequently it

is chosen. Ten exposures to a food in infancy or early childhood can led to established preferences. There is additional evidence that exposure to particular foods extends to preferences for similar foods. However, there is increasing consensus that mere exposure, although necessary, is insufficient for determining food preferences. Exposure facilitates other mechanisms that influence individual food choice. Human and animal studies have demonstrated how conditioning is a major factor in the acquisition of food likes and dislikes. Up to about 2 years of age the human infant will put almost anything in its mouth. What follows is a combination of socially determined appropriate exposure and learning about what to eat and what not to eat. By the age of 10 years most children have knowledge of what is edible and what is not. Individual food acceptance or rejection has been characterized through three basic mechanisms: sensory–affective, anticipated consequences and ideational factors (inappropriateness and disgust). All of these appear to work through Pavlovian conditioning mechanisms.

The essence of Pavlovian conditioning is that an individual is exposed to a pairing of a conditioned stimulus and an unconditioned stimulus, and a subsequent change in behavior towards the conditioned stimulus can be attributed to the pairing (Table 8.4).

It has become reasonably well established that this learning process is central to the acquisition of individual food likes and dislikes. This can occur through direct experience of pairings or through information about the stimuli. Distinctions can be made within Pavlovian conditioning, but such distinctions are not mutually exclusive and may be interrelated.

- Expectancy learning involves a direct causative or predictive relationship between the conditioned stimulus and the unconditional stimulus.
- Affective–evaluative conditioning is a process in which an evaluative response (e.g. hedonic) is transferred

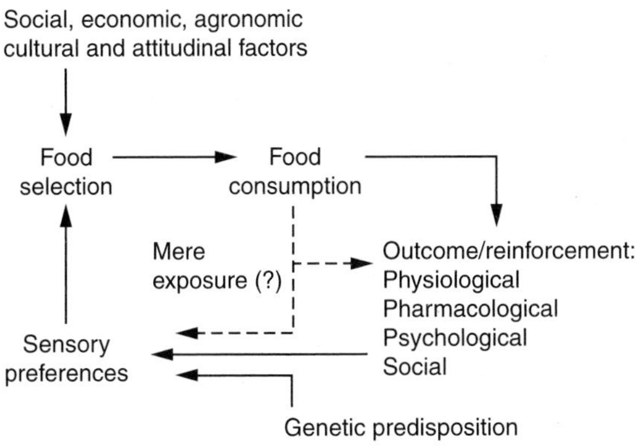

Figure 8.2 Factors influencing food choice. From Mela (1995). Reproduced with permission from The Nutrition Society.

Table 8.4 Simple Pavlovian conditioning applied to food choice

	Unconditioned stimulus	Pairing	Result
Pavlov's original conditioning experiment using a dog as a subject	Food (US) stimulates salivation	Repeated exposure to food (US) paired with a buzzer noise (CS)	Buzzer noise is conditioned (CS), stimulating salivation
Simple example within human food choice	Liked food (US)	Repeated exposure to a liked food (US) paired with a unknown food (CS)	Unknown food is conditioned (CS), stimulating liking

US: unconditioned stimulus; CS: conditioned stimulus.

from the significant stimulus (a liked food) to a previously neutral stimulus (a different food) when they are paired together. Either or both can operate through experiences with food.

- Expectancy learning involves expectations of the consequences of eating food and evaluative conditioning creates a liking for the food. There is an absence of evidence that the latter determines dislike.

Further distinctions are made that consider four types of conditioning mechanisms with regard to the unconditioned stimulus:

- flavor–postingestinal consequences
- flavor–flavor (and additionally pharmacological–flavor) factors
- conditioned compensatory (opponent) responses
- social factors and ideational (cognitive) factors.

Flavor–postingestinal consequences

A vast animal literature exists on hedonic changes (disliking or aversion) to flavors paired with adverse effects such as an electric shock. In humans, experimental evidence is derived from pairing foods with chemotherapy and other nauseous treatments. Other common negative postingestinal consequences include food poisoning, lactase deficiency and allergies; for example, skin rashes, respiratory distress, fever, stomach or gut cramps. Such experiences can therefore be evaluative (a dislike for the food) and/or expectational (the anticipated negative consequences). It is possible that someone likes a food for its sensory (affective) properties, but avoids it because of postingestinal consequences.

Aversions are common, and well described experimentally in both humans and other animals. It has been estimated that 65% of people report a food aversion of some kind, which may last for a lifetime.

The most common effect of food ingestion is satiety. Satiety can be expressed as both gastrointestional (relief of gastric pain, stomach distension, fullness, etc.) and postabsorptive (nutrients, energy). Increased preference for foods of higher energy density has been demonstrated when they are fed to hungry subjects. There is also evidence that flavor preferences increase when associated with carbohydrate and high fat content. Conversely, pairing medicines with physiological benefits did not increase preferences for the flavor of the medicines, suggesting that humans only like flavors paired with some form of satiety. This may not be encouraging for the acceptance of "functional foods"

(nutrient-enhanced foods) or "nutraceuticals", especially when the benefits, in contrast to, for example, a pain-killing drug, may only be apparent in the long term. However, individual beliefs and attitudes, particularly with respect to health, may play a positive role.

Flavor–flavor (sensory–affective) factors

Numerous experiments in both animals and humans have successfully paired liked flavors with neutral or unknown favors and, over time, a positive hedonic shift is recognized. There is some evidence that, in the right social context, information about flavors of new foods can assist with their acceptance. Foods and meals provide simultaneous experiences of numerous flavors that offer, through evaluative conditioning, a partial explanation of how preferences for variety increase and how preferences for new foods are acquired.

As individuals mature they tend to adopt food preferences that oppose basic innate preferences. In particular, bitter beverages and foods (e.g. coffee, tea and alcoholic drinks) and pungent foods (e.g. chili and black pepper) are chosen with increasing frequency as individuals mature. Considerable work has been undertaken on caffeine (itself a bitter substance and innately disliked) and caffeine-containing beverages. As with flavor preferences manipulated by nutrient manipulations, the positive effects on mood derived from the caffeine appear to enhance preferences for flavors paired with caffeine. Results found both negative reinforcement (alleviating caffeine withdrawal symptoms) and positive reinforcement (raising preferences for paired flavors). Caffeine only appears to have a positive effect after long-term frequent consumption. However, pairing of coffee with milk and sugar, at least initially, may facilitate initial preferences for such beverages through a liking for the flavors and tastes of milk and sugar. Similarly, social reinforcing factors may play a role, as tea and coffee are consumed as adult beverages, as rewards or at social rest breaks, and the consequent positive effect on mood may increase preferences for such beverages.

Conditioned compensatory (opponent) responses

One of the greatest mysteries in human food choice is not wondering why people first ate chilies, but why they ate them for a second time. Given that constituents of chilies stimulate oral pain through the trigeminal nerve system, some researchers have hypothesized conditioned opponent or compensatory responses. In simple terms, the chili pain becomes paired with a compensatory biological response (possibly secretion of endorphins, which are endogenous opiates). With continued consumption it is well documented that sensitivity to the chili burn declines. As a result, the compensatory pleasure is hypothesized to exceed the pain. However, once again, the importance of culture and social factors in facilitating this process should be recognized.

Ideational concepts and social learning

Humans are possibly unique with respect to the cognitive or ideational values that they attach to food aversions, in contrast to the postingestinal consequences. Foods are rejected or accepted because of knowledge of what they are, their origins or their symbolic meanings. Differing inappropriateness further distinguishes rejected edible substances. Disgust appears to shape our choice of potential animal foods (in contrast to plants), which are highly selected. For example, in many Western cultures invertebrates (with the exception of shellfish and mollusks) and reptiles are avoided, and only certain mammals selected. Such aversions clearly vary culturally and socially. In some cultures disgust and rejection are strongly influenced by concepts (real or idealized) of contagion. Real contagion issues may be driven by fears of microbiological hazard (a cockroach) or ideational contagion by the associations with objects (a sterilized cockroach). At an individual level, experience of ideational or cognitive aversions of associated disgust may account for one out of five learned taste aversions. Such experiences include disgust, negative information and forced eating in childhood (lack of control over food choice). There is some evidence that cognitive aversions are stronger and longer lasting than other forms of conditioning.

For any individual, all of the above mechanisms take place within a social context and there is evidence of direct social conditioning. For example, seeing a facial expression of someone drinking the same flavored drinks as they were asked to rate could influence young children's preferences. Similar social conditioning with adults increased preferences for the shape of a glass when paired with a positive facial expression, regardless of the color of the beverage in the glass.

Parents would seem to have enormous social influences on their children's food choices. However, the correlations between parents' and children's food preferences are zero to very low (0.3). This has been described as the family paradox, in that the family is powerful for installing culture-wide preferences, but is weak with regard to family-specific preferences. Since there are numerous social influences on children perhaps this is not surprising. Given that learning is a temporal process, high correlations between individuals of differing ages (parents and children) would not necessarily be expected. Such dissimilarities may be an adaptive mechanism resulting in, as an example, lactase deficiency in cultures where dairying was or is not available. Milk provides the nurture and nutrition for an infant's early life, but without commercial dairying cannot be sustained when the child matures.

Personality traits and attitudes

The importance of attitudes and personality traits and their influence on food choice has been well documented. Attitudes have been defined as a very broad concept focusing on an evaluative tendency. Three components of attitude have been described: cognitive, affective and conative. Affective components are often perceived as the central component of attitude. Attitude has also been defined as a tendency or disposition. Whereas tendency can be long or short term, disposition tends to be longer lasting. Tendencies of personalities are described as *traits*. Some food-related traits (dietary restraint, food neophobia and variety-seeking tendencies) are long term and remain stable over a period of years and major lifestyle changes. Such behaviors are typically measured using psychometric questionnaires.

The following section lists some measurable personality traits that have been found to influence food choice.

Externality and dietary restraint

It has been suggested that some people choose foods by strong responses to external cues such as sight or taste rather than the internal cue of hunger, and are consequently predisposed to excessive weight gain.

With the increasing prevalence of overweight and obesity in many Western countries, behavioral explanations have been sought with regard to the influence of food choice. A set-point theory proposed that people had a set point of weight, that society and medical advice challenged such a set weight, and consequently overweight people may feel constant hunger. Although set-point theories have been seriously challenged, it was proposed that high dietary restraint would be a predictor of excessive eating. This would seem to be paradoxical and challenges any physiological control of appetite. However, considerable subsequent work using psychometric scales demonstrated that when highly restrained US consumers broke their restraint (through being given a preload of milkshake, for example) they consumed more food than unrestrained consumers. It is thought that highly restrained consumers become uninhibited once their diet has been broken and eat excessively. This has been described as the boundary model, which proposes an area of biological indifference between hunger and satiety. This area of biological indifference is where cognitive, emotional and other psychological factors are considered to influence food intake. In the model, the restrained eater reaches a cognitively determined boundary before their physiologically determined satiety boundary, and consequently feels dissatisfied. Restrained eaters are thought to have a wider zone of indifference because repeated dieting and weight gain habituates such individuals to extreme sensations of hunger and satiety.

Two other psychometric scales have been developed that predict aspects of restraint. The Three Factor Eating Questionnaire (TFEQ) seeks to identify restraint, disinhibition and hunger. The shorter Dutch Eating Behavior Questionnaire (DEBQ) seeks to identify restraint, emotional eating (e.g. mood, irritation) and external eating (e.g. taste, social influence). There is some overlap between the two and both tend to identify successful dieters successfully, but they differ from earlier measures which tend to identify unsuccessful dieters.

Given that the TFEQ and the DEBQ identify successful dietary restraint, subsequent work has explored restraint further, investigating flexible control of eating, which taps into the ideas of disinhibition. This work suggests that certain individuals have a less rigid approach to restraint, and flexibility may be a successful strategy to maintaining a healthy weight when faced with an abundant food choice. Most work in this area has been restricted to experimental conditions in the laboratory, given the problems associated with underreporting food intake in free-living populations, and the limited work seeking to associate these eating behaviors with free-living dietary choices suggests complex relationships. It has been suggested that low energy requirements due to low levels of physical activity in current Western lifestyles require some kind of dietary restraint to avoid excessive weight gain. The type of restraint chosen by an individual seems to have a profound effect on their success in maintaining a healthy weight.

The role of health beliefs

Differing cultures have variations in their beliefs about the relationship between diet and health outcomes. The emerging consensus about diet–health relationships has filtered down to individual consumers, but there is variation in the strength of these beliefs and how they affect food choice. Many consumers put taste (pleasure) above health concerns. However, considerable work has explored the moderating effect of health beliefs on certain food choices. Different foods are perceived differently as pleasure giving, healthy, rewarding, and so on, and it is important to stress that the moderating effects of health beliefs may only pertain to certain foods. Health and taste attitude questionnaires for assessing consumers' orientations towards the health and hedonic characteristics of foods are useful in segmenting consumers on the basis of general health interests, interest in "light" (low-fat) products, cravings for sweet foods and using food as a reward.

Earlier applications have included health locus of control questionnaires, which seek to understand how much an individual's beliefs about diet and health as internal locus of control affect food choice. Scales of perceived severity and the importance of nutrition have been used, with varying predictive power.

Food variety, "pickiness" and food neophobia

Omnivores faced with a huge and seemingly ever-expanding choice of foods are faced with what has been described as the "omnivore's dilemma". Biologically, we are almost obliged to seek variety and new foods to satisfy nutritional requirements, yet because of fears over poisoning or affective disgust, humans have to be cautious about the foods they choose. This paradox has led to experimental work and population surveys using a scale that measures an individual trait of food neophobia (defined as "a reluctance to eat and/or avoidance of novel foods"). Considerable testing of such a scale has determined that a neophobia–neophilia trait can be predictive of the willingness to try new and novel foods, particularly foods from other cultures. Early studies found that neophobia was particularly predictive of a reluctance to try foods of animal origin. There is some evidence that there is variation in the degree of neophobia across European and North American populations. Experimental manipulations of descriptions of foods and other information have moderated neophobia. Neophilia has been linked to adventurous or sensation-seeking behavior and is used as a screening tool by investigators testing products (neophobes tend to consume less of a food sample, with implications for consumer testing of food products). A study in a large representative sample of the Finnish population found that neophobia predicted willingness to try unfamiliar and familiar foods.

It is possible to distinguish between neophobia and general pickiness. Studies of the tendency to reject any food and novel (fictitious) foods found close relationships between pickiness and food neophobia, moderate relationships with sensation seeking but poor correlation with anxiety traits. These results were inconsistent with other studies of food neophobia and indicate that social and cultural variations may explain the differences. Surprisingly, despite numerous early studies in the mid-twentieth century, pickiness remains a relatively unexplored area of human food choice.

Sensory- or food-specific satiety and variety-seeking tendencies

Sensory-specific satiety has been described as changes in pleasantness ratings after eating specific foods. Experimentally, this has been undertaken by comparing pleasantness scores for foods that were eaten with those for foods that were tasted but not eaten. In the realm of everyday food choice, say within a meal or snack, this means that people tend to tire of a food despite its high palatability. Once again, the exact outcome measure should be questioned, as a food could remain liked, but just unpalatable at the time of eating excessive quantities. Sensory-specific satiety may be a short-lived phenomenon, say within a single meal, but monotony effects can also happen over a longer period (weekly or monthly) when food choice is abundant. As omnivores, individuals tend to cease consumption of a particular food because of postingestive consequences (satiety) and the sensory qualities of the food. A more useful term may therefore be food-specific satiety.

There are also other reasons for seeking variety. Marketing researchers have classified variety seeking behavior into:

- satiation/stimulation
- external situations (e.g. marketing promotions)
- future preference uncertainty.

The satiation/stimulation concept provides additional explanations of sensory-specific satiety, in that individuals seek to satisfy a desire for novelty and complexity, in other words, thrills and sensations. Once again, perceptions of foods are important. Consumers are more likely to become satiated by particular attributes of a food if they relate to the primary aspect, rather than the secondary aspect. For example, if bread is thought of as a food in itself (primary) then consumers are likely to seek variety among breads. Alternatively, if bread is perceived as the outside of a sandwich (secondary) then the attributes of the filling (primary) are likely to be associated with satiation.

Externally, marketing can influence variety seeking through price manipulations and product placement. For example, supermarkets regularly move stock around to break consumers' shopping habits, on the basis that variety is related to increased purchasing.

Preference uncertainty is a less well-explored explanation of variety seeking and could be characterized as expected sensory-specific satiety. Individuals will purchase a variety of foods or flavors to provide options for future satisfaction.

A simple validated variety-seeking scale measures aspects of personality that predispose individuals to seek variety. Such measures may help to explain the acceptance of new foods and there is some evidence that this trait is stable over several years. The need for food sensation has been explored and may further explain certain individuals' need for variety in food choice. Dietary variety may have important implications for choosing "healthy" diets.

The importance of attitudes

Previous discussion of attitudes as long-term dispositions or traits has explored some traits that are thought to be influential with regard to food choice. Attitude can also be considered as a tendency, which can be long or short term, volatile and possibly amenable to change. For the purposes of this section the term attitudes (as opposed to traits) will be used to describe such tendencies. For the public health nutritionist wishing to influence food choice through, for example, social marketing, approaches seeking to understand and attempting to change attitudes are thought to be important. Five behavioral change models have been identified as being correlated with dietary change, of which attitudes play a major role. Attitudes and beliefs about foods should be measured using structured frameworks derived from social psychological theory.

The Theory of Reasoned Action and its extension as the Theory of Planned Behavior have been used extensively in food choice studies. The Theory of Reasoned Action has been used to explain rational behavior under the control (volition) of the individual. Two main factors are attitude and the influence of important others (subjective norm). Attitude is modeled as being the sum of beliefs about a food multiplied by how important that belief is to an individual (outcome evaluations). Subjective norm measures who influences a person's food choice and how motivated that person is to comply. As a modification, the Theory of Planned Behavior adds nonvolitional behaviors (goals and outcomes not under control of the individual) labeled as perceived control. In both models intention is considered to be the best predictor of behavior. Beliefs about foods are often elicited from semistructured interviews, which are converted into survey questions with quantifiable responses (seven-point labeled scales). These and other components of the model provide quantitative data on the importance of attitudes, the influence of other people and an individual's ability to make food choices. These components are used in multiple regression modeling (and, less frequently, structural equation modeling) to predict intention to make certain dietary choices or (reported) behavior (reported dietary intakes).

Metaanalysis of the models' application to consumer choices (including food) found an estimated correlation of 0.53 between intention and behavior, and a multiple correlation of 0.66 between attitudes and subjective norm with intention. On this basis the model is thought to have validity in the study of food choice. Such models can be considered psychosocial in that demographic variables (age, social class, etc.) should influence the food choice through the models' main components and not influence food choice independently.

The methods have been applied to several food choice issues, including healthy eating by pregnant women, reducing fat, increasing fruit and vegetables, and choosing milk, meat and organic foods. Perceived control is important for some foods but not for others. In general, attitude has been found to be the strongest predictor within the model.

Moral and ethical obligations have been included as additional components with regard to foods chosen for someone else, additives to foods and genetically modified foods. Analysis of the differing beliefs about food can help in the understanding of the relative importance of sensory and health factors in choice, for example, milks of differing fat content. Attitudes have been shown to influence the liking of reduced-fat spreads.

Barriers and facilitators of dietary changes have recently been shown to have a role in attitudes and food choice. The importance of barriers to consuming more fruit and vegetables was highlighted in a Dutch study that found that the perceived ability to make dietary changes (self-efficacy) was the most important factor.

These models have been criticized for a modest ability to predict intentions and the lack of studies that seek relationships between intentions and behavior (i.e. consumption). Intentions may be only a desire to eat differently and may not translate into actual food choices. Actual behavior is often omitted because of the survey nature of the methods, the need, for statistical purposes, for large samples (typically 250–1000) and the problem of unreliable dietary measures. The percentage of variation in intention to eat differently or behavior explained by several models has been shown to be about 30% (an R^2, the squared multiple correlation of the model, of 0.3), meaning that 70% of variation in the intention to choose particular foods is explained by other factors. Given the multiplicity of factors involved in food choice, it is perhaps unreasonable to expect more from such models. Researchers have argued that modest effect sizes from medical evidence are given far more weight than social–psychological research, suggesting that however modest attitudinal models may appear, they do make a contribution to understanding of food choice in a public health context. Nevertheless, there is room for improvement.

Expectations and information

Expectations play an important role in individuals' lives, affecting their reactions and decisions. It therefore follows that expectations should play a major role in food choice and acceptance. An individual makes a choice of foods based partially on learnt preferences (social and individual), traits and attitudes. At the point of purchase, an individual visually assesses the food in terms of its appearance, context, information, composition, use attributes, brand and associated advertising. In summary, these informational and visual extrinsic cues can be described as creating expectations of a food. Similarly, attitudes have been shown to have an important independent effect on expectations.

Product name, packaging, nutritional information, cost information and product presentation have all been listed as having a potential effect on the acceptance of new and novel foods. They may not have the same effect on acceptance of familiar foods. With a familiar food, past experience and memories of those experiences may also play an important role.

Expectations can be sensory, in that the expectation can change the perception of the sensory characteristics of a food, and hedonic, in that the expectation can change how much an individual likes a food. Expectation has a sound basis in behavioral theory and four theories describe how an individual might react:

- assimilation
- contrast
- generalized negativity
- assimilation contrast.

It is possible that many of these behaviors are not always conscious.

Assimilation theory (or cognitive dissonance) is based on the premise that an individual minimizes the discomfort felt by discrepancy between the expectation and the experience and therefore changes, for example, the perception or liking of the food to conform to expectations. Contrast theory assumes that an individual will magnify the difference between the expectation and the experience. Generalized negativity supposes that an individual will react negatively (and less favorably than if there was no expectation) to any discrepancy between expectation and experience. The assimilation–contrast approach assumes that there are limits to the size of the discrepancy between expectation and experience that can be tolerated. A large discrepancy may generate a contrast effect or a smaller discrepancy may lead to assimilation.

Application of such theories to food choice has begun to demonstrate the importance of the effects of promotions, information and sensory characteristics of foods. Originating within marketing and psychology, sensory scientists first perceived expectations as confounders in product tests. Today these scientists highlight the importance of sensory expectations at the point of purchase. For example, a study found assimilation (movement in scores in the direction of expected liking) with novel foods and contrast effects when expected bitterness was high. By manipulating the names of branded colas, assimilation effects were also found. An assimilation effect has been shown when regular and low-fat foods were correctly and incorrectly labeled. Other studies found some contrast and assimilation effects with reduced-fat sausages and chocolate.

In general, the existing evidence suggests that individuals tend to assimilate between expected and experienced hedonic or sensory ratings of foods. However, there is some evidence of contrast effects when expectations are pushed too high. These studies have implications for the marketing of products, the labeling of products (e.g. "low in fat" or "high in fiber") and any health claims attached to foods. For food choice to be sustained (repeat purchase) expectation must not be too far removed from the experience.

Food and mood

Anecdotally, there is considerable discussion on how mood affects people's food choices and similarly how food choices affect people's moods. The scientific literature applying mood to food choice is not extensive, with the notable exceptions of two reviews which demonstrate how eating and drinking can have a substantial effect on mood through sensory, predigestive and postabsorptive influences. Some brain chemistry mechanisms are known and may play an important role. Appetite and therefore food choice can also be affected by mood. Such mechanisms are complex and interact with cognitive and basic conditioning mechanisms.

The construct "mood" is multidimensional. In lay terms it refers to how we feel. Definitions of mood and emotion include energy, tension, pleasure and displeasure (hedonics), and general arousal. Moods can be divided into energetic moods (feelings of energy, vigor, liveliness) and tense moods (arousal), which can be feelings of tension, anxiety and fear. Psychologists tend to focus on two main components of mood: depression and anxiety.

Moods are generally measured by self-reported responses on psychometric scales. For example, the evaluation of depression can range from the assessment of clinical depression, (e.g. by the Beck Depression Inventory) to the assessment of depressive symptoms in the normal population (e.g. by the Center for Epidemiological Studies Depression Scale).

Anxiety tends to be viewed as domain specific, that is, relating to something the person is anxious about, such as performance anxiety. More general assessment of anxiety usually focuses on trait anxiety, the extent to which an individual is an anxious person, or state anxiety, the extent to which an individual is anxious at the present time irrespective of their usual anxiety levels. These aspects of anxiety are usually measured by the State–Trait Anxiety Inventory.

These broad aspects of mood are captured in more multidimensional measures of mood such as the Profile of Mood States. This questionnaire covers a number of different mood states: tension/anxiety, anger/hostility, fatigue/inertia, depression/dejection, vigor/anxiety and confusion/bewilderment.

Stress has been defined as an aversive state in which well-being is jeopardized by demands that exceed, or threaten to exceed, coping mechanisms. It is not difficult to conceive of life events such as bereavement, divorce or job loss as being stressful. However, these events can have differing effects on different people, depending on their coping ability, and under different circumstances; for example, divorce could be amicable or unpleasant. In conclusion, individual psychometric self-reports of stress are required. Below, stress and eating behavior in the general population are explored; stress, coping and disordered eating (anorexia nervosa, bulimia nervosa, etc.) have been addressed elsewhere (see the chapter on eating disorders in *Clinical Nutrition*, and Chapter 14 in this textbook).

The most prominent idea concerning food influencing mood was the carbohydrate–serotonin hypothesis. The amino acid tryptophan (Trp) is the precursor of the neurotransmitter serotonin, which potentially has a powerful influence on various cognitive functions and mood. Tryptophan competes for entry into the brain with other large neutral amino acids (ΣLNAA) and the ratio of tryptophan to these other amino acids (Trp:ΣLNAA) was thought to be influenced by the ratio of dietary carbohydrate to protein. Carbohydrate was thought to increase the Trp:ΣLNAA ratio, in contrast to dietary protein, which is a poor source of tryptophan. The hypothesis predicts that a high-carbohydrate (relative to protein) meal will decrease alertness. Numerous experiments have provided mixed results, but have failed to include high-protein treatments. Furthermore, alertness is improved with glucose, so contradicting the theory.

Further hypotheses have been developed that suggest that high carbohydrate could relieve forms of depression, specifically "carbohydrate-craving obesity",

which is itself an unproven hypothesis. Premenstrual syndrome (PMS) and seasonal affective disorder (SAD) have been also been hypothesized to act through the same mechanism. Carbohydrate intake is hypothesized to be self-medication and, if correct, high-carbohydrate–low-protein meals should have different effects on depressed and nondepressed individuals. A few studies have suggested that carbohydrate was less sedating in depressed subjects than in control subjects and that carbohydrate improved mood in PMS sufferers; however, all studies failed to compare such a treatment with high-protein or high-fat meals. Furthermore, dietary records over a 9 day period found a negative correlation between depression and percentage of energy from carbohydrate intake, and a positive correlation between greater feelings of energy and energy from carbohydrate intake.

Further evidence against the hypotheses comes from studies that suggest that only a small amount of protein can block any meal-induced increases in Trp:ΣLNAA (see also the discussion on chocolate in Box 8.3). A comparative treatment study measuring spinal fluid found no influence of dietary carbohydrate on tryptophan or other markers of serotonin. In summary, despite the popularity of the carbohydrate–serotonin hypotheses there is little evidence to support the hypothesis that dietary intakes change brain tryptophan levels or serotonin synthesis. Nevertheless, these hypotheses persist and continue to be explored.

There is little doubt that tryptophan at dosages higher than dietary levels can be a mild but effective antidepressant in PMS and possibly SAD. Similarly, subjects fed diets that were tryptophan free, compared with those on tryptophan supplements, had greater depressed mood, particularly amongst subjects who reported depression or had a family history of depression. However, these studies confirm that usual diets or even manipulations of diets have little effect on serotonergic function.

Serotonin and diet may still have influences upon mood. Cholesterol-lowering diets and dieting per se are linked to serotonin and Trp:ΣLNAA. Despite the high-profile dietary advice to reduce fat and cholesterol, there have been few studies of the effects of lowering fat on psychological well-being. There is increasing evidence that low cholesterol (≤ 4.5 mmol/l) could be linked to poor psychological health, depression and even suicide. Even in healthy populations, in both men and women there appears to be some association between low cholesterol and depression. However, findings are mixed, with some studies finding no differences or even improvements in psychological well-being when subjects were placed on dietary interventions that had significant but modest cholesterol-lowering effects. Inconsistent findings have been attributed to the ratios of n-3 and n-6 fatty acids, and there is a need for further studies given the large implications of dietary advice to lower fat and cholesterol.

The study of dietary fat intakes itself has been relatively little studied in terms of effect on mood. Manipulations of fat:carbohydrate ratios have revealed that ratios close to the subjects' usual intakes resulted in high mood and cognitive performance scores. A small study suggested that fat exerts a greater depression on alertness and mood at breakfast but not at lunch; however, usual fat:carbohydrate intakes were not reported and current eating habits suggest that high-carbohydrate meals are often consumed at breakfast. (For more on the control of food intake see Chapter 15 in *Nutrition and Metabolism*).

It is difficult to isolate the putative biological effects of any food or beverage on mood from the social, contextual, associated attitudes and therefore conditioning mechanisms acquired during the acquisition of preferences for foods. For example, individuals may adjust their intakes of caffeine by choosing strong coffee at breakfast because of associated stimulatory properties and rejecting coffee late at night because of associated beliefs about coffee's ability to prevent sleep. There is also some evidence to suggest that different individuals respond to stimulants such as caffeine differently depending on their personality traits. For example, impulsive individuals appear to benefit more from the performance-enhancing effects of caffeine. Three case studies describing interactions between food and mood are described in Boxes 8.3–8.5.

Stress and food choice

Two basic frameworks have been used in the study of stress and eating. First, the general effect model assessed whether there are general responses to stress, by people eating more (hyperphagia) or less (hypophagia). The evidence reviewed (largely based on animal studies) shows that the findings are mixed. A second set of studies was classified as the individual difference model, which further divided the evidence into those studies that looked at:

- the internal/external paradigm
- eating restraint.

In the internal/external paradigm of the individual difference model, two different possible responses could occur. First, obese individuals, in comparison to normal weight individuals, eat more when stressed (the psychosomatic theory) or, secondly, normal weight individuals, in comparison to obese individuals, eat less when stressed (Schachter's theory). The psychosomatic theory states that obese individuals cannot distinguish between hunger and anxiety, and respond to stress by eating. Schachter's theory is based on evidence that gastric contractions (an internal cue for hunger) decrease when (certain) individuals are stressed. Normal weight people have learnt to recognize these internal cues, whereas obese individuals have not and rely on external cues (sensory or social cues) to eat. What seems to have emerged from numerous studies is the importance of dietary restraint and possible gender differences in response to stress. Most of the evidence for stress-induced hyperphagia has been acquired from cross-sectional laboratory-based studies. However, a longitudinal study of stressed versus nonstressed department store workers demonstrated the effects on eating patterns (energy and macronutrients). Stress was measured predominantly in terms of long work hours and, to a lesser extent, using ratings on a perceived stress scale; and restraint was identified using the restraint scale from the DEBQ. The results revealed that reported appetite and hunger were the same for both long working hours and short working hours, but that stress interacted with high restraint in terms of greater fat, saturated fat, sugar and energy intake (as measured by 24 h recall), with implications for working practices and diet–health relationships.

8.5 Perspectives on the future

Many people have opinions and anecdotes about food choice. The challenge that began in the mid-nineteenth century was to deal with these issues in a scientifically objective way. It has been suggested that too much of what we seek to know about human food choice is derived from laboratory studies. Investigators have been accused of too much emphasis on "artificial" foods (e.g. milkshakes with altered fat content) and meals. Sensory science, physiology, animal models and the study of abnormal eating have all been accused of lacking ecological validity. Consensus is emerging that there is still a vital role for laboratory studies when food

Box 8.3 Case study 1: Chocolate – pharmacological, sensory and social influences on mood

Of all the foods consumed in Western industrialized countries, chocolate is the most emotive and widely discussed. Four main areas of interest in chocolate and mood have been identified:

- chemosensory properties
- psychopharmacological effects and biologically active constituents
- possible self-medication with nutrients or neurochemicals
- cravings, particularly by women in response to hormonal changes.

Although there has been little actual empirical research in this area, it is clear that chocolate has significant effects on mood, generally leading to increased pleasure and reduced tension, although for some individuals increased guilt. Cravings for chocolate can be associated with negative moods such as boredom, tension, anger, depression and tiredness.

The chemosensory qualities of fat (cocoa butter) and sugar, and the "melt in the mouth" texture, together with the rich flavor (found particularly in dark chocolate), make chocolate a highly palatable food. Potential pharmacological components are numerous and include tyramine and most notably, because chocolate contains substantial concentrations, phenylethylamine (PEA), which is considered important in brain chemistry. Several studies have suggested that PEA is an important modulator of mood and that a deficit may induce depression, as administration has been found to be a stimulant. However, other foods such as cheese and sausages have higher concentrations and studies have shown that 200 g of chocolate containing 1 g of PEA had no effects on urinary levels of PEA or its metabolites.

Methylxanthines present in chocolate include caffeine and theobromine; however, chocolate is not a particularly potent source of either and content varies considerably. Little is known about how caffeine and theobromine may interact. Chocolate also contains fatty acids related to the cannabinoid (active in *Cannabis sativa*) anandamide, which is thought to be mood enhancing (heightened sensitivity and euphoria); however, chocolate may not contain sufficient concentrations to produce effects.

To the authors' knowledge, only one published study has attempted to separate the sensory–hedonic from the potential pharmacological properties of chocolate. Dark chocolate, white chocolate (lacking the flavor of dark chocolate) and a capsule of cocoa butter (containing the potential pharmacological properties) were administered to self-identified chocolate "cravers". The dark chocolate gave greatest satisfaction, followed by white chocolate, with no benefit derived from the capsules.

Chocolate has also been implicated in the carbohydrate–serotonin hypothesis (discussed in Section 8.4). However, again the evidence fails to support this controversial hypothesis as chocolate can contain about 10% protein, sufficient to block tryptophan increases. Furthermore, chocolate cravings cannot be appeased by other carbohydrate foods and negative, not positive, moods such as guilt are often reported by chocolate "addicts".

Craving is an emotional state usually associated with drug addiction, but chocolate craving is commonly reported. It is possible that constituents of chocolate act as some kind of self-medication for chocolate cravers. For example, chocolate is a potent source of magnesium. Deficiency of magnesium may play a role in premenstrual syndrome (PMS) as stress depletes magnesium absorption and sufferers of PMS frequently report craving chocolate. Magnesium deficiency depletes dopamine, a neurotransmitter of euphoria and satisfaction, which may play a role in addiction generally. However, other foods such as nuts are also potent sources of magnesium and are rarely craved.

Chocolate cravings in women tend to peak when estrogen is low and progesterone is high (in the menstrual cycle), suggesting an interaction with hormones. The ratios of these two hormones are thought to play a role in regulating food intake (see chapter on the control of food intake in *Nutrition and Metabolism*) as estrogen is related to dopamine and serotonin activity. Other possible craving mechanisms may include the brain peptides galanin and neuropeptide Y, which regulate food intake and may be regulated by progesterone. Preliminary evidence suggests there may be a role for endogenous opiates in the desire for pleasant, sweet, high-fat foods, but the evidence remains mixed. Cravings for highly palatable foods such as chocolate have also been attributed to ambivalence, defined as "opposing emotional attitudes", and subsequent conflict. For example, the sensory–affective properties of chocolate versus the cognitive restraint (or guilt) associated with a high-fat food may lead to the latter suppressing the choice for such a food until the desire for the hedonic aspects of the food become so great as to produce a craving. Such a craving is not within the pharmacological or physiological definitions of craving associated with drug addictions.

In summary, the potential for nutritional or neurochemical mechanisms for the emotive mood-enhancing role of chocolate is promising, but the evidence is, at present, weak and contradictory. Until further work is undertaken it looks as is if the sensory reward plays a dominant role in choosing chocolate. However, given chocolate's position as a food of choice, it is certain that the interaction of the sensory attributes with nutrition and neurochemistry will continue to be investigated.

choice questions can be dealt with in such a setting. However, there is also a need for novel ways of dealing with food choice issues that can account for the influences of the real world in a controlled way. In summary, studies are required that can provide a measure of scientific control and ecological validity.

Social cognitive theory has dominated many recent dietary change programs. This theory posits that the

Box 8.4 Case study 2: Caffeinated beverages – pharmacological, sensory and social influences on mood

Coffee is second only to oil as the world's most traded commodity. Caffeine consumption from coffee, tea, colas and other beverages is prevalent in almost every culture and society. Over 650 caffeine studies exist in the literature. In this chapter, some aspects of conditioning with regard to the acquisition of the liking of caffeinated beverages were explored, and the physiological effects of caffeine are well established. Caffeine is known to block adenosine receptors, and similarly the psychoactive effects of caffeine are well established. Positive aspects of caffeine include quickening reaction times, enhanced vigilance, concentration, alertness and energy. Negative effects include decreased hand steadiness and, in habitual consumers, withdrawal symptoms in the form of headaches, drowsiness, fatigue and anger. So does caffeine provide a true net benefit or, given the ubiquitous presence of caffeine beverages in most people's diets, only provide compensation from withdrawal? The central problem is finding any study subjects who do not have a history of caffeine consumption. Some studies have included deprivation periods, but they may not have been of sufficient duration. Carefully designed studies are required; however, there is some evidence of net benefits, particularly with regard to psychomotor skills and reaction times.

Box 8.5 Case study 3: Alcoholic beverages – pharmacological, sensory and social influences on mood

The effects of alcohol on mood are well known and, on the positive side, moderate consumption has been shown to have antianxiety and euphorgenic properties. Such mood changes cannot be isolated from the social circumstances, expectations and previous experience (associations) of alcoholic beverages. Several studies have found positive effects of moderate alcohol consumption. For example, one placebo-controlled study, administering 8 g of alcohol (approximately half a pint of British beer), found that subjects became less tense and less uncertain. Such a quantity of alcohol is consistent with the apparent physiological health benefits of, for example, moderate consumption of wine. However, the negative mood effects of alcohol are equally well documented and include aggression and other antisocial behaviors. Others have proposed that adverse mood effects are a kind of "alcohol myopia", in which individuals attend to immediate, proximal information while reducing attention to information that is distant. This may explain how social responses become more extreme, well-being is enhanced, and anxiety and depression are alleviated. The complex effects of alcohol probably involve other more basic mechanisms, possibly involving dopaminergic, serotonergic and opioid systems.

environment, an individual's behavior and an individual's personal characteristics interact. While social cognitive theory has been used widely, emerging from the recent US "5-a-Day" literature has been the use of the precede–proceed model, which addresses predisposing, enabling and reinforcing factors associated with changing behavior. The precede–proceed model implements several behavioral models including social cognitive theory. Such nutrition education campaigns therefore utilize cognitive strategies (e.g. increasing knowledge about the health values of fruit and vegetables), environmental strategies (e.g. increasing access to fruit and vegetables in schools) and behavioral strategies (e.g. asking children to self-monitor portions of fruit and vegetables eaten), an approach often referred to as social marketing.

At an individual level, dietetic interventions may rely on a combination of biological factors (e.g. postingestive signs and symptoms), sensory factors (e.g. relative palatability of gluten-free products) and social or cultural position (e.g. low income).

Available research suggests that upwards of 18 000 food products are available in Western supermarkets and yet only around 1 in 10 new products reaches the market and only 1 in 100 actually succeeds. Clearly, consumers are fickle in their choices and the acceptance of a food as measured by market success is likely to be more about consumer perceptions of individual food items and daily life habits than biological or physiological requirements.

Food choice for many individuals has become a "continuous feast". It therefore becomes essential for those studying or working in public health to seek to understand eating as behavior.

Further reading

Fieldhouse P. Food and Nutrition Customs and Culture, 2nd edn, p. 120. London: Chapman & Hall, 1995.

Frewer L, Risvik E, Shifferstein H, eds. Food, People and Society: A European Perspective on Consumers' Food Choices. Berlin: Springer, 2001.

Green LW, Kreuter MW. Health Promotion Planning: An Educational and Ecological Approach, 3rd edn. Mountain View, CA: Mayfield, 1999.

Lawless HT, Heymann H. Sensory Evaluation of Food: Principles and Practice. New York: Chapman & Hall, 1998.

MacFie HJH, Thomson DMH, eds. Measurement of Food Preferences. Gaithersburg, MD: Aspen: 1999.

Marshall DW, ed. Food Choice and the Consumer. Kluwer: Dordrecht, 1995.

Meiselman H, MacFie HJH, eds. Food Choice, Acceptance and Consumption. London: Blackie, 1996.

Meiselman H, ed. Dimensions of the Meal: The Science, Culture, Business and Art of Eating. Gaithersburg, MD: Aspen, 2000.

Mela DJ. Understanding fat preference and consumption: applications of behavioural sciences to a nutritional problem. Proc Nutr Soc 1995, 54: 453–464.

Mela DJ, Rogers PJ. Food, Eating and Obesity. London: Chapman & Hall, 1998.

Murcott A, ed. The Nation's Diet: The Social Science of Food Choice. London: Longman, 1998.

Rozin P. Towards a Psychology of Food Choice. Brussels: Institute Danone, 1998.

The Scottish Health Survey 1995 (Scottish Office Department of Health, 1997, The Stationery Office, Edinburgh).

Shepherd R, Sparks P. Modelling food choice. In: Measurement of Food Preferences (MacFie HJH, Thomson DMH, eds). Gaithersburg, MD: Aspen, 1999.

9
Public Health Aspects of Overnutrition

Jacob C Seidell and Tommy LS Visscher

Key messages

- Chronic excess intake of energy leads to weight gain, overweight and obesity. Foods with a high energy density (high in fat or added sugars and low in fiber) contribute most to this positive energy balance.
- Reduced energy expenditure further increases the positive energy balance.
- The prevalence of overweight and obesity is increasing rapidly, particularly in children and adolescents, in most parts of the world.

- This increasing prevalence of overweight and obesity is associated with a sharp increase in the incidence of type 2 diabetes mellitus.
- Overweight and obesity, particularly when accompanied by a large waist circumference, contribute significantly to the impairment of health, reduction in quality of life and increased health-care costs.

9.1 Introduction

Principles of the assessment of overnutrition

Overnutrition can apply to energy, the individual components of energy and the micronutrients. In the case of individual components of energy, some are considered in the present chapter (sugar and fat), while others are considered elsewhere in this book in relation to diseases such as cancer (Chapter 21) and cardiovascular disease (CVD; Chapter 19). The public health impact of overnutrition in relation to micronutrients is generally confined to voluntary or mandatory fortification of foods or the use of food supplements (see Chapter 16 in *Nutrition and Metabolism*). The primary dietary interest is energy overnutrition and that is the focus of this chapter.

In practice, it is much easier to measure the degree of weight gain and excess weight and the health consequences thereof than to measure directly energy intake in relation to energy expenditure. This is because the methods to assess total daily energy intake and expenditure are usually crude and subject to many forms of bias (see Chapter 10 in *Introduction to Human Nutrition*). Therefore, the degree of overnutrition is usually defined by the degree of overweight or obesity in an individual. Obesity refers to a state where excess fat is stored in adipose tissue but, again, in public health settings this is usually impossible to measure directly and so relatively crude anthropometric measures must be used.

Anthropometric measures are the most commonly used to classify body weight. Alternatives to anthropometry, such as biological impedance measurements or dual-energy X-ray absorptiometry, are sometimes used in population studies and these allow for the measurement of components of body composition such as fat mass and fat-free mass (see Chapter 2 in *Introduction to Human Nutrition*). However, these procedures are certainly not carried out routinely, and internationally accepted criteria for the classification of the degree of obesity measured by these methods do not exist.

Principles of anthropometric classification of overweight and abdominal fatness

International classifications for the degree of overweight are based on the body mass index (BMI) or Quetelet's index (Table 9.1). This measure is calculated by dividing weight (in kilograms) by height squared (height in meters). Definitions of the degree of overweight and obesity allow international comparisons of prevalence rates. Minimal mortality rates are mostly seen in the healthy range of BMI until the age of 60 years. Overweight subjects are at increased risk of morbidity and should avoid further weight gain. Weight loss in this category is recommended when other risk factors for disease are present. Severely overweight or obese subjects are at increased risk of disease irrespective of the presence of other risk factors and weight loss is recommended for all. From an international perspective, it should be noted that the health implications of a given level of BMI with respect to body fatness and fat distribution may vary across populations. Asian populations, for instance, have a higher absolute risk for the onset of type 2 diabetes mellitus than Caucasian populations at the same level of BMI. Therefore, population-specific interpretations of the definitions for obesity remain a possibility.

Other anthropometric measures, based on body circumferences, are also used in this area. One of these measures is the ratio of waist circumference to hip circumference, the waist/hip ratio (WHR), which is an indicator of fat distribution rather than the amount of total body fat. The WHR seems to be difficult to interpret, particularly in the elderly population. A high WHR in the elderly could reflect a high waist circumference but also a decreased hip circumference. The hip circumference could decrease as a consequence of the decreased lean body mass that is often seen with aging. The WHR is often misinterpreted as a measure of abdominal fat only. The amount of abdominal fat is estimated with greater precision by the waist circumference alone. Some researchers have suggested action levels for large waist circumference to replace BMI and WHR (Table 9.1). The waist circumference is measured at the level midway between the lower rib margin and the iliac crest (lateral, upper part of the pelvic bone) with participants in a standing position. The correlation between waist circumference and stature is low enough to ignore adjustment for body height in the age category 20–60 years. The action levels appear to be appropriate for identifying subjects who have cardiovascular risk factors, type 2 diabetes or shortness of breath when walking upstairs. However, others have noted that the criteria underlying the waist action levels have been based on arbitrary levels of the WHR, and that the evaluations with respect to risk have been based on cross-sectional data. Therefore, the cut-off points (or action levels) for the classification of waist circumference are still under debate. Ideally, consensus regarding action levels should be reached by the use of longitudinal data relating waist circumference levels to minimal mortality, morbidity and disability rates. Owing to the relatively recent introduction of the possible use of the waist circumference, such analyses are not widely available.

Prevalence of and trends in overweight

Secular trends in obesity worldwide (BMI $\geqslant 30$) are given in Table 9.2. In every geographical location for which there are data, a rise in the incidence of obesity has been observed. The rise has affected both men and women, and is evident at the extremes such as Japan and China with relatively low levels of obesity and western Samoa with high levels of obesity. Some 10% of women in sub-Saharan Africa are overweight, rising to over 40% in the former Eastern European states and in the Middle East. The extent of overweight and obesity in 10-year-old children in selected European countries is shown in Figure 9.1. The secular rise in

Table 9.1 Definitions of body mass index (BMI)[a] and waist circumference[b] categories

	BMI (kg/m^2)
Underweight	<18.5
Normal weight	18.5–24.9
Moderate overweight	25.0–29.9
Overweight	$\geqslant 25.0$
Preobese	25–29.9
Obesity	$\geqslant 30.0$
Obese class I	30–34.9
Obese class II	35–39.9
Obese class III	$\geqslant 40.0$

	Waist circumference	
	Men	Women
Above action level 1	$\geqslant 80$ cm (~32 inch)	$\geqslant 94$ cm (~37 inch)
Above action level 2	$\geqslant 88$ cm (~35 inch)	$\geqslant 30$ cm (~40 inch)

[a] BMI categories are defined according to the WHO guidelines.
[b] Waist circumference categories are suggested by Lean *et al.*

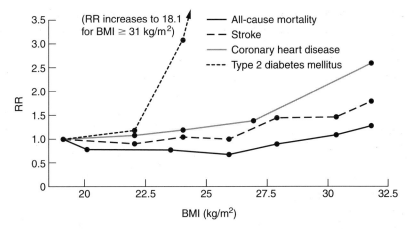

Figure 9.3 Age-adjusted relative risks (RR) by categories of body mass index (BMI) for different end-points among US women from the Nurses' Health Study. Adapted from Visscher and Seidell (2001) with permission from the *Annual Review of Public Health*, Volume 22. © 2001 Annual Reviews (www.annualreviews.org).

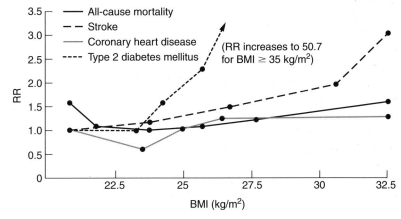

Figure 9.4 Age-adjusted relative risks (RR) by categories of body mass index (BMI) for different end-points among US men from the Health Professionals Study. Adapted from Visscher and Seidell (2001) with permission from *Annual Review of Public Health*, Volume 22. © 2001 Annual Reviews (www.annualreviews.org).

Figures 9.3 and 9.4 show that the age-adjusted relative risk for CHD among men and women was higher than the relative risk of high BMI for mortality. US women from the Nurses' Health Study with a BMI above 30 kg/m^2 had a three-fold higher risk of developing nonfatal myocardial infarction compared with women with a BMI below 21 kg/m^2. Men from the Health Professionals Study with a BMI between 29 and 33 kg/m^2 had a two-fold higher risk of developing CHD and men with BMI higher than 33 kg/m^2 had a three-fold higher risk of developing CHD compared with men with a BMI below 23 kg/m^2. Among these men and women, high BMI was also related to the onset of stroke. The Nurses' Health Study reported that high BMI levels were particularly related to the onset of ischemic stroke. Hemorrhagic strokes, which occurred less often than ischemic strokes, seemed to be less common with high BMI than with low BMI.

It has been estimated that if everyone maintained optimal weight, there would be 25% less CHD and 35% fewer strokes or episodes of heart failure. A 20% weight reduction in the obese should confer a 40% reduced risk of a coronary event.

Obesity and type 2 diabetes mellitus (see also Chapter 20)

Besides being a major risk factor for CVD, obesity, and in particular abdominal obesity, is the most important risk factor in the onset of type 2 diabetes.

Diabetes is by far the most expensive public health consequence of obesity. Countries in economic transition in which a huge obesity-linked diabetes epidemic is expected are unlikely to be able to afford effective medical services to be able to screen, identify and treat diabetes effectively. Consequently, poorly controlled glucose levels will lead to millions of patients developing nephropathy, arteriosclerosis, neuropathy, retinopathy and related disability. The increase in disability due to obesity-induced diabetes will be larger in countries in economic transition than in industrialized countries. Abdominal obesity is now considered to be part of a frequently observed clustering of the major risk factors for CVD and type 2 diabetes. This cluster of risk factors is often described as the metabolic syndrome or the insulin resistance syndrome. Among the other risk factors in this syndrome are elevated glucose concentrations, increased triacylglycerol concentrations, low HDL-cholesterol and hypertension.

Figures 9.3 and 9.4 illustrate the strong association between BMI and the risk of developing type 2 diabetes mellitus. The relative risks in this study were increased more than 10-fold among women from the Nurses' Health Study with BMI higher than 29 kg/m^2 and among men from the Health Professionals Follow-up Study with BMI greater than 31 kg/m^2, compared with the lowest BMI category. The risk of developing type 2 diabetes starts to increase considerably at relatively low levels of BMI. This phenomenon is more pronounced in some ethnic groups, such as among some Asians.

The World Health Organization (WHO) has calculated that about 64% of type 2 diabetes in US men and 74% in US women could be avoided if BMI was maintained at or below 25 kg/m^2. The WHO has also predicted that the number of diabetics will double from 143 million in 1997 to about 300 million in 2025. In Asian countries, the prevalence of type 2 diabetes mellitus will increase more rapidly over time than the increase in obesity. It has been calculated that by 2025, India and China will be the countries, together with the USA, with the largest numbers of diabetics. Recent intervention studies in groups at high risk of type 2 diabetes (i.e. those with impaired glucose tolerance, overweight or obesity, and/or a family history of type 2 diabetes) show that moderate lifestyle changes and relatively minor weight loss may lower the risk of developing type 2 diabetes mellitus by as much as 60%.

Obesity and cancer (see also Chapter 21)

A working group of the International Agency for Research on Cancer (IARC) of the WHO reviewed the association between overweight and cancer. The working group concluded that there is sufficient evidence for a cancer-preventive effect of avoidance of weight gain (prevention of overweight). This evidence has been obtained for cancers of the colon, breast (in post-menopausal women), endometrium, kidney (renal cell) and esophagus (adenocarcinoma). For premenopausal breast cancer, available evidence on the avoidance of weight gain suggests a lack of a cancer-preventive effect. For all other sites the evidence for a causal relationship between overweight and cancer was deemed inadequate.

A possible mechanism for the relationship between high body weight and cancer, mentioned by the IARC and the World Cancer Research Fund, is that high body mass may result in metabolic abnormalities and the metabolic syndrome. This physiological state may promote cell growth in general and also growth of tumor cells owing to their capacity to use glucose and because of up-regulation of receptors for the insulin-like growth factor. Adipose tissue converts androgens into estrogens. In postmenopausal women adipose tissue becomes the most important source of circulating estrogens. Increased levels of bioavailable endogenous estrogen in abdominally obese postmenopausal women may lead to an increased risk of breast cancer. Weight reduction, combined with a program of physical exercise, reduces both estrogen and insulin concentrations, which may have a positive effect on the development of postmenopausal breast cancer. Long-term effects of intentional weight loss on cancer risk are, however, not known.

Obese women have been found to be more reluctant than normal weight women to participate in cervical and breast cancer screening programs. Thus, a delay in the identification of tumor tissue will decrease the chance of therapeutic success. The presence of abundant fat may complicate the detection of a tumor during mammographic screening. Therefore, obesity may not only be a risk factor for these cancers, but also predict later detection and poorer prognosis.

Obesity and musculoskeletal disorders

Obesity is one of the most important preventable risk factors of osteoarthritis in knee and hip joints, and osteoarthritis is an important risk factor for disability.

Osteoarthritis is more common among women than men. The relationship between overweight and osteoarthritis is explained by the high joint pressure in overweight individuals. There may also be a metabolic aspect, as obesity appears to be related to the incidence of osteoarthritis in the hands. A case-controlled study carried out between 1990 and 1993 on women aged 20–80 years found odds ratios of 3.0–10.5 for the incidence of osteoarthritis for the highest tertile of body mass compared with the lowest tertile.

Associations between obesity and herniated lumbar intervertebral disk, low back pain and chronic neck pain have been suggested, but these associations are less strong and predominantly based on cross-sectional studies where it is difficult to separate cause and effect.

Obesity and respiratory disorders

During the 1990s, the role of excess fat on the lungs became an obesity-related public health problem because of its link with shortness of breath, sleep apnea and concurrent psychosocial morbidity. The odds ratios for shortness of breath when walking upstairs in those with a BMI of 30 kg/m^2 or higher were 3.5 in men and 3.3 in women, compared with a BMI below 25 kg/m^2, based on a sample of Dutch adults aged 20–59 years. Furthermore, obese patients are more likely to experience obstructive sleep apnea and concurrent psychosocial morbidity. It has been estimated that the risk of sleep-disordered breathing is around four times higher when BMI is 5 kg/m^2 higher.

A weight-bearing role of body fat on the lungs is indicated by comparing odds ratios for sleep-disordered breathing for girths at different parts of the body. Comparing ratios of girths of the neck, waist and hip, it has been found that the odds ratio for sleep-disordered breathing was lowest for the hip girth and highest for the neck girth. Hypoventilation during sleep leads to nocturnal hypoxia during sleep and extreme sleepiness during the day.

Obesity-induced sleep apnea is an important risk factor for psychosocial morbidity and seems to be associated with some of the components of the metabolic syndrome.

Obesity and work disability

In Finland, disability pensions were granted twice as often to obese men and one-and-a-half times more often to obese women, compared with subjects with a low BMI (Figure 9.5). This study was based on a national survey sample of 31 000 Finns who were followed from 1966/1972 until 1982.

Similarly, 12% of 1300 obese Swedish women aged 30–59 years received disability pensions, compared with 5% in the general population, and the obese women reported 1.5–1.9 times more sick leave during 1 year compared with the normal Swedish population. Obesity

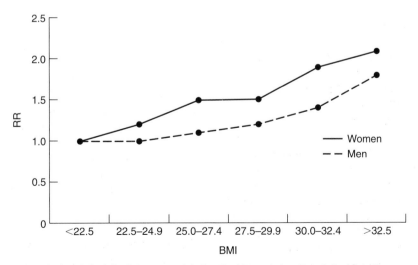

Figure 9.5 Risk of work disability due to overweight in a Finnish population. Data derived from Rissanen *et al.* (1990), with permission from the BMJ Publishing Group. Adapted from Visscher and Seidell (2001) with permission from *Annual Review of Public Health*, Volume 22. © 2001 Annual Reviews (www.annualreviews.org).

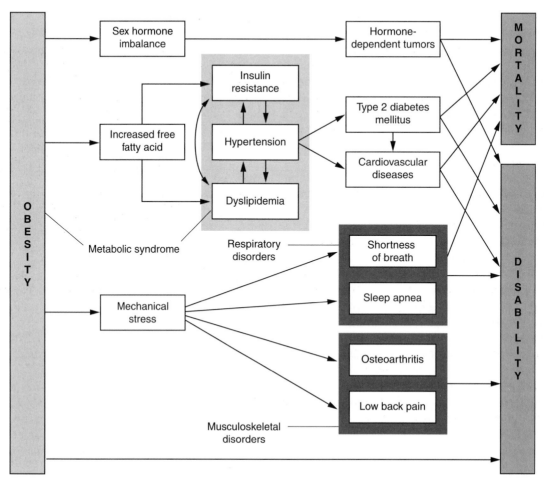

Figure 9.6 Public health impact of obesity. Adapted from Visscher and Seidell (2001) with permission from *Annual Review of Public Health*, Volume 22. © 2001 Annual Reviews (www.annualreviews.org).

is also related to mobility disability, which affects the quality of life and healthy aging.

Summary of the impact of obesity on public health

Figure 9.6 summarizes the links among obesity, risk factors, chronic diseases and mortality. Obesity is related to all-cause mortality and cancer, and even more strongly to the onset of type 2 diabetes, CVD, musculoskeletal disorders, work disability and sleep apnea. Comparisons of relative risks for mortality, CHD, stroke and diabetes were adjusted for age only and on never-smokers and smokers combined. These may not be the most appropriate relative risks to compare the impact of obesity on different end-points.

Direct and indirect costs of obesity are estimated at around 7% of the total health-care costs in the USA and around 1–5% in Europe. These estimations are based on prevalence rates and relative risks. Obesity will increase the number of unhealthy life-years enormously, owing to the closer relationships of obesity with morbidity and disability than with mortality. American researchers have calculated that a weight loss of about 10% of initial body weight would reduce the number of life-years with hypertension by 1.2–2.9 years, and type 2 diabetes mellitus by 0.5–1.7 years. Life expectancy would be increased by 2–7 months. Estimations are again based on calculations using relative risks for the specific outcomes and are theoretical estimates rather than based on empirical data.

Nevertheless, it is very clear that the public health impact of obesity is enormous and will increase rapidly with the increasing prevalence of obesity. Public health-care programs should include in their targets attempts to reduce the obesity epidemic. Countries such as China and India are of particular importance in controlling the obesity epidemic. Every increase in percentage point in these countries involves 20 million more obese subjects.

9.4 Perspectives on the future

Much of the world is facing a sharp increase of the number of obese children and adults. The increasing obesity epidemic points towards the need for urgent strategies that develop multifaceted global and national plans for the adequate prevention and management of obesity. Successful prevention of obesity should be one of the primary targets in public health nutrition. It has been argued that obesity is a normal response to an abnormal environment, rather than an abnormal response to an abnormal environment. Stimulation of physical activity and the promotion of healthy eating habits are essential. Modification of lifestyle habits should not rely on personal advice only, but should also address components of the physical, economic and sociocultural environments in which individuals live.

Further reading

Astrup A, Grunwald GK, Melanson EL *et al*. The role of low-fat diets in body weight control: a meta-analysis of *ad libitum* dietary intervention studies. Int J Obes Relat Metab Disord 2000; 24: 1545–1552.

Hill JO, Prentice AM. Sugar and body weight regulation. Am J Clin Nutr 1995; 62 (1 Suppl): 264S–273S, Discussion 273S–274S.

Lean MEJ, Han TS, Morrison CE. Waist circumference as a measure for indicating need for weight management. BMJ 1995; 311: 158–61.

Rissanen A, Heliövaara M, Knekt P *et al*. Risk of disability and mortality due to overweight in a Finnish population. BMJ 1990; 301: 835–837.

Seidell JC, Visscher TLS, Hoogeveen RT. Overweight and obesity in the mortality rate data: current evidence and research issues. Med Sci Sports Exerc 1999; 31: S597–S601.

Visscher TLS, Seidell JC. The public health impact of obesity. Annu Rev Public Health 2001; 22: 355–375.

Willett WC, Dietz WH, Colditz GA. Guidelines for healthy weight. N Engl J Med 1999; 341: 427–434.

World Health Organization. Obesity: preventing and managing the global epidemic. Report of a WHO consultation. WHO Technical Report Series, No. 894. Geneva: WHO, 2000.

Websites

www.aso.org.uk
www.cdc.gov
www.iaso.org
www.iotf.org
www.naaso.org

10
Public Health Aspects of Undernutrition

Mark J Manary and Noel W Solomons

Key messages

- Undernutrition occurs worldwide, usually in association with poverty.
- Children and the elderly, as well as victims of war and natural disasters, are at greatest risk for undernutrition.
- Chronic and recurrent infections play an important role in promoting undernutrition.
- Public health schemes, led by nutritionists, that draw together a wide range of expertise and partner with the community are necessary to prevent and ameliorate undernutrition.
- Aspects involved in the etiology of undernutrition include interactions between social, demographic, genetic, infectious and societal conditions.

10.1 Introduction

Undernutrition can be found in every society, in every corner of the world. This chapter discusses the public health aspects of undernutrition in free-living people in the community. Children are at greatest risk for undernutrition, but it is important to realize that undernutrition can also be a problem in adults, especially the elderly. As manifest in developing countries, undernutrition can be endemic, affecting up to half of the population. Undernutrition, however, is not unknown in industrialized, developed and affluent countries, occurring in diverse niches of the society for the same and distinct reasons for which it is a concern in the developing world. Undernutrition caused by clinical illnesses or associated with hospitalized patients is beyond the scope of this chapter.

10.2 Definitions of undernutrition

Who is undernourished and the cause of the undernutrition depend on how one defines the term. In its essence, it can be seen as an undernourishing process in which the normal needs for one or several nutrients are not being met, or the nutrients are being lost at a greater rate than they are being acquired. When one envisions the problem in a dynamic sense, that is, as one of accumulating a deficit, then the absolute degree of imbalance is immaterial. Diagnosis becomes problematic, however, because it requires serial monitoring of the individual to detect the negative nutrient balance.

However, undernutrition in a public health context is usually assessed using static, anthropometric criteria or data related to the amount of macronutrients in the diet: protein and energy. Definitions of different types of undernutrition are summarized in Table 10.1. Underweight is the situation of having a less than adequate weight-for-age, derived from an international reference curve based on the growth of a homogeneous group of Caucasian children in southern Ohio in the USA, but generalized by United Nations agencies to a universal growth standard. Having a weight-for-age more than 2 standard deviations (SD) below the median of this reference curve is the criterion for a diagnosis of underweight. Wasting is a deficit of greater than 2 SD to the inferior side of the median of normal

Table 10.1 Definition of different types of undernutrition

Underweight	Weight-for-age <2 SD below the international standard
Marasmus	Weight-for-age <60% of the international standard
Kwashiorkor	The presence of oedema and weight-for-age <80% of the international standard
Marasmic kwashiorkor	The presence of oedema and weight-for-age <60% of the international standard
Wasting	Weight-for-height <2 SD below the international standard
Stunting	Height-for age <2 SD below the international standard
Chronic energy deficiency	Body mass index [weight (kg)/height (m)^2] <18.5

weight-for-height based on the aforementioned sample of children adopted for international reference. Wasting signifies acute protein–energy malnutrition (PEM). Stunting is extreme short stature, exceeding a deficit of 2 SD below the median of the international reference population's length or height. It has been interpreted as a state of chronic malnutrition.

International statistics about rates of undernutrition almost invariably refer to the fraction of children below the appropriate reference weight for their chronological age. However, if they are also of short stature, it is not appropriate on an individual basis for them to carry as much weight. The preferred diagnostic standard would be weight-for-height. Weight-for-age predominates because weight, but not height, is routinely collected and recorded in the health posts around the world from which the prevalence statistics are generated. Past malnutrition (rather than "chronic") might be a more legitimate designation, if a child's height velocity were within normal parameters at whatever his or her age. Whether nutrient availability alone, or in combination with hormonal aberrations resulting from stress, inflammation and infection, is the major determinant of poor longitudinal growth, is not yet understood. Understanding this is important in knowing how to interpret the significance of short stature worldwide.

Anthropometric criteria are used to define undernourished states in all age groups. A commission of the International Dietary Energy Consultative Group defined chronic energy deficiency based on the adult body mass index (BMI). Having a BMI of less than 18.5 kg/m^2 is the diagnostic criterion for this condition. Chronic energy deficiency corresponds to a low weight-for-height, or wasting, rather than simply low weight-for-age. Groups of people with chronic energy deficiency in a community have lower work outputs, lower productivity and compromised ability to respond to physiologically stressful conditions. The robustness of chronic energy deficiency across ethnic and geographical variation has not been

validated, as adult populations of the Indian subcontinent often have 30% of their individuals in the BMI category signifying chronic energy deficiency. The etiology of chronic energy deficiency may be starvation or chronic illness, such as tuberculosis. Chronic energy deficiency does not imply the presence or absence of edema or micronutrient deficiency.

Other biochemical and clinical measures of nutritional status, such as measuring serum albumin or recording food intakes, are not very useful from the public health perspective. They require more time and expense, involve more invasive measurement techniques, and are less accurate than anthropometry.

10.3 Clinical syndromes of undernutrition

There are two clinical syndromes of severe undernutrition (also known as protein–energy malnutrition, PEM): marasmus and kwashiorkor. Marasmus is characterized by extreme wasting; those suffering from marasmus appear to be just "skin and bones". Marasmus is the physiological adaptation to marked restriction of dietary energy. There is marked reduction in fat and subcutaneous tissue, as well as atrophy of visceral tissues. Those suffering from marasmus limit their physical activity and have decreased rates of metabolism and protein turnover in an effort to conserve nutrients. Compared with healthy people, marasmic individuals are more susceptible to infection, and more likely to suffer death or disability from infection.

Kwashiorkor is the clinical constellation of edema and undernutrition. This is most commonly seen in children under 5 years of age and is usually associated with irritability, anorexia and ulceration of the skin. The irritability is a pathological mental status change, making the refeeding of these individuals a challenging task. The metabolic derangements are more severe in kwashiorkor, and the case fatality rate is higher than in marasmus. Kwashiorkor was first recognized in West Africa in the 1930s in children weaned from the breast and was thought of as a milk deficiency state. Subsequently, experts suggested that kwashiorkor was the result of dietary protein deficiency; however, evidence to support this hypothesis was lacking. More recent data suggest that it may result from depletion of antioxidants in association with dietary energy deficiency. The Wellcome Trust Working Party in 1970 defined marasmus as a weight-for-age of less than 60% of the international standard, and kwashiorkor as the presence of edema and weight-for-age of less than 80% of the standard. When severe wasting and edema occur together the condition is called marasmic kwashiorkor, and the prognosis is worse than that of either marasmus or kwashiorkor. The clinical presentation of marasmic kwashiorkor is similar to that of kwashiorkor.

10.4 Micronutrient deficiency: "hidden hunger"

Although undernutrition is generally treated in textbooks in the domain of the deficits of macronutrients (energy, protein), the same factors that compromise macronutrient status also interfere with adequate nutrition with respect to minerals and vitamins. In 1990, the term "hidden hunger" was adopted to refer to micronutrient malnutrition due to substances so small that one could not see them. Endemic deficiencies of iron, iodine and vitamin A, which long headed the list of deficiency states worldwide, have been of principle concern and received major attention. Other micronutrients of growing public health concern are vitamin D, calcium, zinc, vitamin B_{12} and riboflavin. Where macronutrient intake is sufficient to meet energy needs, micronutrient deficiency may still exist as the food consumed is of a low nutrient density. An example of this would be a normal weight woman with iron deficiency on a dietary basis. The magnitude of micronutrient deficiency is thought to be huge, affecting 40% of the world's population, with iron deficiency being the most prevalent, afflicting one-third of the world (see Chapter 13). Table 10.2 lists the principal micronutrients of concern in hidden hunger, the health consequences of deficiency states, the public health magnitude of the problem and examples successful interventions to alleviate the public health problem.

Table 10.2 Micronutrient deficiencies, their consequences and successful strategies to combat them

Micronutrient	Clinical manifestations of deficiency	Public health magnitude of the problem	Effective interventions
Iron (see Chapter 13)	Anemia, poor cognitive development, increased susceptibility to infection	2 billion people worldwide, mostly women and children	Fortification of wheat, administration of supplements and antihookworm treatment
Iodine (see Chapter 12)	Poor cognitive development	43 million worldwide, primarily in areas where soils are iodine poor	Salt iodization programs can eradicate iodine deficiency
Calcium	Decreased bone mineralization	Unknown	Inclusion of dairy products in the diet
Vitamin A (see Chapter 11)	Damage to cornea and retina leading to partial blindness, increased severity of diarrhea and malaria	100 million children, contributory factor in 3 million childhood deaths annually	Single-dose supplementation administered with vaccinations
Vitamin D	Rickets, decreased bone density	About 15% of populations in temperate regions during winter, 50% of veiled Islamic populations	Fortification of margarine
Zinc	Growth failure, increased incidence and severity of diarrhea, pneumonia and malaria	0.5–2 billion people, mostly in developing countries	Supplements, either added to grains or given alone
Vitamin B_{12}	Anemia, neuropathy	Infants breast-fed by strict vegan mothers are at risk, because veg diets contain little vitamin B_{12}	Inclusion of animal products in the diet
Riboflavin	Anemia, sores around the mouth, red and cracked lips	Two small studies showed 40% of children in Nigeria and 50% of the elderly in Guatemala	Inclusion of dairy products in the diet

Descriptions of public health programs that address hidden hunger are presented in Chapters 11–13.

In addition to dietary deficiency of vitamins and minerals, genetic constitution can be an important determinant of micronutrient deficiency. Lower dietary intakes of folate in the periconceptional period have been associated with congenital neural tube defects in Western nations. Additional dietary folate intake by mothers in the periconceptional period is associated with a lower incidence of these birth defects. This is the rationale for national supplementation programs where folate is added public foodstuffs, such as the Canadian policy of adding folate to wheat. These public health interventions have effectively reduced the incidence of neural tube defects. Genetic polymorphism, however, seems to play an important role in individual susceptibility. 5, 10-Methylenetetrahydrofolate reductase is an enzyme that regenerates oxidized folate in the cell so that it can be used again during cell division. A thermolabile genetic variant of this enzyme, which is less effective at regenerating folate, occurs in up to 15% of some Caucasian populations. This genetic variant may result in inadequate cellular proliferation when cell division occurs at an accelerated rate, such as in the developing fetus. The deleterious effect of this variant enzyme can be overcome with additional dietary folate, and this may well explain why folate supplementation reduces neural tube defects in Caucasian populations. Asian populations also seem to respond to enriched exposure to folic acid, with lower rates of congenital neural tube lesions. However, in native American and African ethnicities, the responsiveness of this teratogenic condition to folate status has yet to be determined. This example illustrates how gene–nutrient interactions can explain the basis of important public health interventions, and suggests that public health nutritionists and basic medical scientists can combine their knowledge to improve the health of people worldwide.

10.5 Time trends and contemporary prevalences

The prevalence of underweight, stunting and wasting, and the estimated dietary energy intake for different regions of world in 2000 and 1980 are shown in Table 10.3. The nation with the highest rates of all forms of anthropometric undernutrition is India. Sub-Saharan Africa is the region that has shown the least improvement since 1980. Figures 10.1–10.4 are maps depicting the geographical prevalence of underweight, stunting, wasting and dietary energy consumption in 2000.

10.6 Etiology: determinants and conditioning factors for undernutrition

Physiological mechanisms causing undernutrition

There are five possible mechanisms that result in nutrient deficiency, mechanisms that alone or in combination can reduce nutritional status:

- decreased nutrient intake, e.g. famine or the anorexia of chronic illnesses such as anorexia nervosa
- decreased nutrient absorption, e.g. generalized carbohydrate and amino acid malabsorption in cholera from rapid intestinal transit times or the malabsorption of sugars after diarrhea-induced lactase deficiency

Table 10.3 Prevalence of underweight, stunting and wasting in different regions of the world

Region	% Under-weight		% Stunted		% Wasted	
	1980	2000	1980	2000	1980	2000
Sub-Saharan Africa	23	32	41	41	20	9
North Africa and Middle East	43	18	45	25	9	8
South Asia	66	51	49	52	8	18
East Asia and Pacific	17	22	52	36	5	<5
Latin America and Caribbean	13	10	26	18	10	3
CEE/CIS and Baltic States	na	8	na	16	na	5
Europe, Japan, Australia, USA and Canada	<5	<5	<5	<5	<5	<5

Data from UNICEF.

CEE: Central and Eastern Europe; CIS: Commonwealth of Independent States; na: not available.

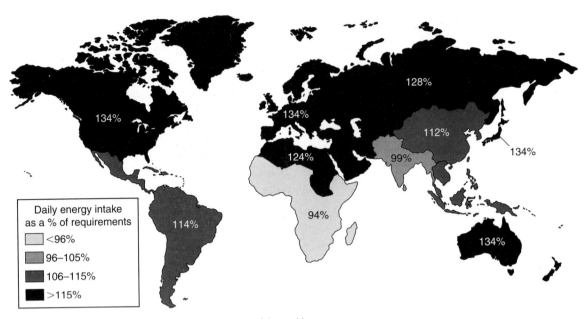

Figure 10.1 Dietary energy consumption in different regions of the world.

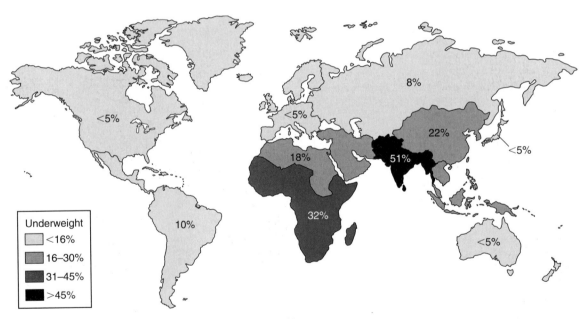

Figure 10.2 Prevalence of underweight in different regions of the world.

- decreased nutrient utilization in the body, e.g. concomitant ingestion of antimalarial drugs which interfere with folate metabolism, and congenital enzyme deficiencies that partially block nutrient metabolic pathways, such as those in phenylketonuria

- increased nutrient losses (most commonly through the gastrointestinal tract, but also through the skin or urine), e.g. the protein-losing enteropathy of inflammatory bowel disease and the loss of nutrients through denuded, burned skin

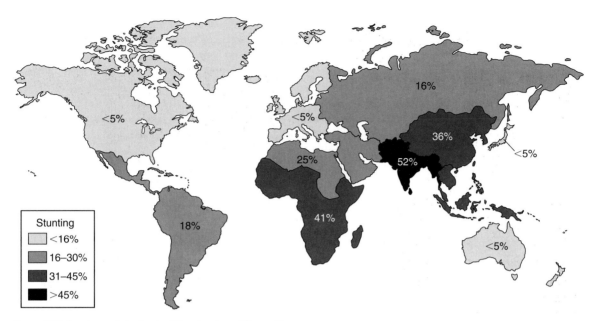

Figure 10.3 Prevalence of stunting in different regions of the world.

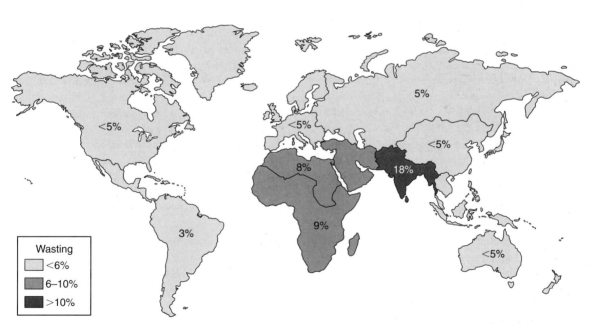

Figure 10.4 Prevalence of wasting in different regions of the world.

- increased nutrient requirements (through pathophysiological states such as chronic inflammation), e.g. the increased metabolic rate with fever or hyperthyroidism.

In a physiological sense, the five mechanisms explain how nutrient balance can become negative.

The elderly, in both low-income and affluent societies, represent a group of added risk for undernutrition.

This derives from the specific vulnerabilities of this group with regard to acquiring and selecting adequate food (immobility, fixed income, infirmity), preparing it (debility, easy fatigue, psychic depression, male widowhood) and consuming it (solitude and depression, chewing problems, medication side-effects). Part of the wasting and micronutrient malnutrition found in community-dwelling elders, however, will be the result of chronic illnesses, either diagnosed or as yet undiscovered, requiring a combination of clinical medicine and public health measures to address the problem of geriatric undernutrition, be it in Chicago or London, or Kolkata or Harare.

Socioeconomic models of undernutrition

Alternatively, mathematical modeling of the national prevalence of childhood malnutrition yields some insights as to which socioeconomic factors are important predictors of undernutrition. Rosegrant and others at the International Food Policy Food Research Institute found five factors that were associated with the prevalence of childhood malnutrition: average dietary energy intake, the fraction of total public expenditure made for social purposes (education, health), the fraction of females with secondary schooling, the fraction of households with access to clean water, and residence in South Asia. These analyses indicate that education of women, access to health services and access to clean water may be very important in decreasing undernutrition. It is interesting to note that other dietary factors, such as amount or quality of dietary protein, micronutrient content or differences in staple cereals, were not predictors of childhood undernutrition. However, the physiological mechanisms and socioeconomic associations are not the primary purview of the public health nutritionist. It is the contextual issues that provoke undernutrition in a given individual, family or community that are most relevant to the public health nutritionist.

Disasters

Natural and unnatural disasters head the list of situations conducive to undernutrition. War displaces large numbers of civilians; those displaced outside the national borders are refugees. There are usually three times as many internally displaced civilians as there are refugees. War routinely causes childhood wasting to increase six- to eight-fold: in northern Mozambique in 1992 wasting was found in 48%, in southern Sudan in 1990 it was found 45% and in Afghanistan in 1993

it was found in 29%. Elderly people were found to be at significant risk during the war in Bosnia in the 1990s, where 16% were found to be wasted. The groups of people that are most dependent on other adults to prepare food and feed them are those that are most likely to suffer from undernutrition in times of war.

Drought results in a failure of most crops in a given geographical area. Severe drought can increase the incidence of childhood wasting by a factor of 2 or 3, as seen in Ethiopia in 1985, where up to 14% of all children were found to be wasted, or in central India in 1966, where childhood wasting was found to be 7%. Drought leads to undernutrition in societies of poor, subsistence farmers, because they lack the means to import and purchase foodstuffs from areas unaffected by the crop failure. The most vulnerable groups of people to undernutrition in drought are the same as those in war: infants, young children and the elderly. The nations most vulnerable to undernutrition caused by drought are the poorest nations.

Other disasters, such as hurricanes, cyclones and floods, are more limited in their impact and duration and thus less likely to result in an undernutrition that presents as a problem of public health dimensions. However, adverse events do compromise nutritional status. In Jamaica in 1988 a severe hurricane struck the island. Even though relief food was plentiful and available in a timely manner, there were associated deficits in height gain for this period among poor populations. This was attributed to an increase in respiratory infections associated with the destructive weather, rather than a food shortage. In Bangladesh in 1994 in the isolated Tendak region a cyclone struck during the harvest month, and the incidence of wasting rose acutely to 35% from 17% the month before. Although war and natural disaster exacerbate undernutrition, often provoking a public health response, most of the world's undernutrition does not occur in these contexts. Poverty, ubiquitous and onerous in its domain, accounts for most of the undernutrition worldwide.

Nutrition and immunity in undernutrition

Sanitation is poor and potable water supplies are precarious in developing societies. Vaccination rates can be low. Both recurrent diarrhea and recurrent respiratory infection have been associated with shorter stature within poor communities in developing countries. The interaction of infection and nutrition is an important paradigm for understanding the etiology of

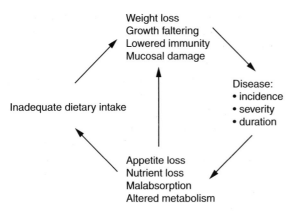

Weight loss
Growth faltering
Lowered immunity
Mucosal damage

Inadequate dietary intake

Disease:
• incidence
• severity
• duration

Appetite loss
Nutrient loss
Malabsorption
Altered metabolism

Figure 10.5 The synergistic cycle of infection and malnutrition.

undernutrition. The interaction between infection and nutrition within an individual has been described as synergistic; during infection, nutritional status declines, and as nutritional status declines the individual is less resistant to infection. The immune response is less effective and less vigorous when the individual is undernourished. The barriers through which microbes must pass to infect individuals, the skin and mucosa of the gastrointestinal and respiratory tracts, are weakened; and the cellular and humoral components of the immune defense system are diminished. This synergism is illustrated in a diagram promoted by the United Nations Children's Fund (UNICEF) (Figure 10.5).

Several aspects of the host response to infection compromise nutritional status. One of the most important is anorexia, the poor appetite associated with most symptomatic illnesses results in energy intakes that are about 20% below the habitual intake. Fever, which accompanies many infections, increases energy expenditure, by about 15% for every 1°C over 37°C. The rate of protein synthesis and breakdown is increased during infection, resulting in increased nitrogen losses and a negative nitrogen balance. Many infections compromise the intestinal absorption of nutrients. In diarrheal illness, absorption of dietary fat is only 58% that of normal, and the absorption of dietary protein only 44% that of normal. Because of this, the absorption of dietary energy is only 71% of normal.

From a public health perspective, infectious epidemics potentiate undernutrition. The classic example of this is measles. This is a viral illness with an attack rate of 95%. Before widespread immunization, in many African countries 5% of all children die from their measles infection. In the wake of a measles epidemic,

rates of childhood wasting will have risen to 35%, even though there was no associated food shortage. Infectious epidemics that affect the agricultural laborers can also affect food production.

The consequences of the synergy between infection and nutrition are also evident in chronic infections such as tuberculosis and human immunodeficiency virus (HIV). Wasting is a common clinical sign in both of these diseases. Wasting is the result of two processes in HIV infection. The first is due to increased energy expenditure by activation of the immune system. It has been observed that the resting energy expenditure is proportional to the number of circulating virus particles (viral load). Secondly, dietary energy intake in HIV-infected populations is below the required amount even when food is plentiful. While increasing dietary energy consumption can ameliorate further loss of lean body mass in HIV, it will not promote complete recovery because of the catabolic response from the chronic infection. The problems impinging on the nutrition of populations with hyperendemic HIV go beyond the physiological ravages of the infected individuals to influence household and community food insecurity, as seen in areas of east and southern Africa. Early mortality of parents leaves children orphaned, often with the financial burden of borrowing for the parents' funeral expenses, and in the care of underemployed or infirm grandparents or at the mercy of a street child existence. Food production for the community also suffers with the acquired immunodeficiency syndrome (AIDS)-depleted loss of the agricultural workforce, and the parent-to-child transmission of the basic skills and know-how of farming and food acquisition are lost with the illness, and then decease, of the parents due to AIDS. The impact on food supply and nutritional status, then, is both immediate and long term.

Social and behavioral aspects associated with undernutrition

Insufficient frequency or duration of breast-feeding is a risk factor for both macronutrient and micronutrient deficiencies in early life. Widespread infant undernutrition has been seen when urban mothers chose to use infant formula instead of breast-feeding. They could not afford to purchase enough formula to provide adequate energy intake for their infants, and undernutrition resulted. In West Africa children are weaned from the breast to a diet of watery, cereal mixtures. This food has a low energy density and very large quantities must be consumed to prevent undernutrition. In southern Africa all family members eat by pulling food from a common pot, rather than receiving individual portions. Young children may not be able to compete for food in this situation as well as older children, and thus this feeding practice places them at risk for undernutrition (see Chapter 16).

Recently, caring strategies of mothers and caretakers have come under scrutiny in terms of determining better or poorer nutritional status. The time at which children are traditionally fed, that is, either before, with or after adults, can be an important determinant of undernutrition. In Ethiopia, one ethnic group fed children before adults and the incidence of stunting was 20%. Another ethnic group in the same geographical area fed the children after the adults had eaten, and the incidence of stunting was 55%. The practice of withholding food when people are perceived as ill is common through the world. Children, with their frequent infections, and the elderly, with their chronic illnesses, may receive less food as a result of this practice. Two recent studies from the International Food Policy Research Institute concluded that investments in the education of women, in both raising literacy and prolonging schooling, have been seen as the most important single interventions to raise the level of nutrition and health in developing countries.

Although the prevalence varies, undernutrition occurs in nations of all economic strata. In wealthier nations undernutrition occurs most commonly among groups of high-risk individuals. For example, recent immigrants have been found to have excessive rates of undernutrition in wealthy and poor nations. This is ascribed to limited access to food and limited facilities for food preparation. Institutionalized elderly individuals are also at risk for undernutrition. This is primarily the result of the inability of the elderly to feed themselves and chew their food, rather than a consequence of limited access to food. To prevent undernutrition, public health measures in the developed world should target these high-risk populations.

Food supply

For hundreds of years, the specter of undernutrition has raised the question: is there enough food in the world to feed everyone? Many policy analysts, including Malthus, have predicted that widespread food shortages would spread to most populations and famine would engulf the world. However, cultural changes, the introduction of new foods and technological advances in agriculture have provided unexpected answers to this question in the past. For example, southern Africa was a primarily a hunter–gatherer society until the seventeenth century, with food being scarce. The introduction of maize and the transition to an agrarian society allowed the land to support four times as many people, providing enough food for a burgeoning population. In the 1960s the green revolution led to dramatic increases in grain production in south Asia. This included supplementing soils with nitrogen and nutrients, irrigating larger tracts of land, and planting breeds of rice that have larger seeds (the edible portion) and smaller stalks. Implementation of these techniques increased rice production in India so much that it became a net exporter, rather than an importer of this dietary staple.

Currently, the answer to the question "is there enough food" is simultaneously both yes and no. The agricultural production of the world is enough to provide adequate dietary nutrients for all people. Almost all of the land that can be agriculturally productive in the world has been cultivated, so the opportunity to increase food production by cultivating more land is limited. Agricultural yields are currently enhanced by addition of nitrogen to the soil (fertilizing) in all areas of the world except for Sub-Saharan Africa. Losses of crops to pests before and after they are harvested account for about 25% of the world's agricultural output. Food is produced in excess in the developed world, primarily in North America, Europe and Australia. Asia and South America produce enough food to be self-sufficient, but cannot export significant quantities. Sub-Saharan Africa produces less food than is needed to meet the nutritional needs of the population.

Distributing food within regions and between regions presents a significant challenge, as often areas in need of food have poor transportation systems. Transport costs are often higher than the food production costs. Measures that increase trade and improve transportation may alleviate food shortages in the future. Biotechnology may be used to develop strains of crops that are drought resistant, grow better in unfertilized or nutrient-depleted soils and are pest resistant; these genetically modified crops may help to meet the world's needs for food in the future. However, biotechnology, like all scientific advances, requires significant investment, which is currently dominated by for-profit corporations. Investment in biotechnology by the public sector may facilitate transfer of its benefits to small-scale, subsistence farmers. Alternatively, significant improvements in agricultural yields in Africa may be possible by better management of small plots of land by traditional farmers. Undoubtedly, the growing demand for food by a growing population, coupled with environmental degradation of agriculturally productive land, is one of the greatest challenges in the future.

10.7 Public health consequences of undernutrition

Beyond having anthropometric measurements below the international reference norms, undernutrition has a series of public health consequences that diminish the individual quality of life and the prospects for social progress.

Susceptibility to mortality

Clinically, undernutrition is associated with greater mortality rates from most childhood diseases. Epidemiological methods have shown that undernutrition accounts for 56% of child deaths worldwide, and that mild, moderate or severe undernutrition increases the risk of death from common childhood illnesses by relative risk factors of 2.5, 4.6 and 8.4, respectively. This understanding has been the impetus for programs to improve the general nutritional status of all children in the developing world, with the hope that this effort will decrease overall child mortality rates. Undernutrition in the elderly is also associated with an increased risk of mortality. The relative risk of death in the elderly is 1.8 when they have a recent history of weight loss of more than 3% of their body weight, even if there is no concurrent wasting illness such as cancer. An increased risk of death is seen with specific nutrient deficiencies as well, such as vitamin A. Accumulating evidence indicates a potential association of zinc deficiency with excess mortality. More than half of the undernutrition and its associated excess morbidity and mortality occurs in children under 5 years of age.

Susceptibility to acute morbidity

Compared with people with adequate nutrition, those with poor nutritional status (determined by anthropometry) are more likely to contract diarrheal, malarial and respiratory infections, and more likely to suffer from these illnesses for a longer duration. They are also more likely to develop debilitating sequelae from these common infections. It is unclear whether specific macronutrient or micronutrient deficiency states result in increased morbidity from infections. In most studies reported, a greater incidence of respiratory or diarrheal diseases could not be attributed to hypovitaminosis A. With respect to iron, its deficiency seems to reduce the chances of contracting or activating various types of intracellular infection, but its interference with phagocyte function raises susceptibility to pyogenic infections. Low zinc status appears to produce higher attack rates for diarrhea, respiratory infections and malaria.

Decreased cognitive development

Associations between taller stature and higher cognitive performance have been found to be robust across ethnic groups and geography, and have been interpreted as better nutritional status during periods of brain development leading to more advanced cognitive development. A study from Kenya demonstrated a positive correlation with all anthropometric indices and developmental testing, which persisted even after correction for socioeconomic status. Figure 10.6 shows

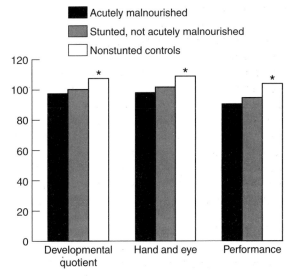

Figure 10.6. Mean score adjusted for age, on the Griffiths Mental Development Scales, in three groups of children. *Significantly greater than the two groups of malnourished children ($p < 0.05$).

data from a case–control study of cognitive development and anthropometric indices in Jamaica. Specific nutrient deficiencies also impair cognitive development; for example, the negative association between iodine deficiency and intellectual impairment has been documented for decades. The occurrence of anemia early in life has been shown in studies in Costa Rica and Chile to leave a permanent residual deficit in learning capacity throughout the school years.

Decreased economic productivity

In agricultural work of intense physical effort, people of larger stature and musculature are more efficient and accomplish more physical labor. In addition, the prompt and complete recovery from infectious diseases that is promoted by adequate nutritional status increases economic productivity. Micronutrient deficiencies, especially anemia, lead to reduced productivity in various kinds of male and female industrial and agricultural labor. All of these lines of evidence suggest that economic productivity is impaired by undernutrition.

Susceptibility to chronic diseases in later life

The most recent concern to emerge for undernutrition in developing countries comes from the epidemiological observations on a cohort of men and women born in the UK. Among this population there is the early appearance and greater prevalence and severity (including mortality) of obesity, hypertension, stroke, cardiac ischemia and diabetes in people with low birth weight and nutritional problems in early life. The working hypothesis is that metabolic programming occurs in early life, maximizing the conservation of nutrients such as energy, sodium and water. This is a rational and protective adaptation in a nutrient-poor environment. According to this theory, this response is never unlearned. When abundant nutrients are present in the diet, the metabolic programming produces excessive retention, tending towards disease. Low birth weight is endemic in developing countries, but ample food is not. With the transition to more plentiful food in emerging developing nations, massive numbers of people deprived in early life may encounter a rising abundance of food supplies, with a consequence of early-onset and widespread chronic disease. (See Chapter 18.)

10.8 Policy and programmatic issues in preventing undernutrition

Preventing clinical malnutrition

Apart from disasters, clinical PEM usually occurs within groups of high-risk individuals, such as young children recently weaned from the breast, or institutionalized elderly people. Prevention schemes should target these high-risk groups with practical, indigenous interventions. This cooperative effort among nutritionists, agriculturists, government agencies, social service organizations and the community should consider the type of food consumed, the availability of such food, and the social practices of food preparation and eating. Schemes should be trialed in small, carefully monitored groups of people to demonstrate their efficacy before being implemented on a wide scale. Growth monitoring of children under 5 years has been advocated as a means of early recognition of undernutrition for decades, and is universally practiced throughout the developing world. The Road to Health chart is a weight-for-age graph on which the child's weights are plotted and compared with the international standards (Figure 10.7). Facilities and programs that use serial weight measurements should have nutritional counseling and support services available to assist those children who are identified as growth faltering. Complementary feeding of breast-fed children is particularly important in preventing growth faltering. For example, in much of Sub-Saharan Africa PEM occurs when 2–3-year-old children who are recently weaned from the breast are served diets of thin, watery cereal mixtures three times a day. These foods have a low energy density and are not served frequently enough. Prevention strategies have focused on increasing the energy density and protein quality of the children's foods, feeding the children more frequently or introducing new foods in the diet. In the developed world, assisted feeding of the elderly and feeding programs for recent immigrants should be given priority to prevent undernutrition.

In the developed world public programs to provide food and subsidize the purchase of food have been effective in improving the nutritional status of vulnerable populations. The Special Supplemental Nutrition Program for Women, Infants and Children (WIC) in the USA, which provides vouchers for certain foods for pregnant women and young children, has demonstrated

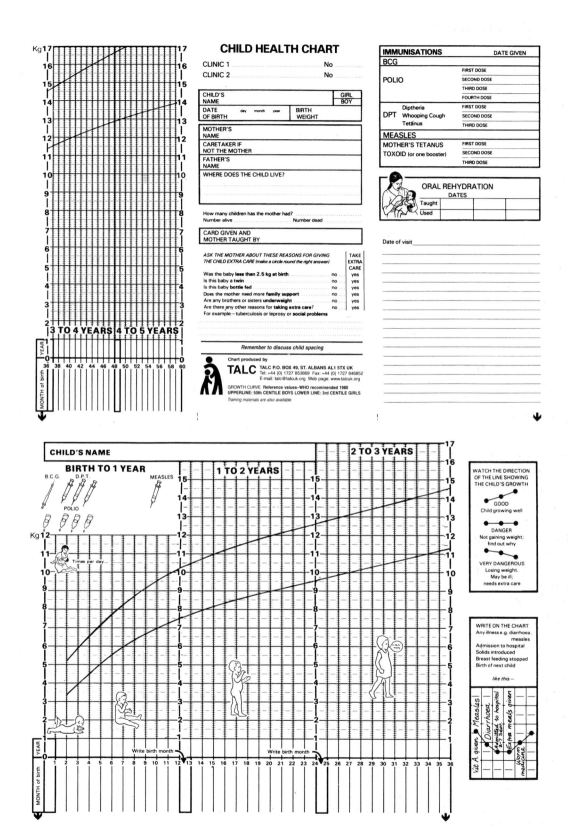

Figure 10.7 Road to Health chart. Reproduced with permission from Teaching-aids at low cost.

lower incidences of low-birth-weight pregnancies, less childhood undernutrition and less iron deficiency in the populations it serves. The program not only prevents undernutrition, but also is estimated to reduce other public social expenditures several-fold for each person it serves.

Preventing short stature

Studies on secular trends in height with migration to more affluent societies, and the growth experience of poor infants adopted into privileged households, suggest that genetic constitution is not the primary determinant of adult stature. Environmental constraints are much more important. Exclusive breast-feeding for the first 6 months optimizes statural growth. Early weaning is clearly detrimental, as can be prolonged breast-feeding without appropriate complementary feeding. It has been speculated, moreover, that assuring micronutrient adequacy during infancy may promote even better longitudinal growth than is seen with maternal milk alone. The logistics of providing supplements through the mother's reserves or directly to the infant as supplements have yet to be worked out.

Safe pure water, hygienic preparation of food and appropriate disposal of waste are essential elements in preventing short stature or chronic undernutrition, but often these are impossible to mobilize in the context of extreme poverty. The chronic asymptomatic carriers of two intestinal protozoal pathogens, *Giardia lamblia* and *Cryptosporidium parvum*, are shorter in stature than their protozoa-free peers. The causal relationship with height deficit is still being explored.

In addition to recurrent, overt infections, the constant exposure to microbes in the environment has been postulated to impair linear growth through immunostimulation. A constant and chronic activation of the acute-phase response directs nutrient metabolism in a catabolic direction, rather than in an anabolic cascade consistent with normal growth. In domestic poultry, for instance, being raised in unsanitary conditions produces poor growth associated with high production of inflammatory mediators (cytokines).

Preventing low weight

Preventing decreased growth velocity in the transition from exclusive breast-feeding to consuming the family diet requires attention to complementary feeding with adequate access to food of suitable energy density and micronutrient content. Moreover, the association of infection with underweight merits prophylactic strategies. Prevention of vaccine-preventable diseases plays a role in reducing the incidence of childhood infections and their adverse consequences on weight (and height) gain. More difficult to prevent, but as important for normal growth, are diarrheal illnesses.

Preventing the adverse nutritional consequences of disaster situations

The most effective intervention for the problem of undernutrition as a consequence of war is an end to the hostilities. Otherwise, programs targeted at vulnerable groups that do not promote further displacement or violence are best. The primary cause of undernutrition in war is the lack of adequate dietary energy and protein, rather than specific nutrient deficiencies. Thus, delivery of staple foods that can be stored without spoilage and easily prepared is the most appropriate intervention. By monitoring agricultural production and weather conditions, poor harvests can be anticipated and relief strategies implemented before famine and population migration ensue.

10.9 Policy and programmatic issues in reversing undernutrition

Posthospitalization rehabilitation of clinical malnutrition

Once the acute refeeding problems and infections have been treated, those suffering from PEM should be offered nutritional support to facilitate their full recovery. This is often done in the home environment. This phase of recovery is characterized by rapid, catch-up growth, requiring energy intakes that are two to three times the habitual requirements. Thus, there should be ample supply of energy-dense food available to those recovering from PEM. Diets that rely on cereals (rice, wheat, maize) for most of the energy may be inadequate because of the low fat content of these foods. Supplements of legumes or animal products are usually necessary to achieve the energy intake required for recovery. In addition, those recovering from PEM may benefit from multiple small feedings. Supplemental foods or food assistance may well be necessary to achieve home-based recovery from PEM.

Can short stature be reversed?

It is well documented in Western countries that stunting secondary to organic disease (e.g. celiac sprue), can be overcome once the disease has been diagnosed and controlled. A major and as yet unanswered question is whether endemic short stature in the community can be reversed, and if so by what measures. A consensus has begun to emerge that the major period of deficit accumulation is from 0 to 3 years, and that once lost, the height cannot be recovered, although children are growing at linear velocities commensurate with their age. Recent data from Filipino children, however, suggest that substantial catch-up growth during the school-age years is possible to achieve.

Correcting low weight-for-age

Low weight-for-age can be corrected just by changing the energy balance during a period in which children consume and retain more energy than they expend. They will move to within the norms of the international reference curves. The shorter is a child is, the greater the risk of producing an unhealthy body composition by correcting the weight for his or her age without taking the short stature into consideration. Surveys in China, Brazil and Mexico have identified short stature as a risk factor for obesity.

10.10 Perspectives on the future

In conclusion, undernutrition is an important problem worldwide. Children and the elderly are most at risk for undernutrition, as well as victims of war and natural disasters. Chronic or recurrent infections also play an important role in promoting undernutrition. Public health schemes led by nutritionists that draw on a variety of participants to partner with the community in effective interventions are necessary to prevent and ameliorate undernutrition.

Undernutrition is not simply a consequence of the lack of affluence of a population, but rather the result of interactions among social, demographic, genetic, infectious and societal conditions. It is likely always to be a problem, since the etiology is so complex. The role of the public health nutritionist in the future involves continued vigilance in wisely monitoring populations and situations, looking for pockets of undernutrition. Effective interventions will be based on advances in understanding human biology, infectious diseases, agricultural science, plant genetics, hydrology, anthropology and sociology. Particular attention should be paid to applying advances in knowledge with a global perspective, and building partnerships between groups of professionals that have not traditionally worked together.

Further reading

Pelletier DL, Frongillo EA Jr, Schroeder DG, Habicht J-P. The effects of malnutrition on child mortality in developing countries. Bull World Health Org 1995; 73: 443–448.

Popkin BM. The nutrition transition and its health implications in lower-income countries. Public Health Nutr 1998; 1: 5–21.

Rosegrant MW, Leach N, Gerpacio RV. Alternative futures for world cereal and meat consumption. Proc Nutr Soc 1999; 58: 219–234.

UNICEF. State of the World's Children 2000. Oxford: Oxford University Press, 2000.

Waterlow JC, Armstrong DG, Fowden L, Riley R, eds. Feeding the world population of more than eight billion people – a challenge to science. Oxford: Oxford University Press, 1998.

11
Vitamin A Deficiency

Faruk Ahmed and Ian Darnton-Hill

Key messages

- Vitamin A deficiency is, after protein–energy malnutrition and iron-deficiency anemia, the most widespread and serious nutritional disease among young children. In the early 1990s, the World Health Organization estimated that globally nearly 14 million children were affected annually by xerophthalmia and 190 million were at risk of subclinical vitamin A deficiency.
- Vitamin A deficiency is the most common cause of childhood blindness. Approximately another 150 million are at increased risk of dying in childhood from infectious diseases due to an inadequate vitamin A status.
- In more industrialized countries over two-thirds of dietary vitamin A is derived from animal sources as preformed

vitamin A, whereas in the developing world, communities depend primarily on provitamin A carotenoids from plant sources.
- Signs of vitamin A deficiency can also occur as a secondary phenomenon to protein–energy malnutrition owing to impairment of the synthesis of plasma retinol binding protein, which normally transports retinol.
- Strategies for the control and treatment of vitamin A deficiency include food-based approaches, supplementation of vitamin A, public health interventions such as immunization and promotion of breast-feeding, and modification of the environment in which at-risk populations live.

11.1 Introduction

Vitamin A deficiency is the most common cause of childhood blindness, causing 250 000–500 000 children to go blind every year, half of whom will die within the year. Approximately another 150 million are at increased risk of dying in childhood from infectious diseases owing to an inadequate vitamin A status. Vitamin A is a generic term used for a group of structurally related chemical compounds known as retinoids that possess qualitatively the biological activity of retinol. Although an essential nutrient needed in only small amounts, it is necessary for normal functioning of a large number of regulatory and other physiological processes of the human body. Vitamin A deficiency disorders occur when body reserves are depleted to the limit at which physiological functions are impaired, even if there is no evidence of clinical xerophthalmia (the pathological eye signs of vitamin A deficiency).

Under normal physiological conditions, nearly 90% of the stored vitamin is found in the liver. Depletion of stored vitamin A is usually seen as the consequence of an inadequate dietary intake of the vitamin itself over a period of time, although losses are increased by associated infection. Vitamin A is extensively recycled between the plasma, liver and other tissues, and the rate of utilization by specific tissues can show some adaptation to diminishing availability. This homeostatic adaptation and recycling serves to maintain a relatively constant level in the blood until body stores become depleted below a critical point.

Sources of vitamin A

Vitamin A in the diets of most human communities comes from a very wide variety of plant and animal sources in order to meet their daily requirements. In the more industrialized countries over two-thirds of dietary vitamin A is derived from animal sources as preformed vitamin A, whereas in the developing world, communities depend primarily on provitamin A carotenoids from plant sources. These latter countries are at higher risk of vitamin A deficiency in their populations, especially where rice is the staple and there is poverty. Common dietary sources of preformed vitamin A are liver, milk and milk products, eggs and fish. The richest sources are liver oils of fish, such as the shark, halibut and cod, and of marine mammals, such as the polar bear. In marine fish, vitamin A_1 alcohol (retinol) is the storage form of vitamin A, while in freshwater fish it is the vitamin A_2 alcohol (3-dehydroretinol), having only about 40% of the activity of retinol. The livers of ox, sheep, calves or chicken also contain vitamin A at concentrations comparable to cod liver oil. Eggs, milk and other dairy products, such as butter and cheese, are all moderate sources. Meat, such as beef, mutton and pork, is a relatively poor source of preformed vitamin A.

Provitamin A carotenoids are found in many plant foods such as yellow and orange fruit and vegetables, and in dark green leafy vegetables such as amaranth and spinach, although the color of fruit and vegetables is not necessarily an indicator of the concentration of provitamin A. Yellow fruits such as papaya, mango and orange, and vegetables such as carrots, yellow pumpkin, orange sweet potato and yellow cassava have appreciable amounts of provitamin A carotenoids. In the tomato, the major constituent is lycopene, a nutritionally inactive pigment. Red palm oil is the richest natural source of carotenoids. Cereal grains, especially when milled, are a poor source.

Bioavailability

Preformed vitamin A from animal foods, which is primarily present in the diet as retinyl esters, is generally assumed to be 70–90% bioavailable when consumed in usual amounts. Bioavailability, which includes absorption and bioconversion, of provitamin A carotenoids in food is much less, depending on the food, preparation, cooking methods and so on. To reflect this substantially lower biological activity of provitamin A carotenoids in foods in the human diet, the current commonly used unit for quantifying vitamin A activity in foods is the retinol equivalent (RE), which is basically $1 \mu g$ of all-trans-retinol. The current useage is that $6 \mu g$ of β-carotene or $12 \mu g$ of other all-trans-carotenoids in foods is equivalent to $1 \mu g$ of vitamin A activity or 1 RE. The total RE value for a given food is calculated by adding the actual amount of retinol to the adjusted equivalent amounts of the provitamin A carotenoids present in the food. The efficiency rate of conversion varies between one-quarter and one-tenth depending on the amount of β-carotene in a meal. It has been set at one-twelfth for all other vitamin A precursors, but this is currently being questioned. Further, all-trans carotenoids have more provitamin A activity than the cis isomers. The conversion process is more efficient in vitamin A-deficient individuals and less efficient in those who are vitamin A replete. However, this conversion ratio is a gross average and recently suggested conversion ratios of carotene to vitamin A in the body range from 26:1 for carrots and green leafy vegetables to 12:1 for fruits.

Evidence indicates that the bioavailability of dietary carotenoids is affected by a large number of factors, including the chemical nature, amount ingested and preexisting nutrient status. The matrix in which a carotenoid is embedded in a particular food appears to be an important determinant of its bioavailability. In green leaves, carotenoids are present within chloroplasts as pigment–protein complexes, whereas in some vegetables and fruits, carotenoids are found in lipid droplets. Cooking can greatly reduce the matrix effect and thus help in the release of carotenoids, but prolonged heating may lead to oxidative degradation of carotenoids. The absorption of carotenoids depends not only on sufficient fat in the diet, but also on sufficient protein and zinc; while a large amount of dietary fiber such as pectin is known to reduce the bioavailability of carotenoids. Systemic or parasitic infection reduces carotenoid bioavailability, and is thus of greater significance in developing countries, where the parasite infection rates may be high. All these factors need to be taken into account when assessing the bioavailability of carotene from various dietary sources. Therefore using dietary tables to estimate the apparent adequacy of dietary intake of vitamin A in the form of carotenoids does not necessarily indicate adequate status in a population.

In the past, the amount of vitamin A was expressed in international units (IU), a system still sometimes used in food composition tables and particularly in labeling vitamin A supplements. One IU equals $0.3 \mu g$ of retinol, $0.344 \mu g$ of retinyl acetate and $0.55 \mu g$ of retinyl palmitate, all in their all-trans isomers. One IU of all-trans-β-carotene is defined as $0.6 \mu g$. Vitamin A concentrations in tissues, including serum and breast milk for analysis, are now expressed in molar terms to conform to the Systeme Internationale (SI units). In SI units, the conversion factor for 1 μg retinol is equal to 0.003491 μmol per liter of fluid or per gram of tissue.

Chemistry and metabolism of vitamin A

All-*trans* retinol is the parent substance of the vitamin A group. Retinol (vitamin A_1 alcohol) consists of a substituted cyclohexene (β-ionone) ring, a tetraene side-chain and a primary hydroxyl group at C15. The hydroxyl group of retinol may be esterified with a fatty acid to form retinyl ester, a major storage form in the body. Retinal (retinaldehyde) is formed by the oxidation of the hydroxyl group of retinol in the body, which may be further oxidized to a carboxylic acid, retinoic acid. In nature, retinol and its metabolites have a number of geometric isomers with specific physiological functions, one of which is 11-*cis*-retinaldehyde, which has a role in vision.

Of over 600 carotenoids that have been isolated from nature, only 50 possess the biological activity of vitamin A, and these are known as provitamin A carotenoids. Of these, the most active and quantitatively important provitamin A in foodstuffs is all-*trans*-β-carotene. For provitamin A activity, carotenoids must contain at least one β-ionone ring that is not hydroxylated and a polyene side-chain. Because of the large number (usually nine to 13) of conjugated double bonds, each carotenoid can form many geometric isomers. For both vitamin A and provitamin A carotenoids, the all-*trans* isomers are the most nutritionally active forms; *cis* isomers show about half, or even less, of the activity of the all-*trans* isomers.

Vitamin A and carotenoids are insoluble in water but are readily miscible with most organic solvents. Because of the structural conjugated double bonds, these compounds when dissolved in solution are sensitive to isomerization, oxidation and polymerization, particularly in the presence of light, oxygen and high temperature. This has important implications for storage of the vitamin in health centers and warehouses. Vitamin A in its natural form, whether present in liver or bound to protein in the plasma, is stable when stored frozen in the dark at a temperature of −70°C. Carotenoids present in the serum or tissue are also stable at −70°C in the absence of light under argon, but tend to be more sensitive than vitamin A to destruction. This stability is important when serum samples are being collected during surveys for later analysis. Vitamin A and carotenoids show a characteristic absorption spectrum, which is used in identification and quantification of vitamin A and carotenoids in biological samples.

Vitamin A and carotenoids are released from protein in the stomach by proteolysis, and then aggregate with other lipids and pass into the small intestine. In the presence of bile salts, essentially all retinyl esters and some carotenoids (xanthophylls) are hydrolyzed, primarily by an enzyme located in the brush border of intestinal mucosal cells and by the pancreatic esterases. The resulting unesterified retinol, xanthophylls and provitamin A carotenoids, in micellar form, are absorbed by the intestinal mucosal cells. Within the mucosal cells, provitamin A carotenoids are oxidatively cleaved by a specific 15,15′-dioxygenase enzyme to form retinal, which binds to a cellular retinol binding protein (CRBP type II), and then is reduced to retinol by retinal reductase. In the mucosal cells, retinol is esterified by two different enzyme systems: lecithin: retinol acyltransferase and acyl-coenzyme A (acyl-CoA) retinol transferase.

Nearly all of the absorbed forms of vitamin A, as retinyl esters with a small amount of retinol, hydrocarbon carotenoids and xanthophylls, are then incorporated into chylomicrons that are rapidly transported from enterocytes via the lymphatics to the systemic circulation. In the circulation, the chylomicrons are hydrolyzed by lipoprotein lipase to form chylomicron remnants, which then clear all vitamin A, including carotenoids, into the liver.

About 90% of the total vitamin A in the body, mainly as retinyl palmitate, is stored in the liver of well-nourished individuals. Vitamin A from the liver store is released into the circulation as retinol bound to a specific transport protein synthesized in liver, retinol binding protein, (RBP) at a ratio of 1:1 to form a complex (holo-RBP). The holo-RBP in the plasma forms a complex with another protein, transthyretin. This holo-RBP–transthyretin complex is then transported to various target tissues for utilization.

11.2 Consequences of vitamin A deficiency

The public health significance of vitamin A deficiency has been redefined since the 1970s, to include its likely association with the deaths of over one million young children each year worldwide. Between 125 and 250 million preschool-aged children are at risk of being vitamin A deficient, with high-risk populations located

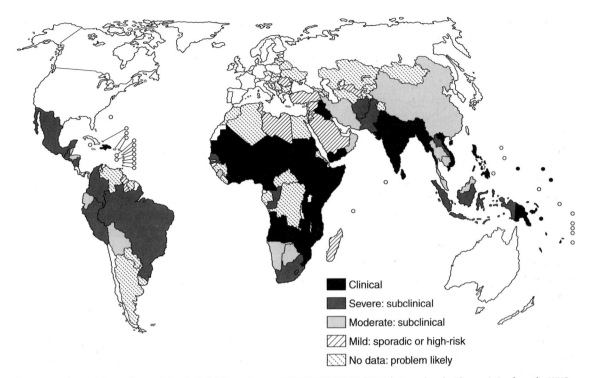

Figure 11.1 The global prevalence of vitamin A deficiency. Source: WHO/UNICEF/IVACG (1995a). Reproduced with permission from the WHO.

mostly in the poorer periequatorial regions of the world (see Figure 11.1 and Section 11.3). It also remains the most common cause of preventable childhood blindness, causing tragic and unnecessary loss of vision in young children. This clinical manifestation (xerophthalmia) reflects likely deficiency in the wider community from which such affected children come. It is now recognized as a condition also affecting women, especially when pregnant or lactating.

Histopathological and physiological effects

The varied expression of vitamin A deficiency represents the many bodily tissues and systems that are affected by a deficiency of the vitamin. While the main impact appears to be on the integrity of the epithelial tissues, there is also involvement of the enzymic, auto-immune, gene regulation and vision systems.

Much of the histopathological information is derived from animal studies, although with some important differences between animals' and humans' systems; for example, the impact on the respiratory system. In the rat, the sequence of the widespread keratinizing metaplasia that follows vitamin A deficiency occurs earliest in the genitourinary tract, then the respiratory tract and then the alimentary tract. Despite eye signs having long defined the deficiency syndrome, the histological changes in the eye actually follow those of the respiratory tract. Atrophy and hypoplasia of glandular ducts usually precede the keratinization of the epithelium, with extreme atrophy of the thymus being universal. Infection commonly follows secondary to the metaplastic changes, suggesting that a keratinized surface provides a conducive substrate for bacterial replication. There are also significant reductions in goblet cell density and secretory granules before any change in the number of ciliated epithelial cells.

In general, the clinical manifestations of vitamin A deficiency depend more on the function of the epithelial surfaces affected than on a functional impact on a particular organ. For example, the dryness of the eye in xerophthalmia is caused by the keratinizing metaplasia of the epithelial tissue of the conjunctiva of the eye, whereas diarrhea is likely to be due to the effect on the lining of the bowel. Nevertheless, the physiological and clinical effects will reflect the many functions of vitamin A in the body, namely, on vision, maintenance of epithelia and immune function. Retinoic acid has also been shown to have a major function in the regulation of gene expression and tissue differentiation.

Clinical and pathological effects

The clinical effects of vitamin A deficiency that are best recognized and described are those affecting the eye (xerophthalmia) and which will lead to irreversible blindness if the deficiency is not corrected, unless death intervenes first. However, as described above, vitamin A deficiency affects virtually all the mucous membranes of the body, and the impact on the eye is later than that on some other organs. These underlying mechanisms are now recognized to affect reductions in immunocompetence, as well as other physiological changes. These lead to increased morbidity and mortality, probably throughout the life cycle, but usually described in infants and young children, and more recently women of reproductive age. The effects are seen most markedly in periods of greatest need: early growth, pregnancy and lactation, and when infections are occurring at the same time. The eye signs making up xerophthalmia will be considered first; then the impact of vitamin A on immunocompetence and infection, morbidity and growth, the associations of vitamin A with malnutrition, and finally its impact on mortality.

Xerophthalmia and keratomalacia

Vitamin A deficiency has long been defined in terms of clinical eye signs, which actually represent a rather more severe manifestation of the deficiency. Xerophthalmia (from the Greek *xeros,* drying, and ophthalmia, of the eye) represents the ocular consequences of vitamin A deficiency that include night blindness (XN), conjunctival xerosis (X1A), Bitot's spots (X1B), corneal xerosis (X2), ulceration (X3A) or necrosis/keratomalacia (X3B). In the early 1980s, it was estimated that half a million children developed corneal xerophthalmia each year in south and south-east Asia alone, but these estimates have improved because of decreasing trends in the incidence of corneal xerophthalmia since the 1980s in these regions, so that the current estimate of global occurrence of corneal disease is likely to be around 500 000 per year at most. Even so, vitamin A deficiency remains the most common preventable cause of childhood blindness in the world. Approximately half of all corneal cases lead to blindness and of these blinded children, half will die within the year.

Conjunctival and corneal xerosis, corneal ulceration and necrosis, and retinal dysfunction leading to poor dark adaptation and night blindness comprise the ocular consequences of vitamin A deficiency. A full description of clinical signs with colored illustrations can be found in the World Health Organization (WHO) guide to vitamin A (WHO, 1995b).

Night blindness (XN)

Night blindness is the earliest specific clinical symptom of vitamin A deficiency and is usually the most prevalent stage of xerophthalmia. Its occurrence reflects a failure in rod photoreceptor cells in the retina to maintain peripheral vision under dimly lit conditions. Opsin, a protein, binds covalently with 11-*cis*-retinal to form rhodopsin (visual purple). Light exposure, even at very low levels, to the back of the eye bleaches rhodopsin. This reaction initiates an electrochemical impulse along the optic nerve to the brain that results in vision. A visual cycle is completed when the vitamin A aldehyde is returned to rods in the outer segment to form rhodopsin. Lack of vitamin A disables this cycle, resulting in poor vision in dim light that, if sufficiently severe, results in night blindness. Typically, a history of night blindness can be elicited using a local term for the condition, often translated as "chicken eyes" (chickens lack rods and, thus, night vision) or "twilight" or "evening" blindness.

A history of night blindness is associated with low-to-deficient serum retinol concentrations in preschool-aged children and pregnant women. Night-blind young children and mothers stumble in poor visibility and stay inactive at dusk and at night. Other nutritional and disease conditions that could contribute to night blindness (e.g. zinc deficiency, wasting, anemia, infection) may be more prevalent in south Asia than in southeast Asia or Africa, where the condition is described less often. Night blindness condition is more readily ascertained in pregnant women than in children for both reasons of reporting and physiology, and may therefore be a better indicator of vitamin A deficiency than by using reports from young children, although there are other, far less common, causes of night blindness in pregnancy besides vitamin A deficiency.

Conjunctival xerosis (X1A) with Bitot's spots (X1B)

The keratinizing metaplasia effect on mucosal surfaces of the body of vitamin A deficiency includes the bulbar conjunctiva. In chronic deficiency, xerosis of the conjunctiva appears as a dry, nonwettable, rough or granular surface, best seen on oblique illumination from a hand-light. It is an unreliable sign because of observer variability and possible environmental causes. On the ocular surface, the tear film breaks up, revealing a xerotic surface. Histologically, the lesions represent a transformation of normal surface columnar epithelium, with abundant mucus-secreting goblet cells, to a stratified squamous epithelium that lacks goblet cells.

In advanced xerosis, grey to yellowish white foamy patches of keratinized cells and saprophytic bacilli, called Bitot's spots, may aggregate on the surface, usually on the temporal conjunctival surface and, in more severe cases, on nasal surfaces as well. Bitot's spots appearing in preschool children generally respond to high-potency vitamin A within 2–5 days and disappear within 2 weeks, although they may persist as smaller aggregates for months and, in some cases, X1B may be refractory to vitamin A and may reflect past rather than present history.

Corneal xerosis, ulceration and necrosis

Corneal xerophthalmia represents an acute decompensation of the corneal epithelium and is a sight-threatening medical emergency. Corneal xerosis quickly responds to vitamin A, usually within 2–5 days of therapy, with the cornea returning to normal without permanent sequellae within 1–2 weeks. Untreated corneal xerosis leads to blindness in one eye or both eyes. Shallow, small corneal ulcers, usually peripheral to the visual axis, can heal with minimal structural damage or risk of visual loss. Ulcers will heal to form an opaque scar (leukoma). Ulcers that perforate are plugged with iris and will, on healing, form an adherent leukoma; as these are often at the periphery of the cornea, central vision of the healed eye is left intact. Corneal necrosis (keratomalacia) must be treated immediately with standard vitamin A therapy, coupled with topical antibiotics and other nutritional measures (see Section 11.4, Treatment) or will result in meltdown of the eye with irreversible blindness in that eye.

Immunocompetence

Effects on the immune system

Not only does vitamin A deficiency reduce the barrier function of mucous membranes, there is also a significantly impaired systemic immune response in marginally deficient children. This improves markedly following vitamin A supplementation. Vitamin A deficiency has been described as a nutritionally acquired immunodeficiency disorder, one characterized by widespread pathological alterations of the mucosal epithelia of the respiratory, gastrointestinal and genitourinary tracts, impaired antibody responses to protein antigens, altered cell-mediated immunity and alterations in T-cell subsets. Vitamin A, through its active metabolite, all-*trans*-retinoic acid, regulates genes through nuclear receptors in the steroid and thyroid hormone superfamily. The genes relevant to immunity that are regulated by vitamin A have not been completely characterized, but probably include those of interleukin-4, interferon-γ, interleukin-2 receptor and others. Growth and activation of T- and B-cells are dependent on vitamin A, and vitamin A supplementation is associated with increases in circulating lymphocytes, including CD4 T-cells and natural killer cells, suggesting that lymphopoiesis is enhanced by vitamin A.

Infection

Vitamin A deficiency predisposes individuals to severe infection and, indeed, vitamin A has long been known as an anti-infective vitamin, given the evidence of numerous synergistic effects with infection on the host. Preschool children with mild xerophthalmia have a two to three-fold higher risk of respiratory infection and diarrhea than their nonxerophthalmic peers. In a prospective study in Indonesia, preschoolers with either diarrhea or acute respiratory disease were twice as likely to have developed xerophthalmia in a subsequent 3 month period than healthier children. Severe diarrhea, dysentery, measles and other severe, febrile illnesses are frequently reported to precede corneal xerophthalmia. Vitamin A deficiency and infection interact within a vicious cycle, whereby one exacerbates and increases the vulnerability to the other.

Infection can induce vitamin A deficiency through a variety of ways, depending on the cause, duration and severity of infection, and the vitamin A status of the host at onset. Serum retinol may be depressed following infection because of decreased dietary intake or absorption due to diarrhea or intestinal pathogens, impaired or accelerated hepatic depletion of retinol reserves, increased retinol utilization by target tissues or increased urinary losses associated with the acute-phase response. Urinary retinol loss, reflecting losses in body stores, depends on the type and severity of infection. In a study in Bangladesh, 6% of children hospitalized with dysentery and 65% with sepsis excreted approximately 10% of a preschool child's estimated metabolic requirement. The interaction of vitamin A deficiency with diarrhea, measles and respiratory disease is well established, and it is increasingly likely with human immunodeficiency virus (HIV) infection and malaria, and to be associated with infectious episodes surrounding pregnancy, birth and the postnatal period.

Morbidity

Early work in Indonesia, particularly by Oomen and colleagues, recognized the high levels of vitamin A deficiency in children in the developing world and its impact on childhood blindness. Community-based observations by Sommer and colleagues in the early 1980s revealed that Indonesian children with mild xerophthalmia (XN or X1B), with no other obvious nutritional stress, were two to three times more likely to develop diarrhea or respiratory infection than those without xerophthalmia. They were also more likely, in a dose–response fashion in relation to eye signs, to die over the ensuing 4 months than children without any xerophthalmic eye signs. The epidemiology of the condition is discussed in greater detail below, but other factors involved in those at risk of vitamin A deficiency and infection, often as indicated by xerophthalmia, include age, gender, and socioeconomic and environmental factors.

In subclinical vitamin A deficiency, the incidence and prevalence of diarrhea may also increase. Mortality in children who are blind from keratomalacia or who have corneal disease is reported to be 50–90%, and measles mortality associated with vitamin A deficiency is increased to 50%. Several meta-analyses provide convincing evidence that community-based improvement in the vitamin A status of deficient children aged 6 months to 6 years reduces their risk of dying by 20–30% on average.

Amidst the consistent overall effects on child mortality, two seemingly incongruent observations exist. First, in contrast to evidence relating vitamin A deficiency to respiratory tract compromise and infection, vitamin A supplementation has not had a consistent effect in reducing the incidence, severity or mortality of acute lower respiratory infection in children. Secondly, vitamin A supplementation of infants under 6 months of age, provided either directly or indirectly through maternal provision, has not been shown to reduce mortality in early infancy (although one study in Indonesian neonates did show a 64% reduction in infant mortality). This apparent lack of effect concurs with a similarly observed lack of effect on early infant diarrheal and respiratory morbidity. Although shown to be safe (at 25 000 IU with immunization contacts in the first 6 months of life), the inconsistency in the effect of vitamin A supplementation on survival in early infancy, in populations at varying risk, has not been resolved. It may be that the amount of vitamin A given has been inadequate, or that other factors are involved. In Section 11.4, it will be seen that a consensus is emerging that, at the very least, it is necessary to ensure that the infant has adequate stores for the second 6 months of his or her life.

Children with severe measles will benefit from vitamin A therapy. Cases should be provided with the same treatment regimen as for children with xerophthalmia, according to the WHO United Nations Children's Fund (UNICEF)/International Vitamin A Consultative Group (IVACG) (1997) guidelines. These have recently been updated (see Section 11.4). Such treatment will, under most conditions, reduce the severity of complications, accelerate recovery and lower case fatality.

A strong dose–risk gradient exists between maternal serum retinol and vertical transmission of HIV and cervicovaginal shedding of HIV DNA, suggesting that maternal vitamin A deficiency may affect pregnancy outcomes in HIV-positive populations. Unfortunately, vitamin A supplementation of HIV-positive pregnant women has shown little effect on outcomes such as low birth weight or perinatal mortality, or in interrupting the transmission of HIV from mother to infant. It seems very possible that low vitamin A levels (and possibly other micronutrients such as zinc) in pregnant women lead to a greater risk of puerperal sepsis.

Growth

Experimental vitamin A depletion in animals causes an initial deceleration in weight gain, which then plateaus as hepatic retinol reserves become exhausted, and eventually loss of weight. It is less clearly seen in children. Corneal xerophthalmia is associated with severe linear growth stunting and acute wasting malnutrition. Mild xerophthalmia (XN or X1B) is associated with moderate stunting and mild wasting, although associated comorbidity and nutritional deficiencies also restrict growth.

Field trials have shown mixed effects of vitamin A on child growth. Several have failed to find an overall effect of vitamin A supplementation on weight or height gain. Others have observed increments in linear, but not ponderal growth, or subgroup increments in both aspects of growth. Additional studies and stratified analyses suggest, however, that vitamin A can improve growth in children for whom vitamin A deficiency is likely to be growth limiting. Seasonal variation can affect the growth response to vitamin A supplementation.

Associations with protein–energy malnutrition and other micronutrient deficiencies

Protein–energy malnutrition

As protein adequacy is a prerequisite for optimal transport and utilization of vitamin A, serum retinol levels are depressed in the presence of wasting protein–energy malnutrition (PEM). Signs of vitamin A deficiency can also occur as a secondary phenomenon to PEM, regardless of whether or not the intake of vitamin A is adequate. This is due to impairment of the synthesis of plasma RBP which is then not available to transport retinol. This contributes to the severely impaired immune response to infection seen, as a result of both the functional vitamin A deficiency and the added impairment of immune responses associated with undernutrition.

Other micronutrients

Several other micronutrients have interactions with vitamin A of public health significance, most notably iron, but also zinc and selenium, and there may be some linked pathway with iodine. A lack of vitamin A can affect iron metabolism when deficiencies of both nutrients coexist and particularly when there is a high infectious disease load. The maximum hemoglobin response occurs when iron and vitamin A deficiencies are corrected together. Vitamin A deficiency appears to influence the availability of storage iron for use by hematopoietic tissue.

Mortality

Infants and children

Since 1986, eight population-based vitamin A–child mortality intervention trials, enrolling more than 165 000 children, have been conducted in south-east and south Asia and Africa (Figure 11.2). Results of meta-analyses based on these trials show that, in areas of endemic vitamin A deficiency, mortality of children 6–71 months of age can be reduced, on average, by 23–34% following vitamin A supplementation. This important effect can be partly explained by an ability of vitamin A to lower case fatality from measles by approximately 50%, as observed in field trials and hospital-based measles trials, mortality from severe diarrhea and dysentery by around 40% and, based on morbidity findings from a recent supplementation trial, possibly *falciparum* malaria. Combining mortality effects with data on the prevalence of vitamin A deficiency, it is estimated that 1.3–2.5 million early childhood deaths each year can be attributed to underlying vitamin A deficiency.

Women of reproductive age

The influence of vitamin A on survival has recently been extended to the reproductive years of women. An estimated 10–20% of women living in rural, malnourished populations of south Asia experience night blindness during pregnancy or lactation. Beyond being symptomatic of vitamin A deficiency, its occurrence during pregnancy appears to reflect a state of chronic vitamin A deficiency, anemia and wasting undernutrition, and an increased risk of infection and reproductive morbidity, and is associated with lower maternal survival during the first 1–2 years following

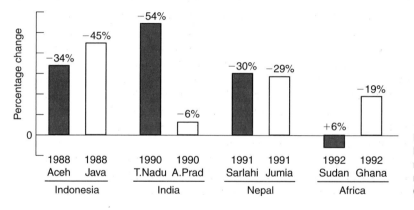

Figure 11.2 Results of eight population-based trials showing vitamin A mortality reduction after supplementation with vitamin A. Adapted from West and Darnton-Hill (2001).

delivery. Thus, in malnourished populations of women of childbearing age, improved vitamin A intake, through supplementation, and presumably by dietary means, may substantially reduce the risk of mortality related to pregnancy.

A study in Nepal, where night blindness is prevalent in pregnant women, pregnant and lactating women who were given 7000 μg RE (~23 300 IU) weekly demonstrated a decrease in prevalence of night blindness and a decrease in maternal mortality. The study is currently being replicated in several centers in Afica and Asia. This recent evidence of relatively high prevalences of vitamin A deficiency in women in the developing world, and the health impact of this situation, has encouraged many in international public health to examine new paradigms in the prevention and control of vitamin A deficiency.

11.3 Epidemiology

Magnitude of the problem

Vitamin A deficiency is, after PEM and iron-deficiency anemia, the most widespread and serious nutritional disease among young children. In the early 1990s, the WHO estimated that globally nearly 14 million children were affected annually by xerophthalmia and 190 million were at risk of subclinical vitamin A deficiency. This estimation was based largely on the appearance of clinical eye signs from which an extrapolation was made to estimate the total at-risk population. In 1994, the WHO updated the information on the magnitude of the vitamin A deficiency problem based on biochemical evidence of subclinical vitamin A deficiency (population-based blood levels of vitamin A $\leq$ 0.70 μmol/l), supported by other biological indicators and ecological risk factors such as poor diet. The 1994 global estimate indicated that 2.8 million preschool children are clinically affected by vitamin A deficiency and 251 million more are subclinically deficient. Thus, a possible 254 million preschool children are at risk in terms of their health and survival. The global distribution of vitamin A deficiency is shown in Figure 11.1, based on the number of preschool children at risk of or suffering from vitamin A deficiency.

Two regions, Asia and Africa, account for nearly 90% of the global problem. Although the prevalence of severe clinical vitamin A deficiency declines with age, less severe forms of vitamin A deficiency are also found in adolescence and young adults and women of reproductive age, where the prevalence of mild xerophthalmia may exceed the rates in preschool children. It is important to note that the estimate of the magnitude of the problem did not include adolescents or women of reproductive age, and it is likely that the size of the problem has been underestimated in this way (although a subsequent estimation has lowered the figure for the number of young children at risk to approximately 140 million).

Risk factors

As a public health problem, vitamin A deficiency occurs within an environment of social, economic and ecological deprivations in which people live in the transitional and developing economies of the world. The relative influence of causal factors at both the macrolevel and the microlevel may vary considerably among countries, and even within regions of countries. It is therefore imperative to understand the local conditions when designing appropriate and effective intervention programs to improve the situation. Nevertheless, there are some underlying risk factors that tend to characterize most situations where vitamin A deficiency is common.

Age

Varying levels of vitamin A deficiency, from subclinical forms to the severe form of blinding malnutrition (keratomalacia), can occur at any age if conditions are sufficiently extreme. However, as a public health problem, vitamin A deficiency, particularly severe deficiency, affects children of preschool age. This is because the requirements for growth in these children are high, while the dietary intake of vitamin A is often low, with the added burden of a greater exposure to infections. The incidence of corneal xerophthalmia is most prevalent among children aged 2–4 years. In children under 12 months of age, corneal disease is relatively a rare event (largely because breast-feeding is protective), but keratomalacia occurs more frequently among infants living in low socioeconomic conditions.

The prevalence of mild xerophthalmia, notably night blindness (XN) and Bitot's spot (XB), increases with age through the preschool years and this relationship is found to be typical among different cultures, regardless of age-specific rates of xerophthalmia. Subclinical vitamin A deficiency is also frequently found among school-aged children, adolescence and young adults in the same communities in which the prevalence in young children is high.

Gender

In healthy human adults, both plasma retinol and RBP are found at levels 20% higher in males than females, although the significance of this physiological difference is not clear. Nevertheless, males have generally been found to be at higher risk of night blindness and Bitot's spot than females during the preschool and early school-age years. This gender difference is less evident with respect to severe xerophthalmia. The differences in cultural practices of feeding and care between boys and girls in some populations may explain the variation with gender when it is observed.

Physiological status

As vitamin A needs are increased during periods of rapid growth, younger children are the most vulnerable group. The demands for vitamin A are also increased during the period of gestation and lactation, and so pregnant and lactating women in underprivileged populations may be unable to meet the increased needs during those periods. Night blindness during pregnancy and lactation is especially common in south Asia, where night blindness may occur in 15–20% of all pregnancies and recur in subsequent pregnancies, and is simply considered a part of being pregnant in some cultures. Studies have also shown that the breast milk of women with poor vitamin A status frequently is low in vitamin A, and could subsequently contribute to increased susceptibility of the infants.

Diet

The basic underlying cause of vitamin A deficiency as a public health problem is a diet lacking adequate amounts of vitamin A, either preformed or provitamin A carotenoids, to meet the requirement. In general, where living conditions are poor, the diet relies on less expensive plant foods, in which the vitamin A (as carotenoids) is much less bioavailable. Populations in which rice is used as a staple food and provides the bulk of the daily diet have proved to be at especially high risk of developing vitamin A deficiency, and thus xerophthalmia is more common in south and east Asia. Subclinical vitamin A deficiency is common wherever diets are of relatively low quality owing to constraints of accessibility and availability, especially to animal foods.

Breast-feeding, the quality of complementary feeding and the quality of the childhood diet are all important factors in maintaining vitamin A status. There is good evidence that children who remain breast-fed are less likely to develop xerophthalmia than children of similar age who are fully weaned from the breast. Furthermore, an increased frequency of breast-feeding also appears to have a protective effect against xerophthalmia.

Numerous epidemiological studies support a progression of appropriate complementary feeding that has been shown to guard children from xerophthalmia through the preschool years. Intake of yellow fruit (mango and papaya) is strongly protective in the second and third years of life. As the influence of breast milk weakens, dark green leafy vegetables play a more important role from the third year onwards. After infancy, routine consumption of animal foods with preformed vitamin A (eggs, dairy products, fish and liver) is highly protective. Conversely, during the first year of life, while weaning, xerophthalmic children have been found to be less likely to be fed vitamin A-rich foods on a regular basis than have nonxerophthalmic children. Consumption of dark green leafy vegetables or yellow fruits and vegetables is associated with a four- to six-fold decrease in the risk of xerophthalmia, while the effect of only infrequent consumption of eggs, meat, fish and milk is associated with a two- to three-fold increase in risk. The dietary patterns of younger siblings in the first 2 years of life have been found to be similar to xerophthalmic cases in the same family, reflecting a chronically poor diet in high-risk households. Vitamin A deficiency is most common in populations consuming most of their vitamin A needs from provitamin carotenoid sources and where minimal dietary fat is available.

Culture-specific food habits and taboos for feeding children, adolescents, and pregnant and lactating women, often restrict consumption of potentially good food sources of vitamin A. However, it has been observed that poor dietary intake of vitamin A-rich food by children is not necessarily synonymous with a lack of availability of such foods in a household. How and with whom children eat their meals may affect their risk of vitamin A deficiency. Detailed ethnographic studies by the Johns Hopkins University group and others have shown that rural Nepalese children are twice as likely to consume vegetables, fruit, pulses, meat or fish, and dairy products when they share a plate with another relative during meals than when left to eat alone. Paradoxically, this suggestive pattern of women ensuring dietary adequacy for children, in some cultures, may predispose mothers to vitamin A deficiency. In Nepal, for example, pregnant women with night blindness were half as likely to consume vitamin A-rich foods, especially in the food-scarce hot, dry and monsoon seasons, and following the Indonesian economic crisis, mothers appeared to sacrifice their egg intake for their children.

Disease patterns

The association between infectious diseases and vitamin A status is a complex issue, and has been extensively reviewed (see Sommer and West, 1996; Semba, 1997). Vitamin A deficiency increases the risk of infectious morbidity and, conversely, infections predispose to vitamin A deficiency. Several infections, such as diarrhea, respiratory infections and measles, are associated with some form of vitamin A deficiency, either a decline in serum retinol levels or an increasing risk of xerophthalmia. Further, the frequency, duration and severity of infectious diseases contribute either directly or indirectly to increased vulnerability for vitamin A deficiency.

The presence of PEM increases the subsequent risk of xerophthalmia by nearly the same order of magnitude as does the presence of diarrhea and respiratory diseases. RBP may be reduced in PEM, reducing the availability of circulating vitamin A. During episodes of infectious disease, the decline seen in serum vitamin A partially represents a nonspecific response to fever when the synthesis of RBP, also a negative acute-phase protein, is reduced. Serum retinol levels return to normal after recovery.

Intestinal worms such as *Giardia* and *Ascaris* have also been reported to lead to reduced absorption of vitamin A and hence may contribute to vitamin A deficiency. One report failed to demonstrate any loss of vitamin A following oral administration of the vitamin A to children with ascariasis. Nevertheless, parasite infections should be treated when dealing with vitamin A-deficient populations.

Some less common diseases, such as cystic fibrosis and chronic small bowel disease, where vitamin A malabsorption is the major cause of deficiency, can be associated with xerophthalmia.

Socioeconomic conditions

In public health terms, poverty is a primary, although not invariable, cause of vitamin A deficiency. In general, vitamin A deficiency is confined largely to relatively impoverished countries. Studies have shown that households with mildly xerophthalmic children have smaller landholdings, poorer housing conditions, fewer draft and grazing animals, and lower economic standing (as measured by having fewer possessions such as radios, watches or bicycles). Although these indicators of lower socioeconomic status were found (in Bangladesh) to be associated with a 1.5–2.3 times higher risk of xerophthalmia, these characteristics do not always, by themselves, predict the occurrence of xerophthalmia. Low education levels of the father, or mother where this can be differentiated, are a further risk factor.

Clustering

The occurrence of vitamin A deficiency tends to cluster rather than be evenly distributed. Data from different countries have shown that clinical signs of deficiency cluster within provinces or districts, subdistricts, villages and even households. Figure 11.3 shows the clustering of vitamin A deficiency by district in Bangladesh. Clustering within countries is basically related to ecological and cultural factors, which are exacerbated by a

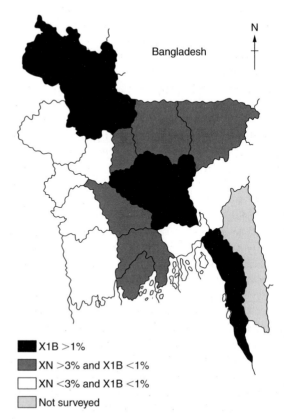

Figure 11.3 Clustering of vitamin A deficiency by district in Bangladesh. Source: Cohen *et al.* (1987).

poorly developed infrastructure, and within households and communities, by common practices and environments unhelpful to adequate diets and health. Evidence indicates that the magnitude of clustering is much greater within households than within villages, and that it is this household factor that explains much of this clustering, rather than infectious diseases. Identifying the vitamin A deficiency clusters can facilitate the implementation of an intervention program and, where a xerophthalmic child is identified, his or her siblings should be treated as being likely to be vitamin A deficient.

11.4 Prevention and control

Strategies for control and treatment

Night blindness as a symptom of vitamin A deficiency is one of the oldest recorded medical conditions. As early as 3500 BC, Egyptians treated night blindness and some eye disorders by the topical application of the juice from cooked animal liver to the eye. Ancient Greek physicians also recommended the ingestion of cooked liver, as well as its topical application, as a cure for night blindness.

Celsus (25 BC to AD 50), a Roman author on medicine, was the first to describe xerophthalmia, but his recommendation for treatment did not mention liver. In 1729, Duddell published a book on diseases of the cornea that first indicated an association between corneal blindness and systemic diseases such as measles, but without suggesting any dietary deficiency. In 1816, the French physiologist Magendie demonstrated that dogs on a diet of wheat gluten, starch, sugar or olive oil developed corneal ulceration, indicating a likely nutritional deficiency cause for the disease. Nearly 50 years later, Hubbenet first described the progression of xerophthalmia and linked it with night blindness and a poor diet. In a study published in 1881, Snell demonstrated that night blindness and xerophthalmia could be cured by giving the patient cod liver oil.

By the end of the nineteenth century, xerophthalmia was recognized in many parts of the world, including continental Europe, the UK, the USA and some tropical countries. In 1904, Mori reported an epidemic proportion of cases of conjunctival xerosis and keratomalacia among preschool Japanese children, and he described an association between xerophthalmia and dietary deficiency of fat. He also demonstrated that cod liver oil could cure the disease.

A major understanding of the nature of vitamin A deficiency and its cure developed during the first two decades of the twentieth century. In 1909, Stepp in Germany identified a small amount of lipid in the diet that was essential for the survival of mice. During the period 1906–1912, Hopkins in England found a growth stimulating factor in the alcoholic extract of milk, which he termed "accessory food factor". In 1913, in the USA, McCollum and Davis in Wisconsin and Osborne and Mendel in Yale showed that the lipid fraction of certain animal fats such as butter, egg yolk or cod liver oil was essential for the growth of rats, and also cured eye disorders. McCollum termed this lipid-soluble substance "fat-soluble A". In 1931, building on the many outstanding discoveries made in the intervening 20 years in relation to vitamin A deficiency and growth, xerophthalmia, abnormal tissue differentiation and resistance to diseases, Karrer and his colleagues in Switzerland elucidated the chemical structure of vitamin A. Subsequently, in 1936, two groups, Fuson and Christ, and Khun and Morris, synthesized vitamin A (retinol).

Treatment

Treatment guidelines were updated in 1997. Children with any stage of xerophthalmia should be treated with vitamin A according to WHO treatment guidelines; that is, with high-potency vitamin A at presentation, on the next day and 1–4 weeks later (Table 11.1). Antibiotic therapy may be needed according to the presenting child's condition. Nutritional and other health education should be offered to the mother or caretaker to try to prevent a return of the same patient later, and because the rest of the family is also likely to be at risk. As both the patient and child are likely to be suffering from, or at risk of, other deficiencies or diseases, an assessment should be made of the whole child, as in integrated management of childhood illness (IMCI) guidelines.

Early childhood night blindness responds within 24–48 h of administering 200 000 IU (6600 mg) vitamin A treatment. Although the WHO guidelines treat pregnant night-blind women with either 25 000 IU (825 mg) each week or 10 000 IU (330 mg) daily for at least 4 weeks, a randomized trial in Nepal reported that long-term, weekly supplementation with approximately 23 000 IU only prevented about two-thirds of maternal night-blindness cases. This recommendation was recently reviewed by the WHO and no change to the current recommendations of maximum safe doses was made.

Table 11.1 Treatment of xerophthalmia and measles in all age groups

Timing of dose[a]	Children aged 0–5 months	Children aged 6–12 months	Children over 12 months, male adolescents and male adults[b]
Immediately on diagnosis	50 000 IU	100 000 IU	200 000 IU
The following day (give to mother to administer at home on the next day if necessary)	50 000 IU	100 000 IU	200 000 IU
At a subsequent contact (at least 2 weeks later)	50 000 IU	100 000 IU	200 000 IU

Source: WHO (1997).
[a] All vitamin A to be given orally and as an oil-based preparation.
[b] Unless in a medical emergency, women of reproductive age should not receive this supplement.

However, xerophthalmic children with severe PEM need to be carefully monitored and given additional doses as needed, usually every 4 weeks, until their nutritional, especially protein, status improves. Individuals with corneal xerophthalmia must be treated according to the schedule shown in Table 11.1, with a topical application of an antibiotic eye ointment in order to prevent a secondary bacterial infection. Improving the nutritional status of a malnourished child, while not correcting vitamin A deficiency, can make greater demands on the already deficient vitamin A stores and produce overt clinical signs of vitamin A deficiency. Children suffering from vitamin A deficiency will most often be suffering multiple micronutrient deficiencies and this should be considered when giving the dietary advice and nutrition education that should always accompany treatment.

In women of reproductive age with night blindness or Bitot's spots, a daily dose of 10 000 IU or a weekly dose of 25 000 IU of vitamin A for at least 4 weeks is the recommended treatment schedule. However, women of reproductive age, whether pregnant or not, who exhibit severe signs of xerophthalmia and thus risk immediate loss of the eye and blindness, should be treated as described in Table 11.1. It has been suggested that in populations with a high prevalence of HIV infection (>10%), neonates should be given an extra dose of 50 000 IU at birth, with particular attention being paid to the vitamin A (and other micronutrients) status of pregnant and lactating mothers.

Prevention

The main causes of vitamin A deficiency in the developing world are insufficient dietary intake of vitamin A, poor bioavailability of provitamin A sources, especially in vegetables, and the lack of vitamin A in the cereal staple (such as rice). Other important contributory factors include the increased requirements at certain stages in the life cycle, increased utilization of vitamin A during infection, especially measles, and sociocultural factors such as intrahousehold distribution and gender. Preventing vitamin A deficiency and its consequences should therefore address vitamin A intake, concurrent infectious diseases and the wider context in which children and families live.

The public health significance of vitamin A deficiency was recognized and acknowledged globally in December 1992, at the Food and Agriculture Organization (FAO)/WHO International Conference on Nutrition (ICN), where representatives of 159 countries agreed to eliminate vitamin A deficiency (and the iodine deficiency disorders) as public health problems by the end of the twentieth century and to reduce substantially the prevalence of iron-deficiency anemia. In 1990 the World Summit for Children, sponsored by UNICEF, had established broader goals for the health and well-being of children, and the nutrition goals, including those for the micronutrients, agreed to at this forum were echoed at the ICN.

The intervention options available for prevention and control of vitamin A deficiency are:

- food-based approaches, including dietary diversification, nutrition education and fortification of staple and value-added foods
- supplementation with vitamin A capsules, with increasing interest in a multimicronutrient supplement and weekly low-dose supplements
- public health interventions such as immunization, adding vitamin A supplementation to national

Table 11.2 Different public health approaches to modifying vitamin A intake used in the prevention and control of vitamin A deficiency

Food-based

Dietary diversification
    Home gardening
    Nutrition education
    Development of high carotenoid content varieties of staple foods

Fortification
    Sugar
    Flour
    Margarine, edible oils
    Noodles
    Condensed milk and other diary products
    Condiments
    Other food vehicles

Supplementation

National distribution to all preschool children
National immunization days and national micronutrient days[a]
Through health system centers, including maternal and child
    health programs
With Expanded Programme of Immunization (EPI)
Postpartum supplementation
Life-cycle distribution to adolescents and young women through
    schools and factories

Complementary public health interventions

Ecological, political and socioeconomic interventions

[a] Can also be combined with other child public health measures.

immunization days, promotion of breast-feeding and treatment of infectious diseases
- change in the possibilities that are available to people by modification of the political, socioeconomic and physical environment; as with so much of public health, those most vulnerable are those who are poorest.

These different approaches (Table 11.2) are complementary, and should generally not be started alone, as they may have different time-frames and differing feasibility depending on local circumstances. Behavioral change to improve the intake of micronutrients is an essential part of whatever method is being used; through communications, social and political facilitation, social marketing and nutrition education.

Food-based approaches

Vitamin A and its precurser carotenoids are found abundantly in many plant foods and animal products. However, poor families usually do not have enough to eat; their diets are not likely to include much nutrient-rich food and so are likely to be low in vitamins and minerals as well as energy. Foods richest in the more

bioavailable vitamin A are animal foods. These foods not only are generally more expensive, but are the first to be eliminated from the diet when income drops, especially in urban settings. This low accessibility to food sources is aggravated by the low bioavailability of the accessible foods, and it is poor dietary quality, rather than quantity, that is considered to be the key determinant of impaired micronutrient status, including vitamin A deficiency. In poorer communities in Africa and Asia, often more than 80% of the diet is of plant origin, with a resulting low bioavailability. Although dietary diversification may be adequate to prevent vitamin A deficiency, it is unlikely to cure it unless animal sources, such as liver, are available.

Dietary diversification

Nevertheless, improving dietary diversification through increasing the variety and frequency of micronutrient-rich food sources through nutrition education and horticultural approaches has been shown to be effective in many settings. Interventions to achieve dietary diversification can include nutrition education concerning available foods, horticultural approaches such as home gardens, and improved methods of food preparation, preservation and cooking that conserve the micronutrient content. There is also increased interest in the genetic manipulation and breeding of staples and other foods to have higher and more available micronutrient content.

Although home gardening is a traditional family food production system widely practiced in many developing countries in the world, anecdotal experience suggests that home gardening (as an intervention method for improving nutrition) has been generally successful at the pilot or local phase, but often has not been scaled up successfully. Recent experience in Bangladesh, by Helen Keller International (HKI) with extensive participation from local nongovernmental organizations (NGOs), has demonstrated a successful example where it has been expanded to a national level and been sustained for over 10 years. Where home gardening is traditionally practiced, using such an approach to increase micronutrient intake is more likely to be successful. It is also recognized that such community-based approaches have other important outcomes, such as empowerment of poor, female home gardeners.

Fortification

Both staple foods and more processed commercial products can be fortified to improve micronutrient (including vitamin A) content and availability in the diet. Micronutrient interventions, and particularly fortification, have been identified by the World Bank as amongst the most cost-effective of all health interventions, and fortification has been a major factor in the control of micronutrient deficiencies in the industrialized world.

There is considerable experience in many countries of Latin America, especially vitamin A in sugar in Guatemala and other Central American countries, and with commercial foods in Asia, with fortification as a prime approach to address micronutrient malnutrition. Other food vehicles, besides sugar, fortified with vitamin A, include fats such as margarine and oils, tea, cereals, flour, monosodium glutamate and instant noodles, as well as milk and milk powder, whole wheat, rice, salt, soybean oil and infant formula. It is interesting to note that vitamin A deficiency in Europe did not disappear until margarine was routinely fortified. In India red palm oil is added to other edible oils, and red palm oil can now be made colorless (an apparent consumer preference) while retaining the β-carotene content. In the Philippines vitamin A is being added to a wheat flour product, pandesal, and the technology of fortifying with both vitamin A and iron has recently been demonstrated. Noodles (or the accompanying sauce and flavorings) are fortified with vitamin A and other micronutrients in south-east Asia. Zambia is working to establish vitamin A fortification of its sugar supply.

Fortification is only one arm of the prevention strategy, but by becoming commercially viable it can reduce the size of the at-risk population needing other measures such as supplementation (Figure 11.4). Where the costs are passed on to the consumer and the food industry routinely fortifies, this approach is potentially very sustainable.

Supplementation

The rationale of supplementation with high doses of vitamin A (usually as retinyl palmitate) rests on the fact that this fat-soluble nutrient can be stored in the body, principally in the liver. Periodic high-dose supplementation (200 000 IU or ~6600 mg every 4–6 months) is intended to protect against vitamin A deficiency and its consequences by building up a reserve of the vitamin for periods of reduced dietary intake or increased needs. Because of the recognized efficacy and effectiveness of vitamin A in deficient populations, supplementation has recently been reemphasized as a prime intervention.

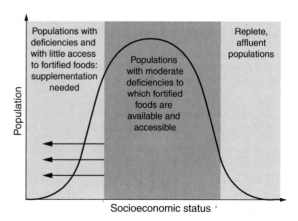

Figure 11.4 Rationale for food supplementation or vitamin supplementation to vulnerable populations. Source: Darnton-Hill (1989). Reproduced with permission from the International Nutrition Foundation.

The currently recommended doses are shown in Table 11.3. With coverage in national immunization days regularly reaching over 85–90%, supplementation is a critical tool in prevention.

A recent review of progress up to 1996 by UNICEF, the Micronutrient Initiative and Tulane University lists 34 countries providing vitamin A supplements during national immunization days or other mass campaigns. These include 10 countries in Asia and the Pacific, nine in Latin America and the Caribbean, 11 in Africa and four in the Middle East providing vitamin A capsules using this approach. Since then, coverage has been consistently maintained in several countries at over 80%. Seroconversion does not appear to be affected. The challenge will be to translate this into micronutrient campaigns (e.g. national micronutrient days), preschooler health days, vitamin A days, and so on, twice a year when the polio national immunization days are discontinued, although other national campaign approaches are planned to be implemented with measles or other vaccines in the future. There is some preliminary experience of success with national micronutrient days in Niger and the Philippines.

Vitamin A capsule coverage of greater than 30–50% of all preschool children has in the past been hard to sustain over time. Nevertheless, supplementation programs have been routine in places such as Bangladesh, India and Indonesia since the 1970s. Supplements sometimes may not reach the children most at risk, such as those in the urban slums, although success has been achieved through the national immunization days. Consequently, other approaches are being used

Table 11.3 Summary schedule for high-dose vitamin A supplementation of postpartum women and infants/children in vitamin A-deficient areas[a]

	At birth	6 weeks (e.g. DTP1)	10 weeks (e.g. DTP2)	14 weeks (e.g. DTP3)	9 months (or any time between 6 and 11 months)	12–59 months
Mother	200 000 IU at delivery and another 200 000 IU during the safe infertile postpartum period[b], at least 24 h after the first dose[c]					
Infant/child		50 000 IU	50 000 IU	50 000 IU	100 000 IU	200 000 IU every 4–6 months

[a] Experimental evidence suggests that in deficient individuals vitamin A stores fall below optimal levels between 3 and 6 months after a high dose. Considerable protection against deficiency (at least sufficient to prevent xerophthalmia and probably most deficiency-related deaths) will generally be obtained by providing supplements at least once every 4–6 months. Twice yearly has become an accepted norm, largely for logistical and resource convenience.

[b] The safe infertile period for breast-feeding mothers to receive high-dose vitamin A is within 8 weeks of delivery; for nonbreast-feeding women it is within 6 weeks of delivery.

[c] At least 24 h apart and preferably longer.

DTP: diphitheria-tetanus-pertussis vaccine.

Table 11.4 Prevention schedule sick and high-risk children (children with severe protein–energy malnutrition or infections such as diarrhea, respiratory disease and chickenpox, or children living in the same vicinity as children with clinical deficiency)

Age group	Vitamin A dose
Children ≥1 year of age	200 000 IU orally
Infants 6–12 months of age	100 000 IU orally
Infants <6 months of age	50 000 IU orally, once

to complement current methods of reaching the most at-risk groups, generally children under 5 and women of reproductive age. Opportunistic supplementation, by targeting sick children when they present to health centers with measles, malnutrition and diarrhea has been widely adopted (Table 11.4). Recommendations for supplementing children at expanded program of immunization (EPI) contacts in the first 6 months (50 000 IU or 1650 mg), and at 9 months (100 000 IU or 3300 mg) with measles, have recently been made following an informal technical meeting convened by the WHO. The guidelines for preventive supplementation have been recently revised, as in Table 11.3, and differing modes of delivery, such as during routine EPI contacts, clarified.

A strategy in line with an increasing emphasis on a life-cycle approach to prevent vitamin A deficiency is to give a supplement to a mother immediately postpartum and strongly encouraging breast-feeding. The poor diets that women in developing countries often consume, because of the poor availability and limited consumption of micronutrient-rich foods, lead to deficiencies of vitamin A and other vitamins and minerals. Such deficiencies have important consequences for women's own health, pregnancy outcomes and their breast-fed children's health and nutritional status. The WHO recommends that women in high-risk populations be given 200 000 IU of vitamin A within 6–8 weeks postpartum as a means to improve maternal status, raise breast milk vitamin A concentrations and improve liver stores of breast-fed infants. A trial in Bangladesh, however, found that this dosage failed to maintain adequate maternal serum and breast milk retinol levels after about the first 3 months postpartum, raising concerns about the adequacy of this regimen in achieving a sustained improvement in the vitamin A status of lactating women. This recommendation has recently been suggested to be increased to 400 000 IU postpartum, but not as a single dose, although within the safe period (8 weeks for breast-feeding mothers, 6 weeks otherwise) (Table 11.3).

Delivering multiple micronutrients, including vitamin A, using existing delivery systems such as those for iron/folate tablets for pregnant women, is also currently being explored. In line with the above-mentioned life-cycle approach, there is some discussion on multimicronutrient syrups for children, and using other delivery systems (e.g. in boarding schools and factories) for adolescents and younger women of childbearing age.

Supplementation coverage has increased markedly with on average, approximately 70% of all eligible young children in affected countries receiving at least one vitamin A supplement in 1996. UNICEF reports that in east Asia and the Pacific over 80% of the population under 5 years of age receive supplements, 75% in south Asia, 33% in Latin America, about 30% in the Middle East and north Africa, and about 25% in the rest of Africa. Out of the 78 countries with recognized vitamin A deficiency, 46 have policies of giving post-partum high-dose vitamin A to mothers within 8 weeks of birth (6 weeks if not breast-feeding). Nevertheless, UNICEF country offices reported only 17 countries where more than 10% of mothers received vitamin A after delivery.

Although the initial optimism that vitamin A supplements might interfere with mother-to-child transmission of HIV seems unlikely, current research suggests that there is a role for vitamin A and multiple micronutrients to improve the vitamin A status of HIV-positive mothers, and perhaps to reduce preterm births. There may also be an effect in infants in reducing the incidence of diarrhea.

Related public health interventions

For maximum impact other public health interventions are essential. The child who is vitamin A deficient is also often at risk of other diseases and malnutrition, and generally comes from a disadvantaged and frequently unhealthy environment. Therefore, the control of infectious diseases, expansion of measles and other childhood immunization interventions, deworming for intestinal parasites (hookworms), malaria control, promotion of breast-feeding, and proper health care such as oral rehydration therapy should be part of the prevention and control of vitamin A deficiency. The coexistence of multiple micronutrient deficiencies and interactions between micronutrients, and because micronutrients are generally ingested as part of the daily diet, make it logical to pursue an integrated approach covering more than one micronutrient. For example, treating iron-deficiency anemia with both iron and vitamin A has a greater effect than treatment with either of the micronutrients alone. A study of pregnant Indonesian women showed that 100% of the anemic women were cured by a combination therapy of vitamin A with iron, in contrast to vitamin A alone (40%) and iron alone (60%).

In affluent populations, newborns are normally born with low liver stores of vitamin A that increase rapidly after about 3 months of age throughout the preschool years. This increase presumably reflects dietary sufficiency from breast milk and complementary foods, and then diet, to provide adequate stores of vitamin A in relation to normal requirements for growth and other needs. However, mothers in countries with high levels of maternal undernutrition often have a low breast milk vitamin A concentration, which can be half that of breast milk from well-nourished populations of women. Nevertheless, breast milk provides a critical dietary source of vitamin A that is critical in poor societies in protecting children from xerophthalmia. In many populations, breast-feeding through the third and even fourth year of life is associated with a 65–90% reduction in the probability of developing xerophthalmia compared with children who have ceased breast-feeding. In Bangladesh, at 20 months, 70% of vitamin A can still come from breast milk. Despite this, in very disadvantaged environments, liver vitamin A stores often fail to accumulate in early infancy, especially if the child is not breast-fed. This is one of the main arguments in favor of supplementing infants and fortifying complementary foods for weaning children aged 6 months and over.

11.5 Assessment of vitamin A status

In public health terms, there are three reasons for the assessment of vitamin A status in populations: to estimate the magnitude of vitamin A deficiency, to identify population groups at risk for developing vitamin A deficiency, and to monitor and evaluate the progress or effectiveness of vitamin A elimination programs.

The vitamin A status of an individual is a continuum from frank deficiency with clinical signs through an adequate state to an excessive body reserve that may lead to toxicity of vitamin A. The risk of infection and increased mortality occurs with milder degrees of vitamin A deficiency without any signs of clinical xerophthalmia (Figure 11.5). Thus, it is important to recognize, even in the absence of obvious clinical signs, that subclinical vitamin A deficiency is a significant public health concern.

Clinical indicators

The standard WHO classification system for eye lesions, based on increasing severity (as above and in Table 11.5), was the traditional way of establishing vitamin

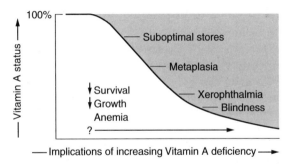

Figure 11.5 Clinical and subclinical implications of vitamin A deficiency. Reproduced from Sommer (1993) with permission from the University of Chicago Press.

Table 11.5 Criteria for assessing the public health significance of xerophthalmia and vitamin A deficiency, based on the prevalence among children less than 6 years old in the community.

Criterion	Minimum prevalence (%)
Clinical (primary)	
Night blindness (XN)[a]	>1.0
Bitot's spot (X1B)	>0.5
Corneal xerosis/ulceration/ keratomalacia (X2, X3A, X3B)	>0.01
Xerophthalmia-related corneal scar (XS)	>0.05
Biochemical (supportive)	
Serum retinol (vitamin A) <0.35 μmol/l (<10 μg/dl)[b]	>5.0

Source: WHO Expert Group (1982) Reproduced with permission from the WHO.
[a] Proposed prevalence of night blindness in pregnant women >5% (IVACG, 2001).
[b] Proposed to be >15% with serum retinol <7.0 μmol/l (IVACG, 2001).

A deficiency as a problem of public health significance. However, the relative infrequency of the eye signs requires large populations in which to detect them, and hence limits how often assessments can be done. Along with the decreasing prevalence of clinical xerophthalmia, this has resulted in greater interest in assessing the magnitude of the problem through other methods that require a smaller sample size.

In 1982, a WHO Expert Group on the Control of Vitamin A Deficiency and Xerophthalmia agreed on a set of prevalence criteria for defining a vitamin A deficiency problem of public health significance based on the clinical signs and symptoms among children under 6 years old in a community (Table 11.5). A prevalence of more than 5% of serum retinol levels below 0.35 μmol/l was defined as corroborative evidence of a public health problem. At the IVACG meeting in Hanoi in 2001, this was modified to more than 15% of under-5-year-olds with serum retinol below 0.7 μmol/l. This criterion was linked with a maternal night blindness rate of over 5% and, in countries without a vitamin A program, an infant mortality rate above 50%. Rapid dark adaptation was recommended for adoption following further testing of appropriate cut-off points.

Subclinical indicators

Vitamin A deficiency can also be assessed using specific biological indicators, with strong support from nonspecific ecological and demographic indicators.

Biological indicators

Biological indicators of vitamin A deficiency can be categorized into biochemical, histological and functional indicators.

Biochemical indicators

A wide variety of biochemical indicators is currently in use to assess subclinical vitamin A deficiency, including serum retinol, breast milk retinol, relative dose response (RDR), modified relative dose response (MRDR) and serum 30 day dose response (+S30DR). This variety reflects the lack of an ideal indicator.

A serum retinol concentration below 0.35 μmol/l (<10 μg/dl) is considered deficient, below 0.70 μmol/l (<20 μg/dl) is classified as low and greater than or equal to 1.05 μmol/l (≥30 μg/dl) is accepted as adequate vitamin A status. However, it is important to note that serum retinol provides reliable estimates of an individual's status only at the two extremes, owing to the concentration of serum retinol being controlled by homeostatic mechanisms. Furthermore, circulating vitamin A concentration is affected by many factors, such as PEM and infection. Nevertheless, serum distribution curves and proportions of individuals below estimated cut-off values are useful in defining the status of a population. The WHO 1996 report recommended the cut-off value of below 0.70 μmol/l for serum retinol as low, the point below which it is considered consistent with the presence of subclinical vitamin A deficiency.

The concentration of vitamin A in breast milk serves as an indicator of vitamin A status of the breast-fed infant. A cut-off value of below 0.35 μmol/l indicates that the infant is at a risk of vitamin A deficiency, with values above 1.4 μmol/l being considered adequate. In a vitamin A-deficient population, average values are below 1.4 μmol/l. Thus, for the status of a particular population, a cut-off value of less than or equal to 1.05 μmol/l or 8 μg/g milk fat has been suggested as deficient.

The RDR assay is based on the release of apo-RBP from the liver in response to a small dose of vitamin A (1.6–3.5 μmol/l of retinyl ester in oil). It measures the change in serum retinol concentration before and 5 h after an oral dose. The RDR, expressed as a percentage, is calculated as the ratio of the difference in serum retinol concentration between the two time-points. A response of more than 20% for RDR is considered to be positive and indicative of inadequate hepatic stores of vitamin A, that is, marginal vitamin A status. A cut-off value of at least 20% for RDR is suggested to define subclinical deficiency in population. The MRDR test is based on the same principle. It uses a dose of 0.35 μmol of 3,4-didehydroretinyl acetate (a metabolite of vitamin A, also known as dehydroretinol)/kg body weight, a single blood sample is taken after 5 h, and serum concentrations of retinol and dehydroretinol are measured. The response is expressed as a molar ratio of dehydroretinol to retinol; a value of 0.06 or above is indicates subclinical vitamin A deficiency and below 0.03 indicates adequate status. The +S30DR test is very similar to that described above for RDR, but the second blood sample is taken 30–45 days after the dosing. A cut-off value of at least 20% is used to identify a deficient individual at baseline.

Histological indicators

In vitamin A-deficient subjects, the epithelial cells of the conjunctiva of the eye become flattened and enlarged, and there is a marked reduction or absence of mucin-secreting goblet cells. Using conjunctival impression cytology or its modification, impression cytology with transfer, it is now possible to identify vitamin A deficiency by evaluating the morphology of the epithelial cells obtained from the conjunctival surface, although the actual impressions are not easy to obtain without training. In both procedures, goblet and epithelial cells are stained differentially and examined using a simple microscope. Subclinical vitamin A deficiency is identified by clearly defined criteria of normal and abnormal cytology; when 20% of a population of children have abnormal conjunctiva cytology in both eyes, there is considered to be public heath problem.

Functional indicators

For night blindness or poor adaptation to the dark, psychophysical (dark adaptation threshold) and electrophysiological (electroretinograms) techniques are available to measure dark adaptation in clinical settings. In populations above 4 years of age, vision restoration time, an objective assessment technique, measures the ability of the bleached eye to recognize a letter under dim light and thus can assess dark adaptation. The scotopic vision test (psychophysical measurement) can be used in children as young as 1 year old and is sensitive enough to detect subclinical vitamin A deficiency. This is based on the fact that the weakest threshold of light visible in the dark-adapted state is approximately of the same intensity needed to cause pupillary contraction. This technique measures the pupillary contraction in low illumination. However, these tests still need to be standardized and reference data established before being useful as functional indicators of subclinical vitamin A deficiency in a population.

In field conditions, a history of night blindness has been recommended for use as a functional indicator of subclinical vitamin A deficiency in a population. A history of the symptoms of night blindness, using a local term to describe the symptoms characteristic of the condition, can be obtained from the mother or responsible adults for a child who is at least 24 months of age. Questioning about night blindness is not consistently a reliable assessment measure where a local term is absent, and there are no clearly defined blood retinol levels that are directly associated with occurrence of the symptom. A cut-off point of prevalence of night blindness above 5% indicates a severe public health problem in a population (Table 11.6). As night blindness in women of reproductive age, especially during pregnancy, is increasingly recognized as being prevalent in developing countries (levels of 1–3% or even more), a prevalence greater than 5% is considered to demonstrate a vitamin A deficiency problem of public health significance.

Given the current understanding of the significance of vitamin A deficiency in the context of general health and survival, in 1996 the WHO recommended a set of biological indicators with cut-off levels that define subclinical deficiency. Also developed was a set of minimum prevalence criteria to define a public health problem in a community (Table 11.6). However, these recommendations still need to be validated through field studies, especially in relation to identifying degrees

Table 11.6 Criteria for assessing the severity of a public health problem using various biological indicators of subclinical vitamin A deficiency in children 6–7 months of age

Indicators (cut-off)	Prevalence below cut-offs to define the level of public health problem		
	Mild	Moderate	Severe
Functional			
Night blindness (present at 24–71 months)	>0 to <1	≥1 to <5	≥5
Biochemical			
Serum retinol (≤0.70 μmol/l)	>2 to <10	≥10 to <20	≥20
Breast milk retinol (≤1.05 μmol/l or ≤ 8 μg/g milk fat)	<10	≥10 to <25	≥25
RDR (≥20%)	<20	≥20 to <30	≥30
MRDR (ratio 0.06%)	<20	≥20 to <30	≥30
+S30DR (≥20%)	<20	≥20 to <30	≥30
Histological			
CIC/ICT (abnormal at 24–71 months of age)	<20	≥20 to <40	≥ 40

Source: WHO (1996). Reproduced with permission from the WHO. RDR: relative dose response; MRDR: modified relative dose response; +S30DR: serum 30 day dose response; CIC: conjunctival impression cytology; ICT: impression cytology with transfer.

Table 11.7 Criteria for assessing the area or population at risk of vitamin A deficiency using ecological indicators

Indicator	Suggested prevalence
Nutrition and diet related	
Breast-feeding pattern	
<6 months of age	<50% receive breast milk
≥6–18 months of age	<75% receive vitamin A-containing foods in addition to breast milk, at least three times/week
Nutritional status (<−2SD from WHO/NCHS reference for children <5 years of age)	
Stunting (height-for-age)	≥30%
Wasting (weight-for-height)	≥10%
Low birth weight (<2500 g)	≥15%
Food availability	
Market	Dark green leafy vegetables unavailable for ≥6 months/year
Household	<75% of households consume vitamin A-rich food at least three times/week
Dietary pattern	
6–71-month-old children, pregnant and lactating women	<75% consume vitamin A-rich food at least three times/week
Semiquantitative/qualitative	
Food frequency	Foods of high vitamin A content eaten less than three times/week by ≥75% of vulnerable groups
Illness-related (children 6–71 months of age)	
Immunization coverage at 12–23 months of age	<50% fully immunized or <50% immunized for measles
Measles case fatality rate	≥1%
Reported diarrhea disease rate (2 week period prevalence)	≥20%
Reported fever rates (2 week period prevalence)	≥20%
Helminthic infection rates, particularly ascaris	≥50%

Source: WHO (1996). Reproduced with permission from the WHO. NCHS: National Center for Health Statistics.

of severity. There is now a tendency to define a problem as one of public health significance rather than trying to define levels of severity (although these can be useful for advocacy purposes). When the prevalence in a population for at least two of the biological indicators of vitamin A status is below the recommended cut-off, it is said to indicate a public health problem.

Ecological and demographic indicators

The WHO 1996 report recommended a set of indicators associated with the risk of vitamin A deficiency, termed ecological and related indicators (Table 11.7). These indicators should not be used alone for determining the vitamin A status of a population and cannot replace biological indicators. However, a composite based on these indirect indicators can be used as supportive information for more direct biological indicators to identify a public health problem.

Nutritional status and diet-related indicators

Information on the breast-feeding patterns of infants up to 18 months, vitamin A-containing complementary foods (including continued breast-feeding to infants aged

6–18 months), the prevalence of low birth weight and the prevalence of stunting (<−2 Z-scores for height-for-age) and wasting (<−2 Z-scores for weight-for-height) among children under 5 years of age can all be used to identify populations at risk of vitamin A deficiency.

Dietary information is also useful in assessing the risk of vitamin A deficiency in a population. The availability or otherwise of vitamin A-rich foods in the home and the market is indicative of risk of vitamin A deficiency in a community. The dietary pattern, assessed using food frequency or 24 h recall (e.g. the HKI 24-VASQ), of consumption of vitamin A-rich foods by the vulnerable groups, such as pregnant and lactating women and children 6–71 months of age, can also be used as a risk indicator. The WHO 1996 report suggested prevalence cut-off levels for each of the above indicators to assess the risk of vitamin A deficiency in a population (Table 11.7).

Illness-related indicators

Measles case fatality, diarrheal disease prevalence, fever and helminthic infection rates may be useful in identifying populations at risk of vitamin A deficiency, and the WHO 1996 report recommended prevalence cut-off values beyond which a population would be considered to be at high risk of vitamin A deficiency (Table 11.7).

Socioeconomic indicators

Socioeconomic indicators can also provide supportive information to identify or rank areas or populations by risk of having a vitamin A deficiency problem. It has been suggested that when over half of women 15–44 years of age are illiterate, or urban households having no regular income spend more than 70% of income on food, or more than half of households spend more than 50% of income on food, then those households are at risk. Communities at risk of vitamin A deficiency include those where more than half of households have no safe water supply, poor villages over 10 km from health services, or those with inadequate access to land or agricultural services and inputs.

The WHO 1996 report proposed that when one biological indicator of deficiency (as in Table 11.6) is supported by at least four ecological indicators, two of which are nutrition and diet related, then the composite picture of demographic and ecological indicators indicates that the population is likely to have a public health problem. In practice, most surveys have used serum retinal levels to confirm and quantify a suspected problem. Any cases of xerophthalmia in a community are indicative of a wider subclinical problem.

11.6 Monitoring and evaluation

Indicators for monitoring and evaluation

Monitoring systems are designed to track the progress of a program, and to assess and improve program management and performance, by identifying where

Table 11.8 Examples of process indicators for monitoring vitamin A deficiency control programs

Vitamin A capsule supplementation program

Percentage coverage of at-risk population by program, e.g. number of capsules received and delivered/year per target population

Percentage of health centers, institutions, etc., with sufficient supplements for coverage of the target populations for a 4–6 month distribution cycle

Fortification program

Number of vitamin A-fortified foods available in selected markets

Percentage of fortified foods available in market that meet specified levels of vitamin A

Percentage of households containing a specific vitamin A-fortified food selected as suitable for consumption by target groups

Percentage of target group consuming specific fortified food

Nutrition education/social marketing program

Number of contacts for message delivery per week

Knowledge, attitudes and practices indicators of messages delivered and understood at the household level

Percentage awareness of consequences of vitamin A deficiency and local vitamin A-containing foods

Percentage of infants <24 months old consuming the recommended dietary intake of vitamin A from foods or supplements

Feeding patterns for vitamin A-rich foods, e.g. percentage of children <3 years of age eating vitamin A-rich foods three times a week

Horticulture program

Percentage of homes in a district with a garden growing provitamin A-containing foods

Percentage of schools in a district with a garden growing provitamin A-containing foods

the problems are occurring. This also allows managers to take timely corrective action. Evaluation measures the impact of the program, that is, the extent to which the programs inputs and activities change the conditions in the targeted communities.

The indicators of the effectiveness of vitamin A deficiency control programs, often referred to as process indicators, measure the functioning of program activity necessary to have an impact on vitamin A status. Table 11.8 provides some examples of process indicators that might be used in vitamin A deficiency control programs. Serum retinol, breast milk retinol and night blindness have been recommended by a WHO/UNICEF technical consultation as core indicators for assessing progress towards achieving the goal of virtual elimination of vitamin A deficiency. As shown in Table 11.9, the threshold prevalence levels of serum retinol with a cut-off level of 0.70 μmol/l or

Table 11.9 Core indicators for assessing the progress of vitamin A deficiency control programs

Indicators	Prevalence goal
Functional indicators	
Night blindness (children 24–71 months of age)	<1%
Biochemical indicators	
Serum retinol ≤0.70 μmol/l or	<5%
Breast milk retinol ≤1.05 μmol/l or ≤8 μg/g milk fat	<10%

below is set at less than 5%. A level of less than 5% of younger children with serum retinol levels 0.70 μmol/l or below is characteristic of affluent societies and children with adequate vitamin A status. When diets are adequate in vitamin A, very few mothers have breast milk retinol concentrations below 1.05 μmol/l. It is likely that the night blindness prevalence in women of reproductive age will be used as a monitoring indicator when it has been better validated.

Tracking global distribution and magnitude

Vitamin A deficiency has been identified as a major public health problem in approximately 78 developing countries, largely spanning periequatorial regions of the world (Figure 11.1), where vast numbers of rural and periurban poor are exposed to inadequate dietary vitamin A and frequent infections. The extent and severity of deficiency are most widespread where diets generally lack preformed vitamin A, such as across large areas of south and south-east Asia and Sahelian and sub-Saharan Africa.

Monitoring the undoubted progress in the control of vitamin A deficiency, and evaluating the success of programs, has only become possible since improved data became available. In 1964, Oomen, McLaren and Escapini completed a 46-country review of national health and nutrition institutions for extant reports and data on xerophthalmia, for the FAO/WHO, which indicated the global significance of this problem throughout the developing world at that time. Later preliminary estimates, published by the WHO in 1995, gave global figures for the first time but commented on the lack of available data, especially on national prevalences. Many of the data in the 1995 WHO Monitoring and Data Information System were based on small samples or localized information, and hence extensive extrapolations were made. Although these were informed and based on the best available data, they could only be estimates.

At the same time, the prevalence was certainly falling in some countries, and new problems were being identified in many African countries, or finally recognized, for example in Micronesia. These figures, which are in the process of being updated by the WHO, are probably overestimates of the true current figures. A later estimate was developed for UNICEF using a different methodology and is about half the WHO estimate, at approximately 125 million. However, these figures do not include women of reproductive age, who are now recognized as having a considerable problem in some countries. The current figures used for largely advocacy purposes are 125–240 million.

Programs to improve the intake, absorption and utilization of micronutrients in people's diets, especially in poor people, have an impact, but this must be measured to convince policy makers and governments. This is an important role for monitoring and evaluation. With the institution of international and national goals, attention has turned to the monitoring of progress and evaluation of successful, and less successful, interventions. Where an impact has not been shown in the past, for example in evaluating some of the food-based approaches, it has often been that the measurement tools used were insufficiently sensitive, or in many cases, failed to measure a less obvious behavioral or societal change that was also taking place along with the dietary change.

Part of evaluation and monitoring is some measure of sustainability. The HKI experience using local NGOs to train households, often those headed by single females, in improved home gardening, and the further experience with local nurseries, are examples of clear sustainability, and this intervention has been rigorously evaluated. Sustainability in a programmatic sense has seen supplementation in Bangladesh and India maintained for over 30 years, with reductions in clinical xerophthalmia to below WHO cut-off points. Indonesia, the Philippines and Thailand all buy their own capsules, which is one important measure of sustainability.

With efficacy being repeatedly shown for supplementation, effectiveness will reflect differences in programs under real-life circumstances. The theoretical effectiveness, or the expected reduction, is the product of efficacy and coverage, which is why increased attention is being paid to the remaining hard-to-access groups in terms of improving coverage and hence effectiveness. Effectiveness was relatively low with supplements before the success of polio national immunization days, although Indonesia has shown a coverage of around 65% through routine distribution channels. A concern already expressed is how this effectiveness will be maintained after these have been completed, although there has already been some success with micronutrient days, national child health weeks and other variants of a campaign approach.

It is often presumed that up to 30% of the population is not reached by conventional methods, and that they are also those most at risk. More careful analysis, for example in Bangladesh, suggests that at least 10% of that population is not consistently reached. One of the current challenges is to identify more exactly those who are not being reached by existing supplementation and are unlikely to be reached by fortification. It may be that some of these, presumed to be among the poorest of the poor, can only be reached by home gardening approaches, or by outreach, safety-net supplementation programs.

Progress towards elimination

There has been definite progress in reducing vitamin A deficiency, and this can only be recorded and observed if good baseline data exist. Evidence of impact has enormous implications for funding that countries commit to such programs, and for funds available from bilateral and other donors. A significant motivator has been the global goal agreed to by virtually all concerned at several international forums. The risk of vitamin A deficiency can also shift over long periods that reflect systemic improvements in economic development, food consumption, health services and the environment. Although time trend data are absent, the past century has witnessed the virtual disappearance of xerophthalmia from industrialized Western Europe, North America and Japan.

Indonesia has been declared xerophthalmia free, although it is recognized that a problem of subclinical deficiency persists, especially in rural areas. Indonesia, the Philippines and Vietnam have all seen national prevalences drop to below levels designated by the WHO as constituting a public health problem, although pockets of high prevalence exist, particularly in poorer provinces. India and Bangladesh have demonstrated a decline in prevalence, particularly of severe xerophthalmia. As Africa accumulates more prevalence data, such as the national surveys in Morocco and South Africa, it is becoming clear that most of Africa has a significant public health problem of subclinical vitamin A deficiency. National programs are now being put into place in most of these countries. Adding vitamin A to polio national immunization days has been successful in some of the poorest countries in the world, in sub-Saharan west Africa.

It is estimated that there has been a 40% decline in the prevalence of clinical signs of vitamin A deficiency since the 1990s. Similarly, subclinical vitamin A deficiency is declining. If the current rates ($\sim$70%) were maintained, the goal of eliminating clinical vitamin A deficiency as a public health problem would be reached in many countries by around 2010–2020. Subclinical deficiency elimination would take longer, but is thought to be feasible within three decades. Analyses of both the Bangladesh and Vietnam experience show that the reduction in vitamin A deficiency in those countries has been mainly an effect of the vitamin A supplementation program. This suggests that the underlying cause of lack of vitamin A in the diet (through fortification or through foods in the diet) has still not been solved, although households with home gardens were at reduced risk. Complementary approaches of nutrition education, fortification, dietary diversification and supplementation are together most likely to ensure sustainability.

11.7 Perspectives on the future

The virtual elimination of vitamin A deficiency has been endorsed as an achievable goal by virtually all countries in the world. While severe vitamin A deficiency is declining in all regions of the world, subclinical deficiency still affects between 140 and 250 million preschool children in developing countries, with associated high rates of morbidity and mortality. As these numbers do not take into account older children, adolescents and adults, these estimates probably seriously underestimate the total magnitude. The cost-effectiveness of most micronutrient interventions (including for vitamin A deficiency) continues to need advocacy to policy makers: overall, it has been estimated by the World Bank that for less than 0.3% of their gross domestic product (GDP), nutrient-deficient countries could rid themselves of these entirely preventable diseases, which now cost them more than

5% of the GDP in lost lives, disability and productivity. Given the recent success of many of the vitamin A deficiency prevention and control programs in many parts of the world, the chance of achieving the internationally agreed goal of the elimination of vitamin A deficiency and its consequences seems possible for many affected countries.

Further reading

Cohen N, Jalil MA, Rahman H, Matin MA, Sprague J, Islam M, Davison J, Leemhuis de Regt E, Mitra M. Landholding, wealth and risk of blinding malnutrition in rural Bangladeshi households. Soc Sci Med 1985; 21: 1269–1272.

Cohen N, Rahman H, Mitra M, Sprague J, Islam S, Leemhuis de Regt E et al. Impact of massive doses of vitamin A on nutritional blindness in Bangladesh. Am J Clin Nutr 1987; 45: 970–976.

Darnton-Hill I. Overview rationale and elements of a successful food-fortification programme. Food Nutr Bull 1989; 11: 92–100.

Food and Agriculture Organization/World Health Organization Expert Consultation. Requirements of vitamin A, iron, folate and vitamin B12. Food and Nutrition Series No. **23**. Rome: FAO, 1988.

Huffman SL, Baker J, Shumann J, Zehner ER. The Case for Promoting Multiple Vitamin/Mineral Supplements for Women of Reproductive Age in Developing Countries. LINKAGES/PSI/USAID. Washington, DC: LINKAGES Project, AED, 1998.

Institute of Medicine (Howson CP, Kennedy ET, Horwitz A, eds). Prevention of Micronutrient Deficiencies: Tools for Policy Makers and Public Health Workers. Summary and Key Elements. Committee on Micronutrient Deficiencies, Board of International Health, Food and Nutrition Board of the Institute of Medicine, National Academy of Sciences. Washington, DC: National Academy Press, 1998.

International Vitamin A Consultative Group (IVACG). A Brief Guide to Current Methods of Assessing Vitamin A Status. Washington, DC: LSI, Nutrition Foundation, 1993.

McGuire J, Galloway R. Enriching Lives. Overcoming Vitamin and Mineral Malnutrition in Developing Countries. Washington, DC: World Bank, 1994.

McLaren DS, Frigg M. Sight and Life Manual on Vitamin A Deficiency Disorders (VADD). Switzerland: Task Force Sight and Life, 1997.

Micronutrient Initiative/United Nations Children's Fund/Tulane University. Progress in Controlling Vitamin A Deficiency. Ottawa: Micronutrient Initiative, 1998.

Oomen HAPC, ten Doesschate J. The periodicity of xerophthalmia in South and East Asia. Ecol Food Nutr 1973; 2: 207–217.

Semba RD. The impact of vitamin A on immunity and infection in developing countries. In: Bendich A, Deckelbaum RJ (eds). Preventative Nutrition: the comprehensive guide for health professionals. Totowa, NJ: Humana Press, 1997; 489–99.

Sommer A. Nutritional blindness, xerophthalmia and keratomalacia. New York: Oxford University Press, 1992.

Sommer A, West KP Jr. Vitamin A deficiency: Health, Survival and Vision. New York: Oxford University Press, 1996.

Sommer A. Vitamin A, infectious disease, and childhood mortality: a 2 solution? J Infect Dis 1993 May; 167(5): 1003–7.

West KP Jr, Darnton-Hill I. Vitamin A deficiency. In: Preventive Nutrition, Vol. 3, Nutrition and Health in Developing Countries (Semba RD, Bloem MW, eds), pp. 267–306. Totowa, NJ: Humana Press, 2000.

Wolf G. A history of vitamin A and retinoids. FASEB J 1996; 10: 1102–1107.

World Health Organization. The global prevalence of vitamin A deficiency. WHO, Micronutrient Deficiency Information System (MDIS) Working Paper No. 2. WHO/UNICEF. Document WHO/NUT/95.3. Geneva: WHO, 1995a.

World Health Organization. Vitamin A and its Consequences A Field Guide to Their Detection and Control, 3rd edn. Geneva; WHO, 1995b.

World Health Organization. Indicators for Assessing Vitamin A Deficiency and Their Application in Monitoring and Evaluating Intervention Programmes. Geneva: WHO, 1996.

World Health Organization/United Nations Children's Fund/International Vitamin A Consultative Group. Vitamin A Supplements: A Guide to Their Use in the Treatment and Prevention of Vitamin A Deficiency and Xerophthalmia, 2nd edn. Geneva: WHO, 1997.

World Health Organization Expert Group. Control of vitamin A deficiency and xerophthalmia. Report of a Joint WHO/UNICEF/USAID/HKI/IVACG Meeting. Technical Report Series No. 672. Geneva: WHO, 1982.

12
Iodine and Iodine-deficiency Disorders

Clive E West, Pieter L Jooste and Chandrakant S Pandav

Key messages

- The ocean is the main source of iodine, and hence seafood is a rich dietary source. In areas where seafood is not regularly consumed and where iodized salt is not available, iodine intake depends, for the large part, on the iodine content of the soil.
- Iodine deficiency is prevalent in mountainous areas and areas where leaching of the soil occurs, as well as very inland areas such as central Africa.
- In 1999 the World Health Organization estimated that 740 million people had goiter: 13% of the world's population.

- An insufficient dietary supply of iodine results in suboptimal synthesis of thyroid hormones and hypothyroidism, which is responsible for a wide range of abnormalities collectively known as iodine-deficiency disorders (IDD).
- Before commencing a public health program to combat IDD in a country, the prevalence and distribution of the IDD should be known.
- Programs for increasing iodine consumption include iodized salt, iodination of drinking water and fortification of foodstuffs.

12.1 Introduction

The epidemiology of iodine deficiency disorders (IDD) is currently in a transitional phase because of the great progress seen during the 1990s in the battle against IDD, mainly in the form of national salt iodization programs. In 1999, the World Health Organization (WHO) estimated that, of its 191 member states, 130 had a significant IDD problem, with a total of 740 million people affected by goiter, or 13% of the world's total population. In 1999, of the 130 countries with IDD, 98 (75%) had legislation on salt iodization in place, and a further 12 had it in draft form. Following the promulgation of legislation on salt and the sensitization of the salt industry, there has been an enormous increase in the consumption of iodized salt, leading to a reduction in the goiter rates. The latest available data on the magnitude of IDD is indicated by the goiter rates in the different regions: 20% in Africa, 5% in America, 12% in south-east Asia, 32% in the eastern Mediterranean, 15% in Europe and 8% in the western Pacific. In 1999, the number of people at risk of iodine deficiency had probably been reduced to approximately 500 million.

12.2 Definition of iodine deficiency

The diagnosis of iodine deficiency should be seen as a group, community or population diagnosis rather than an assessment on the individual level. Although the relevant measurements are done on individuals, the summary data of the group are used for interpretation of IDD status. It is well known that biological variation, due to varying levels of hydration, could occur in the concentration of urinary iodine of different individuals. It is also known that interobserver variation is likely to exist where more than one observer performs palpation of the thyroid glands of a group of individuals. To reduce the effect of interindividual and intraindividual observer variation, sufficient sample sizes and thorough training of observers are required for valid estimates of prevalence rates.

At a consultation by the WHO, the United Nations Children's Fund and the International Council for Control of Iodine Deficiency Disorders (ICCIDD), held in May 1999 in Geneva, the following outcome indicators were recommended for the assessment of IDD and their elimination.

Table 12.1 Definition of iodine status of a population based on median urinary iodine concentration

Iodine status	Median urinary iodine concentration (μg/l)
Severe iodine deficiency	<20
Moderate iodine deficiency	20–49
Mild iodine deficiency	50–99
Ideal iodine intake	100–200
More than adequate iodine intake: may pose increased risk of iodine-induced hyperthyroidism	201–299
Excessive iodine intake	>300

Urinary iodine excretion

Urinary iodine excretion provides a good indication of recent dietary iodine intake. A sample size of at least 30 individuals will compensate for the individual variation in iodine concentration that may occur. A casual or spot urine sample should be taken in an iodine-free container, tightly sealed and stored until analysis. Great care should be taken to avoid contamination during the whole sample collection and analysis procedure.

Most laboratories use the Sandell–Kolthoff reaction in the analysis of urinary iodine, and it is advisable for laboratories to participate in quality assurance programs to ensure accurate results. It is not necessary to relate the urinary iodine to creatinine excretion. The cut-off points for defining the iodine status of a population according to the median urinary iodine concentration are given in Table 12.1.

As urinary iodine values from populations are usually not normally distributed, the frequency distributions are necessary for correct interpretation of data, and the median value should be used rather than the mean value.

For the elimination of iodine deficiency it is required that the median urinary iodine concentration should be 100 μg/l or more and not more than 20% of samples should be below 50 μg/l.

Thyroid size

The size of the thyroid gland changes inversely in response to alterations in iodine intake, with a lag interval which varies from a few months to several years depending on factors such as the severity and duration of iodine deficiency, the effectiveness of iodine intervention and possibly goitrogenic factors.

For many years thyroid size has been determined by inspection and palpation. This method appears attractive because it enables observers to examine a large number of people in a short time without the use of expensive equipment. However, there is concern about the accuracy of diagnosis with this method. Ultrasonography provides a more accurate and objective method of determining thyroid size, but it requires expensive equipment and thorough training, and the measurement takes more time.

It is important to choose an appropriate target group for determination of thyroid size. Because of the small size of the thyroid gland of neonates and preschoolers, it is neither feasible nor practical to assess goiter in this group, not even by ultrasonography.

The preferred target group is school-aged children between 6 and 12 years, and if possible, 8–10-year-old children, to avoid the rather small thyroid glands of the young children and pubertal effects in the older ones. Schoolchildren are often used for goiter studies because of their accessibility and vulnerability to iodine deficiency (Figure 12.1). Pregnant women are a prime target group for IDD control activities because they are especially sensitive to marginal iodine deficiency and are relatively accessible given their participation in antenatal clinics.

Thyroid size by palpation

Determination of thyroid size by palpation requires careful training and initial collaboration with an experienced observer. After visual inspection of the thyroid gland, the gland is palpated by gently sliding the finger along the side of the trachea (windpipe) between the cricoid cartilage and the top of the sternum. Both sides of the trachea should be palpated. The size and consistency of the gland are carefully noted. If necessary, palpation may be slightly enhanced by asking the subject to swallow to make the thyroid move up. A thyroid gland with lateral lobes each having a volume greater than the terminal phalanges of the thumbs of the subject being examined will be considered goitrous.

The size of the thyroid gland is categorized into one of the following grades:

- grade 0: no palpable or visible goiter
- grade 1: a mass in the neck that is consistent with an enlarged thyroid that is palpable but not visible when the neck is in the normal position, but moves upwards in the neck as the subject swallows; nodular alterations

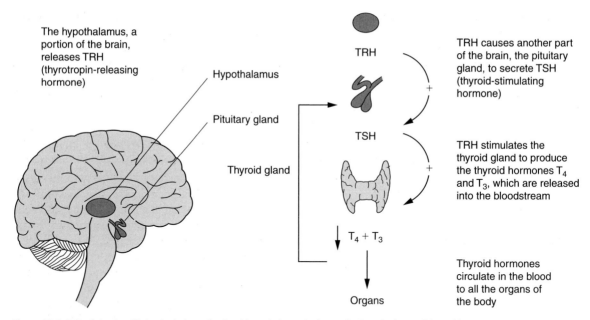

Figure 12.1 Role of the thyroid gland, pituitary gland and hypothalamus in the synthesis and release of thyroid hormones.

can occur even when the thyroid is not visibly enlarged
- grade 2: a swelling in the neck that is visible when the neck is in a normal position and is consistent with an enlarged thyroid when the neck is palpated.

This classification system based on grades replaces one based on stages. In that system grade 1 was divided into stage Ia (detectable only by palpation) and stage Ib (visible when neck fully extended; can also include nodular glands even if not goitrous), while grade 2 was divided into stage II (visible with neck in normal position) and stage III (very large goiter recognizable at a considerable distance). The total goiter rate is calculated as the sum of grades 1 and 2. When this rate exceeds 5% in 6–12-year-old schoolchildren the population is said to have a public health problem, except in the short term after the introduction of an iodization program. Usually the iodine deficiency is corrected rapidly with an effective iodization program, but the goiter rates take longer to return to an acceptable level.

Thyroid size by ultrasonography

Ultrasonography is a safe, noninvasive, specialized technique, which provides a more accurate measurement of thyroid volume than palpation. The increased accuracy of ultrasonographic measurement is particularly useful in distinguishing between goiter grades 0 and 1, in situations where the prevalence of visible goiter is small, and in monitoring iodine control programs where thyroid volumes are expected to decrease over time.

Portable instruments are available on the market and should be used with a 7.5 MHz transducer by a trained and standardized operator. No universal normative values for the thyroid volume of iodine-replete children are available, except for thyroid volumes in European schoolchildren aged 6–15 years as a function of age, gender and body surface area. Normative values for populations under investigation should be established.

Thyroid-stimulating hormone and thyroglobulin

Thyroid-stimulating hormone (TSH) and thyroglobulin can be used as indicators to assess IDD, or as surveillance indicators, under certain circumstances. Blood spots on filter paper or serum samples can be used to measure TSH, using the highly sensitive analytical assay. TSH concentrations increase in iodine deficiency as part of the feedback system involving the thyroid-related hormones. However, the increase is not great unless the deficiency is moderate or severe. Therefore, the TSH concentration in school-aged children and adults is not a good indicator for iodine deficiency, and its use in school-based surveys is not recommended. Blood-spot TSH in neonates is a valuable indicator for iodine deficiency because the neonatal thyroid has limited iodine stores and even mild iodine deficiency may increase TSH secretion. Blood can be taken either from the cord at delivery or by heel prick after birth (usually after 72 h). Usually the primary purpose of screening for neonatal TSH is to detect congenital hypothyroidism, but it can also be used as an indicator of community iodine nutrition. For this reason the screening must be universal, and must not omit children born in remote or low socioeconomic areas.

When the thyroid is enlarged in iodine deficiency larger amounts of thyroglobulin are released, increasing the thyroglobulin levels in the circulation. The laboratory technique is similar to that for TSH and other immunoassays. It has been successfully applied to blood spots, but not yet developed commercially.

Other indicators of iodine deficiency

Cretinism provides an indication of the magnitude of the IDD problem only when it is severe. The condition is comparatively rare and difficult to diagnose (particularly the more subtle cases), cases are often hidden away, and since the life expectancy of cretins varies, incidence data may be more appropriate than prevalence data.

Determining serum concentrations of the thyroid hormones thyroxine (T_4) and triiodothyronine (T_3) as indicators of iodine deficiency is usually not usually recommended as these tests are cumbersome, more expensive and less sensitive than other indicators. In iodine deficiency the serum T_4 concentration is typically lower, and the serum T_3 concentration higher, than in normal populations, but the overlap reduces the usefulness of these hormones in assessing IDD.

12.3 Clinical features

A suboptimal dietary supply of iodine results in insufficient synthesis of thyroid hormone and in hypothyroidism, which is responsible for the wide range of abnormalities collectively known as IDD.

An enlarged thyroid, or goiter, is the most apparent manifestation of iodine deficiency, and serves as a biological marker for the potential existence of other IDD.

A person is regarded as having goiter when the thyroid gland is enlarged to such an extent that the lateral lobe is bigger than the terminal phalanx of the thumb of the individual being examined. A goiter of this size is not visible but can be palpated.

When the thyroid gland is further enlarged, it becomes visible and it is estimated that in 1990 over 200 million individuals, mostly in developing countries, had visible goiter. The prevalence and severity of goiter increase with increasing severity of iodine deficiency, and become almost universal in populations where iodine intake is less than 10 μg/day. In general, goiter is not particularly serious. If the thyroid gland is large, it may be regarded as unattractive, with such consequences that is difficult to find a husband or wife. Fashions change: in the past in Europe, goiter was regarded as somewhat attractive, just as obesity was. Large goiters sometimes develop nodules, which can exert undue pressure on the trachea and esophagus, thus causing difficulty with breathing and swallowing.

12.4 Iodine metabolism

The only known function of iodine in the body is for the synthesis of thyroid hormones, which occurs in the thyroid gland. These hormones play an important role in the regulation of metabolism. Iodine is rapidly absorbed from the gut and then circulated in the form of plasma inorganic iodide (PII). From the circulation this iodide is taken up by the cells of the thyroid gland by an iodine pump (a sodium/iodine symporter) under the control of TSH, which is released from the pituitary gland. This is an active transport mechanism, which maintains a gradient of 100:1 between the thyroid cells and the extracellular fluid. This gradient can increase to 400:1 in iodine deficiency. Of the 15–20 mg of iodine in the body, 70–80% is found in the thyroid gland.

Once taken up by the thyroid cells, the iodine is released into the colloid of the thyroid gland where it is oxidized by hydrogen peroxide derived from the thyroid peroxidase system. The iodide is then incorporated into tyrosine of thyroglobulin to form monoiodotyrosine (MIT) and diiodotyrosine (DIT) (Figure 12.2). When a DIT molecule is coupled to another DIT, tetraiodothyronine or thyroxine (T_4) is formed, and when an MIT and a DIT are coupled, triiodothyronine (T_3) is formed. The thyroglobulin is then taken up by the thyroid cells by a process known

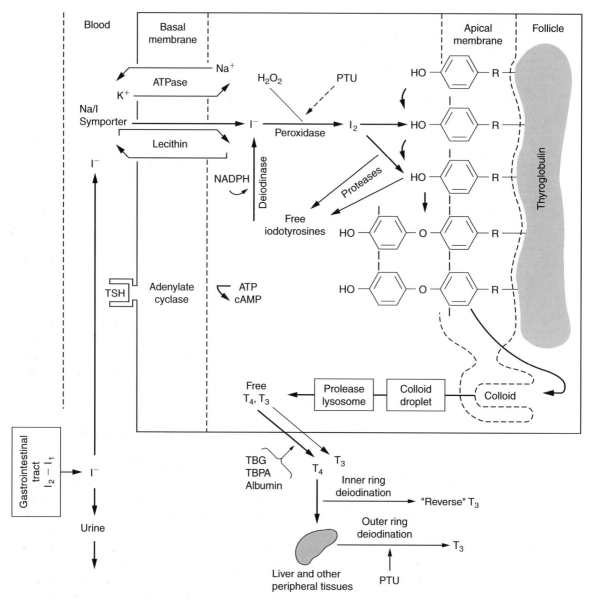

Figure 12.2 Synthesis of thyroid hormones (with formulae). H_2O_2: hydrogen peroxide; PTU: propylthiouracil; TSH: thyroid-stimulating hormone; TBG: thyroxine-binding globulin; TBPA: thyroxine-binding prealbumin.

as pinocytosis. In the thyroid cells, T_4 and T_3 are released from the thyroid gland by a process of proteolysis. The secretion of T_4 and T_3 from the thyroid gland is under the influence of TSH, the secretion of which is stimulated by thyrotropin-releasing hormone (TRH) from the hypothalamus. There is a feedback mechanism in which increased levels of T_4 inhibit the secretion of TSH directly and antagonize the action of TRH (Figure 12.3).

Thus, as the concentration of T_4 in the blood falls, TSH secretion increases and vice versa. In severe iodine deficiency, T_4 remains low and TSH is raised, and this picture of a low T_4 and raised TSH is indicative of hypothyroidism. Raised TSH can be due to iodine deficiency or can be due to congenital defects in the synthesis of thyroxine, the incidence of which is 1:4000 births. The increased TSH in iodine deficiency stimulates

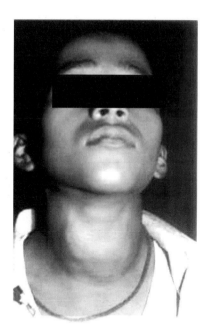

Figure 12.3 Child with a goiter.

Table 12.2 WHO/UNICEF/ICCIDD recommended dietary intake for iodine (2001)

Category	Intake (μg/day)
Infants, 0–59 months	90
Schoolchildren, 6–12 years	120
Children >12 years and adults	150
Pregnant and lactating women	200

Reproduced with permission from the WHO.

the activity of the thyroid cells, resulting in hypertrophy and hyperplasia of thyroid cells to produce the enlargement of the thyroid gland, which is called a goiter.

When the iodine supply to the thyroid gland is limited, it produces more T_3 (which is more active than T_4) and less T_4 is produced. When T_4 levels are low, target tissues also convert T_4 to T_3. However, it should be noted that the brain can take up T_4 but not T_3, so brain function is affected when T_4 levels are low even though there may be sufficient T_3 to carry out the function of thyroid hormones in other organs and tissues. When the iodine supply to the thyroid gland is limited, the gland releases thyroglobulin into the circulation, some of which contains no thyroid hormone (T_4 or T_3). Thus, an elevated thyroglobulin level is a candidate indicator of iodine deficiency that has lasted for months or years.

After 12 weeks of gestation, the thyroid and pituitary, which are responsible for the production of T_4 and TSH, respectively, have developed. The hypothalamus, responsible for the production of TRH, develops from the 10th to the 30th week. Thus, up to about 20 weeks, the fetus is dependent on the mother for the supply of T_4. After this time, the fetus produces its own TSH, which can stimulate fetal production of T_4. The concentration of the usual form of T_3 remains low because the 5-deiodinase present (type III or ID-III) results in the formation of reverse T_3. (Reverse T_3 lacks an iodine

atom in the inner ring of the molecule, as opposed to the normal form of T_3 which lacks an iodine atom in the outer ring; see Figure 12.2. Reverse T_3 is inactive, while normal T_3 is more active than T_4.) Just before birth, there is a change from ID-III to 5′-deiodinase (type I deiodinase or ID-I), which produces the normal form of T_3.

Selenium is a component of the 5′-deiodinases (ID-I and ID-II) and 5-deiodinase (ID-III). There is evidence from the Democratic Republic of Congo (formerly Zaire) that selenium deficiency may precipitate IDD in areas where both iodine and selenium are deficient.

12.5 Reference intakes for iodine

Requirements for and sources of iodine

The recommended dietary intakes for iodine for different age categories and for pregnant and lactating women are given in Table 12.2.

The ocean is the main source of iodine, and hence seafood such as fish, shellfish and edible seaweed is a rich dietary source. An ecological iodine cycle in nature starts in the form of evaporation of seawater (containing iodine), which is carried by wind and clouds to land areas. This falls as rainwater which partly replenishes the losses of iodine in the topsoil, but snow, rain, floods and rivers again leach the iodine to the sea. Some iodine derived from the soil finds its way into drinking water and in very small amounts to plants and animals and their products such as cereals, legumes, fruit, vegetables, meat, milk and eggs. Therefore, in areas where seafood is not regularly consumed and where iodized salt is not available, the intake of iodine depends, to a large extent, on the content of iodine in the soil where people live.

Iodine deficiency is prevalent in mountainous areas and in other areas where leaching of the soil occurs and where the level of iodine in the soil and water used for drinking and irrigating crops is low. Iodine deficiency also occurs in lowlands, far from the oceans, such as the central part of Africa. In industrialized countries, the iodine content of the soil is less important because the food supply is more diverse, it comes from a much wider area and iodized salt is widely available.

Dietary sources of iodine

The uptake of iodine by the thyroid gland and subsequent release of thyroid hormone from the gland are inhibited by three types of goitrogens.

Those which produce substances that compete with iodine uptake by the gland include the cyanogenic glycosides present in cassava, maize, bamboo shoots, sweet potatoes, lima beans and millet. The cyanogenic glycosides release cyanide, which forms thiocyanate, which competes with iodine for uptake by the gland. Substances derived from coliform bacteria also seem to compete with iodine uptake by the gland and incorporation into thyroid hormones.

Those which produce substances that block (non-competitively) the uptake of iodine by the gland are goitrins (5-vinyl-2-thiooxazolidones). They inhibit not only the incorporation of iodine into thyroid hormones but also the coupling processes to produce T_4. Because the inhibition is noncompetitive, it cannot be overcome by increasing the intake of iodine in the diet. Goitrins are produced by the genus *Brassica* (cabbage, rape and mustard) of the family Cruciferae, which also produce thiocyanate, which has a similar effect to that produced from cyanide, as described above.

Those which produce substances that block the proteolysis of the thyroid hormones from thyroglobulin include excess iodide and substances from some seaweeds. When the bioavailability of iodine is low because of the presence of goitrogens in the diet the daily intake of iodine needs to be increased by 50–100 µg.

12.6 Public health aspects to iodine deficiency

Public health implications of iodine deficiency

From a public health point of view the manifestations of iodine deficiency, at all ages, are considered extremely important because they are preventable. The most critical period of iodine deficiency is during fetal life and early childhood when the developing brain is particularly vulnerable to iodine deficiency and the consequent insufficient thyroid hormones. The spectrum of IDD at the different stages of life is shown in Table 12.3. The net result of these disorders on societies can be seen in their lower productivity and higher demand for social services.

Whereas the attention in iodine deficiency was previously focused on endemic goiter in the early years, it has now shifted to the effects of hypothyroxinemia in the development of brain and central nervous system between the 15th week of gestation to 3 years of life. These changes are irreversible and may lead to permanent neurological defects and deficient learning abilities. The result of the neurological effects can also be seen in the lower intelligence quotient, between 10 and 15 points, of children in iodine-deficient areas, and in poor school performance. Moreover, some studies have reported improved performance on tests of intellectual functioning of school-aged children given iodine supplementation.

Iodine-induced hyperthyroidism (IIH) is the most important side-effect that may develop in a few

Table 12.3 Spectrum of iodine-deficiency disorders at the different stages of life

Life stage	Iodine-deficiency disorders
Fetus	Abortions, stillbirths, congenital anomalies Increased perinatal and infant mortality Neurological cretinism (mental deficiency, deaf–mutism, spastic diplegia, squint) Myxedematous cretinism (dwarfism, mental deficiency) Psychomotor defects
Neonate	Neonatal goiter Neonatal hypothyroidism Increased susceptibility to nuclear radiation
Child and adolescent	Goiter Juvenile hypothyroidism Impaired mental function Retarded physical development Increased susceptibility to nuclear radiation
Adult	Goiter with complications such as impaired breathing and swallowing Hypothyroidism Impaired mental function Iodine-induced hyperthyroidism Increased susceptibility to nuclear radiation

susceptible individuals as a result of the rapidly increased intake of iodine. IIH is therefore considered one of the IDD. Following the introduction of iodization of salt or bread, or the use of iodized oil in the 1920s, IIH has occurred in many countries, including the USA, the Netherlands, Austria, Brazil, Australia (Tasmania), Ecuador and, more recently, in Zimbabwe and the Democratic Republic of Congo.

Additional iodine over and above the basic or usual intake, even at usual physiological concentrations, carries a risk of inducing IIH in susceptible people. Iodine from any source, whether it is derived from iodized salt, drinking water, medication, iodized oil, Lugol® solution, iodine-containing food or iodine in almost any chemical form, carries a risk of causing hyperthyroidism. Endemic IIH appears to be a temporary phenomenon, related to the rapid introduction of iodized salt into areas formerly affected by severe IDD. In Switzerland, it was shown that long-term supplementation of iodine ultimately reduces the incidence of hyperthyroidism. Because the benefits of salt iodization programs on whole populations far outweigh the risk of IIH in a few individuals, the current approach is to continue iodization programs while alerting and informing physicians about the diagnosis and treatment of IIH.

Hyperthyroidism occurs, in contrast to the reverse situation in hypothyroidism, when excessive amounts of the thyroid hormones T_4 and T_3 are in the circulation. Focal areas, or more commonly single or multiple nodules in the thyroid gland, become autonomous and produce an excess of hormones. Therefore, the critical event in the development of IIH is autonomy of thyroid function.

Autonomy can be defined as the functioning of the thyroid follicular cells in the absence of the normal physiological stimulatory effect of TSH. Despite the inhibitory effect of the elevated thyroid hormones on the pituitary resulting in depressed TSH secretion, uncontrolled thyroid hormone secretion continues as long as sufficient iodide is available. IIH occurs mostly, but not exclusively, in older people, particularly women, with preexisting multinodular goiter (toxic nodular goiter) and in people with Grave's disease who live in areas where severe iodine deficiency is treated with any form of iodine fortification or supplementation. Euthyroid people with autonomously functioning foci may also develop hyperthyroidism when sufficient amounts of iodine become available.

Thyrotoxicosis refers to the clinical effects resulting from an excess of thyroid hormone, irrespective of its origin. These effects may include nervousness, anxiety, palpitations, weight loss, muscle weakness, fatigue, sweating and heat intolerance. The most severe manifestations of IIH are cardiac, of which palpitations are probably the most common cardiac symptom. Other consequences of IIH include tachycardia, systolic hypertension, atrial fibrillation, heart failure and cardiomyopathy. The clinical diagnosis of IIH is often subtle because of the similarity between some of the signs and symptoms of IIH and some infectious diseases, or of aging and chronic illness. When the clinical effects of thyrotoxicosis are observed in patients with goiter or in people whose iodine intake increased in the recent past, it would be advisable to pursue biochemical tests such as the highly sensitive TSH assay, and free and total T_4 and T_3. Other biochemical tests are the T_3 resin uptake test, thyroglobulin and thyroid antibodies. If available, thyroid imaging consisting of ultrasound with a 5 MHz transducer (or higher frequency), and radioactive scans (scintigraphy) are very useful in distinguishing the underlying type of thyroid disease, and the structure and function of the thyroid.

Once positively diagnosed, IIH patients are usually treated with antithyroid drugs, radioiodine or surgery, with long-term follow-up.

12.7 Management of iodine deficiency

Depending on the severity of IDD, the accessibility of the target population, the availability of a universal iodine carrier and the resources available for combating the IDD problem, one or a combination of strategies may be decided upon to eradicate iodine deficiency in a particular country. Strategies decided upon depend on:

- the severity of IDD
- the accessibility of the target population
- the resources available.

Programs may include one or both of the following strategies:

- food-based approaches
- use of natural foods.

Because iodine deficiency is generally the result of the lack of iodine in drinking water and in the soil and water on which crops for human and livestock consumption are grown, the selection of natural foods either to increase iodine intake or to reduce the consumption of goitrogens is not generally regarded as an effective way of combating iodine deficiency. Increasing iodine consumption is usually much more effective.

Use of iodized salt

For many years iodized salt has been the most effective way to combat IDD in a large number of countries. A joint policy from the WHO, UNICEF and the ICCIDD recommends that in order to provide approximately 120–140 μg/day of iodine the iodine concentration in salt at the point of production should be within the range of 20–40 mg of iodine per kilogram of salt. This recommendation assumes that 20% of the iodine will be lost from the production site to the household and another 20% lost during cooking, and that the average salt intake is 10 g per person per day.

Either potassium iodate or iodide may be used for fortification, but iodate is more suitable in hot and humid climates because of its greater stability. The iodine losses and requirements under local conditions should be determined, and health officials should ensure that proper monitoring of iodized salt is regularly conducted. Salt designated for specific purposes can be targeted for iodization. For example, in the Netherlands the salt used in the baking of bread has been iodized since 1942, but availability of iodized table salt was only promoted in a limited way until recently. The iodine levels in both bread and table salt were increased in 1982 and in 1998 in response to a decrease in the average consumption of bread.

Iodination of drinking water

This approach, using different kinds of iodinators, has proved to be successful in some areas, provided the iodine concentration is not too high. In an iodine-deficient area of China iodination of irrigation water has increased the iodine status of women and decreased neonatal and infant mortality.

Fortification of infant formulas

In view of information on the thyroid function and physiology of preterm babies, the iodine content of many infant formulas seems to be inadequate. As premature babies in many countries are iodine deficient, ICCIDD recommended in 1992 that the level of fortification for preterm formulas and starting formulas, in terms of the final concentration in the prepared formulas, should be 200 μg/l and 100 μg/l, respectively.

Fortification of other foods

In a number of countries, for example the UK, iodine deficiency was eliminated fortuitously (that is, by accident) through the use of iodophores (iodine-containing detergents) in cleaning milking machines and through iodine supplementation of feed for dairy cows. When the use of iodophores has been controlled, iodine deficiency has also been reported to reappear. Other foods have also been investigated as carriers for iodine, for example fish paste in Thailand and sugar in Sudan.

Fortification of foods consumed by farm animals

IDD in animals are receiving increasing attention because increasing the iodine status of farm animals has been shown to improve their health and economic productivity. Improving the iodine status of animals would also lead to increased iodine status of humans consuming animal products such as meat, dairy products and eggs. Thus, iodine deficiency control programs should also address the problem of iodine deficiency in farm animals. Care should be taken to ensure that the level of iodine provided, usually added to salt, is sufficient to overcome deficiency without being excessive.

Nutraceutical approach

Use of iodized oil

In some developing countries with moderate or severe IDD iodized salt is not universally available or does not reach remote areas. Under circumstances where other iodine supplementation strategies have failed or are not practical, treating iodine deficiency with iodized oil is very effective. Large quantities of iodine are administered intramuscularly or orally in the form of slowly resorbable iodized oil. The effectiveness of orally administered iodized oil appears to be enhanced with the use of monounsaturated oil such as rapeseed oil and peanut oil compared with the traditionally used poppyseed oil. Intestinal parasites have been found to inhibit the absorption of iodized oil. Thus, when using iodized oil to control iodine deficiency, deworming before dosing will increase the duration of effectiveness of iodized oil. No studies have been carried out to assess the effect of worm load or deworming on increasing iodine requirements or reducing the effectiveness of iodized salt in controlling iodine deficiency.

Use of potassium iodide solution

A 10% potassium iodide solution is an easily prepared, readily available, simple and cheap alternative approach when the main methods (iodized salt and iodized oil) used to prevent and control iodine deficiency are not immediately available. Iodide doses of approximately 30 mg every month or 8 mg every 2 weeks can be delivered conveniently as a simple solution using a dropper bottle.

12.8 Assessment and elimination of iodine deficiency disorders

Indicators used for assessing IDD and their elimination may be subdivided into process indicators and outcome indicators. In the temporal sequence of events, the process indicators measure the factors that are likely to play a causal role in the response of the outcome indicators. Ideally, both process and outcome indicators should be included as variables in the assessment of the IDD situation in a community or country.

Process indicators

Several public health strategies have been implemented globally to eliminate IDD on a community and on a population basis. The most universal strategy is the iodization of salt, and this section will therefore focus on the process indicators assessing national salt iodization programs.

Salt is iodized by the addition of fixed amounts of potassium iodide or iodate either as a dry solid or an aqueous solution at the point of production. The actual availability of iodine from iodized salt at the consumer level can vary over a wide range as a result of several factors. These factors include the varying amounts of iodine added during the iodization process, uneven distribution of iodine in the iodized salt within batches or individual bags (owing to inefficient mixing), the extent of loss of iodine due to salt impurities, packaging and environmental conditions during storage and distribution, and the loss of iodine during food processing and cooking in the household. The loss of iodine from iodized salt stored in porous packaging may range from 30 to 80% within a period of 6 months in a hot and humid climate.

In the assessment of the IDD situation it is therefore appropriate to measure the iodine content of iodized salt. Potentially, the assessment of iodine content of salt

can be performed at one or more of three levels: at the production site (or at the entry point when salt is imported into a country), at the retail level and at the household level.

Factors such as the objectives of the assessment, logistics and accessibility will determine at which level the assessment should be done. Usually the most useful information is obtained at the point of production and at the household level. The most accurate results are obtained by the titration method, but for monitoring purposes at the household level, the rapid test kit may be used as a qualitative indication of whether or not household salt is iodized. The test kits currently in use do not provide an accurate quantitative measure of iodine concentration in salt.

In addition to measuring the iodine concentration of salt, it is necessary to establish the coverage of iodized salt at household level in a representative sample of a community or population. Coverage refers to the proportion of households using adequately iodized salt, that is, household salt with an iodine concentration of more than 15 mg/kg. Ideally, this percentage should exceed 90%. This process indicator provides a measure of the extent to which a salt iodization program has been successfully implemented, and also indicates whether or not favorable observations in outcome indicators could be expected.

Observations on the iodine concentration of salt, and on the proportion of households consuming adequately iodized salt, would be interpreted more accurately if the amount of salt consumed per person were known. In general, it is assumed that the daily consumption of salt varies between 5 and 10 g per person in most populations. However, this assumption may not be valid in some populations who, owing to cultural nutritional habits, consume considerably more salt, or other populations who, as a result of low socioeconomic conditions, consume less salt. Although it is difficult to establish the daily salt consumption in a population, this information would not only assist in the interpretation of process indicators, but also be useful in determining the appropriate level of iodization.

Outcome indicators

Before commencing a public health program to combat IDD in a country, the prevalence and the distribution of the IDD should be known. A national survey is the usual way to define the magnitude of an IDD problem in a country. In the absence of a national survey, proxy information may also be useful, such as regional IDD data or data from some geographical areas that indicate the existence of IDD.

Outcome indicators recommended by the WHO/UNICEF/ICCIDD consultation for the assessment and elimination of IDD are described in detail in Section 12.2. These include:

- urinary iodine secretion
- thyroid size, TSH and thyroglobulin
- cretinism
- T_4 and T_3 levels.

Other sources of data, such as the knowledge that cretins were born, information obtained through a national screening system for TSH, historical data that IDD existed in specific areas and information about IDD in neighboring countries, may also be indicative of IDD.

12.9 Perspectives on the future

Unlike the situation for infectious diseases that may be cured, and even permanently eradicated, the fight against IDD must continue indefinitely. Once iodine deficiency is diagnosed in an area, it is likely that iodine intervention will be required indefinitely. Several examples have shown a return of IDD during lapses in iodine prophylactic measures. Sustainability of IDD elimination programs is absolutely critical and requires continuous political support, administrative backup and the generation of scientific data to maintain the fight against IDD.

Further reading

Dunn JT, ed. IDD Newsletter. Obtainable free of charge for those interested in iodine deficiency disorders from: Dr JT Dunn, Box 511, University of Virginia Medical Center, Charlottesville, VA 22908, USA.

Dunn JT, van der Haar F. A practical guide to the correction of iodine deficiency. Technical Manual No. 3. ICCIDD, 1990. Canada.

Hetzel BS, Pandav CS, eds. S.O.S. for a Billion: The Conquest of Iodine Deficiency Disorders. Delhi: Oxford University Press, 1994.

Jooste PL, Weight MJ, Lombard CJ. Short-term effectiveness of mandatory iodization of table salt, at an elevated concentration, on the iodine and goiter status of schoolchildren with endemic goiter. Am J Clin Nutr 2000; 71: 75–80.

World Health Organization/United Nations Children's Fund/International Council for Control of Iodine Deficiency Disorders. Assessment of Iodine Deficiency Disorders and Monitoring their Elimination. WHO/NHD/01.1, 2001.

World Health Organization/United Nations Children's Fund/International Council for Control of Iodine Deficiency Disorders. Progress towards the elimination of iodine deficiency disorders (IDD). Report of a Joint WHO/UNICEF/ICCIDD Consultation. WHO/NHD/99.4. Geneva: World Health Organization, 1999.

13
Iron-deficiency Anemias

Kamasamudram Vijayaraghavan

Key messages

- Iron-deficiency anemia (IDA) is the most common nutritional disorder in the world. The numbers are staggering: as many as 4–5 billion people, 66–80% of the world's population, may be iron deficient; 2 billion people, over 30% of the world's population, are anemic, mainly as a result of iron deficiency, and in developing countries, frequently exacerbated by malaria and worm infections.
- Iron deficiency and anemia reduce the work capacity of individuals and entire populations, bringing serious economic consequences and obstacles to national development. Conversely, treatment can raise national productivity levels by 20%.

- Nine out of 10 IDA sufferers live in developing countries; on average, every second pregnant woman and four out of 10 preschool children are anemic.
- For children, health consequences include premature birth, low birth weight, infections and elevated risk of death. Later, physical and cognitive development is impaired, resulting in lowered school performance. For pregnant women, IDA contributes to 20% of all maternal deaths.
- There are four main approaches to the prevention and control of IDA: iron supplementation, food fortification, nutrition education and agricultural approaches to improve the iron availability of common foods.

13.1 Introduction

Iron-deficiency anemia (IDA) is the most common nutritional disorder in the world, constituting a public health condition of epidemic proportions. It particularly affects women in the reproductive age group and young children in tropical and subtropical regions. The World Bank estimates that the direct contribution of IDA to global burden of disease is 14 disability-adjusted life-years per 1000 population. It has the greatest overall effect in terms of ill-health, premature death and lost earnings.

Prevalence

IDA affects over 2 billion people in the world. In the developing countries alone, 370 million women suffer from IDA. The average prevalence is higher in pregnant women (51%) than in the nonpregnant women (41%). The prevalence among pregnant women varies from 31% in South America to 64% in south Asia (Figure 13.1). South and south-east Asia combined contribute to 58% of the total anemic people in the developing world. In North America, Europe and Australia IDA during pregnancy is less common. Even in the USA, about 5% of young children and 5–10% of women of reproductive age suffer from IDA. About 20–30% of pregnant women in low socioeconomic strata in the USA exhibit iron deficiency during the third trimester of pregnancy. Surveys from North America and Europe indicate that, among pregnant women, the prevalence of anemia ranges between 10 and 30%. In the developing countries, the problem of iron deficiency is high. In India about 88% of pregnant women are anemic and in other parts of Asia almost 60% of women are anemic; in China, however, the prevalence does not exceed 40%.

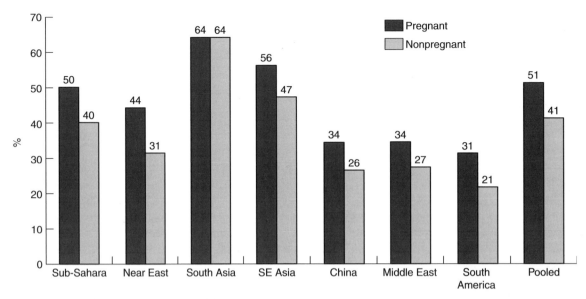

Figure 13.1 Prevalence of anemia in women in different regions.

13.2 Definition and clinical features of iron-deficiency anemia

Anemia occurs when hemoglobin production is considerably reduced, leading to a fall in its levels in the blood. The World Health Organization (WHO) recommends cut-off values to determine IDA in different age, gender and physiological groups (Table 13.1).

Although most anemia is due to iron deficiency, the role of other causes (such as folate and vitamin B_{12} deficiency or anemia of chronic disease) should be distinguished.

Iron depletion can be categorized into three stages of varying degrees of severity ranging from mild to severe (Figure 13.2).

- The first stage involves a decrease in iron stores, which is diagnosed by a decreased serum ferritin level. Although not associated with adverse physiological consequences, this represents increased vulnerability from long-term marginal iron balance that could lead to severe iron deficiency.
- The second stage is characterized by biochemical changes reflecting a lack of iron for normal hemoglobin production. There is decreased tranferrin saturation or increased erythrocyte protoporphyrin, and increased serum transferrin receptor levels.
- The third stage of iron deficiency is anemia. In severe IDA the levels of hemoglobin are less than 7 g/dl.

Table 13.1 Cut-off points for hemoglobin values for the diagnosis of anemia

Population group	Hemoglobin (g/l)
Adult men	<120
Nonpregnant and nonlactating adult women	<120
Pregnant women	<110
Lactating women	<120
Children <6 years	<110
Children >6 years	<120

Source: WHO (1972). Reproduced with permission from the WHO.

Iron nutritional status can be assessed by the following biochemical and hematological tests.

Serum iron concentration

In IDA, serum iron may either be low or even normal. It is regulated by reticuloendothelial release. The normal values vary between 50 and 175 μg/dl. There is a considerable diurnal variation; the levels are highest in the morning and lowest during the night. It is reduced in inflammation and malignancy and during menstruation. Therefore, this test cannot be really considered as of real diagnostic value.

Total iron binding capacity

Total iron binding capacity (TIBC) and transferrin saturation indicate iron supply to tissues. The normal value

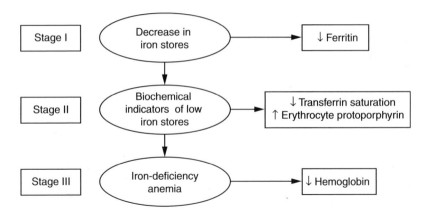

Stage I	Decrease in iron stores	→	↓ Ferritin
Stage II	Biochemical indicators of low iron stores	→	↓ Transferrin saturation ↑ Erythrocyte protoporphyrin
Stage III	Iron-deficiency anemia	→	↓ Hemoglobin

Figure 13.2 Stages of iron depletion.

is about 300 µg/dl. TIBC is lowered in chronic disease and raised in iron deficiency.

Transferrin saturation

This is a ratio (expressed as a percentage) of serum iron and TIBC. The normal value is 33%. In iron deficiency, there is a decreased saturation, while in chronic diseases the saturation is normal.

Protoporphyrin

Protoporphyrin is the precursor of heme. Free red blood cell (RBC) protoporphyrin is raised when there is an insufficient supply of iron for heme synthesis. It is also high in IDA, caused by lead toxicity and other sideroblastic anemias.

Serum ferritin

Serum ferritin reflects the status of total body iron stores. It is generally considered as the test of choice for estimating iron stores. A value below about 10 ng/ml is considered as diagnostic of iron deficiency. However, its levels are raised in inflammation, infections and liver disease. The effect of infections on serum ferritin often limits the usefulness of serum ferritin as a sensitive indicator of iron stores, particularly in areas where the incidence of infections is very high, as in the developing countries of south-east Asia. The criteria generally used to diagnose iron deficiency are listed in Table 13.2.

Transferrin receptors

Transferrin receptors become elevated on cell surfaces and in plasma whenever there is insufficient iron supply to cells or iron depletion. The ratio of transferrin to ferritin may be a good discriminator between iron deficiency and anemia of chronic inflammation.

Table 13.2 Diagnostic criteria for iron-deficiency anemia

Indicator	Cut-off guideline
Serum iron (µg/dl)	<60
Total iron binding capacity (µg/dl)	>300
Transferrin saturation (%)	<15
Erythrocyte protoporphyrin (µg/dl)	>100
Serum ferritin (µg/l)	<12

Because of the cost implications for multiple biochemical tests, the parameter used to indicate iron status in population studies of IDA is measured by hemoglobin.

Clinical features of iron-deficiency anemia

The symptoms of IDA depend on the rate at which anemia develops in an individual. Symptoms may relate to rate of fall in hemoglobin. Since lowering of hemoglobin affects oxygen carrying capacity, in IDA, any physical exertion leads to shortness of breath. Initially, most patients complain of increasing lethargy and fatigue. More unusual symptoms are headache, tinnitus and disturbance in taste. There is often a poor correlation between hemoglobin level and symptoms. As the severity of deficiency increases, the patients develop pallor of the conjunctiva, tongue, nailbeds and soft palate. In IDA of longer duration, there may be papillary atrophy of the tongue and, the nails may become spoon shaped (koilnychia). There may also be enlargement of the spleen (splenomegaly). In children, chronic IDA may lead to behavioral changes; they may have impairment of cognitive function and short attention spans and appear withdrawn.

13.3 Iron metabolism

The human body requires iron for the synthesis of the oxygen transport proteins, hemoglobin and myoglobin in the body, and other iron-containing enzymes that participate in electron transfer and oxidation–reduction reactions. An active process in the duodenum absorbs iron. The iron thus absorbed is mobilized across the mucosal and serosal membranes into the blood where the plasma transport protein (transferrin) transports it to the cells or the bone marrow for erythropoiesis. Transferrin delivers iron to the tissues by transferrin-specific cell membrane receptors. The cell receptors bind the transferrin–iron complex at the cell surface and carry it into the cell to release iron.

In the human body, iron is distributed in six compartments (Box 13.1). Total body iron in men is about 3.8 g, while in women it is 2.3 g. In men, about one-third of the total body iron is storage iron, whereas in women it forms only about one-eighth. Approximately two-thirds of the total iron is functional, serving either a metabolic or an enzymic function. Almost all of this is in the form of hemoglobin, circulating within the RBC. Myoglobin and other iron-containing enzymes constitute about 15% of functional iron.

The factors influencing iron balance are intake of iron, iron stores and iron loss. Adult males require about 1 mg of absorbed iron daily to replace the losses in gut secretions, epithelial cells, urine and skin. In menstruating females this can increase to 1.4 mg.

Iron homeostasis, as with the most of the other metals, is maintained by controlling absorption, which increases during deficiency and decreases when erythropoisis is depressed. The body can excrete iron in a limited capacity and the excess is stored either as ferritin or as hemosiderin in the liver, spleen and bone marrow.

Inadequate iron intake will:

- enhance absorption of dietary iron
- mobilize the body's iron stores

> **Box 13.1** Storage sites for iron in the body
>
> - Hemoglobin (2–2.5 g of iron)
> - Storage iron as ferritin and hemosiderin (1 g in men; 600 mg in women)
> - Myoglobin in skeletal and cardiac muscle (130 mg of iron)
> - Labile iron pool (80–90 mg iron)
> - Tissue iron consisting of heme and flavoproteins (6–8 mg of iron)
> - Transport iron forming (3 mg of iron)

- reduce the transport of iron to the bone marrow
- lower the hemoglobin levels, leading finally to IDA.

Hemoglobin plays a crucial role in the transport of oxygen. With moderate IDA, there is a compensatory mechanism by biochemical changes to compensate for the reduced oxygen carrying capacity of blood. In contrast, in severe IDA, the markedly reduced hemoglobin content decreases the oxygen carrying capacity, leading to chronic tissue hypoxia.

Iron absorption

The primary regulatory mechanism of iron balance is iron absorption through the gastrointestinal tract. Since humans have no physiological pathway for the excretion of iron, the regulation of the intestinal absorption of iron is crucial. As duodenal crypt cells mature into absorptive enterocytes, their capacity for iron absorption reflects the iron status prevailing at the time of maturation. The low pH of gastric juice helps in dissolving the ingested iron and facilitates enzymic reduction of ferric iron to the ferrous form by a brush-border ferrireductase. However, the mechanism by which the iron absorption is regulated is still not very clear.

Body iron stores and the hemoglobin status of individuals determine the percentage of iron absorption. Since women and children have lower iron stores, they absorb a higher proportion of dietary iron. In pregnancy, as iron stores decline with gestation, iron absorption gradually and steadily becomes more efficient. Conversely, the higher iron stores in males reduce the percentage of iron absorbed, thereby protecting against iron overload. About two-thirds of the total body iron is contained in RBC. Destruction or production of RBC accounts for most of iron turnover. Most of the iron of destroyed RBC is recaptured for the synthesis of hemoglobin.

Iron is widely distributed in meat, eggs, vegetables and cereals, but the concentrations in milk, fruit and vegetables are low. The iron content per se of individual foods has little meaning as iron absorption varies considerably. There are two types of food iron: nonheme iron, which is present in both plant foods and animal tissues, and heme iron, coming from the hemoglobin and myoglobin in animal products. Heme iron represents 30–70% of the total iron in lean meat and is always well absorbed. Nonheme iron from meat and vegetable foods enters a common nonheme iron pool in the gastric juice, from which the amount of iron absorbed depends to a large extent on the presence of enhancing and inhibiting substances in the meal and on the iron status of the individual.

Heme iron is obtained mostly from meat, poultry and fish, and is at least two to three times better absorbed than nonheme iron. Nonheme iron is derived mostly from plant and dairy products and accounts for more than 85% of dietary iron. Several factors are known to enhance or inhibit iron absorption. The absorption of nonheme iron is strongly influenced by the presence of iron absorption inhibitors and enhancers of iron solubility in the upper part of the small intestine. Factors affecting iron absorption are listed in Box 13.2.

Iron absorption enhancers

The best known enhancer of iron absorption is ascorbic acid (vitamin C), which can increase nonheme iron absorption significantly. Thus, amla, guava and citrus fruits increase iron absorption from plant foods. Factors present in meat also enhance nonheme iron absorption. Lactoferrin, a milk glycoprotein present in breast milk, binds iron, enabling the optimal use of iron by delivering iron during deficiency and preventing its availability for intestinal bacteria. Although the iron content of breast milk is same as that of cow's milk, in view of better absorption, breast milk is a better source of iron than either cow's milk or nonfortified milk substitutes.

Iron absorption inhibitors

The inhibitors of iron absorption include calcium phosphate, bran, phytic acid and polyphenols. Phytic acid, which is extensively present in cereals and legumes, is the major factor responsible for the poor bioavailability of iron in these foods. Since fiber per se does not inhibit iron absorption, the inhibitory effect of bran is solely due to the presence of phytic acid. Soaking, fermentation and germination of these food grains improve absorption by activating phytases to degrade phytic acid. Polyphenols (phenolic acids, flavonoids and their polymerization products) are present in tea, coffee, cocoa and red wine. Tannins present in black tea are

the most potent of all inhibitors. Calcium, consumed in dairy products such as milk or cheese, can inhibit iron absorption. Other components, particularly the enhancers of iron absorption, and especially in a complex meal, however, can offset the inhibitory effect of the polyphenols and calcium.

Iron storage

Iron is stored as ferritin or hemosiderin primarily in the liver, reticuloendothelial cells and bone marrow. In the liver it is stored in parenchymal cells or hepatocytes, while in the bone marrow and spleen it is stored in reticuloendothelial cells. The stored iron is mainly a reservoir of iron to supply cellular needs for hemoglobin production. It is important to note that the iron bound to ferritin is more readily mobilized than that bound to hemosiderin. The total amount of storage iron varies considerably without any apparent impairment of body functions. Storage iron may be totally depleted before the appearance of IDA. Under conditions of long-term negative iron balance, the stores are depleted before the onset of iron deficiency in the tissues. When there is positive balance, iron stores increase slowly even when the absorption of iron is lower, as in postmenopausal women.

Iron losses

Iron losses in healthy individuals occur primarily in feces (0.6 mg/day), bile and desquamated mucosal cells, and in minute quantities of blood. Urinary losses are small. Women of reproductive age, in addition to the basal losses, lose iron in menstruation. The median menstrual blood loss is about 30 ml/day, which is equivalent to an additional requirement of 0.5 mg of iron per day. This daily blood loss is computed from the iron content of blood lost during the menstrual period over a month. About 10% of women lose as much as 80 ml of blood, corresponding to a loss of 1 mg of iron per day. Adopting the higher value (1 mg/day), the total (basal plus menstrual) loss of iron in women would be 30 μg/kg per day (>1.5 mg/day). Such women cannot maintain positive iron balance if iron requirements are based on median menstrual loss of 30 ml. In the tropical countries, hookworm infestation is a major cause of gastrointestinal blood loss contributing to iron deficiency in older children and adults. In the developed world, among adults, chronic use of drugs such as aspirin, bleeding tumors and ulcers contribute to iron losses.

Box 13.2 Factors influencing iron absorption

- Type of food consumed
- Interactions between foods
- Regulatory mechanisms in the intestinal mucosa
- Bioavailability (utilization of ingested iron for metabolic functions)
- Amount of iron stores
- Rate of production of red blood cells

13.4 Reference intakes for iron

The concept of dietary reference values is covered in detail in Chapter 7 of *Introduction to Human Nutrition* and more information on iron can be found in Chapter 9 of the same book. The following is an outline of the principles involved in coming to these recommended values.

Daily (absorbed or physiological) iron requirements are calculated from the amount of dietary iron necessary to cover basal iron losses, menstrual losses and growth needs. They vary according to age and gender, and in relation to body weight they are highest for the young infant. An adult man has obligatory iron losses of approximately 1 mg of iron daily, largely from the gastrointestinal tract (exfoliation of epithelial cells and secretions), skin and urinary tract. Thus, to remain replete with regard to iron, an average adult man needs to absorb only 1 mg of iron from the diet on a daily basis. Similar obligatory iron losses for women amount to around 0.8 mg daily. However, adult women experience additional iron loss owing to menstruation, which raises the median daily iron requirement for absorption to 1.4 mg (this covers 90% of menstruating women: 10% will require daily absorption of at least 2.4 mg iron to compensate for their very high menstrual losses). Pregnancy creates an additional demand for iron, especially during the second and third trimesters, leading to daily requirements of 4–6 mg. Growing children and adolescents require 0.5 mg iron daily in excess of body losses to support growth. Physiological iron needs can be translated into dietary requirements by taking into account the efficiency at which iron is absorbed from the diet. A full-term healthy baby is born with iron stores adequate for the first 6 months of life. For this reason, iron deficiency is rarely seen in breast-fed babies before 6 months of age. After 6 months, solid foods should be gradually added to the baby's diet to meet their increased requirements for iron and protein (see Chapter 16).

Current RDA values for iron are summarized in Table 13.3. An important aspect that requires consideration while computing requirements for iron is the percentage of iron absorbed from the diet. While a value of 5% is assumed for cereal–legume-based diets, about 10–15% is used for diets containing meat and animal products.

13.5 Public health implications of iron-deficiency anemia

In the developing countries, IDA is associated with poor reproductive performance, a higher proportion of maternal deaths (10–20% of the total deaths), a high incidence of low birth weights (<2.5 kg weight at birth) and intrauterine malnutrition. IDA in children impairs scholastic performance. The available evidence indicates impaired psychomotor development and intellectual performance, and changes in behavior following IDA (see Chapter 15). There is also evidence of decreased resistance to infections in iron deficiency. IDA substantially reduces the work capacity of individuals; even a mild degree of IDA can reduce performance during brief but intense exercise. Studies among men working in rubber plantations in Indonesia and women working in tea plantations in Sri Lanka indicate reduced productivity of iron-deficient individuals compared with healthy subjects.

Risk factors for anemia

Poor iron stores
The iron stores of Asians are negligible as evidenced by low bone marrow hemosiderin levels and low liver stores. When the infants are born with poor iron stores iron, deficiency is aggravated in infants who are solely breast-fed for prolonged periods.

Dietary inadequacy
The major determinant of IDA, particularly in the developing countries, is inadequate dietary consumption.

Table 13.3 RDA values for different age groups[a]

	Age and gender	Iron (mg/day)
Infants	First 6 months	0.27
	7–12 months	11
Children	1–3 years	7
	4–8 years	10
Teenage boys	9–13 years	8
	14–18 years	11
Teenage girls	9–13 years	8
	14–18 years	15
Adult men	≥19 years	8
Adult women	19–50 years	18
Adults	≥51 years	8
Pregnant women		27
Lactating women	<18 years	10
Lactating women	19–50 years	9

[a] Recommended by the US Food and Nutrition Board in 2001. Reproduced with permission from the WHO.

Many people are dependent on plant-based foods in which the iron absorption is poor and several substances in the diet interfere with iron absorption.

Increased demands

There is increased demand for iron during pregnancy. Rapid growth during infancy and childhood increases iron requirements. Iron requirements increase considerably during puberty; in girls the onset of menstruation imposes a double burden.

Malabsorption and increased losses

Repeated episodes of diarrhea, resulting from unhygienic practices, can result in malabsorption. The incidence of diarrhea is particularly high in most of the developing countries. Infestations, especially hookworm infestation and ascariasis, result in iron losses and malabsorption of iron. In endemic areas repeated attacks of malaria can lead to IDA. In women, postpartum hemorrhage due to poor obstetric care, repeated and closely spaced pregnancies, prolonged periods of lactation and the use of intrauterine contraceptive devices for birth control are important contributory factors.

Hemoglobinopathies

Abnormal formation of hemoglobin, as in thalassemia and sickle cell anemia, is an important non-nutritional factor.

Drugs and other factors

Drug idiosyncrasy, leukemia, radiation therapy, anticancer and anticonvulsant drugs are some of the risk factors. Among the elderly, IDA is associated with chronic inflammatory conditions such as arthritis, gastrointestinal blood loss from long-term use of drugs such as aspirin, and tumors.

Prevention and control of iron-deficiency anemia

The basic principles in the prevention of IDA are to ensure regular consumption of iron to meet the requirements of the body and to increase the content and bioavailability of iron in the diet. There are four main approaches:

- provision of iron supplements
- fortification of commonly consumed foods with iron
- nutrition education
- horticulture-based approaches to improving the iron bioavailability of common foods.

Iron supplementation

The essential principle of management of IDA is iron replacement therapy and treatment of the underlying cause, such as parasitic infections or gastrointestinal bleeding. Oral iron therapy is the preferred form of treatment. Ferrous sulfate is the most inexpensive and widely used oral iron preparation. Other preparations such as ferrous gluconate or ferrous fumerate may also be given. A total dose equivalent to 60 mg of elemental iron (300 mg of ferrous sulfate) per day is adequate for adults, and should be given between meals either in the morning or at bedtime. In the case of infants and young children, 30 mg/day of elemental iron would be adequate. In general, over a period of 4 weeks a hemoglobin rise of about 2 g/dl would be expected. It is important to remember to continue iron therapy for about 3 months, even after the hemoglobin level becomes normal. In very severe IDA with hemoglobin in the range 5–7 g/dl, packed-cell transfusion is recommended. The common side-effects of iron supplementation are nausea, constipation, black stools and even diarrhea. The risk of side-effects is proportional to the iron dose. Poor compliance is the major reason for failure to respond to iron therapy, so simultaneous and appropriate counseling of the individuals may be required.

In the developing countries, where IDA is widely prevalent, universal iron supplementation of women and children would be appropriate. In segments of the population of higher socioeconomic groups, selective provision of iron supplements only to anemic individuals would be preferable. This approach, however, requires screening of individuals for IDA, requiring suitable skilled staff and laboratory facilities.

Oral iron is the treatment of choice for prevention of IDA. In general, daily supplements providing about 100 mg of elemental iron are recommended for a period of about 100 days to the most vulnerable groups of population, such as pregnant women. The dosage is fixed, taking into consideration the biological effectiveness and the side-effects. The common side-effects of oral iron therapy are gastrointestinal disturbances such as constipation and the passing of dark stools. Prolonged use may lead to joint pains. The success of such a program depends on the distribution of adequate quantities of iron supplements and adherence to treatment. As far as possible, the delivery should be done through the existing delivery systems. The experience in India is an example of the shortcomings of such programs when attempted on a large scale. In 1970, India adopted a national program of supplementation of daily iron and folic acid tablets (for 100 days) to pregnant women, lactating mothers and young children. Evaluation of this program indicated that, owing to inadequate and irregular supplies of the supplements, there was no change in the prevalence of IDA in the country. Similarly, in Indonesia, even after 10 years of distribution of 120 mg of iron daily for 3 months to all pregnant women, the prevalence of IDA remained high.

Unfortunately, under the present socioeconomic conditions in which the current dietary intakes are not adequate, pregnant women in developing countries will continue to require iron supplementation to meet their iron needs. For this reason, there is a need for alternative approaches to supplementation such as the use of small-dose iron supplementation and slow-release iron preparations. Slow-release iron preparations can achieve the same benefit as the lower dose iron with very few side-effects. Weekly iron supplementation in place of daily iron distribution has also been suggested; this may result in greater absorption of the iron dose, but may only be effective under supervised conditions.

Fortification

Fortification of some commonly consumed foods with iron is an attractive option to tackle the problem of inadequate dietary intakes in the community. The food fortificant and food vehicles should be safe and effective. Foods successfully used as vehicles for food fortification are wheat, bread, milk powder, salt, infant formula and sugar. Sweden has a long history of fortifying wheat flour with iron, at a rate of 65 mg/kg. In the USA wheat flour is also fortified with iron (44 mg/kg). In India, multicentric field trials indicate that iron-fortified common salt has been effective in reducing the prevalence of IDA in rural communities.

Nutrition education

Extensive and persuasive efforts are required to bring about behavioral changes in the community for people to adopt dietary diversification. Ultimately, the only sustainable solution to IDA is to help the communities to consume regularly foods that are rich in iron, to encourage intake of promoters of iron absorption such as vitamin C and to discourage high consumption of inhibitory factors.

The following approaches are considered as important in preventing and controlling nutritional anemias in general:

- promotion of the consumption of iron-rich foods, e.g. pulses, green leafy vegetables, other vegetables and meat products
- encouraging regular consumption of foods that are rich in vitamin C, e.g. citrus fruits, guava and amla
- promotion of the addition of iron-rich foods to weaning foods
- discouraging consumption of foods that inhibit iron absorption, particularly by women and children.

Person-to-person communication still remains an effective method of communication in most of the developing countries. Group talks, slide shows, folk plays, street plays, television and radio are the other methods of nutrition education. Social marketing, which applies marketing principles to improve nutrition awareness by involving communication experts, may be one of the strategies to be adopted.

Agriculture and horticulture approaches

Horticulture strategies to encourage production of iron-rich vegetables and fruits are an important component of any long-term approach to control and prevent IDA in the developing countries. It is paradoxical that IDA is widely prevalent in countries where a wide variety of iron-rich foods and iron absorption promoters are already available. At the government level, there is a need to add nutrition components to all horticulture and social forestry programs, while at the household level, efforts should be made to encourage production of vegetables. Home gardening is one of the sustainable approaches to control IDA in poor rural communities. It is rather paradoxical that communities involved in agriculture require extension and education to raise nutritious foods in their backyards. An advantage of home gardening is that it facilitates consumption of multiple nutrients. In the case of IDA, in addition to providing iron-rich foods, it facilitates inclusion of iron absorption promoters in the diet.

13.6 Perspectives on the future

Genetically modified (GM) foods use biotechnological techniques to increase the micronutrient content of foods by genetic manipulation. Foods such as carotene-rich canola oil and vitamin A-rich golden rice are being produced in some countries. A similar strategy would help to increase production of iron-rich foods in the countries where per capita availability of iron rich foods is very low. However, there is a need to develop proper monitoring mechanisms to protect against any deleterious effects due to the use of such GM foods. Proper labeling is needed in the case of use of processed foods based on GM ingredients. Multisectoral and integrated approach will be required to eliminate IDA in the poorer communities. The cooperation of the sectors of health, education, agriculture and industry is essential.

Further reading

Bruce M. Small, Iron Metabolism and Deficiency. Buffalo: State University of New York, 1998.

Charlton RW, Bothwell TH. Iron absorption. Ann Rev Med 1983; 34: 55–68.

National Research Council. Recommended Dietary Allowances, 10th edn. Washington, DC: National Academy Press, 1989.

Peters TJ, Raja KB, Simpson RJ, Snape S. Mechanisms and regulation of intestinal iron absorption. Ann N Y Acad Sci 1988; 526: 141–147.

Viteri FE, Torun B. Anaemia and physical work capacity. Clin Haematol 1974, 3: 609–626.

World Health Organization Expert Group Nutritional Anaemias, WHO Technical Report Series No. 503, Geneva: WHO, 1972.

World Health Organization. The Prevalence of Anaemia in Women: A Tabulation of Available Information, 2nd edn. WHO/MCH/MSM/92.2. Geneva: WHO, 1992.

World Health Organization/United Nations Children's Fund. Report on Consultations on Indications and Strategies for Iron Deficiency Anaemia Programme. Geneva: WHO, 1994.

14
Fear of Fatness and Fad Slimming Diets

Mary AT Flynn

Key messages

- Fear of fatness and fad dieting carry serious implications for public health owing to associated unhealthy slimming practices, which include smoking and dietary restraint, which may cause growth stunting among nutritionally vulnerable groups such as children and pregnant women.
- Fear of fatness and fad dieting represent a major barrier to public health nutrition programs because fad diets do not reflect population-based dietary guidelines, which are designed to address the specific nutritional inadequacies and chronic diseases of the population.
- Fear of fatness and fad dieting present an enormous challenge to obesity prevention programs and necessitate

- sensitivity and a multistrategic approach, which includes effective techniques to build self-esteem and reduce stigma associated with fatness.
- In the face of rapidly rising obesity levels and the prioritization of obesity prevention in public health, caution is needed to ensure that no harm is done in terms of the development of body image concerns and fad dieting among previously unaffected groups.
- Priority research needs include the development and evaluation of programs that are effective in the long term at preventing fear of fatness and fad dieting, especially among children and adolescents.

14.1 Introduction

Fear of fatness (body dysphoria) may be described as a culture-bound syndrome in that it appears to be limited to a number of cultures with similar psychosocial features. In the modern world the factors that foster fatness phobia appear to prevail in Western cultures or cultures strongly influenced by them. Nonetheless, several reports suggest that fatness phobia is not a modern phenomenon, while others propose that Mary Queen of Scots (b. 1542, d. 1587) and the Empress Elisabeth of Austria (b. 1837, d. 1898) may be included among the many women affected. Fatness phobia can be largely explained by the stigmatization of obesity and this is not exclusive to modern Western societies. For example, during medieval times, fatness was considered to be the Karmic consequence of a moral failing in the Buddhist context, while in Europe such a stigma was based on the Christian deadly sin of gluttony. Furthermore, cases of anorexia occurring in the sixteenth century and earlier have been referred to as holy anorexia because such

dietary restraint was predominantly associated with religious life. Indeed, such origins may explain the severely abstinent and self-denying characteristics of modern-day anorexia nervosa and the "good" connotations of dietary restraint as opposed to the "sinful" connotations of breaking a diet.

From 1600 up to our own times anorexia has been described as becoming more of a concept that depends upon, and reflects, the changing directions of medical fashion from physical, psychiatric and sociocultural viewpoints. The importance of cultural and societal factors for defining pathological eating behaviors can be appreciated by considering how the typical eating behaviors of bygone days would be viewed today. For example, the everyday eating habits of the Romans during the first two centuries AD, including the bulimic behaviors of the Roman emperors Claudius and Vitellius, were not considered abnormal at the time, but would certainly be considered pathological nowadays.

Anorexia nervosa and bulimia are recognized eating disorders requiring clinical and psychological management. Fear of fatness is a necessary precursor of these eating disorders, but the majority of people obsessed with body image and exhibiting this fear of fatness do not go on to develop clinically manifest eating disorders. Because it is so widespread, fear of fatness is a very significant public health issue and is the primary focus of the present chapter.

14.2 Epidemiology

Fear of fatness affects far more women than men, which explains why the quest for slenderness is largely regarded as a female matter. Fear of fatness and fad dieting may persist even during pregnancy. After controlling for body weight, white women living in Western societies, or cultures strongly influenced by these, have been shown to be the most vulnerable to fear of fatness. However, other studies have shown that among women who diet within the vulnerable societies, unhealthy eating attitudes and practices may be similar regardless of their ethnic background. Apart from Japan, there are very few quantitative studies on eating disorders from Asian, Middle Eastern, Hispanic or African countries.

Adolescent girls are recognized as being most at risk and in vulnerable societies it is estimated that up to 70% may be affected. Fear of fatness is so pervasive among adolescent girls that is has been referred to as "a normative discontent" for this age and gender group. However, fatness phobia starts well before adolescence and studies indicate that children as young as 9 years try to lose weight, with roughly double the number of girls affected compared with boys.

After adolescence, the lasting effects of fear of fatness were described in a 10-year follow-up study of American college students. Although this study showed that women experienced an overall decline in body weight concerns as they matured into adulthood, many of those who were dissatisfied with their bodies continued dieting and engaging in disordered eating. While few women who were satisfied with their weight and shape in college developed weight phobia and eating problems in adulthood, quite a different picture emerged for the men involved in the study. More than half of these men gained more than 4.5 kg (10 lb) in the 10 years after leaving college and their body weight concerns, eating-disordered attitudes and behaviors were found to increase accordingly.

During adulthood, the largest natural fluctuations in body weight and body fatness occur during pregnancy. In general, slenderness does not seem to be important for female appearance during pregnancy and this condition has been shown to legitimize increased food intake. Nevertheless, although studies suggest that fear of fatness and associated unhealthy slimming behaviors diminish for many women during pregnancy, this is not a universal trend. There are reports to suggest that a significant minority of pregnant women continue to control their weight gain by restraining their food intake, purging and smoking. Such behaviors during pregnancy have been associated with the delivery of babies who are small for gestational age. Although women having a past history of an eating disorder are more likely to restrain food intake during pregnancy, studies have shown that this background does not predict intrauterine growth retardation. Therefore, the possibility of restrained eating owing to fear of fatness should be considered in cases where intrauterine growth is of concern, even among women without a history of pathological eating behavior.

At any age men, compared with women, are generally more positive about their body physique and figure, and are less affected by fear of fatness. Studies comparing older and younger women indicate that although those in younger age categories are the most vulnerable, elderly (60 to over 65 years old) women continue to have body weight concerns and share the same trait of wanting to be thinner despite being of normal weight.

14.3 Life-cycle fatness trends

It is only during the first year of life that males and females are similar in terms of body fatness levels. Both genders experience significant changes in fatness levels over the life cycle. An understanding of these variations in body fatness levels helps to provide some insight into fear of fatness and why some age and gender stages are more vulnerable than others.

The Ten State Nutrition Survey of 1970 measured triceps and/or subscapular fatfolds in more than 40 000 individuals, generating a database covering nine decades of life in both white and black Americans. A report from this study included a graphical description of trends in fatness over the life cycle given as median triceps skinfold for the white participants in this study ($n = 15 260$). This graph, plotted on a

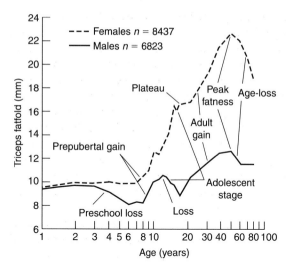

Figure 14.1 Life-cycle fatness trends in females (*broken line*) and males (*solid line*) as shown for more than 15 000 white participants in the Ten State Nutrition Survey. From Garn and Clark (1976). Reproduced with permission from *Pediatrics,* volume 57. ©1976.

semilogarithmic scale to emphasize changes during the first two decades, is included here as Figure 14.1. Overall there were similar trends in fatness levels over the life cycle evident for the black participants in the study (data not shown). The slight differences between white and black people that emerged at particular stages are discussed below. As illustrated in Figure 14.1 males at all ages are leaner than females; however, these differences are more significant during certain stages of development. While fatness levels in girls remain stable until the prepubertal gain, boys experience a reduction in fatness during the preschool period. However, it is during adolescence that the most significant gender differences in fatness develop. Under the influence of the sex hormones, these differences not only affect body composition, but also affect body shape as gender differences in how fat is distributed over the body occur. While a surge in body fatness is characteristic of female adolescence, boys tend to experience some depletion in levels of body fatness during this time. Testosterone in boys influences the development of lean tissue, while estrogen and progesterone in girls promote the deposition of body fat and the development of new fat stores in the gluteal and femoral regions. As they mature these fat stores will form the typical pear-shaped body fat distribution of adult women. At all life stages, the adult male remains

significantly leaner than his female contemporary. A comparison of black and white people, in this study found that from the third year of life onwards, white males tended to be fatter than black males. White females were found to be fatter through adolescence, after which the difference was reversed, and after the age of 17 years black females tended to be considerably fatter than white females.

The fact that women are significantly fatter than men throughout life explains to some extent why preoccupation with body fatness levels and fear of fatness is predominantly a female issue. Consideration of the physical changes that girls undergo during adolescence compared with those experienced by boys provides some insight into their particular vulnerability to fear of fatness. The marked increase in fatness levels during female adolescence is rapid in onset and permanently alters body shape. Psychosocial adjustment to such dramatic physical changes, which occur within a short timeframe, can be very difficult, especially for girls living within societies where slenderness is highly valued. At the same time, the tendency towards leanness in boys during this growth phase indicates why, in general, body fatness is not an issue for them. Furthermore, boys cannot be directly compared with girls of the same age during adolescence because they develop later and in biological terms tend to be 2 years behind girls of similar chronological age. Other factors that impact on these life-cycle fatness trends to cause fatness phobia and fad slimming diets are explored in Section 14.5.

14.4 Definitions and descriptions

Fear of fatness

Definition

Fear of fatness is a general term used to describe aversion to fatness accompanied by weight-loss attempts that are unrelated to body size and which do not meet the criteria for diagnosis of a defined eating disorder.

Description

There is a spectrum of pathological eating behaviors associated with fatness phobia. Anorexia and bulimia represent the severe end of the scale. Although those affected by these serious eating disorders and those who are more mildly obesity phobic may indulge in similar unhealthy slimming practices, there are significant differences in the severity of their symptoms. The slimming behaviors of relatively few of the many individuals affected fulfill the strict diagnostic criteria for diagnosis of anorexia or bulimia nervosa. Therefore, the more prevalent milder variants of these serious eating disorders tend to be collectively described by the general term "fear of fatness". In general, this describes aversion to body fatness or dissatisfaction with weight and/or shape that is unrelated to body size and which is accompanied by unhealthy weight-loss attempts.

A feature of fear of fatness is that many of the individuals affected perceive themselves to be significantly fatter than they actually are (body image disparagement), while the remainder continue to slim despite recognizing that they are not overweight. This results in inappropriate slimming behaviors among those who are of normal weight or are even underweight. Typical unhealthy weight loss behaviors include random avoidance of staple foods such as meat and dairy, skipping meals, fasting, taking diet pills, smoking, inducing vomiting, abusing laxatives and diuretics.

Fad slimming diets

Definition
Fad slimming diets involve patterns of food and fluid intakes that are promoted as having the ability to induce rapid or permanent weight reduction owing, it is usually claimed, to some intrinsic components which are based on unscientific principles. Such fads may or may not be accompanied by special nutritional or herbal supplements. Fad diets have also been defined as any plan failing to match the needs of the person.

Description
To describe fad slimming diets it is reasonable to start by considering the factors that distinguish fad and sound approaches to the dietary treatment of obesity. Program checklists to aid avoidance of fad slimming diets have been developed and an example is given in Table 14.1. This checklist includes 10 crucial questions whereby the soundness of a slimming diet or program can be assessed. A description of the different domains covered by this checklist is outlined in the text that follows. While many of these questions cover distinct areas, the scope of others target similar concerns but from different angles.

Sound slimming diets: a checklist
The first question, which obligates the dieter to seek medical advice before following the diet, concerns safety.

A medical opinion helps to ensure that the special needs of individuals, such as growing children and pregnant and nursing mothers, are protected. Other examples include individuals with chronic conditions, which may or may not be related to their obesity. For example, in association with increasing fatness trends growing numbers of people are being diagnosed with type 2 diabetes. Although these individuals will benefit from weight loss, their weight-reducing diets and medication regimens (where appropriate) require careful adjustment to avoid fluctuations in blood sugar levels. Gout is another example of an obesity-related condition that may be exacerbated by weight loss that is too rapid.

The second question, concerning the involvement of a suitable qualified health professional in the design of the diet or program or for follow-up consultation, is another endeavor to ensure that health is not compromised while following the diet. The involvement of a professional who is specially trained in nutritional science is necessary to ensure that the diet provides all micronutrients adequately and is balanced to maximize fat loss while preserving lean tissue.

The third question concerns using established standards to define weight loss goals. This is important to protect those who do not need to lose weight and to set realistic goals for those who do. Although the body mass index (BMI) is usually the standard of choice, care must be taken that it is used appropriately; for example, the standard $20–25 \, kg/m^2$ does not apply to children, adolescents or some athletes, and may be unsuitable for those over 65 years of age. Finally, sound programs involve weight loss goals that are realistic, which may involve some flexibility in the standards used; for example, the BMI goal may exceed $25 \, kg/m^2$ for very obese individuals.

The fourth question concerns the maximum rate of weight loss. Although weight loss may be rapid during the first 2 weeks of a reducing diet, after this initial period a maximal rate of 1 kg (2 lb)/week is recommended. This relates to safety, because faster rates of weight loss are associated with greater losses of lean body tissue, especially in those who are only mildly overweight. In addition, faster rates of weight loss usually involve limiting food intake more drastically, making it difficult to ensure an adequate intake of all nutrients, which may lead to nutritional deficiencies.

The fifth question concerns ensuring that the program is in line with healthy eating guidelines. There are three reasons why this is important.

Table 14.1 How to avoid fad diets: a program checklist that should be considered when choosing a weight-reducing diet. Adapted with permission from Dietitians of Canada website www.dietitians.ca, FAQS and Factsheets, Winning at the game of losing

Ten crucial questions	Ten correct answers (with reasons)
1. Does the diet recommend consulting a physician?	YES – A medical opinion will ensure that special needs arising from medical conditions are met. In particular, the special needs of children, teenagers and pregnant/nursing mothers will be protected
2. Has a registered dietitian/nutritionist helped to design the program or is one available for consultation?	YES – Registered dietitians/nutritionists are specially trained in the science of nutrition to design a plan that will safeguard health during weight loss
3. Does the program use BMI, with or without body fat distribution parameters, to help you set realistic goals?	YES – Because of fear of fatness many dieters are already within the healthy BMI range (20–25) and do not need to lose weight. Realistic weight goals for obese individuals goals may, however, exceed the ideal BMI range. Finally, BMI does not apply to growing children, athletes or those over 65 years
4. Is the recommended weight loss approximately two pounds (1 kg) *or less* per week?	YES – Although weight loss rate may exceed this in the initial 2 weeks, it should stabilize at a rate not exceeding 2 pounds (1 kg) per week. Greater rates of weight loss increase the risk of lean tissue depletion and nutritional deficiencies
5. Is the program based on selecting foods from all of the food groups as advised by the healthy eating guidelines of client's country of residence?	YES – Any weight-reducing program should be based on a variety of foods from the food groups as this represents the best way of meeting all nutritional requirements and preventing nutrition-related disease
6. Does the program provide at least 1200 kcal (5 MJ) per day for women and 1500 kcal (6.5 MJ) per day for men.	YES – Women or men eating less than these amounts of energy will have difficulty in meeting all of their nutritional requirements
7. Does the program allow for personal eating styles as well as your individual nutritional needs?	YES – Individual nutritional needs must be catered for, e.g. premenopausal women require more iron. Likes, dislikes, lifestyle and beliefs (vegetarianism) need to be accounted for if the plan is to be long-lasting and successful
8. Does the program encourage regular physical activity which is suited to client's lifestyle and physical condition?	YES – Regular exercise that suits the physical condition of the dieter helps loss of fat tissue while sparing lean tissue and, in addition, carries significant benefits for overall health and well-being. A medical opinion on fitness level is important
9. Does the program depend on special products, special foods, supplements or treatments?	NO – A permanent change in eating habits is what will enable permanent weight loss. Strange food combinations and supplements will not aid weight loss. Vitamins and minerals do not enhance weight loss and will not be necessary if a balanced diet is eaten – this is achieved through eating the recommended amounts of foods as advised in general healthy eating advice
10. Are magical claims or high-pressure salesmanship involved in any part of the program?	NO – If it sounds too good to be true then it probably is. Resist strong pressure to buy something; take time instead to consider the "magic cure" in the light of this checklist and only lose weight the healthy way

- The first is about the adequacy of the resulting diet. If the program advises lower amounts from a recommended food group or, worse still, that the food group is left out altogether, it is unlikely to deliver an adequate intake of all nutrients. For example, it is nearly impossible to maintain calcium intakes while following a diet that excludes all dairy foods.
- Secondly, national dietary guidelines are formulated to address the particular nutrition-related diseases that are prevalent in the country. Therefore, following a dietary pattern that deviates from these guidelines exposes the dieter to higher risk of disease.

- Finally, this question is also about the importance of achieving a permanent change in eating habits in order to maintain weight control in the long term. Sound programs involve food intakes that are in agreement with the normal cultural and traditional context of the individual, so that some aspects can remain permanent when the individual has achieved his or her desired weight.

The sixth question on the minimal energy content of weight reducing programs for healthy men and women concerns the same issues addressed in question 4 on maximal weight loss rates. Both questions guard against rapid weight loss, which may lead to lean body tissue depletion, and nutritional inadequacies.

- The seventh question concerns personal eating styles and nutritional needs. This question covers the same issues outlined above in the first and fifth questions. The importance of having individual nutritional needs catered for (question one) and the need for long term adoption of some aspects of the program for successful weight maintenance (described in the second part of the fifth question).
- The eighth question concerns the importance of physical activity. Apart from obvious benefits in terms of weight loss, physical activity is important for the other health benefits it confers. Recommended physical activity should not be excessive, should fit with the individual's lifestyle and should be safe. A medical opinion is especially important for those who are unfit.
- The last two questions (nine and ten) attempt to protect the dieter from the many fad approaches that exist. Stating that special products, foods and supplements/treatments are not necessary constitutes a warning that strange food combination and special products/supplements will not aid healthy weight loss. Finally the weary truth – if it sounds too good to be true, it most likely is!

Slimming diets: what makes them faddish?

Diets that are promoted freely to the public at large need to be in line with the general dietary recommendations for the population and should provide adequate amounts of all nutrients. Energy intakes need to be restricted for weight loss, but to remain adequate to preserve lean tissue. Just to meet these goals alone, the varying requirements of the general population necessitate a versatile approach to the treatment of obesity. However, most fad diets are inflexible and are not amenable for adaptation to meet individual needs.

Novelty, simplicity and observed weight loss are important factors in obtaining compliance with a weight-reducing diet. The popularity of a novel approach that induces a rapid weight loss is almost guaranteed. Consequently, owing to market demands, fad diets are usually characterized by all three of these factors. Compliance with many of these approaches to weight loss requires considerable commitment in terms of time and lifestyle. As time progresses the novelty value wears off even the most bizarre diets, greater efforts are required to comply with the more restrictive

diets (everyday commitments of normal life get in the way) and the rate of weight loss diminishes. These treatments do not resemble normal life, so causative factors for the weight problems are not specifically addressed, which leads to relapse on stopping the novel diet plan.

The appendix (p. 370) gives are some common features of popular fad slimming diets and the reasons why these approaches to weight-reducing should not be used. With the exception of nutritionally complete single food or beverage diets, a sound scientific basis is lacking for the diets listed. Nutritionally complete single food or beverage diets are specifically designed for certain conditions which if not observed will represent a 'fad' in that the needs of the dieter will not be met.

Nutritionally complete very low-energy formula diets [less than 3.4 MJ (800 kcal) per day] have been shown to be helpful in the treatment of obesity, particularly in the initial stages. Research has shown that compliance may be enhanced by the novel value of these single-food regimens and repeated intakes of the same food or drink may lead to earlier satiety (sensory-specific satiety). However, it is recommended that these diets should provide a protein intake of at least 0.8–1.5 g/kg of ideal body weight per day, and only be used under medical supervision in individuals with a BMI greater than 30 kg/m^2 for a period not exceeding 4 weeks. The inappropriate use of these specialized weight-reducing programs is included in the list of fad slimming diets as an example of how the improper use of a sound regimen represents a fad approach.

In conclusion, the numerous options for weight reduction at any given time are a testament to the enormous market potential for weight-reduction therapies that claim to be effective. This is mostly due to the socioeconomic pressures associated with fatness, especially in females (see below), which fuel weight phobia in obese, overweight and even normal weight individuals. The popularity of fad slimming diets is further enhanced by the ineffectiveness of current approaches in the treatment of obesity, a situation that encourages each new fad to claim to be the elusive cure. A significant increase in such fads can be expected to accompany the spiraling increases in obesity prevalence.

14.5 Etiology

Socioeconomic prejudice against fatness, particularly female fatness, represents the key etiological factor in fear of fatness and fad dieting in Western societies. Other important pressures include the relentless promotion of slenderness as an integral part of physical beauty by the media and, as discussed in Section 14.3, periods of increasing fatness due to growth.

The stigma associated with fatness is apparent even in young children. Studies have repeatedly shown that very young children regard obesity in their peers as being synonymous with "ugliness", "selfishness", "laziness" and "stupidity", and they would "least like to be friends with" an overweight child. Thus, long before they reach adolescence children have a clear impression that being fat is socially unacceptable. Not surprisingly, a desire to weigh less is prevalent among prepubertal girls and boys, including those of normal weight.

During adolescence this fear of fatness increases substantially in girls and fad slimming behaviors become prevalent, while among boys fatness phobia diminishes. Reasons for this certainly include the gender differences that develop in fatness trends during the adolescent growth phase (see Section 14.3). Teenage girls are generally under the care of adults and are not financially independent. In this situation weight-loss efforts often include the random avoidance of staple foodstuffs, meal skipping, vegetarianism and purging. Investigation of the slimming habits of prepubertal children indicates that while a desire to weigh less is prevalent, fortunately active slimming and purging are relatively uncommon.

The strong prejudice against overweight women in modern Western societies represents further fuel for the weight phobia of adolescent girls, and ensures the maintenance of such fears and slimming practices for adult women. Several long-term studies, carried out relatively recently, have shown that overweight women tend to earn less money, are less likely to marry and spend less time in education than their leaner peers. Although this stigmatization of fatness did not affect the overweight men in these studies to anything like the same extent, there is evidence that men are not immune. It seems that, in a similar way to overweight women, severely obese young men live with a social handicap that is independent of social class, intelligence and education.

14.6 Consequences for public health

The use of smoking as a slimming strategy represents the most overwhelming reason for urgent and effective action to address the issue of fear of fatness. This

Table 14.2 Public health consequences associated with fear of fatness and fad slimming diets

Issues	Consequences for public health
The use of smoking as a slimming strategy	Affects more women than men May explain increased numbers of smokers among teenage girls Has disastrous consequences for women's future health Represents a far greater threat to health than obesity
Fear of fatness and fad slimming diets represent a significant challenge to obesity prevention programs	Urgent need to effectively address the rising levels of obesity Obesity prevention strategies may exacerbate fear of fatness Complicates screening for overweight among schoolchildren Obesity prevention programs need to address fear of fatness
Increased risk of developing eating disorders	Dieting adolescent girls at higher risk of developing eating disorders Fear of fatness may be as intractable as clinical eating disorders
Nutritional deficiencies associated with dietary restraint	Dietary restraint will exacerbate existing nutritional inadequacies Risk of growth failure in children affected Inadequate dietary intakes impact negatively on bone health Reduced physical and mental capacity due to anemia (iron)
Impact of fear of fatness and fad dieting during pregnancy and lactation	Intrauterine growth retardation in offspring Lower rates of breast-feeding among affected women Adolescent mothers reject contraceptives owing to weight concerns
Challenge to public health nutrition programs	Fad diets prevent compliance with healthy eating guidelines Challenge to nutrition programs addressing the needs of a population Fear of fatness leads to underreporting of dietary intakes and interferes with assessment of nutritional status and goal setting

is more of an issue for women than for men, and it has been suggested that this may be due to the greater propensity for weight gain in women compared with men on smoking cessation. The numbers of teenage girls who are becoming regular smokers have been increasing and studies suggest that fear of fatness may be an important factor. This is a difficult problem to deal with because teenage girls are likely to be far more concerned about the immediate possibility of weight gain than the remote probability of serious disease and premature death from smoking-related illnesses.

The second most important implication of fear of fatness and fad dieting is the challenge that it presents for obesity prevention. The sharp and continuing rise in obesity prevalence is also reflected in trends for children and adolescents. Because of the refractory nature of obesity many consider that prevention represents the only effective strategy and that children and adolescents should be targeted in particular. However, owing to the negative connotations associated with obesity, even surveillance processes involving the measurement of weight and height to monitor obesity trends may increase fear of fatness and fad dieting. The issues of fear of fatness and fad dieting need to be addressed as part of obesity prevention programs. This will almost certainly involve effectively dealing with the stigma associated with fatness.

The public health consequences associated with fear of fatness and fad slimming diets are shown in Table 14.2.

The purging behaviors associated with fear of fatness reveal the vulnerability of individuals affected to the development of clinically defined eating disorders. Most of the information available is derived from studies involving adolescent girls, who are the most vulnerable population group for the development of eating disorders. More than 10% of healthy Irish and American adolescent girls report purging behavior involving self-induced vomiting, or laxative or diuretic abuse. A 3 year follow-up study reported that adolescent girls who dieted at a severe level were 18 times more likely to develop an eating disorder than those who did not diet (Patton et al., 1999). It is not known whether the same vulnerability to the development of eating disorders exists for older women or males affected by fear of fatness. It has been estimated that clinically determined eating pathology (anorexia, bulimia and binge-eating disorder) affects 1–3% of young women, while probably twice as many are affected by clinically important variants. Research indicates that these clinically defined disorders are chronic for many individuals affected.

The dietary restraint and the fad slimming practices associated with fear of fatness raise several nutritional concerns. Children and adolescents, owing to their continuing growth, have higher nutritional requirements, and dietary inadequacy during these developmental stages can have far-reaching effects. It has been documented that dieting during childhood and adolescence, even in the absence of clinically defined eating disorders, can lead to growth failure and delayed puberty. Furthermore, there is evidence of reductions in growth velocity even in situations where weight control diets have been closely supervised and well balanced for micronutrient adequacy. It remains unknown whether such interference with normal growth patterns carries any long-term adverse consequences.

Apart from insufficient energy to support growth, the restricted food intakes of restrained eaters can lead to specific micronutrient deficiencies. Low-energy diets mean lower food intakes, and thus such diets usually provide fewer vitamins and minerals, unless food intakes are well planned and include nutrient-dense food choices. However, many fad diets are not well balanced for nutrient adequacy, particularly those that involve the exclusion of staple foodstuffs or food groups. Thus, fad diets generally exacerbate inadequacies for those micronutrients that are prone to be deficient in Western diets. This is of particular concern for population groups who are especially vulnerable because of their high requirements as a consequence of growth or ill health, such as children, adolescents, pregnant or nursing mothers and the elderly. Women, as a population group, are most vulnerable to iron deficiency. Yet they comprise the group that, because of fear of fatness, is most likely specifically to avoid red meat, an excellent sources of absorbable (heme) iron, owing to their misconception that this food is fattening. The public health cost of iron deficiency is enormous where reduced work capacity and cognitive function, lowered resistance to infection and increased risks for pregnant women are the consequences of anemia. The significance of the more prevalent condition of iron deficiency without anemia is less well established, but there is some evidence of reductions in work capacity, resistance to infection and intellectual performance. In a similar way, the avoidance of calcium-rich foods through fad dieting has implications for bone health, particularly if this occurs during the dynamic period of bone development during adolescence. Other factors associated with fear of fatness and disordered eating that impact very negatively on bone health include low body weight, amenorrhea, reduced levels of insulin-like growth factor-1 and hormonal imbalances.

Finally, fear of fatness represents a major barrier to public health nutrition programs because fad diets rarely reflect population-based dietary guidelines, which are effectively public health initiatives to address the specific nutritional inadequacies and chronic diseases of the population. Furthermore, because weight consciousness is associated with underreporting of dietary intakes by women of all ages, this interferes with the assessment of nutritional adequacy and confounds the setting of realistic goals in nutritional guidelines. In relation to this, such dietary assessment not only is complicated by periods of dietary restraint, but also must consider periods of disinhibition and bingeing and try to untangle the relative importance of each to overall assessment of nutritional adequacy.

14.7 Prevention strategies

Research in the area of preventing fear of fatness and fad slimming behaviors is limited. Strategies that have been developed mainly focus on the prevention of eating disorders and target adolescent girls or young women in their educational settings. Evaluation of these interventions indicates that while they appear to be somewhat effective in preventing the development of unhealthy slimming practices, they have limited value for young people who already engage in drastic efforts to control their weight. Therefore, there is growing interest in the development of programs that focus on prevention and target younger children who have not yet developed fatness phobia.

Another factor stimulating interest in this area concerns the global increases in obesity prevalence observed in recent years. The lack of success in treating obesity when it is established, and the steadily accumulating evidence that fatness levels are increasing dramatically among the youngest population age groups, have focused attention on obesity prevention. Many public health programs are now committed to developing strategies that prevent childhood and adolescent obesity. Concern has been raised that many of the obesity prevention activities, especially those that involve the collection of information on fatness levels in young people for evaluation purposes, may exacerbate fear of fatness and unhealthy slimming practices. It has been pointed out that some of the frantic slimming efforts associated with fear of fatness, such as smoking, may impact more negatively on public health than a continued rise in obesity levels. This has led experts in public health to acknowledge the necessity of adding tactics that prevent fear of fatness and the development of eating disorders to strategies aimed at obesity prevention.

Eating disorder prevention programs commonly aim to reduce unhealthy slimming behaviors through the promotion of positive body image and self-esteem. Positive body image is important for self-esteem, which is, in turn, protective against many risk behaviors in youth. Many programs foster skills that will empower the target population critically to analyze their environment for pressures to be thin and will help them to develop a realistic outlook regarding their own body size and shape. Practical strategies involved in these programs include the development of media literacy skills, which enable the target population to reject unrealistic messages and images portrayed in the media. In addition, activities carrying other health benefits, such as components on active living, which also benefit self-esteem, are commonly involved.

Not surprisingly, the programs that enjoy most success are interactive and include issues and role models that are current for the target audience The involvement of families, schools and communities provides crucial support.

In general, intervention programs to reduce fear of fatness and eating disorders have been short term, with evaluation occurring within a limited follow-up period. The evaluation of these programs often indicates effectiveness in achieving direct goals such as enhancing media literacy. However, only minimal to moderate success has been reported in attaining the main indirect goals of improving body size acceptance and dieting behaviors. More promising results for these outcomes are generally most apparent immediately after completion of the intervention programs. It has been suggested that this indicates a need for longer term interventions, involving the entire community, to counteract the constant barrage of media and social messages celebrating the ultrathin ideal. Finally, evaluation of fear of fatness prevention programs needs to include the assessment of undesirable outcomes such as an increase in body size dissatisfaction and unhealthy slimming practices. This recognizes the danger involved in emphasizing healthy body images, where programs may lead to a preoccupation with body size that was not there in the first place.

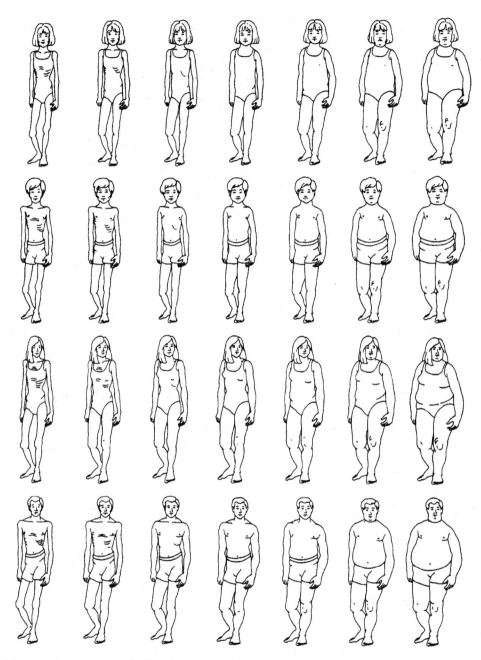

Figure 14.2 Child and adult figures. From Collins (1991). Reprinted with permission of John Wiley & Sons. © 1991.

14.8 Assessing body image

With the current emphasis on obesity prevention and the need for monitoring, there is a growing interest in information on current weight status and dietary intakes of children, adolescents and adults. In addition, an assessment of how body size is perceived, compared with actual body size, is recognized as providing valuable information. However, fear of fatness and fad dieting are so pervasive that nutritionists and public health personnel need to be aware of sensitivities around the assessment of body size and dietary intakes.

Assessment of body image may involve simply asking the target group how they perceive themselves (underweight, normal weight or overweight). Satisfaction with perceived body image entails further questions to identify whether the subjects would like to be heavier, lighter, taller or smaller. Figure line drawings, depicting a range of body sizes from very underweight to very overweight for children and adults of both genders (Figure 14.2), are often used to assess perceived body image. By means of questions such as "which one looks most like you?" and "which one would you most like to look like?" these figure line drawings can provide valuable information on self-perceptions of body size, which may then be compared with some actual measures of body size. Assessment of actual body size involves measuring weight and height, and may involve body circumference and skinfold measurements.

14.9 Perspectives on the future

The global increase in obesity prevalence and the shift within public health organizations to prioritize the development of obesity prevention programs may signal significant increases in fear of fatness and fad slimming diets. It is sobering to consider the possibility that such issues, with all the accompanying adverse health outcomes, may become more manifest in young children and males as fatness levels increase among these groups.

In the meantime there is growing awareness among health professionals of the many serious health consequences associated with unhealthy slimming practices and fad dieting due to fear of fatness. For example, it is recognized that periods of high blood sugar levels among young insulin-dependent diabetics may be due to their purposely reducing their insulin doses below their requirements in order to achieve weight loss. In addition, in cases of intrauterine growth retardation, there is increasing awareness that fear of fatness and fad dieting during pregnancy need to be considered as possible causes.

Any inflation of this situation carries serious implications for health, and women's health in particular. There is growing recognition that to be sure of doing no harm obesity prevention programs must integrate the prevention of fear of fatness and fad dieting. Such programs will certainly include successfully tackling the enormous stigma associated with obesity if they are to be effective. There is some hope in the growth of community-based obesity prevention programs, which aim to increase capacity within communities to deal with obesity. Consultation and involvement of the community in the development of such programs are critical for long-term success and endurance. The involvement of target populations is unlikely to miss out the importance of psychosocial issues concerning fear of fatness and fad dieting.

Further reading

Austin SB. Prevention research in eating disorders: theory and new directions. Psychol Med 2000; 30: 1249–1262.

Bemporad JR. Cultural and historical aspects of eating disorders. Theor Med 1997; 18(4): 401–420.

Collins ME. Body figure perceptions and preferences among preadolescent children. Int J Eat Disord 1991; 10: 199–208.

Crichton P. Were the Roman emperors Claudius and Vitellius bulimic? International Journal of Eating Disorders 1996; 19(2): 203–207.

Flynn MAT. Fear of fatness in adolescent girls: implications for obesity prevention. Proc Nutr Soc 1997; 56: 305–317.

Franzoi SL, Koehler V. Age and gender differences in body attitudes: a comparison of young and elderly adults. Int J Aging Hum Dev 1998; 47: 1–10.

Garn SM, Clark DC. Trends in fatness and the origins of obesity. Pediatrics 1976; 57(4): 443–456

Gortmaker SL, Must A, Perrin JM et al. Social and economic consequences of overweight in adolescence and young adulthood. N Engl J Med 1993, 329: 1008–1012.

Heatherton TF, Mahamedi F, Striepe M et al. A 10-year longitudinal study of body weight, dieting and eating disorder symptoms. J Abnorm Psychol 1997; 106: 117–125.

Hill AJ, Draper B, Stack J. A weight on children's minds: body shape dissatisfaction at 9 years old. International Journal of Obesity 1994; 18: 383–389.

O'Dea J. School-based interventions to prevent eating problems: first do no harm. Eating Disorders 2000; 8: 123–130.

Patton CG, Seizer R, Coffey C, Carlin JB, Wolfe R. Onset of adolescent eating disorders: population based cohort study over 3 years. British Medical Journal 1999; 3 18: 765–768.

Summerbell C, Watts C, Higgins JP, Garrow JS. Randomized controlled trial of novel, simple and well supervised weight reducing diets in outpatients. British Medical Journal 1998; 317: 1487–1489.

Wiseman CV, Gray JJ, Mosimann JE, Ahrens AH. Cultural expectations of thinness in women: an update. Int J Eat Disord 1992; 11: 85–89.

15
Nutrition and Child Development

Helen Baker-Henningham and Sally Grantham-McGregor

Key messages

- There is considerable evidence that young children exposed to poor nutrition have poorer development than adequately nourished children both concurrently and in later childhood.
- There is some evidence implicating the following nutritional conditions: intrauterine growth retardation, failure to breast-feed, early childhood stunting and wasting, short-term food deprivation, and micronutrient deficiencies including iron, iodine and zinc.
- Children with nutritional deficiencies usually come from disadvantaged environments and are likely to be exposed to multiple biological risks.

- These disadvantages may have independent effects on children's development and modify the effects of undernutrition, thus demonstrating causal relationships is difficult and requires randomized controlled treatment trials.
- The effect of poor nutrition on child development depends to some extent on severity and duration of the deficiency and stage of development of the child. There may be sensitive stages which vary by the particular deficiency, but nutrition can have an effect throughout life.
- Integrated programming involving health and nutrition and psychosocial stimulation interventions is required to combat the detrimental effects of poor nutrition on child development.

15.1 Introduction

Since the 1950s, there has been concern that poor nutrition may affect children's development. There is now a considerable amount of research on the association between nutritional deficiencies and children's development and cognition and mood in adults. The main nutritional conditions studied include intrauterine growth retardation (IUGR), the benefits of breast-feeding, early childhood undernutrition (moderate and severe stunting, underweight and wasting), short-term hunger and school feeding, and micronutrient deficiencies, including iron, iodine, zinc and vitamin A. Although these conditions are usually more prevalent and severe in developing countries, in developed countries most of them still occur and iron deficiency in particular remains common.

Poor nutrition can affect development prenatally from early gestation and throughout childhood. Nutrition may also affect adult functioning, at least transiently.

However, it is likely that certain periods are more vulnerable than others and these periods may differ according to the type of deficiency. For example, the first two trimesters of pregnancy are the most sensitive to iodine deficiency, whereas the first two postnatal years are probably the most sensitive to undernutrition.

Child development is multidimensional and comprises several interrelated domains including motor, cognitive, social and emotional development. Investigators studying the effect of nutrition have traditionally focused on children's motor and cognitive development and less often on school achievement. There is relatively little information on social and emotional development and mental health.

Children with nutritional deficiencies usually come from disadvantaged environments and are likely to be exposed to multiple biological risks. These disadvantages may have independent effects on children's development and may modify the effects of nutritional deficiencies. Thus, demonstrating an association between a nutritional deficiency and poor development is insufficient to infer a causal relationship and randomized controlled trials (RCTs) of nutritional supplementation are required, but may not always be feasible.

Development in children under 3 years has usually been assessed with infant development scales such as the Bayley Scales for Infant Development, which were standardized in the USA, or the Griffiths Scales, which were standardized in England. The Bayley gives a global mental score of general cognitive and language development and a motor score. The Griffiths has more subscales. In the first year of life infant development scales have very limited predictive value, although the predictive ability increases with age. There are now more efforts to use tests of recognition memory, problem solving and attention, which may have better predictive ability, at least in the first year. Intelligence tests such as the Weschler Intelligence Scales for Children (WISC) have been used in older children and adults to assess intelligence. Batteries of cognitive tests have been used to assess specific cognitive functions, mainly in older children and adults, and school achievement tests used to assess school subjects such as reading and arithmetic. Parental and teacher reports have usually been used to assess behavior, which may suffer from some bias in that parents of malnourished children are generally less educated and have lower intelligence quotients (IQs) than those of adequately nourished children. Behavior observations are probably a more valid way of assessing behavior, but they are time consuming and require considerable training. A problem with many tests, especially infant assessment scales and IQ tests, is that they are not standardized for most developing countries and may not be culturally appropriate. Therefore, the best approach depends on having a local control group and only making within-population comparisons. It is important to have some measure of the validity of the test within the population that is being studied.

This chapter briefly discusses the effect of the environment on child development and possible mechanisms linking nutritional deficiencies to poor child development, then describes for each of the conditions mentioned above the evidence for an effect on child development.

15.2 Child development and the role of the environment

It is important to understand how children develop and the context of undernutrition in order to evaluate the effects of undernutrition. Children's development is multifactorial, being influenced by a multitude of factors including genetics, child characteristics (e.g. temperament), the biological state of the child (e.g. health and nutritional status), the proximal environment (e.g. level of stimulation in the home, quality of maternal–child interaction) and the distal environment (e.g. parental education, culture, urban or rural residence, type of neighborhood). Some factors are protective, whereas others make the child more vulnerable. For example, high levels of maternal education and intelligence and good stimulation in the home may act as protective factors, which reduce the detrimental effect of low birth weight or early childhood undernutrition on child development. Conversely, the same nutritional conditions are likely to have worse effects on child development when mothers are illiterate, and the family lives in a poor home with inadequate levels of stimulation. Risk and protective factors continue to affect development throughout childhood and the long-term effects of nutritional deficiencies in early childhood depend to some extent on previous, current and future experiences.

15.3 Possible mechanisms linking undernutrition to poor development

There are two main hypotheses explaining how nutritional deficiencies could affect mental development. One theory is the functional isolation hypothesis. In this theory, the behavioral characteristics of undernourished children lead to reduced interaction with the environment and this in turn leads to poor developmental outcomes. Young children who are underweight, stunted, iron deficient, small for gestational age (SGA) or, to a lesser extent, zinc deficient have been found to show altered behavior, which concurs with this hypothesis. They have reduced activity, increased fussiness and unhappiness, and less exploration than adequately nourished children. These behaviors are believed to impede development. Caregivers may also be affected by the child's altered behavior. For example, caregivers of children with nutritional deficiencies have been described as having poorer quality vocalizations, to hold and carry their child more, to be less responsive, and to give their child less praise and affection. Poor maternal–child interactions further exacerbate the child's poor developmental progress. It is not clear whether the mothers are less stimulating before the onset of undernutrition or become less stimulating as a response to the children's altered behavior following the onset of malnutrition. It is likely that both occur.

Another hypothesis is that undernutrition results in structural and functional alterations in the brain. Animal studies have shown that prenatal and early postnatal malnutrition in rats leads to many changes in brain structure, although some of these changes are reversible on refeeding. However, several alterations are thought to be irreversible, including a reduction in myelin and the number of cortical dentrites in neural spines and an increase in neuronal mitochondria. Evidence of changes to brain structure and function in children is limited, although severely malnourished children have small heads and abnormal auditory-evoked potentials, which remain abnormal after recovery from the acute stage. In addition, stunted children have small heads, and head circumference in early childhood has been shown to predict IQ in later childhood. Changes in brain structure have been described in animals with protein–energy malnutrition (PEM), iron deficiency and zinc deficiency. Marked changes also occur when the fetus is exposed to severe iodine deficiency, which results in cretinism.

There is less evidence for a third possible mechanism, which is that an altered stress response could contribute to undernourished children's behavioral differences and poorer development. In one study in Jamaica, stunted children aged 8–10 years were more inhibited in a stressful situation and had increased salivary cortisol levels and urinary adrenaline (epinephrine) and higher heart rates than nonstunted children. The finding of an altered stress response in stunted children needs replicating and further exploring in other populations to determine whether it plays a role in the etiology of poor development.

15.4 Prevalence of nutritional deficiencies

Low birth weight

In developing countries low birth weight (LBW) babies are more likely than those in developed countries to have had intrauterine growth retardation (IUGR) secondary to poor maternal nutrition and increased infections. Sixteen per cent of infants worldwide are born with LBW (<2500 g) and 95% of these are in developing countries. The prevalence ranges from around 50% in Bangladesh to 6% in developed countries.

Stunting and wasting

Stunting and wasting are diagnosed by anthropometry. The child's weight and height are expressed in standard scores of the median of internationally accepted references for their age and gender. Moderate underweight indicates weight for age below −2 standard deviations (SD) below the median of the National Center for Health Statistics (NCHS) international references, moderate stunting indicates height for age below −2 SD, and moderate wasting indicates weight for height below −2 SD. Below −3 SD indicates a severe condition. Another form of severe undernutrition is kwashiorkor, in which edema occurs in association with underweight. Undernutrition was previously referred to as PEM. However, when children are undernourished as a result of low dietary intakes of energy and protein their diets are usually also deficient in many micronutrients. Although there has been some decline in the prevalence of childhood undernutrition it remains extremely high. In developing countries, 29% of children under 5 years are moderately underweight, 33% are moderately stunted and 10% are moderately wasted. In least developed countries, 40% of children under 5 are underweight and 45% are stunted. The prevalence of moderately and severely underweight children is estimated to have declined globally from 38% in 1980 to 30% in 1997 and 29% in 2001. However, several countries in sub-Saharan Africa are showing an increase in the prevalence of childhood undernutrition. Undernutrition thus remains a very important public health issue in the twenty-first century.

Iron deficiency anemia

The prevalence of anemia is used as a proxy indicator for iron deficiency in the public health setting. The prevalence of anemia is determined by the level of hemoglobin in the blood. The cut-off points for blood hemoglobin to define anemia differ by age and are 110 g/l for children aged 6–59 months, 115 g/l for children aged 5–11 years and 120 g/l for children aged 12–14 years. There are no recent comprehensive data on the prevalence of anemia in children, but in 1985 the estimated prevalence of anemia (hemoglobin <110 g/l) in children under 5 years of age was 46–51% in developing countries and 7–12% in developed countries. Iron-deficiency anemia (IDA) is often found in poor neighborhoods and immigrant populations in England. It is the most common cause of anemia and is most prevalent in children from 6 to 24 months of age.

Zinc deficiency

The prevalence of zinc deficiency is not known, but it is common in populations that consume little meat and high levels of phytate and fiber, which reduce zinc bioavailability. This diet is highly prevalent in many developing countries. Zinc is also lost from the body during episodes of diarrheal disease. Requirements for zinc increase during periods of rapid growth, for example, infancy and pregnancy. Therefore, in many developing countries, where young children have poor diets and frequent diarrhea, it is likely that zinc deficiency is present.

Iodine deficiency

The indicators for assessing iodine-deficiency disorder (IDD) are the median urinary iodine and the prevalence of goiter. The normal median value for urinary iodine is 100–200 μg/l. Values of 50–99 μg/l indicate a mild deficiency, 20–49 μg/l indicate a moderate deficiency and below 20 μg/l indicate a severe deficiency. The presence of goiter is examined by inspection and palpation and the goiter is graded according to size. The criterion for elimination of IDD as a public health problem is a goiter prevalence of less than 5% of the population. School-aged children are usually the target group for surveillance. According to the World Health Organization (WHO), 13% of the world's population (740 million people) are affected by IDD and a further 30% are at risk. Nearly 50 million people are believed to suffer from some form of neurological or cognitive deficits related to IDD. Iodine deficiency is prevalent in areas in which the soil is low in iodine content owing to leaching caused by high rainfall, flooding, melting snow and glaciation, and thus mountainous areas are particularly at risk.

Vitamin A deficiency

Vitamin A deficiency is diagnosed by the concentrations of serum retinol. Serum retinol below 20 μg/dl (0.70 mol/l) is classified as moderate vitamin A deficiency and levels below 10 μg/dl (0.35 mol/l) are classified as severe. The WHO states that vitamin A deficiency is a public health problem in 118 countries worldwide and is especially prevalent in Africa and south-east Asia. Some 100–140 million children are vitamin A deficient and between one-quarter and half a million of these children become blind every year, with half of them dying within 12 months of losing their sight.

15.5 Intrauterine growth retardation

In developing countries, the majority of LBW infants are born at term and have suffered from IUGR as a result of maternal stunting and inadequate nutrition before and during pregnancy, and/or frequent infections such as malaria.

In contrast, in developed countries, biomedical causes such as multiple pregnancy and prematurity are responsible for a higher proportion of LBW infants. Cigarette smoking also contributes to LBW. Although at present cigarette smoking by women is not common in developing countries it is on the increase in some countries.

The effects of SGA on child development have been investigated in many studies. However, there are many problems in interpreting the results. First, different definitions of SGA have been used. The WHO recommends using the 10th centile of birth weights for gestational age from a standard population as the cut-off point. However, this cut-off may be too high to represent a risk for development.

In addition, there is a greater incidence of perinatal and neonatal complications in LBW babies that may also detrimentally affect development. Some studies have omitted children with complications, while others have included them.

Particularly in low-income countries, LBW is associated with poor environments, which may independently affect child development. Many studies have failed to control adequately for the effects of these environments.

Further problems include the fact that LBW babies are also less likely to be breast-fed and that many studies have had high dropout rates of between 30 and 50%, which are likely to be biased. For example, in a Brazilian study, LBW infants who were lost to follow-up at 12 months of age had significantly lower developmental levels at 6 months than those who were located.

The effect of being small for gestational age on child development

The majority of studies on the effects of being low birth weight born at term (LBW-T) or SGA on child development have been conducted in developed countries. Most studies have found no significant differences between SGA term babies and normal birth weight babies in the first year of life, although a few have found differences. Traditional infant developmental tests were generally used in the first year of life and may not be sensitive to some cognitive functions. However, in a study in Brazil, normal birth weight infants scored significantly higher than SGA infants on tests of both motor and mental development at 6 and 12 months. By the second year of life, most studies found significant developmental deficits for SGA children, although the differences were largely found in particularly vulnerable subgroups. These groups included male children, black children, children with congenital abnormalities and children with birth weight below 2300 g.

Studies in early childhood (2–7 years of age) have generally shown differences in development between SGA and normal birth weight infants, favoring the latter. SGA children have been found to have lower IQ, poorer language skills, lower reading readiness scores and poorer school achievement, and to be more likely to be retained at grade level or to be in a special class. These differences have been detected even when there was no difference detected in the same study sample in the first year of life.

Studies investigating the effects of SGA into adolescence have consistently found developmental deficits including lower IQ, higher placement in special education classes and poorer school achievement. These differences usually remained after controlling for socioeconomic variables, but in some studies they were no longer significant.

A few studies have examined the effects of SGA into late adolescence and adulthood and most, but not all, have found that small deficits in attained educational levels or cognitive abilities persist. Several studies have found that the relationship between cognition and birth weight is also present across the normal birth weight range.

Nearly all of the above studies were from developed countries. Two studies on the medium- or long-term development of children born SGA were identified from developing countries. In India, early childhood malnutrition had a greater effect than SGA on child development, and in Guatemala, there was no evidence of a cognitive deficit in SGA children. It may be that the poor health, poor nutrition and low levels of stimulation often experienced by children living in poverty in developing countries overwhelm the effect of SGA on child development.

Children born SGA have also been found to have different behavior than normal birth weight children. They have been described as less active, less vocal, less responsive, less happy and less cooperative in the first 2 years of life, and more fidgety, more anxious, less happy and having a poorer attention span at school age.

SGA interacts with other risk factors for development. For example, in Brazil, the development of SGA children was shown to be detrimentally affected by low levels of stimulation in the home, maternal illiteracy and frequent diarrhea, whereas the development of normal birth weight children was not. This heightened vulnerability of SGA children has implications for developing countries in that most SGA children come from disadvantaged homes which will put these children at further risk for poor development.

Recommendations for public health interventions

Children born LBW are at risk not only for poor development, but also for poor health and nutrition, and often come from poorer homes. An integrated program approach combing health, nutrition and child development activities is most appropriate. Programs involving early stimulation for LBW children in developed countries (primarily in North America) have shown benefits to children's mental development and behavior, and similar programs are likely to be beneficial in developing countries.

15.6 Breast-feeding and its influence on child development

How breast-feeding benefits development

There are several mechanisms by which breast-feeding may benefit child development. First, breastmilk is a rich source of long-chain polyunsaturated fatty acids (LCPUFA), which are not only a source of energy, but are also the predominant molecules found in myelin, and are particularly concentrated in the retina. LCPUFA are therefore important in brain development. Humans cannot make certain LCPUFA (n-6 and n-3), and acquire them from the mother mainly in the last trimester of pregnancy and postnatally from their diet. In formula milk the concentration of LCPUFA is thought to be insufficient to meet infant requirements, particularly for preterm infants. However, it is controversial whether this insufficiency has long-term developmental consequences. Many studies have investigated the effects of LCPUFA supplementation on visual acuity. Most studies with formula-fed preterm infants have shown that supplementation improves their visual acuity in the first few months. However, some studies have shown that the nonsupplemented infants catch up on weaning. Fewer studies have looked at visual acuity in term infants and they have had inconsistent findings.

Fewer studies have examined the effects of supplementation on general development and results have again been inconsistent. In preterm infants effects were found on motor but not mental scores of the Bayley test in one study, and on Bayley mental but not motor scores in another study. In a third study no effect on Bayley scores was found. Results for term infants show less effect than for preterm infants.

Speed of processing (habituation) or problem solving has also been improved with supplementation in a few studies. There is a need for longer term studies as there is little information after the second year and most tests of infant cognition have only low predictive ability for future intelligence. In addition, the results may depend on the relative amounts of the different LCPUFA and the duration and timing of supplementation. Excessive amounts or imbalances among the PUFA may cause problems.

Secondly, breast-feeding may increase infant immunity to disease, as shown by studies in which breast-feeding is associated with a decrease in levels of diarrhea, chronic constipation, gastrointestinal illness, and respiratory tract and ear infections. Through promoting improved health of the infant, it is likely that breast-feeding will indirectly benefit psychomotor development, as a sick child is less able to explore and learn from the environment. There is some evidence that even small amounts of breast milk can increase an infant's immunity, with a dose–response relationship between breast-feeding and reduced infection.

Finally, breast-feeding may benefit the maternal–child interaction and facilitate the development of a secure attachment, which is thus likely to benefit the child's development and behavior.

Short-term effects of breast-feeding

There are many studies on the concurrent effects of breast-feeding on child development, involving children from birth to 2 years. Most studies were conducted in developed countries (with only two studies identified from developing countries) and used the Bayley Scale of Infant Development as the outcome measure. Studies investigated differences between breast-fed and nonbreast-fed infants at 6, 12, 18 and 24 months, and at all points in time breast-feeding was generally associated with higher scores on developmental tests, although the differences were not always significant. However, more significant differences were found in the second year of life and it may be that the Bayley test is not sensitive enough to detect small differences in the first year of life. There is some evidence that the longer the infant is breast-fed, the greater the gains in psychomotor development. Breast-feeding appears to benefit all children, regardless of social class. The benefits are usually reduced after controlling for the effects of socioeconomic variables, although they generally remain significant.

In two recent randomized trials in Honduras, infants who were exclusively breast-fed for 6 months crawled sooner in both studies and were more likely to be walking by 12 months in one of the studies than infants who were exclusively breast-fed for 4 months.

Studies investigating the long-term effects of breast-feeding have examined the association between breast-feeding and mental development from 4 years until 50 years of age. All studies identified were conducted in developed countries and showed a small but consistent benefit to mental development in breast-fed individuals. In the majority of studies, the differences in mental development between breast-fed and nonbreast-fed children remained significant after controlling for socioeconomic variables. A metaanalysis of 20 longitudinal studies of the effects of breast-feeding on cognitive development included children from infancy to adolescence and found a benefit of 3.2 IQ points after controlling for measured covariates. This small but significant difference may have implications at the population level. Breast-feeding has also been associated with fewer emotional or behavioral problems and fewer minor neurological problems later in life.

Problems in the evaluation of studies on breast-feeding and child development

Most longitudinal studies comparing breast-fed with nonbreast-fed children have shown small benefits to the breast-fed children's later development up to adolescence or adulthood, but the studies have several problems. First, investigators have used different definitions of breast-feeding, and studies vary in the length and exclusivity of breast-feeding. In addition, the milk given to nonbreast-fed infants has differed across studies and has included different types of formula milk, cow's milk and condensed milk. A third factor is that studies vary in the exclusion criteria used, with some studies excluding infants with LBW, preterm and perinatal complications, and infants with health problems. As the health of the neonate will affect the likelihood of successful breast-feeding, inclusion of infants at high biomedical risk will probably introduce bias into the study design. Fourthly, and most importantly, breast-feeding is associated with a large number of family background characteristics that are themselves related to child development, such as parental education level, maternal age, socioeconomic status, family size, maternal smoking and crowding. It is extremely difficult to control for all confounding variables. Thus, because of the observational nature of these studies causal inferences cannot be made with certainty.

In conclusion, despite the observational nature of the majority of the studies on breast-feeding and the limitations of such studies, the consistency of the data is impressive. Furthermore, the two randomized trials on early or late weaning did show benefits. Thus, the findings suggest that breast-feeding confers a small beneficial effect to children's development.

Promoting breast-feeding

The WHO and the United Nations Children's Fund (UNICEF) recommend exclusive breast-feeding for at least 4 months and if possible for 6 months. Exclusive breast-feeding is defined as no other food or drink (not even water) except for breast milk. The WHO maintains a Global Data Bank covering 94 countries and 65% of the world's infant population, and estimates that 35% of infants are exclusively breast-fed from 0 to 4 months. UNICEF and WHO have a joint venture designed to promote breast-feeding in maternity hospitals worldwide called the Baby Friendly Hospital Initiative (BFHI), which outlines 10 steps to successful breast-feeding (see Chapter 16). A randomized trial in Belarus in which maternity units were assigned to an intervention modeled on the BFHI or a control group showed that infants at the experimental sites were more likely to be exclusively breast-fed at 3 and 6 months, were more likely to be breast-fed at 12 months, and had a significant reduction in the risk of gastrointestinal tract infections and atopic eczema.

The greatest effects of breast-feeding on mental development are found for children classified as high risk owing to pregnancy complications or LBW, or both, suggesting that breast-feeding is particularly important for infants at biomedical risk. For example, in the metaanalysis mentioned above, LBW infants showed a larger benefit of breast-feeding (5.2 IQ points) than normal birth weight infants (2.7 IQ points). This may be partly explained by the high concentration of LCPUFA in breast milk, as discussed earlier. There is very little information on the association between breast-feeding and mental development in developing countries, but it is likely to have an important influence on child development in such countries, where alternative feeds are often infected and nutritionally inadequate and many children are at significant socioeconomic and biomedical risk.

15.7 Wasting, stunting and severe clinical malnutrition

Short-term effects

Stunting represents longer term undernutrition and takes some time to develop and recover, whereas wasting may be due to a relatively brief period of undernutrition and can improve rapidly. Underweight represents a combination of wasting and stunting. A large number of cross-sectional studies has shown an association between moderate or severe stunting or underweight, poor motor and mental development in early childhood, and poor cognition and school achievement in later childhood. Associations between moderate wasting (low weight for height) and development have also been found, but less often. The development of children who are admitted to hospital with clinical malnutrition (kwashiorkor and marasmus) is particularly poor.

It is well recognized that severely malnourished children in hospital exhibit marked behavioral changes in the acute stage. They are more apathetic and less active, but irritable when disturbed. They explore their environments less, using fewer types of manipulation than better nourished children. When in hospital, they show less active distress than well-nourished children and have low-amplitude, abnormal cries. They also show a reduced orienting response to auditory stimuli. Most of these behaviors return to normal quickly with recovery, except for the quality of exploration. In contrast, they still have poor levels of development.

Moderately underweight and stunted children also show altered behavior. In young children, this behavior includes increased fussing and crying, lower activity level, less amount of and enthusiasm for play and exploration, fewer vocalizations, less positive affect, and a tendency to stay closer to the mother and be more apathetic.

The main problem with cross-sectional observational studies is that the children's disadvantaged backgrounds may have confounded the findings. In addition, the temporal relationship, with undernutrition preceding poor development, cannot be established. Longitudinal studies give a better idea of the type of functions affected in the long term and relationships over time.

Long-term effects

Follow-up of children with stunting in early childhood

Children who are stunted in early childhood continue to have poorer performance in a wide range of cognitive functions and poorer school achievement than nonstunted children through to 12 years of age. They also have behavioral problems and have been found to be more inhibited and less attentive and to have more conduct disorders. There is little available information for older ages.

Several studies have found an association between linear growth and change in development in the first 3 years of life. In Guatemala, change in height from 6 to 24 months of age was associated with change in development. In Jamaica, stunted children were enrolled between 6 and 24 months and change in height over the subsequent 24 months of the study was associated with change in mental age. Furthermore, change in height in the first 12 months predicted change in mental age in the second 12 months, even after controlling for height change in the second year. Change in weight for height has also been significantly related to change in development, but less frequently.

Follow-up of children with severe clinical malnutrition in early childhood

In developing countries many follow-up studies have been conducted of older children who were hospitalized for severe malnutrition in early childhood. At 4–5 years of age, children were observed to play less, to stay closer to their mothers and to be less responsive when given a task. In general, school-aged children who return to poor environments have deficits in cognitive development and school achievement, compared with matched controls. The children also have poorer behavior in school, including attention deficits and poorer social skills, than children with no history of malnutrition. They are also more aggressive and distractible at home. Developmental deficits have been found up to puberty, but there are few data from adults.

Studies using siblings for comparison were less likely to show significant differences, but the siblings were likely to have been moderately undernourished themselves. In general, there was no association between level of function and age of admission to hospital, which ranged from 6 to 36 months.

It appears that the long-term outcome of undernourished children is modified by the subsequent environment. Undernourished children who have been adopted by middle-class families have shown marked improvements. Similarly, stimulation programs have shown significant benefits that last at least through childhood. Severe malnutrition in early childhood is less likely to affect the development of children from middle-class homes than the development of children living in poverty. In developed countries children who suffered from severe or moderate underweight, secondary to illness, have shown smaller and less consistent deficits. In addition, nutritional supplementation in developing countries has been shown to have a greater benefit on the long-term development of children from poorer homes.

Supplementation studies

Because of the difficulty in controlling for the multitude of factors that affect children's development, intervention studies are needed to establish causal relationships. Several supplementation studies with developmental outcomes have been conducted. They may be divided into preventive studies, which began in pregnancy or at birth, and remedial studies, which targeted children who were already undernourished. A few studies also included stimulation.

Preventive supplementation

A randomized trial in Taiwan involved supplementing high-risk women in pregnancy and lactation alone, but not their offspring. Benefits were found on children's motor development at 8 months of age, but there was no evidence of a benefit on their IQ at 5 years.

In Colombia, Mexico and Guatemala, pregnant women at risk for undernutrition were supplemented in pregnancy and subsequently the children were supplemented for at least 3 years. In all three studies, supplementation was associated with concurrent and longer term benefits on children's development. These studies provide some of the best evidence of a causal relationship between nutrition and development. There were, however, problems with design of some of the trials. The Mexican study was not a randomized trial, and in Guatemala only four villages were randomized to high-calorie and protein or low-calorie supplements. In addition, as all of the studies involved supplementation of mothers, it is possible that the benefits to the children could be ascribed to the effects of supplementation on maternal behavior.

Remedial supplementation

There is limited evidence that supplementation beginning after the age of 3 years has no concurrent or long-term benefits, although when combined with stimulation benefits occur. However, benefits have been found from supplementing undernourished children under 2 years of age. Concurrent benefits were obtained in three studies beginning before the age of 24 months. Two of these studies were conducted in Indonesia and one was conducted in Jamaica. Two studies reported long-term follow-up. In Indonesia, some benefit was sustained at 9 years, but only for children supplemented before the age of 18 months and in one test of memory. In Jamaica, children were evaluated at 7–8 years on a battery of tests assessing cognitive function, fine motor skills and school achievement, and children who had received supplementation outperformed the control group on 14 out of 15 tests. At 11–12 years of age, benefits of supplementation were no longer detected.

Supplementation in the first 2 years of life more consistently benefited motor development than mental development. It may be that longer periods of supplementation are required to benefit mental development; for example, in Jamaica, stunted children on supplementation aged 9–24 months had improved motor performance only in the first year, but in the second year benefits in mental development also appeared.

In conclusion, concurrent benefits occurred from nutritional supplementation beginning at any age from pregnancy up to 24 months. Supplementation begun after 24 months had no or very little effect, although there were extremely few studies. The evidence suggests that supplementation benefits are more likely to be sustained if begun in late pregnancy and continued with the child for at least the first 24 months.

Evidence for a sensitive period

Evidence from observational studies indicates that undernutrition (severe clinical undernutrition or stunting) any time in the first 36 months of age is usually associated with long-term effects. Longitudinal analyses of findings from a Jamaican study reinforce the importance of early childhood. Measurements of height and head circumference between 9 and 24 months, and head circumference 2 years later, predicted IQ at 11 years, whereas these measurements at older ages did not. However, the severity of undernutrition probably also plays a role and the children's nutritional status was worst between 9 and 24 months. Two other studies had similar findings. In the Philippines, children who became stunted by 6 months of age had poorer IQ scores at 11 years than children who became stunted by 24 months. However, when severity of stunting at 24 months was considered, early stunting was no longer significant. Ethiopian children whose weights fell below the third centile of the NCHS references by 4 months of age had poorer developmental levels at 24 months than children whose weights fell below this point by 10 or 12 months. However, when weight at 2 years of age was controlled, the groups were not different. Both groups had poorer development than children whose weights were never below the third centile at these ages. Supplementation studies generally have design problems; however, they should give more precise estimates of sensitive periods. The findings from the supplementation studies discussed below indicate that supplementation in pregnancy alone, with or without the first 6 months, had concurrent but no sustained benefit. In contrast, supplementation in the last trimester of pregnancy and for the first 2 or 3 years of life resulted in concurrent and sustained benefits. Remedial supplementation in undernourished children usually had concurrent benefits under 2 years of age, but the evidence is inconsistent as to whether benefits are sustained. Supplementing children over 3 years has failed to produce benefits, but the data are extremely limited. In conclusion, there are insufficient data from which to draw firm conclusions, but they point to development being most sensitive to nutrition in the first 2 years.

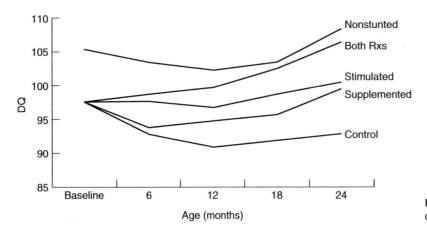

Figure 15.1 Interventions with stunted children (Grantham-McGregor *et al.*, 1991).

Psychosocial stimulation

Several intervention studies involving psychosocial stimulation (with or without supplementation) with undernourished children have had success and most have produced concurrent and long-term benefits for children. A Jamaican study with stunted children showed that both food and stimulation had independent benefits on the children's development and the effects were additive. Only the group that received both caught up with a comparison nonstunted group (Figure 15.1). This demonstrates the need for integrated programs if undernourished children are to return to normal.

It is often difficult to separate macronutrients from micronutrients in the above supplementation studies, because several of them (Colombia, Mexico, Jamaica) gave micronutrients as well as food, whereas the controls received nothing. In two studies (Taiwan and Guatemala) both supplemented and placebo groups received some micronutrients. In Indonesia, no micronutrients were given to either group, so the supplemented group only received the micronutrients naturally present in the food.

A recent Indonesian study of supplementing undernourished children was probably the only study to compare the effects of micronutrients with micronutrients combined with macronutrients. Children were enrolled at 12 and 18 months and randomized to receive condensed milk with micronutrients, skimmed milk and micronutrients or skimmed milk alone. The children receiving condensed milk and micronutrients performed better than those receiving skimmed milk and micronutrients on motor milestones and on a test of object permanence in the 12 month cohort, and in the 18 month cohort on the Bayley scale of mental development. These findings suggest that energy has an effect on development.

Recommendations for public health interventions

The evidence for a causal association between childhood undernutrition and poor development is reasonably strong. Although the disadvantaged backgrounds of undernourished children contribute to their poor development, poor nutrition almost certainly plays a role. Thus, in areas with a high prevalence of stunting, programs to improve children's nutritional status are urgently needed. These programs should target children in the first 2 years of life and should be combined with health care, psychosocial stimulation and parental education activities. The effect of supplementation with energy and protein in pregnancy on child development needs more research before policy implications are clear.

15.8 Iron-deficiency anemia

The main cause of anemia in developed countries is inadequate dietary intake of bioavailable iron. In developing countries inadequate dietary intake is also a major cause, but consumption of inhibitors such as tea, and parasitic infections, particularly malaria and hookworm, also play a role.

Many studies have shown an association between IDA in children and poor concurrent cognitive and motor development and behavioral problems. Similarly to underweight children, anemic children have been shown to be more fearful and withdrawn, unreactive to stimuli, more solemn, less involved and more unhappy during the developmental test session, and to stay closer to their mothers, show less pleasure, be more wary and tire more easily in a free-play situation. The caregivers of anemic children have also been shown to demonstrate altered behaviors. For example, in one study, the mothers of iron-anemic children were judged to show less affection, and even the developmental testers presented fewer tasks and made fewer attempts to elicit responses during the test session. In addition, several longitudinal studies have followed up children who were anemic in the first 2 years of life, at 4–14 years of age. The children were found to have poorer cognitive and motor development, minor neurological deficits and poorer school achievement than children who were not anemic. Even when the anemia was successfully treated in infancy the deficits remained. Behavioral deficits were also evident, with anemic children displaying more anxiety and depression and increased social and attentional problems. Although these studies suggest that IDA may have irreversible effects on child development, it remains possible that the myriad of other disadvantages experienced by anemic children may be the cause of the poor developmental prognosis.

Severity and duration

The duration of anemia has also been found to be linked with developmental levels. In Chile, infants who suffered from anemia for long periods had poorer developmental levels than those who had anemia for a short period. Developmental levels are also associated with severity of anemia, with hemoglobin levels below certain levels being associated with poorer development. However, the level of hemoglobin at which the association with development appears varied in different studies, from 8 g/dl in Zanzibar to 10.9 g/dl in Chile. It is difficult to explain this variation, but it may be due to different causes of anemia or differences in confounding variables such as poverty.

Treatment trials

Preventive or therapeutic RCTs provide the best evidence for causal relationships. In preventive trials, nonanemic children who are likely to become anemic are assigned to iron supplementation or placebo. It is anticipated that children in the placebo group will become anemic, whereas those in the treatment group will not. The development of the children in each group is then compared. In therapeutic trials,

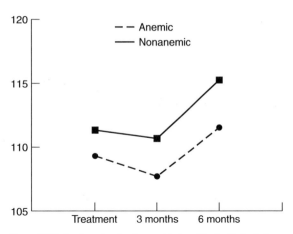

Figure 15.2 Psychomotor development index of Bayley Scales in iron-deficient anemic and nonanemic groups during treatment. Reprinted from Lozoff et al. (1996) with permission from Elsevier.

children who already have IDA are randomly assigned to receive iron treatment or placebo. In this case the findings will show whether any developmental deficit is reversible with iron treatment. There have been few rigorous treatment trials with iron supplementation. Many of the therapeutic trials have used nonanemic, iron-replete children as controls and there has been no placebo anemic group. Causality cannot be shown in these trials as the anemic children are likely to have more disadvantaged backgrounds and may develop differently to nonanemic children. These studies can show, however, whether anemic children catch up with nonanemic ones. In the following sections evidence from treatment trials with children over and under 2 years of age will be discussed, follow by evidence from preventive trials.

Short-term trials of iron supplementation in which children are supplemented for 2 weeks or less have generally shown no benefits from iron supplementation. However, the studies lacked statistical power as the samples were usually small, and hence no firm conclusions can be drawn. Longer term trials in which anemic children have been compared with nonanemic controls have usually shown that anemic children failed to catch up with iron supplementation (Figure 15.2). This suggests that either iron deficiency was not responsible for the poor development, or it has irremediable deleterious effects on child development. However, differences in home backgrounds make complete catch-up unlikely.

Only two randomized trials (in Zanzibar and Indonesia) have shown clear improvements in

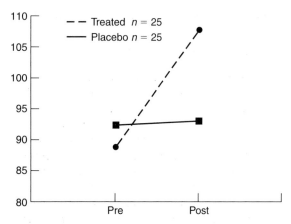

Figure 15.3 Mental development in iron-treated and placebo iron-deficient anemic children. Reprinted from Idjradinata and Pollitt (1993) with permission from Elsevier.

development of anemic children. In Indonesia, anemic children receiving iron supplementation showed marked improvements in mental and motor development measured on the Bayley scales of infant development compared with anemic children in the placebo group (Figure 15.3). However, this was an extremely small study.

In Zanzibar, anemic children with hemoglobin levels under 8 mg/dl improved in motor milestones, whereas all anemic children improved in language milestones compared with the placebo group. Many of these children were infected with malaria or other parasites and came from extremely poor families, so caution should be applied in extrapolating to less disadvantaged children.

In a third RCT of iron supplementation of anemic children in the UK, no treatment effect was observed on the Denver screening test. However, this test was designed to screen for developmental delay and hence may lack sensitivity to small developmental differences. It is unknown whether benefits from iron treatment are sustained. There is little information on the effects of anemia in vulnerable groups, such as children born LBW or stunted children, because they have usually been excluded from the studies. Children at socio-economic and/or biomedical risk may be more vulnerable to the effects of IDA than are low-risk children.

There are several RCTs with iron treatment in anemic iron-deficient or nonanemic iron-deficient older children and adolescents. Most but not all of them have found benefits in cognitive function, but investigators often analyzed the data without allowing for initial differences. Thus, the evidence from treatment trials with

anemic children over 3 years of age is reasonably strong that iron supplementation benefits cognition. Furthermore, anemic children have frequently caught up with nonanemic children in their levels of cognition.

Improvements in school achievement are probably more difficult to achieve and are likely to take longer as the treated anemic children would need to have the opportunity to catch up. The results have been inconsistent, but there is too little information on the effects of iron supplementation on school achievement to draw any conclusions.

Preventive trials of iron supplementation

Prophylactic treatment trials are more expensive than treatment trials as only a proportion of the placebo group will become anemic; thus, much larger samples are required. Only a few preventive treatment trials of iron supplementation have been conducted and the results have been a little disappointing. Transient benefits were found in a Canadian trial, while small benefits were reported in two trials in England and Chile. In an RCT, Canadian children were supplemented starting from the first 2 months of life until 15 months. Differences in motor development between treated and placebo children were found at 9 and 12 months of age, but there was no longer a significant difference at 15 months, suggesting that the benefits are transient. No differences were found in mental development.

In the English study, benefits of treatment were not found during treatment, but were present 6 months after the cessation of treatment, when the children were 24 months old. However, a problem with this study was that the treatment group was given iron-fortified formula while the placebo group received cow's milk. Formula differs from cow's milk in more than the iron content and other micronutrients or constituents may have been responsible for the differences in development. In a Chilean study, no benefits of iron supplementation were evident on the Bayley test, but children in the treatment group performed better on a measure of attention and ability to encode stimuli. Three other preventive trials have failed to find benefits. Hence, there is some evidence, albeit limited, that preventing IDA benefits development in young children.

Recommendations for public health interventions

Interventions to control IDA involve iron fortification of food staples and fortification of complementary foods in both developed and developing countries. Nutrition education is another public health measure, but the effectiveness has not been well evaluated. In developing countries the control and treatment of malaria, hookworm infection and schistosomiasis is also important. Long-term iron supplementation can also successfully reduce the prevalence of anemia, although to be effective at least weekly supplementation is required and daily supplementation is preferable, although compliance is often low. However, it is uncertain whether giving an iron supplement to non-iron deficient children has side-effects. As children with anemia usually come from disadvantaged backgrounds, an integrated approach is necessary which includes access to health care and child development activities as well as attention to nutrition.

15.9 Iodine deficiency

Iodine is a constituent of thyroid hormones which are important for skeletal maturation and the development of the central nervous system. Iron-deficiency disorders (IDD) include goiter, endemic cretinism, increased prenatal and postnatal mortality, and cognitive, sensory and motor deficits. Iodine deficiency has severe socioeconomic implications as iodine-deficient individuals have reduced work capacity and are less productive. In the following sections, observational studies and intervention studies investigating the effect of iodine deficiency on mental development will be reviewed.

Children living in iodine-deficient areas usually have poorer mental and motor development than those living in nondeficient areas. A metaanalysis of 18 studies investigating the relationship between iodine deficiency and cognition in children and adults found an average deficit of of 13.5 IQ points in the iodine-deficient individuals compared with controls. This is a very large deficit. However, the control of family and community background factors that may also affect development was generally poor. Iodine-deficient areas tend to be isolated and poorer and to have fewer facilities than nondeficient areas. However, the result does concur with the hypothesis that iodine deficiency affects child development.

Supplementation studies

Several supplementation trials have been conducted involving giving iodine to individuals living in iodine-deficient areas and comparing their development with that of nonsupplemented controls, also in iodine-deficient areas. Supplementation studies have mainly been conducted with women before and during pregnancy, and with children.

Supplementation studies with women

These studies involved giving iodized oil to women either before or during pregnancy and investigating the effects on their children's mental development. Several studies were reported on a single population in Ecuador and involved supplementing women in one iodine-deficient village and comparing children born to these women with children born to women in a matched iodine-deficient village. These studies found that iodine supplementation before conception or early in pregnancy was associated with increased IQ and a reduction in the number of children with cretinism or severe learning disability. Supplementation before conception was found to be most effective, whereas iodine prophylaxis after the fifth month of pregnancy had little or no effect on child cognition. The study design was, however, not rigorous as no placebo was provided for the controls and only two villages were involved in the study which, despite being matched for gross socioeconomic indicators, are unlikely to have been the same in all factors affecting child development (e.g. the quality of schooling).

Two RCTs have provided good evidence of a causal link between iodine deficiency and increased cretinism and decreased mental development. It is therefore no longer considered ethical to withhold iodine treatment from women of fertile age. The first study was conducted in 14 villages in Papua New Guinea, where women of childbearing age received injections of either iodized oil or a placebo. Children born to these women were followed until they reached 15 years of age. Iodine supplementation prevented endemic cretinism, and children in the treatment group had better cognitive development and better fine motor skills than children born to mothers who received a placebo. Mortality was also reduced in the treatment group.

The other trial was conducted in Zaire. Pregnant women were supplemented with iodized oil at a mean of 28 weeks into pregnancy and compared with pregnant women supplemented with vitamins in oil. Children's development was tested from 4 to 25 months of age and significantly higher developmental quotients were found in the treated group.

Supplementation studies with children

Several studies have compared children supplmented with iodine in one village with unsupplemented children in a control village. Results were inconsistent, with one study finding a treatment effect in girls only, another reporting poorer hearing in the iodine-deficient area that improved with treatment, and a third study finding no differences on tests assessing manual dexterity and reaction speed. However, the villages were not well matched so the results are difficult to interpret.

Several RCTs have been conducted on the effects of iodine supplementation on the cognitive development of children. In Bolivia and Bangladesh the treated children failed to show benefits in cognition; however, in Bolivia, the iodine intake of the control group also increased during the study, making interpretation of results difficult. A treatment trial in Malawi found significant benefits of iodine supplementation in 6–8-year-old children on mental and motor development. However, the pretest scores were invalid and hence it is not possible to know whether differences between treatment and control were present before supplementation.

Recommendations for public health interventions

The evidence points to the critical importance of iodine supplementation before conception and in the first two trimesters of pregnancy for women living in iodine-deficient areas. The research on the effect of iodine supplementation for children and the effect on cognition is inconsistent, although iodine supplementation remains important to reduce the incidence of goiter and is particularly important for girls of reproductive age. The easiest and most cost-effective method of iodization is the fortification of salt for all human and animal consumption. Iodized oil may also be used where it is not possible to fortify salt. The WHO recommends the use of iodized oil in situations where the prevalence of IDD is moderate or severe, cretinism or neonatal hypothyroidism is present, or universal salt iodization would not reach women of reproductive age in 1 or 2 years.

15.10 Zinc deficiency

Zinc deficiency is associated with reduced immunity to infection, increased severity and duration of diarrhea, and growth retardation. There is some evidence that zinc deficiency also affects children's cognitive and motor development and behavior.

For example, zinc-supplemented infants and toddlers have been found to be more active, and to sit and play more often and lie down less often than unsupplemented children. In a study in Canada, very LBW children ($<1500 \, g$) supplemented with zinc and copper for the first 6 months of life had improved motor development compared with nonsupplemented children. There were no differences in mental development. However, in two recent studies in Bangladesh, zinc supplementation given to undernourished children or pregnant women had a very small detrimental effect on infant development. In the first study, infants were supplemented from 1 month to 5 months of age, and the children receiving placebo scored 3.7 points (0.25 SD) higher on mental development than the children receiving zinc at 13 months of age. In the second study, pregnant women were supplemented from the fourth month of gestation until birth, and the infants of the women receiving zinc supplementation scored 3.3 points (0.33 SD) lower on mental development and 5.1 points (0.33 SD) lower on motor development at 13 months of age. It may be that in undernourished populations mononutrient supplementation interferes with the nutrient balance and increases other micronutrient deficiencies by inhibiting absorption.

Studies on the effects of zinc supplementation on the cognitive function of schoolchildren have had inconsistent results, with two RCTs showing no cognitive benefits and two other studies in China and Mexico showing improved cognitive performance. As it is difficult to assess zinc deficiency at a population level, it may be that in some of the studies the samples were not zinc deficient initially.

In conclusion, it appears that zinc affects children's development, but it is unknown at present which populations will benefit from supplementation. It is uncertain whether multinutrients would provide more benefits and be safer than zinc supplementation alone. It is likely that children who are undernourished and deficient in energy and proteins should be given macronutrients and micronutrients.

15.11 Vitamin A deficiency

Vitamin A deficiency is a major public health problem, particularly in Africa and south-east Asia. It is the main cause of preventable blindness and severe visual impairment in young children, and increases the risk of severe illness and death from childhood infections such as diarrhea and measles. The WHO estimates that 100–140 million children are vitamin A deficient and between one-quarter and half a million children become blind every year as a result of vitamin A deficiency. Although, to the authors' knowledge, no studies have looked at the effect of vitamin A deficiency on child development, blindness will obviously impact on a child's development, especially in areas with limited facilities for blind children, and there is also evidence that repeated childhood infections detrimentally affect development.

Recommendations for public health interventions

The effect of vitamin A deficiency on child mortality and morbidity and the importance of vitamin A in blindness prevention make vitamin A deficiency a major public health problem. Vitamin A deficiency is often linked to the nature of the foods available and feeding practices used. Interventions to combat vitamin A deficiency include promoting breast-feeding, fortifying foods (e.g. sugar), improving dietary diversity (e.g. through home gardens) and administering a high-dose supplement of vitamin A every 4–6 months.

15.12 Studies on the effects of short-term hunger and school feeding

There is some evidence of the effects of short-term hunger on cognition and behavior from studies on giving or missing breakfast. Studies on school feeding also provide information on the effect of school meals on school achievement, classroom behavior, attendance and nutritional status. Studies have been conducted in both developed and developing countries.

Effects on child cognition

Probably the best approach to investigate the effect of short-term hunger is using RCTs of giving or missing breakfast. The most rigorous studies investigating the effects of missing breakfast on child cognition have ensured dietary control by admitting the children into a residential facility overnight and providing a standardized meal. In these studies, cross-over designs were used in which a children's performance was compared in the late morning when they received breakfast and when they received a placebo; thus, the children acted as their own control. Four such studies were identified,

two in the USA, one in Jamaica and one in Peru. In the US studies, adequately nourished children performed better on tests of visual perception and problem solving after receiving breakfast than when they received a placebo. In the studies in both Jamaica and Peru, children who were undernourished were detrimentally affected in their performance on several cognitive tests when they missed breakfast, whereas adequately nourished children showed no adverse effects. It is unclear why well-nourished children in Jamaica and Peru were not affected by missing breakfast, whereas well-nourished children in the USA were affected. One possible explanation could be that the children from Jamaica and Peru were poorer and may have developed a tolerance for the effects of short-term hunger, in contrast to their more affluent counterparts in developed countries.

Several laboratory studies in the UK and USA have shown that glucose drinks given to children who missed breakfast benefited cognition or behavior, or both.

Evidence from less rigorous studies based in schools is more mixed. In Sweden, children who received adequate breakfasts performed better in tests of addition and creativity, and persevered more in physical exercises than when they received inadequate breakfasts. In another Jamaican study, children had better performance on a similar test of creativity on days they were given breakfast at school than when they were not given breakfast.

In contrast, in two studies, in India and Chile there was no effect of missing breakfast on the cognitive function of primary schoolchildren. In the latter study there was no control over what the children ate the night before and as many as 23% of the children admitted to eating breakfast at home on the morning of the study.

Effects on school achievement and attendance

Several observational studies have shown that a history of missing breakfast or feeling hungry in school is associated with poor school achievement. However, similarly to the nutritional deficiencies discussed above, there are many confounding factors that are difficult to control for. Most evaluations of large-scale programs suggest that school attendance improves if meals are provided. Although these evaluations were not usually randomized trials, some had control schools from other neighborhoods or regions and others had data before and after the introduction of school meals.

One evaluation showed that when school meals were stopped attendance declined.

Stronger evidence of the beneficial effects of providing breakfast comes from research studies of school feeding. However, school studies are usually less rigorous than the laboratory-controlled studies mentioned above, as there is no control over what children are eating at home. However, these studies are important to determine whether providing breakfast in schools is an appropriate public health measure. In the USA, a 3 month breakfast program resulted in benefits for the participating children in a test of school achievement measuring language, mathematics and reading, and decreased absenteeism and lateness. A study in Peru showed benefits of a 1 month breakfast program on children's school attendance and vocabulary scores, but not on mathematics or reading comprehension. In Jamaica, two studies have been conducted on giving a school breakfast and school achievement. In one study, breakfast was provided for one school term. Children in the treatment group had better attendance and higher scores in a test of arithmetic than children in a matched school class receiving a placebo. The second study was an RCT with children assigned to breakfast or a small piece of fruit within the same school for one school year. The children receiving breakfast improved in school attendance and scores in arithmetic, as well as in nutritional status.

In conclusion, there are surprisingly few well-evaluated studies on the effect of providing breakfast in schools in either developed or developing countries. Most have been shown to increase school attendance and attainment in at least one school subject. However, very few well-designed studies have examined attainment levels.

Effects on behavior

Providing breakfast has also been found to have beneficial effects on children's behavior. For example, in South Africa a 6 week breakfast program reduced the occurrence and duration of off-task and out-of-seat behavior. However, other studies have demonstrated that the effects of school breakfast on child behavior depend on other factors in the environment. For example, a study in the USA showed that the level of improvement in on-task behavior after being given breakfast varied according to the task the children were doing. In Jamaica, the effect of eating breakfast on child behavior varied as a function of the quality of the school: in a well-organized school the children's behavior improved, whereas in two overcrowded schools with poorer facilities the children's behavior deteriorated after they were given breakfast. The biological status of the child therefore interacted with the quality of the school to produce different effects.

Mechanism of how breakfast benefits educational outcomes

There are several potential mechanisms by which the provision of breakfast may benefit educational outcomes. First, as providing breakfast has been shown to increase school attendance the amount of time children spend in school will be increased. Secondly, by alleviating short-term hunger, attentiveness, working memory and speed of information processing may improve, hence enabling children to benefit more from instruction. Thirdly, in the long term, breakfast may improve children's nutritional status and correct micronutrient deficiencies, thus affecting child cognition.

In conclusion, there is a need for more well-controlled trials of school feeding in both developing and developed countries. The limited results suggest that school breakfast can have important benefits on attendance, school attainment and classroom behavior when children are not having adequate breakfasts at home or are undernourished. There are few data regarding the provision of lunch.

15.13 Perspectives on the future

There is now a wide range of nutritional conditions associated with children's development. There are extremely consistent data from observational studies linking breast-feeding with better development and reasonably consistent data linking SGA to poor development. However, the evidence from RCTs linking these conditions causally to poor child development is limited owing to problems of conducting such studies. Very few studies of supplementation with macronutrients in pregnancy only have been conducted and have generally had disappointing results. Only two studies were identified (both in Honduras) in which infants were randomized to exclusive breast-feeding for 6 months or weaning at 4 months, and in each case the late weaning group demonstrated benefits to their motor development.

The evidence from randomized trials linking other conditions to poor development is reasonably strong for concurrent effects of stunting and underweight and strong for iodine deficiency *in utero*. The evidence of a causal relationship is also reasonably strong for iron deficiency in school-aged children, but less robust for children under 2 years. More data are needed on zinc deficiency to be able to draw conclusions with confidence. It is clear that vitamin A deficiency causes blindness.

Missing breakfast affects cognition in the late morning and school meals benefit school attendance, but their effect on school achievement needs more study.

There are consistent data from longitudinal observational studies linking stunting, underweight, iodine deficiency *in utero* and iron deficiency to poorer cognition and behavior in later childhood. However, the evidence of long-term effects from randomized trials is good for iodine deficiency *in utero*, limited for stunting and underweight, and not available for iron or zinc deficiency.

It is likely that there are other nutritional deficiencies, yet to be studied, that affect development. It is obvious from existing information that the development of children with poor nutrition is in jeopardy. Considering the large numbers of children affected, urgent interventions are needed, as well as further research.

Further reading

Anderson J, Johnstone B, Remley D. Breastfeeding and cognitive development – a meta-analysis. Am J Clin Nutr 1999; 70: 525–535.

Grantham-McGregor S, Ani C. The role of micronutrients in psychomotor and cognitive development. Br Med Bull 1999; 55: 511–527.

Grantham-McGregor S, Ani A. Review of studies on the effect of iron deficiency on cognitive development in children. J Nutr 2001; 131: 649S–668S.

Grantham-McGregor S, Powell C, Walker S, Himes J. Nutritional supplementation, psychosocial stimulation, and mental development of stunted children: the Jamaican Study. Lancet 1991; 338: 1–5.

Idjradinata P, Pollitt E. Reversal of developmental delays in iron-deficient anemic infants treated with iron. Lancet 1993; 341: 1–4.

Lozoff B, Wolf A, Jimenez E. Iron-deficiency anemia and infant development: effects of extended oral iron therapy. J Pediatr 1996; 129: 382–389.

Pollitt E, ed. Undernutrition and behavioral development in children. J Nutr 1995; 125S.

Pollitt E, Schurch B, eds. Developmental pathways of the malnourished child: results of a supplementation trial in Indonesia. Eur J Clin Nutr 2000; 54 (Suppl 2): S1–S119.

Scrimshaw N, Schurch B, eds. Causes and consequences of intrauterine growth retardation. Eur J Clin Nutr 1998; 52 (Suppl 1).

Stanbury J, ed. The Damaged Brain of Iodine Deficiency. New York: Cognizant Communication Corporation, 1994.

Stoltzfus RJ, Kvalsvig JD, Chwaya HM *et al*. Effects of iron supplementation and anthelmintic treatment on motor and language development of preschool children in Zanzibar: double blind, placebo controlled study. BMJ 2001; 323: 1–8.

16
Infant Feeding

Anna Coutsoudis and Jane Bentley

Key messages

- Exclusive breast-feeding is the best way to feed an infant in the first 6 months. Mothers need active encouragement, and emotional support from the health-care practitioners and family members to be able to breast-feed successfully.
- Several misconceptions about breast-feeding exist, providing barriers to successful feeding.
- Health-care workers need to ensure that their conduct is in line with the Baby Friendly hospital guidelines and the Code of Marketing of Breastmilk Substitutes to ensure that breast-feeding has a chance of success.
- There are situations where a mother cannot breast-feed her infant, but this is uncommon.
- During illness, or with physical difficulties, the mother should receive additional support and encouragement from the health-care team to enable her to provide optimal nutrition to her infant.
- Breast milk from human immunodeficiency virus (HIV)-positive women contains HIV: the risk of transmission is 5–8% during the first 6 months in mixed breast-fed infants.
- In developing countries HIV-positive women should be well informed before having to make a decision on how to feed their baby.
- Introduction of solids is a vulnerable period for the infant. A wide variety of foods should be introduced to the infant to ensure adequate micronutrient intake.
- Intake and growth should be closely monitored to enable the health worker to detect difficulties early.

16.1 Introduction

Breast-feeding has always been acknowledged as the optimal way to feed an infant, although recommendations regarding practices have changed as more information has become available. Many early studies on the beneficial effects of breast-feeding were seriously flawed in terms of study design, as well as in the definition of breast-feeding. This led to debate as to whether breast-feeding was advantageous in industrialized countries, where hygiene conditions significantly reduced the incidence of infectious diseases. The discovery that the advantages of breast-feeding are dose related has led to more thorough definitions of breast-feeding patterns and better controlled studies. In 1991, a joint meeting of international World Health Organization (WHO) and United Nations Children's Fund (UNICEF) representatives culminated in the Innocenti Declaration on the Protection, Promotion and Support of Breastfeeding, defining optimal infant feeding as exclusive breast-feeding from birth to 4–6 months, and continued into the second year of life, with appropriate complementary foods added at about 6 months. Subsequently, the WHO convened an Expert Panel meeting which reviewed over 3000 research papers and concluded that as a population recommendation, 6 months was the optimum age for exclusive breast-feeding. This was then adopted as a World Health Assembly Resolution in May 2001.

Recent evidence has shown that the benefits of breast-feeding over formula feeding are also obvious even in developed countries where there is presumably good access to clean water and sufficient resources to make up formula safely.

- In the UK, low birth weight (LBW) infants in particular have been found to benefit from breast milk, where formula feeding has been found to increase the risk of necrotizing enterocolitis by a factor of at least six-fold.

- In Scotland, long-term benefits for children 7 years of age, who were exclusively breast-fed for at least 15 weeks from birth, included a significantly reduced probability of ever having a respiratory infection or wheeze, and a lower systolic blood pressure.
- Swedish infants who were formula fed have been found to have significantly higher risk of otitis media in the first year of life compared with predominantly breast-fed infants.
- Swedish preschool infants who were breast-fed for less than 13 weeks were found to have a significantly increased risk of *Haemophilus influenzae* meningitis, the risk decreasing with every additional week of exclusive breast-feeding.
- In America, formula-fed infants faced double the risk of diarrheal disease and 19% more otitis media in the first year of life, compared with fully breast-fed infants.
- Not only does breast-feeding influence health in infancy and early childhood, but it also appears to have long-term benefits, reducing the incidence of asthma in 6-year-old children from Australia.

It is now becoming clear that not all breast-feeding is equal in terms of health outcomes in the infant and that exclusive breast-feeding carries significant advantages over mixed breast-feeding. There are examples of this from around the world.

- In the Gambia, children who were given prelacteal feeds were 3.38 times more likely to die.
- Similarly, in Peru, infant mortality was associated with mixed breast-feeding as well as with never having been breast-fed.
- In Latin America, it has been estimated that 13.9% of all infant deaths could be prevented by exclusive breast-feeding, translating into 52 000 preventable deaths for that area.

This chapter discusses the importance of breast-feeding, reviews trends of infant feeding in different countries over the past century, particularly in relation to socioeconomic status and includes the challenges to optimum breast-feeding. Consideration will be given to breast-feeding difficulties and in particular the issues around breast-feeding by human immunodeficiency virus (HIV)-infected women. Finally, infant feeding after 6 months will be discussed, as well as the importance of monitoring the child's growth in the first few years.

16.2 Role and importance of breast-feeding

The goal of good nutrition is adequate growth and development. It is well known that this depends not only on adequate dietary intake but also on psychosocial well-being and health (Figure 16.1). Breast-feeding is thus a unique practice, which offers not only adequate nutrient and energy intake, but also psychosocial care through bonding with the mother and health through the immunological properties of breast milk. Breast-feeding in the first 6 months is the one time when infants of rich and poor mothers are on equal footing, as mentioned by James Grant, a past director of UNICEF (Box 16.1).

Several factors affect lactation in a positive and a negative way. These include environmental, psychological and pharmacological factors, and are summarized in Table 16.1.

Advantages of breast-feeding

Human milk is constituted to provide all of the infant's nutrient requirements for a period of about 6 months,

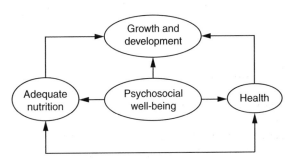

Figure 16.1 Adapted UNICEF framework describing the interdependence of nutrition, psychosocial well-being and health to promote the growth and development of a child.

Box 16.1

"Breast-feeding is a natural 'safety net' against the worst effects of poverty. If a child survives the first month of life (the most dangerous period of childhood) then for the next four months or so, exclusive breast-feeding goes a long way towards cancelling out the health difference between being born into poverty and being born into affluence ... it is almost as if breast-feeding takes the infant out of poverty for those first few months in order to give the child a fairer start in life and compensate for the injustice of the world into which it was born."

James Grant, past Director of UNICEF

except if the mother is severely malnourished. The composition of the milk changes in line with the infant's requirements.

The presence of antibodies and macrophages in the colostrum and breast milk confers protection against certain infections (Table 16.2). Immunity against enteral, and to a lesser extent parenteral infections, is derived from the antibodies. As a result it is uncommon for a fully breast-fed infant to contract infective diarrhea or necrotizing enterocolitis. Respiratory and ear infections also occur less frequently in breast-fed babies.

The incidence of allergies in infants who are breast-fed is decreased compared with those who have been fed cow's milk. The delayed introduction of foreign proteins may also be beneficial in reducing the chances of developing autoimmune reactions such as occur in the development of insulin-dependent diabetes mellitus.

The incidence of sudden infant death syndrome is lower in breast-fed babies, although the reason for this is not clear.

Breast milk is hygienic, inexpensive, convenient and readily available for the infant. It requires no preparation or sterilization. These factors are likely to outweigh the possible disadvantages of restricted activities or temporary unemployment for the mother and therefore need serious consideration. Breast-feeding is less expensive than any substitute, even if the mother has to eat slightly more. An additional factor to consider is that the breast-fed infant's ration does not have to be shared by other members of the family.

One study found that significantly higher scores for cognitive development were associated with breast-fed children compared with those who were formula fed. This effect was sustained until 15 years of age and those breast-fed for the longest showed the most difference. (see Chapter 15). Breast-feeding strengthens the psychological bonding process between mother and child. There is anecdotal evidence that this is especially important in the later development of the child's personality and in the socialization of the child. Ovulation is suppressed by demand breast-feeding. Decreased fertility due to lactational amenorrhea, associated with regular continued breast-feeding, differs between individual women, but may continue for 12 months or longer. This should not be considered a reliable method of contraception, as 3–7% of breast-feeding women do become pregnant. The relative risks of disease in formula-fed infants are summarized in Table 16.3.

Table 16.1 Factors affecting lactation

	Favorable	Unfavorable
Environment	Calm, relaxed	Noisy, stressful
Frequency of feeds	Frequent	Infrequent
Breast contents		Engorged
Emotional state	Relaxed	Anxious
Physical state	Comfortable	Pain, tense
Drugs	Metoclopramide	Estrogen
	Oxytocin (sublingual)	Testosterone
		Bromocriptine
		Sedatives (large doses)

Table 16.2 Immune factors in breast milk

Immune factor	Functions
B-lymphocytes	Give rise to antibodies targeted at specific microbes
Macrophages	Kill microbes in the infant's gut; produce lysozyme; activate other components of the immune system
Neutrophils	Ingest bacteria in the infant's gut
T-lymphocytes	Kill infected cells, send chemical messages to mobilize other defences
Immunoglobulin A antibodies	Bind to microbes in the infant's gut, preventing them from passing through the mucosa
B_{12} binding protein	Binds B_{12}, preventing use by bacteria for growth
Bifidus factor	Promotes growth of *Lactobacillus bifidus*
Fatty acids	Disrupt membranes surrounding certain viruses, destroying them
Fibronectin	Increases antimicrobial activity of macrophages; facilitates repair of damaged tissues
Gamma-interferon	Enhances antimicrobial activity of immune cells
Hormones and epithelial growth factor	Stimulate epithelial maturation, reducing vulnerability to microorganisms
Lactoferrin	Binds iron, reducing availability for bacteria
Lysozyme	Kills bacteria by disrupting cell walls
Mucins	Adhere to bacteria and viruses, preventing attachment to mucosa
Oligosaccharides	Adhere to microorganisms, preventing attachment to mucosa

Table 16.3 Relative risks of disease in formula-fed infants highlighted by individual studies

Diarrhea	In Brazil, formula-fed infants are 14.2 times more likely to die from diarrhea than breast-fed babies
Ear infection	Formula-fed infants have twice the number of ear infections of exclusively breast-fed infants
Bacterial infections	In the USA, formula-fed infants are 10 times more likely to be admitted to hospital for any bacterial infection, and four times more likely to have meningitis
Cancer	Formula-fed infants are twice as likely to develop cancer by 15 years of age compared with breast-fed infants
Sudden infant death syndrome	Formula-fed infants are almost three times more likely to die from sudden infant death syndrome than breast-fed infants
Crohn's disease and ulcerative colitis	These diseases are more common in formula-fed infants
Eyesight	Formula-fed infants have poorer vision at 4 and 36 months compared with breast-fed infants
Pneumonia	In Brazil, infants fed only formula milk were 3.9 times more likely to die from pneumonia than breast-fed infants
Urinary tract infections	Formula-fed infants are five times more likely to contract urinary tract infections than breast-fed infants
Necrotizing enterocolitis	Infants born at 30 weeks of gestation, who are formula fed, are 20 times more likely to develop necrotizing enterocolitis
Diabetes	Infants who are formula fed before 2 months of age are twice as likely to develop diabetes
Celiac disease	Formula-fed infants show accelerated development of celiac disease
Dental caries	Children who have been formula fed have more dental caries than breast-fed children
Cognitive development	Formula-fed infants show lower scores on mental ability tests

Table 16.4 Relative risks of not breast-feeding for the mother highlighted by individual studies

Breast cancer	Women who have not breast-fed for at least 3 months have double the risk of developing premenopausal breast cancer
Child spacing	Formula feeding increases the risk of a second pregnancy, which adversely affects the mother's health
Ovarian cancer	Women who have not breast-fed for at least 2 months per child have a 25% increased risk of epithelial ovarian cancer
Osteoporosis	The risk of hip fracture is doubled in women over 65 if they have never breast-fed

Breast and ovarian cancer occurs less frequently in women who have breast-fed. The relative risks of not breast-feeding to the mother are summarized in Table 16.4.

Researchers have not always used the same definitions of breast-feeding, making comparisons of different studies difficult. To standardize research, and thereby obtain a better understanding of the benefits of breast-feeding, the definitions now used are summarized in Box 16.2.

Secular trends in infant feeding

In the 1920s, breast-feeding rates began to decline rapidly in industrialized countries, from approximately 50–70% of newborns breast-feeding on discharge from hospital, to the 1970s, where only 10–25% of newborns were breast-fed in the first week of life. This decline was associated with the increased availability of infant formulas, the aggressive marketing of replacement formula and the introduction of many conveniences associated with formula feeding. Since the 1970s, there have been many programs aimed at increasing the rate of breast-feeding.

Box 16.2 Definitions of commonly used terms

Exclusive breast-feeding: the infant receives only breast milk from his or her mother or expressed breast milk, and no other liquids or solids with the exception of drops or syrups consisting of vitamins, mineral supplements or medicines. The infant who receives only expressed breast milk in a cup whilst the mother works outside the home is still deemed to be exclusively breast-fed.

Prelacteal feeds: any food, solid or liquid, other than breast milk given to an infant before the initiation of breast-feeding.

At the beginning of the decline, disadvantaged mothers were more likely to breast-feed than advantaged mothers. Advantaged mothers, with a higher educational level, led the decline, but subsequently also led the upward trend. The increase in breast-feeding among disadvantaged women has been much slower. In the USA, the mother least likely to breast-feed is a young African–American, with no college education, living in a rural area, who has an LBW infant: possibly the infant who would most benefit from breast-feeding. Similar findings from the UK, where inner-city mothers, with less than 18 years of education, delivering at the hospital with the regional neonatal high-care unit, experienced the sharpest decline in breast-feeding between 1979 and 1988. In the Philippines, delivering in a hospital was associated with a significantly lower incidence of breast-feeding.

Wide differences exist in breastfeeding initiation and duration both between and within developed countries. For example, in Europe, rates of exclusive breast-feeding at 6 months vary from as much as 46% in Austria and 42% in Sweden to 21% in the UK and 10% in Germany. However, it should be noted that data on exclusive breast-feeding are scarce and unavailable in many countries. Reliable surveillance systems across Europe using a common harmonized methodology need to be developed. In addition to this intercountry variability in breast-feeding rates, wide within-country differences exist. A strong relationship between duration of breast-feeding and socioeconomic status has been shown, with a pattern of shorter duration of breast-feeding among lower social classes. For example, in the UK 48% of women from the highest social class were still breast-feeding at 6 months compared with just 22% from the lowest social class.

Because of this association between breast-feeding (initiation and duration) and social class, it is important when examining the relationship between breast-feeding and childhood morbidity that social class is controlled for in the analyses. This is generally done through stratification of the data or through the use of multivariate analysis. While most studies correct for social status, few studies actually represent the differences in morbidity for different socioeconomic levels. An example of this may be seen in a study examining the impact of breast-feeding on admission for pneumonia during the postneonatal period in Brazil. The study found that infants who were not being breast-fed were 17 times more likely than those being breast-fed to be admitted to hospital for pneumonia. Since social class was associated both with the outcome (admission to hospital for pneumonia) and the variable of interest (feeding method) it was controlled for in this multivariate analysis. Table 16.5 outlines the risk for admission to hospital for pneumonia according to socioeconomic status (defined in this study by economic status). The higher social classes (professionals and owners of large businesses) had the lowest risk for admisssion to hospital, while the lowest category of social class (unemployed/casual workers) had the highest risk for hospital admission.

Table 16.5 Risk of hospitalization for pneumonia according to socio-economic status in Brazil

Social class represented by employment	Odds ratio
Professionals large business owners	0.2
Small business owners and shopkeepers	1.49
Nonmanual, regularly employed	1
Manual, regularly employed	1.78
Unemployed/casual workers	3.5

Reproduced from Cesar (1999) with permission from the BMJ Publishing Group. The lower the odds ratio, the less protective effect breast-feeding has on the risk of diarrhea.

In developing countries, the effect of socioeconomic status is reversed. More affluent mothers with a higher level of education are less likely to breast-feed. An inverse relationship has been found between maternal education and the mean duration of breast-feeding. Again, a strong inverse relationship was found between births attended by health-care workers and mean duration of breast-feeding.

While breast-feeding rates are increasing in many developed countries, the decline in breast-feeding is still obvious in the developing countries, especially in urbanized areas. Various scenarios operate to perpetuate this situation. Artificial feeding is regarded as a status symbol by many, partly because of the marketing of breast-milk substitutes, and partly because replacement feeding has been commonly practiced by affluent women. Working mothers frequently have to leave their babies in the care of others and institute cessation of breast-feeding very early. This is often due to a lack of, or inadequate facilities at their place of work which, if available, would allow mothers to continue to breast-feed. Many of these mothers are unaware of how to maintain lactation.

16.3 Barriers to successful breast-feeding

Many unsubstantiated beliefs and attitudes about breast-feeding mean that mothers may not choose to breast-feed exclusively in the first 6 months. Common reasons why mothers do not breast-feed exclusively include:

- mother's unfounded fear that the milk is insufficient and/or of poor quality
- delay in initiating breast-feeding, and discarding colostrum
- poor breast-feeding technique

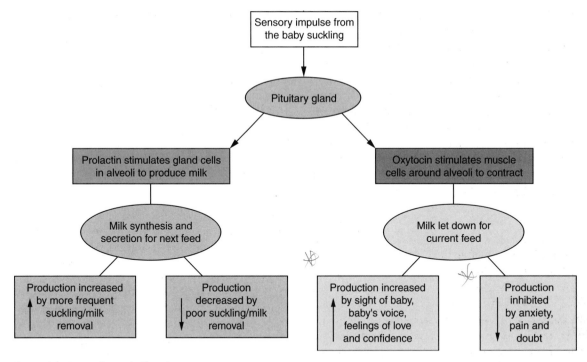

Figure 16.2 Hormonal control of lactation.

- mistaken belief that infants become thirsty and need extra fluid
- lack of support from the health services
- marketing of breast-milk substitutes.

Mother's unfounded fear that the milk is insufficient and/or of poor quality

This can be linked to the appearance of the foremilk, which is thin and watery. The mother needs to understand that changes in milk composition occur with suckling. The foremilk is thin and watery, but high in protein and antibodies. The foremilk will satisfy the infant's thirst, while the hindmilk, rich in fat, will satisfy the infant's hunger.

Breast-milk quantity can be kept up by frequent suckling at the breast. Hormonal control of breast-milk production is represented in Figure 16.2. Breast-milk production cannot be increased by dietary changes. The relatively small stools of the breast-fed infant are due to the minimal amount of indigestible material present in the milk and the stools of exclusively breast-fed infants are normally loose and yellow. The mother should be reassured and supported to continue breast-feeding as long as the infant is gaining at least 500 g per month,

appears satisfied and passes a normal amount of urine (approximately six to eight wet nappies per day or a wet nappy after each feed, provided the infant does not receive any fluid other than breast milk).

Delay in initiating breast-feeding, and discarding colostrum

In many developing communities traditional beliefs are firmly entrenched and colostrum may be regarded as poisonous, or it may be felt that affliction or bewitchment can occur through breast milk. Such traditional beliefs have to be handled tactfully and with discretion. Mothers who initiate breast-feeding early are more likely to breast-feed exclusively, and breast-feed for longer.

Poor breast-feeding technique

Breast-feeding is a learned art. Both mother and infant need to learn how to breast-feed successfully. If the infant is not well attached or appropriately positioned, the mother is likely to experience nipple pain, nipple fissures, and possibly engorgement and mastitis as the infant may not effectively remove milk from the breast. This is likely to lead to cessation of breast-feeding.

The 10 points for successful breast-feeding are summarized in Box 16.3. For comfortable, relaxed breast-feeding, the mother should lean on a backrest and hold the baby securely in her arms. The infant should face the mother, with the infant's whole body turned towards the mother, and the buttocks should be well supported. Head and body should be straight. The infant should be brought up to the mother's breast. For the infant to be well attached, the mouth should be wide open, with more areola visible above the mouth than below, the lower lip should be turned out and the infant's chin should be touching the breast (Figure 16.3).

Box 16.3 Ten steps to successful breast-feeding

Every facility providing maternity services and care for newborn infants should:

1. Have a written breast-feeding policy that is routinely communicated to all health-care staff
2. Train all health-care staff in the skills necessary to implement this policy
3. Inform all pregnant women about the benefits and management of breast-feeding
4. Help mothers to initiate breast-feeding within half an hour of birth
5. Show mothers how to breast-feed and how to maintain lactation even if they should be separated from their infants
6. Give newborn infants no food or drink other than breast milk, unless medically indicated
7. Practice rooming-in: allow mothers and infants to remain together 24 hours a day
8. Encourage breast-feeding on demand
9. Give no artificial teats or pacifiers to breast-feeding infants
10. Foster the establishment of breast-feeding support groups and refer mothers to them on discharge from the hospital or clinic.

In addition, facilities should refuse to accept free and low-cost supplies of breast-milk substitutes, feeding bottles and tests.

Mistaken belief that infants need extra fluids

Recent research has demonstrated that giving young infants supplementary fluids such as water and tea in addition to breast milk is associated with a significant increase in the risk of diarrheal disease.

Young infants who receive these supplementary fluids have a lower intake of breast milk than if they are exclusively breast-fed and are also more likely to be breast-fed for shorter periods. In Brazil, for example, infants who were offered water and tea in addition to breast milk in the first days of life were twice as likely to stop breast-feeding before the age of 3 months as those who were exclusively breast-fed.

The average daily fluid requirement of a healthy infant ranges from 80–100 ml/kg in the first week of life to 140–160 ml/kg for the first 6 months, depending on the concentration of the feeds, energy consumption, and environmental humidity and temperature. Consumption below the required level will lead to dehydration, with increases in serum and urine osmolarity.

With the low concentrations of sodium, chloride, potassium and nitrogen in breast milk, only a relatively small amount of the fluid intake is needed for the excretion of resulting waste products. Calculations indicate that healthy infants who consume enough breast milk to satisfy their energy needs receive, with a considerable safety margin, enough fluid to satisfy their fluid requirement, even in hot and dry environments.

To check the validity of these calculations, six studies were performed in settings with a high environmental temperature and varying degrees of humidity to measure the urine osmolarity values of healthy, exclusively breast-fed infants. The studies were summarized by the WHO, and are presented in Table 16.6. Results from these studies support the theoretical

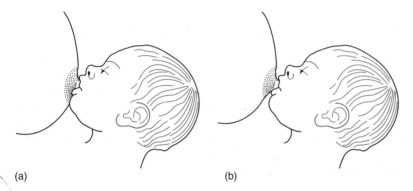

(a)   (b)

Figure 16.3 Attachment of a child to the breast for successful breast-feeding. (a) well-attached infant; (b) infant suckling nipple, not breast. From WHO: Breastfeeding: A Counselling Course. Reproduced with permission from the WHO.

Table 16.6 Summary of studies on the water requirements of exclusively breast-fed infants

Country	Year	Temperature (°C)	Relative humidity (%)	Number of infants	Age (months)	Number of samples	Urine osmolarity (mOsm/l)
Argentina	1979	20–39	60–80	8	<1–2	24	105–199
Israel	1983	32–37	13–41	15	1–5	15	55–320
India	1990	27–42	10–60	31	1–5	63	66–1234
India	1991	34–41	9–75	23	1–4	23	99–703
Jamaica	1978	24–28	62–90	16	<1–4	48	103–468
Peru	1986	24–30	45–96	40	<1–6	40	30–544

calculations: osmolarity values were maintained well within the normal concentration capacity of the kidney, even under extremely hot and dry conditions.

Supplementation in the form of water and tea in early infancy is a common practice because it is believed that infants become thirsty. However, on both theoretical and empirical grounds it is concluded that these supplementary fluids are not needed to maintain water balance in healthy infants younger than 6 months who are exclusively breast-fed. Their use should therefore be actively discouraged, as they are associated with significantly increased risks of diarrhea morbidity and mortality. Therefore, exclusive breast-feeding should be promoted as the ideal feeding practice during the first 6 months of life.

Lack of support from the health services

Evidence has shown that where the UNICEF-initiated Baby Friendly Hospital Initiative (www.unicef.org/bfhi) is practiced, exclusive breast-feeding practices are improved. For example, in Sweden, 100% of hospitals with maternity facilities were designated baby friendly and the rate of initially breast-fed babies is 100%, whereas in the UK (1996–1997) just two out of 202 hospitals were designated baby friendly and their breast-feeding initiation rate was 66%.

Marketing of breast-milk substitutes

The marketing of breast-milk substitutes has led to the belief that they are superior to breast milk, thereby undermining breast-feeding practices. To counteract this problem, in 1981 the WHO Assembly developed the Code of Marketing of Breastmilk Substitutes, the aim of which is to control the promotion of artificial feeds. Its essence is to protect children from the abuse or misuse of such products. All health personnel, especially those involved with infant nutrition, should be

Box 16.4 Principles of the code of marketing of breast-milk substitutes

- There should be no advertising or other forms of promotion to the general public of products within the scope of the Code.
- Manufacturers and distributors should not provide free samples or gifts to the public.
- There should not be any contact between the marketing personnel and mothers.
- There should be no promotion to induce sales directly to the consumer at retail level, such as special displays, discount coupons, premiums, special sales, loss-leaders or tie-in sales for the products.
- Neither the container nor the label should have pictures of infants or text which may idealize the use of infant formulas.
- No health care facility should be used for the promotion or advertisement of infant formulas or other products within the Code.
- No financial or material inducement should be offered to health workers or marketing personnel for the promotion of the products.

familiar with the Code. In particular, the aim of the Code is to contribute to the provision of safe and adequate nutrition for infants by the protection and promotion of breast-feeding, and to ensure the proper use of artificial feeds. The scope of the Code applies to infant formulas, other milk products, foods and beverages, and feeding bottles and teats. The principles of the code are summarized in Box 16.4.

16.4 Breast-feeding challenges

There are some situations where breast-feeding is contraindicated and breast-milk substitutes are required, but these are very rare. The contraindications are summarized in Table 16.7. If breast-milk substitutes are to be used it is important that they are prepared safely (Box 16.5). The difficulties experienced by a mother can be physical and cultural, and can affect the initiation and duration of feeding.

Table 16.7 Contraindications to breast-feeding

	Absolute	Relative
Mother	Psychosis	Late pregnancy
	HIV in developed countries	Infections:[b]
	Serious systemic disease	Typhoid
	Carcinoma of the breast	AIDS
		Herpes
		Septicemia
		Pneumonia
Drugs[a]	Radioactive iodine	
	Cytotoxins	
	Thioracil	
Infant	Galactosemia	Lactose intolerance[b]
	Phenylketonuria	

[a] Alternative drugs should be considered before introducing artificial feeds.
[b] The severity of the illness will determine whether breast-feeding should be terminated or continued.

Box 16.5

Safe preparation includes:

- Readily available, clean water
- Adequate facilities to boil water
- Adequate facilities to sterilize equipment
- Appropriate utensils for measuring accurately
- Adequate sanitation
- Clear understanding of importance of hygiene, mixing and storage directions

---

Physical difficulties experienced by the mother

Mothers do experience difficulties during breast-feeding which, without appropriate help and support, commonly result in cessation of breast-feeding. These include:

- engorgement
- sore or cracked nipples
- blocked milk ducts
- mastitis or breast abscess
- *Candida albicans* infection
- flat and inverted nipples.

The causes and presentation of these conditions are summarized in Table 16.8, while their treatment, management and prevention are summarized in Table 16.9.

Breast-milk expression

Mothers going back to work frequently initiate cessation of breast-feeding owing to the period of separation from the infant. Mothers can continue to breast-feed successfully, and exclusively, in the first 6 months, and continue breast-feeding for at least 2 years even while working.

A mother can choose to express her milk in different ways:

- hand expression
- using a breast pump
- using the warm bottle method.

Table 16.8

	Causes	Presentation
Engorgement	Delayed initiation of breast-feeding postpartum	Both breasts are full and painful
	Inadequate removal of milk	Breasts look tight and shiny owing to edema in the tissues
		Milk may stop flowing
		Mother may feel feverish for 24 h
Sore or cracked nipples	Poor attachment	One or both breasts are red and sore
	Poor positioning	There may be visible fissures on or around the nipple
	Candida albicans infection	
Blocked milk ducts	Inadequate removal of milk	Painful lump in one area
	Pressure on one side of the breast (such as tight clothes)	Woman feels well
Mastitis or breast abscess	Inadequate removal of milk	Usually only one breast affected
	Infection of the breast	Red, hot, swollen and very painful area of the breast
		Mother feels feverish and generally unwell
Candida albicans infection	More common if skin not intact	Persistent pain, even between feeding
	Common in hot, humid climates	Itchy, or sharp, like needles going into breast
	Mother can often be infected by infant, and vice versa	Areola may have white spots
		Areola may be red, shiny and flaky
Flat and inverted nipples		Nipple may be short, flat on the skin or inverted

Table 16.9

	Treatment/management	Prevention
Engorgement	Infant should feed on demand Correct positioning and attachment if necessary If infant cannot latch well owing to fullness of breast, express enough milk to soften the breast If the infant cannot suckle at all, feed expressed breast milk Before feeding, place a warm cloth on the breast to help milk flow After feeding, place a cool cloth on the breast to reduce pain and swelling	Initiate breast-feeding within half an hour of delivery Assist mother with positioning and attachment on the first day Allow the infant unrestricted breast-feeding: feed on demand
Sore or cracked nipples	Correct positioning and attachment Continue breast-feeding if possible Express breast milk if too painful to breast-feed, and cup-feed infant Smear some hind milk onto the breast and allow to dry Expose breasts to sun and air Do not put creams and lotions onto the breast If *Candida* infection suspected, treat appropriately	Assist mother with positioning and attachment on the first day Nipples should not be washed with soap, and only need to be washed once daily Allow the infant to finish feeding and release the breast; do not pull the breast out of the infant's mouth
Blocked milk ducts	Infant should feed on demand Correct positioning and attachment if necessary Before feeding, place a warm cloth on the breast to help milk flow Feed on the affected side first Massage the lump towards the nipple during allow easy access for the infant to feedfeeding	Assist mother with positioning and attachment on the first day Allow the infant unrestricted breast-feeding: feed on demand Encourage women to wear loose-fitting clothes, and tops that allow easy access for the infant to feed
Mastitis or breast abscess	Infant should feed as often as possible; the milk is not harmful to the baby HIV-positive women should express and discard milk from the affected area; infant should not be breast-fed on affected side Before feeding, place a warm cloth on the breast to help milk flow If too painful to feed, milk should be regularly expressed Antibiotics and painkillers should be prescribed Mother must rest Abscess must be drained	Assist mother with positioning and attachment on the first day Allow the infant unrestricted breast-feeding: feed on demand
Candida albicans infection	Nystatin cream Need to treat mother and baby if baby has oral thrush	
Flat and inverted nipples	The mother should be given encouragement that she will be able to breast-feed successfully The mother will require extra encouragement as she will have been told that she cannot breast-feed with inverted nipples The infant latches onto the breast, not the nipple, so attachment will not be a problem The infant must not be given any other teat to suckle as this will cause confusion, leading to breast refusal A nipple shield is not recommended Preparing nipples during pregnancy has not been found to be helpful and should be avoided	Expose nipples to sun and air

Hand expression

Hand expression is the most simple method of expressing breast milk.

1. Wash hands and container well.
2. Sit comfortably, holding the container near the breast.
3. Place the thumb on the breast above the areola, and the first finger below the areola, opposite the thumb. Support the breast with the other fingers.
4. Press thumb and first finger towards the chest wall, at the same time pressing the thumb and first finger inwards, towards each other.
5. Press and release, press and release, developing a rhythm.
6. Press the areola in the same way on the sides to ensure milk is expressed from all lactiferous sinuses.
7. If there is any pain, the technique is not correct. Expressing is not painful if done correctly.
8. Avoid rubbing or sliding the fingers along the skin. The fingers should roll.
9. Avoid squeezing the nipple itself.
10. Express one breast for 3–5 min, until the flow of milk slows, then change to the other breast.
11. Expressing takes between 20 and 30 min.

Warm bottle method

1. Find a bottle with a wide opening, at least the size of the areola.
2. The bottle should hold at least 750 ml.
3. Clean the bottle well.
4. Pour boiling water into the bottle.
5. When warm, wrap a cloth around the bottle and pour the water out.
6. Cool the neck of the bottle by holding under running water.
7. Test the warmth of the neck on the inside of your arm: it should be cool.
8. Hold the bottle over the areola, allowing a seal to develop.
9. Milk will flow freely into the bottle as it cools.
10. This process may have to be repeated to obtain sufficient milk.

Storing and using expressed breast milk

Expressed breast milk can be safely stored in a cool place, out of the refrigerator for 8–10 h or in a refrigerator for 3 days. It can be stored in a fridge–freezer for 3 months, or in a chest freezer for 6 months. If the milk needs to be warmed before use, it should be held under warm, running water, or stood in a pot of hot water. The milk must never be heated directly or in a microwave.

Maintaining breast-milk production

Expressing must take place at least three or four times during the day to maintain breast-milk supply. If breast milk can be refrigerated, this milk can be kept until the following day. If refrigeration is not possible, the milk must be discarded. Working mothers should breast-feed their baby when they arrive home, and continue night breast-feeds on demand.

16.5 Potential feeding difficulties

Low birth weight

LBW infants frequently are too weak to suckle effectively, so cannot feed directly from the breast. Development of the suckling reflex, and coordination of suckling and swallowing, depend on the age of the infant. Infants less than 1500 g usually require the addition of protein, energy and other micronutrients. They should be assessed individually. Infants not fed breast milk are at an increased risk of developing necrotizing enterocolitis.

Breast milk produced by the mother of an LBW infant differs from milk produced by the mother of a full-term infant. Preterm milk has a higher protein content, more antibodies and a lower lactose content. Most mothers of LBW infants need to learn to express and cup-feed. Although the infant may not suckle, they can be put to the breast very early. The infant may lick the nipple and learn the smell of the mother. This is facilitated by "kangaroo care", which refers to holding the infant on the mother's chest under her shirt, allowing skin-to-skin contact. This close contact facilitates milk production and bonding. Infants cared for in this manner are often discharged earlier and grow more rapidly.

Although each mother–infant pair needs to be treated individually, the following serves as a general guideline.

- An infant with a gestational age of <30–32 weeks:
  - should be fed via a nasogastric tube
  - can suckle the mother's finger during feeding to develop the suckling reflex.
- For a gestational age around 30–32 weeks:
  - a small cup can be used to feed the infant in addition to the nasogastric tube

– as the infant drinks more effectively from the cup, nasogastric feeds can be decreased and cup feeds increased.
- An infant with a gestational age of 32–34 weeks:
  – can be put to the breast to suckle
  – will suckle for short periods and rest for long periods in between
  – may have slightly uncoordinated suckling
  – will still need to be cup fed as well.
- At a gestational age of 34–36 weeks:
  – the infant should be able to breast-feed successfully, but cup-feeds may need to be added.

Cleft palate

Infants born with a cleft palate can be breast-fed successfully. The mother may need some extra help and encouragement.

- The breast may close over the cleft if the infant is suckling in a good position.
- The infant should be held in a more upright position to reduce the risk of choking.
- The mother could obtain a plate to put into the mouth to facilitate feeding.
- If breast-feeding is not possible, the mother can express breast milk and feed via a cup or nasogastric tube.

Diarrhea

When an infant develops diarrhea, it is important to ensure that the infant does not dehydrate. Rehydration is important if the mother has not managed to keep the infant well hydrated.

- Usually infants become anorexic, only accepting breast milk and rejecting other feeds.
- Mothers who are breast-feeding should continue to breast-feed frequently.
- The infant should be breast-fed at least after every stool passed.
- If the infant is not breast-feeding well, the mother should express breast milk and cup-feed.

Mothers frequently start giving oral rehydration solution (ORS) and neglect breast-feeding. This is not advisable, as ORS is not very palatable, so infants usually do not drink sufficient quantities. Frequently, ORS is usually not mixed correctly, which can lead to further complications. Stopping breast-feeding negatively

> **Box 16.6** How to cup-feed
>
> - Hold the infant on your lap, in a semiupright position.
> - Hold the cup to the infant's lips, and tilt the cup until the milk just touches the lips.
> - Rest the cup gently on the lower lip:
>   – a low birth weight infant will start to take the milk into his mouth with his tongue
>   – a full-term infant will suck the milk, and may spill.
> - DO NOT POUR the milk into the infant's mouth – this will cause choking.
> - When the infant is finished, he will close his mouth, and not take any more.
> - Be sure to measure intake over a 24 h period, as the infant may not always consume the same amount of feed.

affects the nutritional intake of the infant. It is therefore more advisable to encourage mothers to continue breast-feeding frequently, rather than to recommend oral rehydration therapy. Breast milk contains all the appropriate micronutrients in oral rehydration, and provides additional antibodies and nutrition as well. Continued breast-feeding results in less severe diarrhea, of shorter duration.

Breathing difficulties

Infants with breathing difficulties frequently do not feed well. Usually in the choice between feeding and breathing, the latter wins. The mother should be encouraged to express breast milk and cup-feed. Small, frequent feeds will most probably be necessary. The method of cup-feeding is described in Box 16.6.

Jaundice

A mild jaundice is fairly common in infants. It is more common in LBW infants and those that are not breast-fed, as colostrum has a laxative effect and clears the meconium effectively. Giving glucose water or other fluids reduces the effectiveness of colostrum and is therefore not recommended. If an infant has jaundice, the infant should be breast-fed frequently. If under phototherapy and cup-feeding, an extra 20% should be added to the fluid allowance to prevent dehydration.

16.6 Breast-feeding and human immunodeficiency virus transmission

Transmission of HIV through breast-feeding was first described in 1985 in women newly infected after

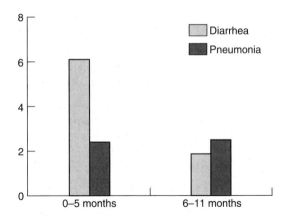

Figure 16.4 Findings of the WHO metaanalysis of relative risk of mortality from diarrhea and pneumonia in nonbreast-fed children compared with breast-fed children. Reproduced with permission from the WHO.

delivery through blood transfusion or heterosexual exposure. An early metaanalysis estimated that breast-feeding by women with established infection may increase the rate of transmission by an additional 14%. The risk of transmission increases for the mother with a newly acquired infection in the breast-feeding period estimated as 29%. Two large trials in Kenya and South Africa have confirmed that breast-feeding for about 2 years carries a risk of transmission of about 15%. It is therefore desirable that women should breast-feed for shorter periods: it is estimated that breast-feeding for about 6 months carries a 5–8% risk.

The obvious response to the observation that breast-feeding by HIV-infected women resulted in HIV transmission to infants was for women not to breast-feed and instead feed the infant formula milk. This may not be a serious problem in developed countries which have the resources to compensate for increased morbidity from formula feeding, but in developing countries this is a major concern as formula feeding from the day of birth will considerably increase child morbidity, malnutrition and mortality. A WHO-conducted metaanalysis of data from developing countries showed that mortality from diarrhea, acute respiratory infections and other infectious diseases is five or six times higher in infants who are not breast-fed than in those who are breast-fed for the first 2 months of life (Figure 16.4). The authors of this WHO collaborative study concluded: "Our results suggest that it will be difficult, if not impossible, to provide breast-milk substitutes to children from underdeveloped populations."

In 1997, a joint statement by WHO, UNICEF and UNAIDS read as follows:

"When children born to HIV-infected women can be assured of uninterrupted access to nutritionally adequate breast-milk substitutes that are safely prepared and fed to them, they are at less risk of illness and death if they are not breast-fed. However, when these conditions cannot be met – in particular in environments where infectious diseases and malnutrition are the primary causes of death during infancy – then artificial feeding substantially increases children's risk of illness and death. The policy objective must be to minimize all infant feeding risks and to urgently expand access to adequate alternatives so that HIV-infected women have a range of choices. The policy should also stipulate what measures are being taken to make breast-milk substitutes available and affordable; to teach the safest means of feeding them to infants; and to provide the conditions which will diminish the risks of using them."

Influence of pattern of breast-feeding on transmission

There has been much controversy over breast-feeding and HIV infection. In developed countries, the decision to formula feed to reduce mother-to-child transmission is an easy one. In developing countries, where sanitation is poor, clean water not readily accessible and fuel for boiling water limited, the infant will run a higher risk of dying from infectious disease, than from HIV transmitted by the mother during breast-feeding. Mothers should be given as much relevant information as possible to enable them to make a well-informed decision regarding how to feed their infant.

There is some evidence that exclusive breast-feeding, as defined by the WHO, carries no more risk of HIV transmission than formula feeding during the first 6 months of life. In a prospective study conducted in Durban, South Africa, involving HIV-infected pregnant women, breast-feeding women were counseled and encouraged to practice exclusive breast-feeding for up to 6 months. The rate of transmission at 6 months (19.4%) was the same in the infants who were formula fed and those who had been exclusively breast-fed for at least 3 months. Transmission in the mixed breast-feeding group was much higher, at 26.1%. At 15 months the transmission rate remained lower among those

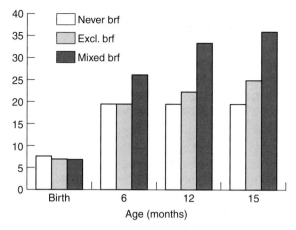

Figure 16.5 Risk of transmission of HIV according to feeding practice. brf: breast-feed; Excl: exclusive.

who exclusively breast-fed for at least 3 months than among other breast-feeders: 24.75% versus 35.9% (Figure 16.5). If confirmed in future studies, this observation has important implications for public health policy. New studies specifically designed to test this hypothesis on exclusive breast-feeding are planned at a number of sites in Africa (South Africa, West Africa, Ethiopia and Zambia).

Support for exclusive breast-feeding has also come from preliminary results from a study in Kisumu, Kenya. In this study, the incidence of HIV infection was greater for infants who started mixed breast-feeding before 30 days than for infants who started mixed breast-feeding after 30 days. Similarly, the incidence of HIV infections was greater for infants who started mixed breast-feeding before 120 days compared with those who started after 120 days. However, the effects of viral load and severity of maternal illness were not factored into the results. Potential mechanisms accounting for the protective effect of exclusive breast-feeding are summarized in Box 16.7.

Several factors increase the risk of transmission of HIV through breast-feeding and are summarized in Box 16.8. Guidelines on making breast-feeding safer for HIV-infected women are summarized in Box 16.9.

16.7 Infant feeding after 6 months

After 6 months, breast milk alone no longer provides sufficient energy and nutrients to promote optimal growth and development of the child, and complementary foods need to be added to the child's diet in addition to breast-feeding. This period of addition of complementary foods (traditionally referred to as the weaning period) is a particularly vulnerable time in the life a child for a number of reasons, including:

- an inadequate energy and nutrient intake
- the ingestion of contaminated weaning foods

- reduced immunity to infections
- children putting many items into their mouths during exploration of the environment.

Insufficient intake and frequent infections result in stunting and wasting. Although weight can be regained, stature is affected permanently. The long-term consequences for females include difficult childbirth owing to small pelvic size, risk of maternal morbidity and mortality, and increased risk of an LBW baby.

The period between 6 and 24 months has been described as a critical transition period when the exposure to environmental pathogens is most intense, the likelihood of inadequate nutrient intake most probable, and the emotional trauma of less intimate maternal–infant contact most stressful.

As far as possible, complementary foods should be:

- energy and nutrient dense
- easily obtained and prepared by the family
- culturally acceptable
- of an appropriate consistency for the age and development of the child
- clean and safe for consumption.

Breast-milk intake

Although other foods are being introduced, breast milk still provides a significant amount of energy and nutrients for the infant. Frequent, on-demand breast-feeding should continue throughout the day and night. In Bangladesh, breast milk was found to provide half the protein, and 60% of the energy and vitamin A consumed. When complementary foods are low in fat, breast-milk fat may be essential for the utilization of vitamin A. Breast milk continues to reduce the risk of infection, and is particularly important during illness, when an infant often refuses other feeds.

Care should be taken that complementary foods do not replace breast milk, but provide additional nutrients. Breast milk should be offered first, with solids after the feed, or in between, to ensure that the infant continues to receive sufficient breast milk. Breast-feeding before a meal will also extend the use of lactational amenorrhea as a form of contraception, as long as menses have not returned.

Introducing solids

Solids should be introduced slowly, one at a time, to ensure that there are no adverse reactions to the new food.

- The amount offered initially should be small, and should be gradually increased:
  - Initially 1–2 teaspoons per meal, should be given, increasing to about 1 cup per day by 8 months.
  - At 6–8 months of age, the child should be fed two or three times per day.
  - At 9–11 months of age, the child should be fed three or four times per day.
  - At 12–24 months of age, the child should be fed four or five times per day.
- Consistency should be increased, adapting foods to the infant's requirements and abilities:
  - Initially, food should be mashed to a smooth paste, preferably softened with expressed breast milk.
  - Between 7 and 9 months, foods should be mashed, gradually adding more texture.
  - "Finger foods" that the child can hold should be introduced at about 8 months of age.
  - After 10 months, foods can be chopped, not mashed.
  - By about 12 months of age, the child should be able to eat family foods.
- A variety of nutrient-dense foods should be provided:
  - Fruit and vegetables, especially vitamin A-rich vegetables, should be given to children daily.
  - Animal proteins should be eaten as often as possible, unless unacceptable (e.g. in a vegetarian family). Mothers should be encouraged to chop these proteins into small pieces, rather than giving the child a piece to suck, or just the gravy.
  - Where meat, poultry and fish are unavailable, cheaper sources of protein should be given, such as eggs, beans and lentils. Vitamin C-rich foods should be combined with legumes to improve absorption of nonheme iron.
  - Starches can be softened with expressed breast milk to increase the energy density.

The developmental stages of infant feeding are summarized in Table 16.10.

An infant's iron stores are depleted within 6 months. Breast milk is still an important source of iron for an infant, but is inadequate as the only source. Mothers should be encouraged to include adequate quantities of iron-rich foods in the diet. Heme iron is far more readily absorbed than nonheme iron. Vitamin C and heme-iron-containing foods, consumed at the same meal, increase the absorption of nonheme iron in foods. Other micronutrients that are frequently

Table 16.10 Developmental stages

Learner eater (6 months)	Exploring eater (7–9 months)	Confident eater (10–12 months)
Sits unaided	Starts to be able to chew	Can eat family foods chopped into small pieces
Munching pattern begins	Can hold food in palm of hand	Can hold small pieces of food between finger and thumb
Eating from a spoon is a very different action with the tongue compared with suckling from the breast and has to be learnt	Encourage the baby to feed him/herself by giving soft finger foods	Introduce smaller pieces of food
	Foods need to be mashed/minced with a fork	Let the baby feed him/herself with a spoon
The baby may spit out food, but this is because forward tongue movement is all the baby knows and he/she has to learn how to take food to the back of the mouth to swallow	Never leave the baby alone with food as he or she may choke.	Let the baby drink from a cup unaided
Give milk feed first	Give milk feed first	Give solid foods first and milk as snacks
Then offer very soft, semiliquid foods for the baby to suck off a spoon	Then offer mashed/minced food with a spoon	Chop family foods into small pieces
Give 1–2 teaspoons/meal at first and build up gradually	Give finger foods as snacks between meals	Give finger food as snacks
Take time and don't rush or force-feed the baby	Practice active feeding	Practice active feeding
Practice good hygiene	Practice good hygiene	Practice good hygiene

Table 16.11

Nutrient	Sources
Vitamin A	Liver, carrots, sweet potatoes, pumpkin, mango, papaya, apricots, spinach, green leafy vegetables
Vitamin C	Oranges, guavas, papaya, tomatoes, strawberries, lemons, grapefruit, raw cabbage, broccoli, spinach
Heme iron	Liver, red meat, poultry, fish
Nonheme iron	Egg, dried beans, dried peas, lentils, cereals, green leafy vegetables
Zinc	Oysters, liver, eggs, beef, pork, chicken, turkey

inadequate in the diet are vitamin A, zinc, calcium if little milk is consumed and vitamin C, which is often only seasonally available. Good dietary sources of these foods are summarized in Table 16.11.

Guidelines for the active feeding of a young child are summarized in Box 16.10, and factors improving the hygiene level of weaning foods are summarized in Box 16.11.

Since HIV-positive mothers who choose to breast-feed exclusively to 6 months of age will also be introducing solids at 6 months, an alternative milk source should be found, if possible. The mother may consider:

- using formula milk
- expressing and heat-treating breast milk
- using an alternative milk, such as cow's milk
- asking a wet nurse to continue feeding her child.

Box 16.10 Active feeding

Practice active feeding:

- Children who are not actively encouraged to feed are more frequently malnourished.
- Caregivers should feed infants directly, and assist older children to feed themselves.
- Adequate time should be allowed for feeding.
- Talk to the infant while feeding.
- Minimize distractions during meals.
- Offer favorite foods when children have poor appetites.
- Mix poorly accepted foods with favorite foods to encourage intake.
- Experiment with different textures, colors and food combinations.
- Do not force children to eat.
- If a meal is refused, offer food again within an hour.
- Siblings can eat at the same time. All children should have their own bowls of food to ensure that the slower eating younger child is not deprived of food by older family members.

Active feeding during and after illness:

- During illness, increase the frequency of breast-feeding.
- Patiently encourage favorite foods.
- After illness, feed at least one extra meal per day, and encourage a larger helping to be taken at each meal.

If the mother does not have sufficient income to purchase alternative milk or to have a healthy, varied diet, it will be more beneficial to the child to continue breast-feeding, in addition to solids. In communities where prolonged breast-feeding is expected, the mother would have to develop stories to explain why she has stopped breast-feeding, and would have to learn other ways to deal with a baby who is crying, as well as ways to reduce her breast-milk production so that she does not develop any breast difficulties such as mastitis.

Formula feeding

Although formula milk would be the milk of choice in developed countries, in most developing countries this milk is prohibitively expensive. The mother would need guidance on hygiene, mixing feeding and storing.

Heat-treating expressed breast milk

This method is useful if the mother does not have enough money to purchase alternative milks, but has money for fuel and wants to stop breast-feeding. The procedure for heat-treating is as follows.

1. Express 150 ml milk into a clean 450 ml glass container with a lid.
2. Boil 450 ml of water.
3. Take the water off the heat, and stand the glass jar of milk in the water for 30 min or until water is comfortable to touch.
4. Allow to cool before feeding the baby.

Adapted cow's milk

Cow's milk is not appropriate to be given to infants undiluted as it has a very high protein and electrolyte content. Dilution of the cow's milk reduces the energy content, so sugar needs to be added to increase the energy. Hygiene, mixing and storage would need to be carefully discussed with the mother. To make

150 ml of adapted cow's milk, 100 ml full-strength cow's milk, 50 ml boiled water and 10 g sugar are mixed together.

Wet nursing

A wet nurse would have to be very carefully selected. This woman would need to be HIV-negative, and lead a life that would not expose her to HIV infection. If she became infected with HIV while breast-feeding, the risk of transmitting HIV to the infant would be high, as her viral load would be very high.

16.8 Monitoring the child's growth: the road-to-health chart

Regular monitoring of the child's weight plays an important role in ensuring optimal health and nutritional status, and preventing growth faltering and failure. The weight is plotted on a road-to-health chart. The exact position of the child's weight on the graph is less important than whether the line plotted follows the same general direction as the curves on the growth chart. It is vital that the procedure of weighing is not seen as an end in itself: weighing is not an intervention. The data should be used by the health worker in conjunction with the mother to reinforce behaviors that promote good growth or to discuss behaviors that could be adopted to correct growth faltering or failure. These must relate to the age of the child and will revolve around ensuring consumption of adequate amounts of safe and appropriate food, preventing and treating infections, and proper care of the child. Some examples of possible abnormal growth responses are illustrated in Figure 16.6. The growth chart should not be seen as a tool to be used solely by the health worker. It is important that the mother understands what the lines on the card represent. The growth chart can become a valuable teaching aid to reinforce and assess the effectiveness of growth-promoting behavior, as well as for health and nutrition education. Referral to other levels of services (including health) will depend on the age of the child (growth failure within the first 6 months of life is far more serious than in the second year), as well as the underlying causes. Inadequate household food security is better dealt with in the long term in a community-based development program than by a health worker, whereas a parasitic infestation obviously needs medical treatment, as well as perhaps support in a social program to prevent recurrence of the infestation.

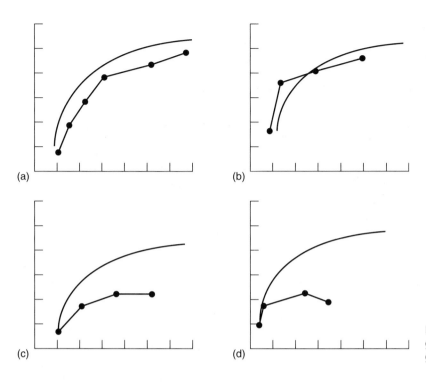

Figure 16.6 Examples of (a) adequate growth, (b) growth faltering, (c) poor growth and (d) negative growth.

The following situations require further investigation:

- growth failure over a period of 1 month in a child under 6 months of age:
- in a child 6–15 months of age: 3 months of faltering or failure
- in a child 16–60 months of age: 3 months of faltering or failure below the road-to-health area and/or loss of more than 1 kg in a month
- any time that a child's weight is below 60% of the median.

Regular weighing, and discussion regarding appropriate complementary foods will help to ensure that early signs of growth faltering are immediately detected and actions taken to remedy this potentially dangerous situation.

16.9 Perspectives on the future

Data on exclusive breast-feeding are scarce and unavailable in many countries. Reliable surveillance systems across Europe using a common harmonized methodology need to be developed.

More information is required in other areas of maternal and child health with regard to HIV, including the impact of breast-feeding on the disease progression, morbidity and mortality of the mother, and the effect of maternal health on HIV transmission. Although poor breast health has been found to increase the transmission of HIV through breast milk, there has been no research prospectively looking at the impact of good breast-feeding practices, nutritional interventions and antibiotic treatment on clinical and subclinical mastitis, and therefore on breast-feeding transmission. There is early evidence that breast-feeding transmission may be reduced by antiretroviral prophylaxis to the infant, mother or both during breast-feeding, but further research is required.

Breast-feeding is well established as a major contributor to infant survival, and the impact of national policies recommending breast-milk substitutes to HIV-positive women on HIV-negative and untested women (spill-over effect) needs to be urgently assessed to influence policy development, especially in developing countries. The effect of not breast-feeding, or early cessation of breast-feeding, on infant morbidity and mortality in infants born to HIV-positive women needs to be assessed, as well as the role of breast-feeding on the clinical outcome of HIV-infected children. Options of expressing and heat-treating milk, and breast-milk banks should be investigated for acceptability and feasibility.

Further reading

Anderson JW, Johnstone BM, Remley DT. Breast feeding and cognitive development: a meta-analysis. Am J Clin Nutr 1999; 70: 525–535.

Coutsoudis A, Pillay K, Kuhn L *et al*. Method of feeding and transmission of HIV-1 from mothers to children by 15 months of age: prospective cohort study from Durban, South Africa. AIDS 2001; 15: 379–387.

Latham M, Preble E. Appropriate feeding methods for infants of HIV infected mothers in sub-Saharan Africa. BMJ 2000; 320: 1656–1660.

Lawrence RA. Breastfeeding: A Guide for the Medical Profession, 4th edn. St Louis, MO: Mosby, 1994.

World Health Organization. Breastfeeding: A Counselling Course. WHO/CDR/93.3–5. Geneva: WHO, no date.

World Health Organization. Complementary Feeding: Family Foods for Breastfed Children. WHO/NHD/00.1. Geneva: WHO, 2000.

World Health Organization Collaborative Study Team. Effect of breastfeeding on infant and child mortality due to infectious diseases in less developed countries: a pooled analysis. Lancet 2000; 355: 451–455.

World Health Organization Division of Child Health and Development. Evidence for the Ten Steps to Successful Breastfeeding. Geneva: WHO, 1998.

Websites

www.childinfo.org
www.iapac.org
www.lalecheleague.org
www.waba.org.br

17

Adverse Outcomes in Pregnancy: The Role of Folate and Related B-Vitamins

John Scott and Helene McNulty

Key messages

- The folate cofactors provide carbon (formyl or methylene) groups for the biosynthesis of purines and pyrimidines and thus DNA.
- They also provide the methyl ($-CH_3$) groups that are used in this methylation cycle to modify the structure and function of a wide range of proteins, lipids and DNA.
- Deficiency of folate results in anemia, but even modest reduction in its status greatly increases the risk of spina bifida and other neural tube defects (NTD).
- Most NTD can be prevented by the mother taking extra folic acid via fortified foods or supplements, but increasing dietary folate sufficiently to do this is very difficult.
- Such intervention must be before the neural tube closes (21 days after conception), at which point most women do not realize they are pregnant.

- Because of this, efforts to make women take folic acid periconceptionally have failed badly everywhere, leading the USA to fortify flour with folic acid as an alternative.
- For safety reasons because of the range of exposure, a nonoptimal amount of folic acid has been used for fortification, resulting in only a 20% reduction in NTD since it began.
- Increasing the level of folic acid in flour to achieve an optimal response is unlikely for safety reasons and thus a dual policy of fortification and advice to take supplements should be continued.

17.1 Introduction

The importance of maintaining good nutrition during pregnancy is well established, as reflected in the increased dietary recommendations for many micronutrients which are considered necessary to cover the extra nutrient demands of pregnancy and lactation. However, since the 1980s there has been more recognition of the importance of ensuring a good nutritional status in the mother, not only during pregnancy and lactation, but also before conception and in the very early weeks of pregnancy. In particular, maternal folate status is now known to have a major impact on early development of the embryo up to the first 4 weeks of pregnancy, a time when many women will not be aware that they are pregnant. There is now conclusive evidence with respect to the benefits at this time of optimal maternal folate status in the prevention of neural tube defects (NTD). Although this knowledge is universally accepted across the scientific and medical communities, it is less clear how best the official recommendations can be translated into public health policy to optimize folate status in women who may become pregnant. What is evident is that the diet currently consumed by most women of childbearing age in European countries fails to provide levels of intake of folate and the metabolically related B-vitamins that are associated with optimal maternal folate status in early pregnancy and therefore the lowest risk of NTD.

As pregnancy progresses, folate continues to play an important role, but after the early weeks the emphasis is focused on protecting the mother from developing folate deficiency of pregnancy. Maternal folate deficiency not only has consequences for the mother's own health, but has also been shown to result in fetal growth retardation, low birth weight (LBW) and neonatal folate deficiency, with important implications for the health of the neonate and infant. Thus, throughout pregnancy, folate plays key roles in terms of maternal, fetal and neonatal health. The public health challenge now facing policy makers and others is how best to achieve optimal folate status in women of reproductive age.

This chapter will focus on the role of folate and metabolically related B-vitamins during preconception and pregnancy in protecting against adverse outcomes for both the mother and the baby.

17.2 Biochemical basis for the role of folate in adverse outcomes of pregnancy

As discussed above, there is conclusive evidence that any reduction in folate status has an associated increased risk of an NTD and possibly also other birth defects. How this reduced status increases risk, and its correction by extra folic acid/folate reduces risk, is not understood. However, to avail of this potentially substantial public health benefit in an optimal way it is important to increase our understanding of the event or events involved and how they are modulated by folate and related nutrients. To make this possible, a comprehensive understanding of the biochemistry of this area, which is largely understood, is an essential starting point.

Metabolic role of folate cofactors and metabolically related B-vitamins

The folate cofactors exist in cells as their metabolically active tetrahydro forms (Figure 17.1). Their metabolic role is as cofactors to the several folate-dependent enzymes found in all cells (Figure 17.2). This role consists principally of the metabolic transfer or donation of carbon-1 units. As such, they are involved in two cycles in cells, the DNA biosynthesis cycle and the methylation cycle. The source of these carbon-1 units is directly from the carbon-3 of serine via serine hydroxymethyltransferase, leading to the synthesis of 5,10-methylenetetrahydrofolate. A more significant source of carbon-1 units is from serine, but after its uptake and metabolism

by mitochondria. The result is that formate is produced in the mitochondria from cytoplasmic serine. This formate emerges from the mitochondria and is used by the trifunctional enzyme to make folates with carbon-1 units, namely 10-formyltetrahydrofolate and 5,10-methylenetetrahydrofolate. Thus, there are two possible ways of making these carbon-1 folate cofactors in cells. These go on to be the carbon-1 donors in purine and pyrimidine biosynthesis, respectively, as discussed below (Figure 17.2). They can also be converted to 5-methyltetrahydrofolate.

The DNA biosynthesis cycle

The biosynthesis of purine involves two enzymes that are folate dependent. The folate cofactor 10-formyltetrahydrofolate is involved in the synthesis of purines and the folate cofactor 5,10-methylenetetrahydrofolate is involved in pyrimidine synthesis (Figure 17.2). It is important to recognize that the folate cofactor conversions are part of these two cycles with the continuous regeneration of tetrahydrofolate, which can then accept a further carbon-1 group, as described above. Folates are present in only tiny amounts in cells and the different forms are continuously recycled. Anything that interrupts their recycling, be it a deficiency of folate, a major inborn error of metabolism or a less significant change in metabolism due to a polymorphism in any enzyme involved in these or other cycles, will quickly reduce or even stop folate-related biosynthesis and affect purine and pyrimidine biosynthesis. This, in turn, will diminish DNA biosynthesis and with it cell division. While this will affect all replicating cells it will be most apparent in those cells with rapid replication rates such as the erythroid series making red cells, with a reduction in their rate of cell division progressing to a macrocytic anemia. This anemia is further characterized by the arrest of red cell maturation in the bone marrow. These abnormal red cell precursors, called megaloblasts, only arise when the rate of purine and pyrimidine biosynthesis is decreased so as to compromise the normal rate of mitotic cell division. This, in turn, results in an abnormally large, poorly differentiated nucleus, which is characteristic of a megaloblast. These megaloblasts are unique to impaired purine and pyrimidine biosynthesis. They only arise directly through folate deficiency or indirectly through interrupted folate metabolism which occurs consequent to vitamin B_{12} deficiency. The only other cause of megaloblastic anemia is the use of drugs which either directly (cytosine

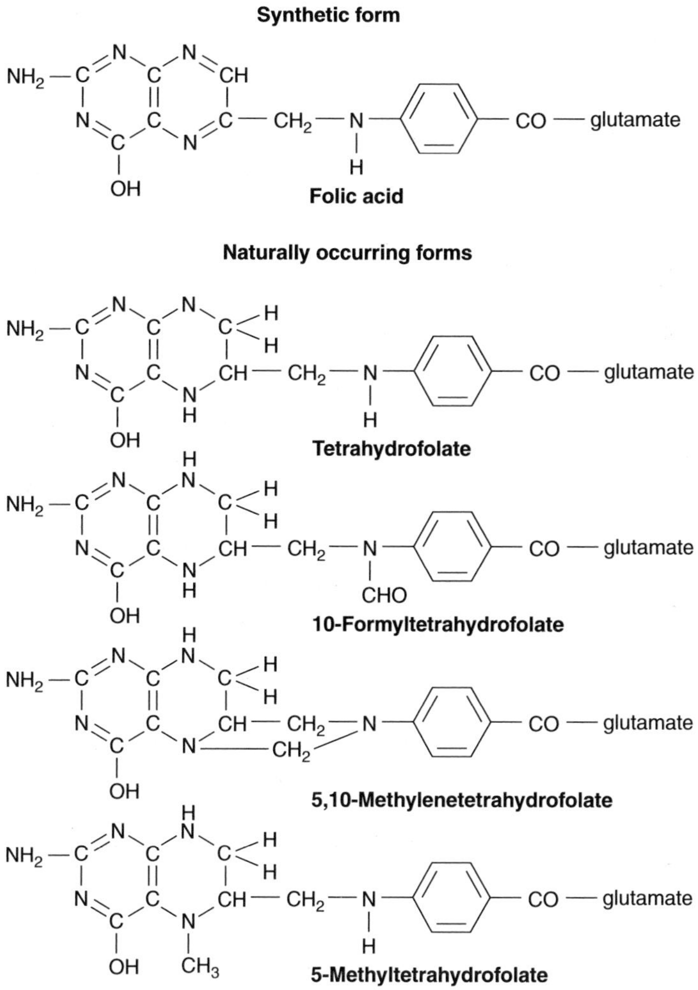

Figure 17.1 Synthetic and naturally occurring forms of the folates.

arabinoside) or indirectly (methotrexate) inhibit DNA biosynthesis. Thus, folates are essential for DNA biosynthesis and cell replication and could be said to participate in the DNA cycle.

The methylation cycle

The other role of the folates is less obvious but no less important. All cells contain a range of enzymes called methyltransferases. As this name suggests, their function is to transfer a methyl (—CH₃) group. The range of substrates for these methylations is very wide indeed. They include:

- methylation of the hormone dopa to methyl-dopa, as one of its methods of inactivation
- methylation of the phospholipid phosphotidyl-ethanolamine via methyltransferase

- methylation of cytosine residues of DNA, which has the important functional effect of preventing the replication of such methylated DNA
- methylation of proteins, changing their stability (e.g. myelin basic proteins) or their function (isoprenoid methyltransferase changes the function of a G-protein involved in cell signaling).

All methyltransferases must have the methyl group presented to their active site in a high-energy activated form. This is the methionine derivative S-adenosyl-methionine (abbreviated to SAM or AdoMet). It and its related structures are shown in Figure 17.3. A product of the methyltransferase reactions is SAM minus its methyl group, namely S-adenosylhomocysteine (SAH or AdoHcy). This product, SAH, is subject to

Methylation cycle

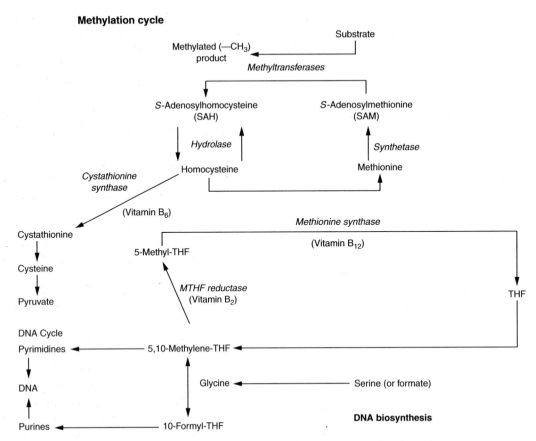

Figure 17.2 Metabolism of the folate cofactors and their role in **DNA biosynthesis** and in the **methylation cycle**.

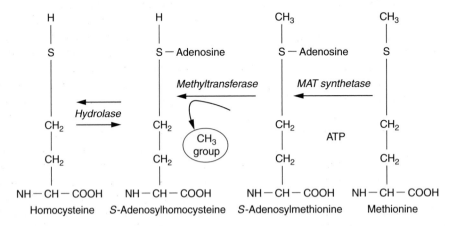

Figure 17.3 Chemical conversions involved in the methylation cycle resulting in the utilization of a methyl (—CH_3) group by the cellular methyltransferase.

only one fate: it is rapidly hydrolyzed to homocysteine and adenosine, the kinetics of which result in the level of SAH being kept extremely low in all cells except in abnormal circumstances. This is important functionally because SAH is a potent inhibitor of all methyltransferases, with one exception. Different methyltransferases may be switched off at different levels of accumulation of SAH, depending on their functional importance. If for any reason, such as during deficiency of folate, vitamin B_6 or vitamin B_{12}, homocysteine accumulates in the cell, it will inevitably lead to an elevation of intracellular SAH with a consequence of inhibition of several methyltransferases. Depending on the methyltransferase that is being inhibited, this could have a range of consequences discussed below under clinical and subclinical signs of folate or vitamin B_{12} deficiency.

The link between the DNA and methylation cycles

To maintain the activity of the methyltransferase, each cell would have two options. It could continue to take up methionine from the plasma, activate it to SAM and use its methyl group for a methylation reaction. This would leave it with the burden of generating an SAH and a homocysteine every time this happened, with the necessity of either degrading or perhaps wastefully exporting this homocysteine back into the plasma. The alternative, which is used by most cells, is to remethylate the homocysteine back to methionine, thus completing the cycle. Cells carry out this methylation of homocysteine back to methionine using the vitamin B_{12}-dependent enzyme methionine synthase. The immediate source of this methyl group is 5-methyltetrahydrofolate. This cosubstrate with homocysteine must be supplied on a continuous basis in all cells. Thus, the methylation cycle continuously uses or consumes methyl groups by donating them to the dozens of methyltransferases in the cell. The input of these methyl groups requires that they are presented attached to the folate cofactor as 5-methyltetrahydrofolate. The origin of these methyl groups is an enzyme, 5,10-methylenetetrahydrofolate reductase (MTHFR), which links the DNA cycle with the methylation cycle. This key enzyme can direct carbon-1 groups away from DNA biosynthesis and supply them instead to the methylation cycle. The carbon-1 that is pulled off is the folate cofactor, 5,10-methylenetetrahydrofolate, which is directly involved in the biosynthesis of DNA. The enzyme MTHFR reduces 5,10-methylenetetrahydrofolate to 5-methyltetrahydrofolate. This enzyme is thus a key link between these two important cycles. It is highly controlled. Its activity in all cells except for those of the liver is controlled by intracellular level of SAM. As the intracellular level of SAM begins to drop there is a consequent increase in the activity of the enzyme. The resultant increased level of 5,10-methyltetrahydrofolate

facilitates the methylation of homocysteine to methionine by methionine synthase. Once the methionine and consequently the SAM level has been restored in the cell, its rising level progressively inhibits MTHFR.

This method of control and the fact that MTHFR is irreversible *in vivo* have profound consequences if the activity of methionine synthase is compromised owing, for example, to vitamin B_{12} deficiency. In that circumstance the interruption of the methylation cycle at the point of this enzyme inevitably leads to the cell running low in SAM to supply its methyltransferases. The proper response is that the resultant reduction in the inhibition of MTHFR will cause diversion of carbon-1 units from the DNA cycle into the methylation cycle by increasing levels of 5-methyltetrahydrofolate as a result of increased activation of MTHFR. However, the only enzyme capable of utilizing this cofactor is methionine synthase, the activity of which is decreased or absent because it requires vitamin B_{12}. Thus, as suggested by the methyl trap hypothesis, 5-methyltetrafolate becomes metabolically trapped in this form. Surprisingly, the cell seems to have no metabolic response or only a wrong metabolic response to such vitamin B_{12} deficiency. Instead of recognizing that no amount of 5-methyltetrahydrofolate can restart the methylation cycle in the absence of vitamin B_{12} and methionine synthase, the cell continues to respond to the ever-decreasing SAM level by further increasing the activity of MTHFR. The resultant continuing drawing of the folate cofactors away from the forms found in the DNA cycle into the methodically trapped 5-methyltetrahydrofolate form quickly depletes the former pools of 5,10-methylenetetrahydrofolate and 10-formyltetrahydrofolate and reduces the cells' capacity to synthesize pyrimidines and purines, and thus DNA. The cell thus has its folate in a form that cannot be used and undergoes a sort of pseudo-folate deficiency, where there is folate in the cell but it cannot be used for DNA biosynthesis or cell replication. The consequence in such circumstances, such as in patients with the vitamin B_{12} deficiency condition pernicious anemia, is that a macrocytic megaloblastic anemia develops which is indistinguishable from that which occurs in folate deficiency. In addition, even though the level of 5-methyltetrahydrofolate is high in such vitamins B_{12}-deficient cells, it cannot be used to maintain the methylation cycle. This is because its use has an absolute requirement for a functioning methionine synthase. Thus, there is also a progressive reduction in the level of SAM and a reduction in the activity of all of the methyltransferases in the cell. This is probably further exacerbated by the fact that the level of SAM also controls the activity of the enzyme cystathionine synthase, which initiates the catabolism of homocysteine. Low SAM levels effectively shut down this enzyme, decreasing homocysteine catabolism. This accumulated homocysteine cannot be remethylated to methionine. As already mentioned, the equilibrium of SAH hydrolase will favor this homocysteine being converted to SAH. An elevation of SAH would have the additional effect of inhibiting all of the methyltransferase in the cell. Thus, methylation reactions will be compromised in two ways, by a lack of SAM and by inhibition by SAH.

Clinical and subclinical signs of folate or vitamin B_{12} deficiency

As discussed above, when there is insufficient folate in the diet the level of the folate cofactors necessary to maintain the DNA cycle is insufficient. This, in turn, compromises DNA biosynthesis, causing an arrest in cell division. This is most easily seen in cells that are replicating rapidly, not only because they have a high demand for *de novo* purine and pyrimidine biosynthesis to maintain DNA biosynthesis, but also because as such cells divide they halve their folate content. The two resultant daughter cells need to reestablish the level of folate to an optimal amount if these new cells are to continue to make DNA at an unhindered level. This is the case for all rapidly dividing cells, such as those of the bone marrow, red cells, granulocytes, lymphocytes and megakaryocytes. One would thus anticipate that folate deficiency, if severe enough and prolonged enough, would lead, respectively, to anemia, infection, a reduced immune response and decreased clotting as a result of a reduction in platelets. Other rapidly dividing cells such as those lining the gut will also be affected, causing malabsorption if the deficiency is severe and prolonged.

Cells that divide are affected, and the degree to which this will happen will depend on their rate of cell division. For example, hepatocytes turn over slowly and thus do not have the joint requirements to make lots of purines or pyrimidines and also to keep reestablishing new folate levels as a result of cell division. In contrast, during embryonic and fetal development and neonatal development, the demand for purines and pyrimidines and the need to take up new folates will be extremely high. Thus, developing structures would

be particularly susceptible to reduced folate status. They would also be vulnerable to anything that interfered with the recycling of the folate cofactor, such as reduced vitamin B_{12} status or a polymorphism that affected a folate-dependent enzyme such as exists for C→T677 MTHFR.

The effects of reduction in the DNA cycle are predictable: decreased purine and pyrimidine biosynthesis followed by reduced DNA biosynthesis and an impaired rate of cell replication most easily seen in the development of characteristic megaloblastic anemia. The consequence of reduction in the methylation cycle, as would be expected also to occur in both folate deficiency and vitamin B_{12} deficiency, are much more difficult to predict. All methyltransferases in the cell will be compromised.

Thus, there are well-recognized circumstances in which either the DNA cycle or the methylation cycle is compromised. In folate deficiency one would expect both to be compromised and this is most clearly seen in the arrest of cell division causing megaloblastic anemia. One would also expect the methylation cycle to be compromised, and consequently one would expect folate deficiency to lead to the same type of demyelination seen in vitamin B_{12} deficiency. However, peripheral neuropathy, ataxia and subacute combined degeneration, well-established consequences of vitamin B_{12} deficiency, are not usually seen in folate deficiency. The reason for this is unclear. A possible explanation is that the central nervous system concentrates folate by a specific transporter, resulting in a higher level in cerebrospinal fluid than exists in the circulating plasma. Perhaps this ensures that nerve tissue continues to have a sufficiency of folate even though there are overt signs and symptoms of deficiency in other tissues and organs. It may be the case that in practice the level of folate usually does not fall to sufficiently low levels in neural tissue to produce a reduction in the methylation cycle sufficient to cause demethylation. In this context, one study found the classical signs associated with vitamin B_{12} deficiency in subjects who were apparently vitamin B_{12} replete, but who had chronically extremely low folate levels.

A high level of interest in MTHFR is being generated because a polymorphism for it exists where there is a base change at base pair 677 from a thymidine to a cytosine. This, in turn, changes an amino acid at residue 244 from a glycine to an aspartate. This results in a structural alteration in the resultant enzyme, whereby it loses its cofactor flavin adenine dinucleotide (FAD) from its active site, resulting in instability and an irreversible loss of activity of the enzyme. The resultant phenotype is that those homozygous for the C→T677 variant of MTHFR have significantly reduced levels of the activity of the enzyme *in vivo*, resulting in a significant elevation of plasma homocysteine. This is greatest in those homozygous for the variant, but also elevated in those heterozygous for the variant. There is a further difference in phenotype with respect to both plasma and red cell folate, with an increasing gradient between those homozygous, heterozygous and wild-type for the variant. The expression of the elevation in plasma homocysteine in those homozygous for the C→T677 variant of MTHFR is very dependent not only on folate status, but also on riboflavin (vitamin B_2) status. It has been shown that only those who have the variant accompanied by a reduced riboflavin status show an elevation in plasma homocysteine. It would appear that a sufficiently good supply of riboflavin in the diet produces an amount of its cofactor derivative FAD in the cell that is sufficient to keep the active site of MTHFR with the cofactor bound to it. This, in turn, protects the enzyme from the inactivation that it would experience were the active site to lose its FAD group.

The clinical consequences of this variant are also of great interest. Numerous studies have examined whether it increases the risk of cardiovascular disease (CVD) as would be predicted because of its concurrent elevation in plasma homocysteine, which a body of evidence suggests is associated with CVD. While the results of these studies were mixed, two metaanalyses concluded that the variant does indeed increase CVD risk. As discussed below, it has also been shown conclusively to increase the risk of spina bifida and probably all NTD.

How might reduced folate status increase the risk of neural tube defects?

As discussed above, the metabolic role of the folate cofactors can be divided into two main areas: the DNA cycle (and cell division) and the methylation cycle (and methylation).

Neural tube defects and DNA cycle reduction

The reduced synthesis of DNA associated with reduced folate status or with genetic variants that affect this cycle would be expected to prevent cells dividing at the correct rate. It should be borne in mind that all dividing cells are particularly vulnerable to reduced folate status, not only because of the essential role of folate in making DNA, but also because as cells grow and divide they halve their folate content on each occasion. Thus, for the two daughter cells to work properly they must take up folate from the plasma or their supporting milieu to reinstate the correct level of folate before a further cell division reduces the intracellular folate concentration yet again. If, because of a poor folate supply or an impaired enzyme, this uptake did not keep pace with cell division, such replicating cells would have an increasingly inadequate level of folate and thus be metabolically compromised. This would affect the rate of cell division. Cell division during the early stages of the development of the embryo is extremely rapid. A series of structures is growing in a synchronized manner to bring about the various phases of development. Specifically, the neural plate undergoes a transformation beginning on day 21 postconception and finishing on day 27, with complete closure to form the neural tube. At the same time a protrusion is sent out from this developing structure to form what ultimately becomes the cranium.

An inadequate rate of cell division brought about by an inadequate amount of the necessary folate cofactors could compromise this normal development, resulting in an imperfect closure of the neural tube, causing spina bifida, or a lack of completion of the cranium, causing anencephaly. Similarly, in a pregnancy with inadequate vitamin B_{12} status some metabolic trapping of folate as 5-methyltetrahydrofolate may occur. The resultant reduction in the forms of folate that participate in purine and pyrimidine, 10-formyltetrahydrofolate and 5,10-methyltetrahydrofolate, respectively, may produce an impaired rate of cell division and a resultant embryo with spina bifida or anencephaly. The effect of increased folate (be it dietary folate or folic acid supplied in supplements and fortified food) would produce higher levels of intracellular folates, thus facilitating DNA biosynthesis and cell division. Similarly, if it is confirmed that vitamin B_{12} status is a maternal risk factor for NTD, improving intracellular vitamin B_{12} levels would also ensure that trapping of 5-methyltetrahydrofolate was not an issue.

Because this discussion is about dividing cells, in some instances, very rapidly dividing cells, it must be reemphasized that after each cell division there is a need quickly to reestablish the intracellular folate level halved by this division to its original level. Cells with adequate circulating levels of folate and/or vitamin B_{12}

would be in a position to do this in an optimal way. Similarly, in embryos homozygous for the C→T677 variant of MTHFR adequate riboflavin status would be desirable not only in the cell but also in the circulation, again to replenish the intracellular level after cell division. This polymorphism has been established as contributing a percentage of the population attributable risk for NTD in the order of 13%. A further polymorphism, in the trifunctional enzyme MTHFD-1, has been shown to be a maternal risk factor for an NTD-affected birth, contributing 9% of the population attributable risk. As discussed earlier, the anticipated reduction in the activity of the enzyme would reduce the flow of carbon-1 units from the formate exiting the mitochondria on their way to being converted to 10-formyltetrahydrofolate (for purine biosynthesis) and 5,10-methylenetetrahydrofolate (for pyrimidine biosynthesis). This latter cofactor is also known to be channeled up to the methylation cycle, since radioactive-labeled formate is formed into methionine and methylated cellular derivative in cells in tissue culture. Thus, the polymorphism in MTHFD-1 may also affect methylation. This polymorphism has been shown to be a maternal risk, but there is no increased risk if the embryo is homozygous for this variant. One can only speculate as to how compromising this enzyme in the mother may affect the closing neural tube in the embryo: the mother may supply the embryo with a structure or a metabolite involved in neural tube closure, or she may metabolize an embryonic or a fetal product.

Neural tube defects and methylation cycle reduction

As discussed earlier, the methylation cycle supplies SAM to dozens of methyltransferases. The resultant methylations have an equal number of metabolic effects. Reduced folate status would directly (and reduced vitamin B_{12} status would indirectly) potentially compromise a whole range of cellular processes. The two risk polymorphisms identified to date, namely C→T677 and MTHFD-1, could also compromise the supply of methyl groups to the methylation cycle.

It is not known which methyltransferases are important in the closure of the neural tube. An attractive candidate is the cytosine methyltransferase that methylates that base in existing DNA. This has the effect of silencing it or preventing this DNA from replicating. Studies on various animal models show that the development of the neural plate into the neural tube and cranium

involves switching on and off a series of genes in a strict order and to a strict time-frame. This controls the supply of protein gene products that go to make up these new structures. Methylation and demethylation are the principal ways in which genes are inactivated and activated, respectively. A reduced level of SAM with a probable concurrent increased level of the potent methyltransferase inhibitor SAH would thus produce a lack of synchrony in this complicated sequence of events. This would lead to an imperfect closure of the neural tube or inadequate development of the cranium. Another candidate methyltransferase would be the one that methylates phosphotidylethanolamine to phosphotidylcholine. This latter phospholipid is known to be involved in cell surface receptor function. Other methyltransferases can methylate the side-chain of the amino acids arginine and lysine when they are in proteins. Such methylations are known to affect function and stability. The reduction in the activity of the isopenoid methyltransferase associated with vitamin B_{12} deficiency has been mentioned as causing an inflammatory response in neural tissue. Such a reduction in function could also affect the developing embryo. As mentioned already, there are dozens of other methyltransferase in all cells, all of which are dependent on an optimal methylation cycle. Thus, reduction in any of these could potentially cause a birth defect.

17.3 Evidence that folate and other related vitamins play a protective role against adverse outcomes of pregnancy

For many years the prevalence at birth of NTD or other birth defects was thought to be due to some genetic predisposition interacting with an environmental factor or factors. Significant genetic involvement was indicated by the 10–20-fold increased risk of recurrence, that is, once a parent had one affected child (an occurrence) there was a high increase in risk of a subsequent affected baby (a recurrence). Further evidence for a large genetic role came from consistent differences in prevalence between different ethnic groups. However, if these defects were purely genetic, their rate would be relatively constant within any particular ethnic group. This does not happen: there are well-recognized cycles where prevalence rises and falls. Such rises in prevalence were often associated with periods of nutritional deprivation, such as after the Dutch famine at the end of World War II and during the Depression in the USA in the 1920s. Although the environmental factor was long thought to be nutritional, the fact that it was largely or solely due to folate only emerged in the 1980s. The involvement of folate status in NTD is now proven, but its role in other birth defects is less certain, as discussed below.

Neural tube defects

Failure of the proper closure of the neural tube, producing spina bifida or other NTDs, is the most common birth defect.

At day 21 postconception the neural plate begins to close and form the neural tube, which will eventually becomes the spinal column in the embryo and the fetus. A protrusion is sent out to encompass the cranium. Incomplete closure of the spinal column results in spina bifida with various levels of disability, from an almost normal life to severe disability, including paralysis of the lower limbs and bladder. Incomplete closure of the cranium results in an anencephaly, which is incompatible with life. Spina bifida and anencephaly make up about 50% and 40% of NTD, respectively, with the remaining 10% comprising encephalocele and inencephale. It is generally agreed that all of these NTD have a common etiology. The principal basis for this is that the increased risk of a recurrence applies to any one of the conditions. Furthermore, increased ethnic risk is for the group of conditions. It was long recognized that NTD resulted from an underlying genetic predisposition that was influenced by an environmental factor, which was very probably nutritional. The evidence for a genetic etiology was the high recurrence rate in mothers with a previously affected pregnancy, the difference in prevalence in different ethnic groups and studies on twins. However, if NTD were purely genetic their prevalence would be constant; furthermore, there was ample evidence that NTD rates went through cycles, frequently increasing after times of nutritional deprivation. This suggests that one or more nutrients may be involved.

Epidemiological evidence and randomized trials

An involvement for folate was first suggested by the British obstetrician Bryan Hibbard in 1964. The observation that urinary formiminoglutamic acid (a not very good marker for folate status) was elevated in women with pregnancies affected by an NTD birth compared with a normal control population added some

experimental support. There followed a series of studies, some supporting the contention that folate deficiency was involved, but several finding no obvious difference in folate status in affected pregnancies compared with normal pregnancies. Most of these studies were too small to demonstrate a difference given the small reduction in status that is now known to have an influence on the prevalence of NTD pregnancies.

Richard Smithells should be credited with generating the first real evidence that NTD could be prevented with a multivitamin preparation that contained folic acid (Smithells *et al.*, 1980). The original intention was to conduct a double-blind placebo intervention, but one of the three ethics committees to which the proposal was submitted refused permission to give a placebo to half of the women, all of whom had had a previous pregnancy affected by an NTD, as this was a recurrence trial. At the time such periconceptional vitamin and mineral preparations had no proven or even suggested therapeutic role in prevention of NTD, so the view of this ethical committee may be considered to have been misguided. It caused a great number of problems down the line and probably delayed the effective prevention of NTD on a wide scale by one or two decades. This was because, in response to the decision of the ethics committee, Smithells and his colleagues changed the design of the trial to be one of intervention, whereby all women who were enrolled received the treatment. They used for comparison, as a control group, women who for various reasons had not been recruited into the trial. The intervention seemed subsequently to lower the recurrence prevalence of NTD by one-half or perhaps as much as three-quarters. The problem was that the majority of the medical community would not accept the result because of the recognized intrinsic differences between people who enter clinical trials and those who either refuse to enter or are not recruited in the first place. Indeed, Smithells *et al.* (1983) argued that the treated and untreated pregnancies were the same. Wald and Polani (1984) pointed out that differences between the two groups existed that could have given the treated group an intrinsically lower risk of an NTD-affected birth.

A properly designed intervention trial had been undertaken previously by Laurence and his colleagues, working in Wales. They compared the effect of 4.0 mg folic acid per day given periconceptionally to 60 women compared with a placebo given to 51 women all of whom had a previous history of an NTD-affected pregnancy.

The results of this recurrence trial were negative in that two women in the treatment group had a child with an NTD. Some time later, one of these women confessed to not having taken the folic acid tablets; therefore, Laurence *et al.* (1981) felt justified in saying that she was not treated by virtue of noncompliance and thus transferred her to the control group. The other mother in the treatment group with an NTD child remained adamant that she had taken the tablets. However, Laurence observed that she had the lowest serum folate of anybody in the treatment group. By virtue of this, they determined that she could also be added to the control group, at which point the result of the effect of folic acid in preventing NTD became statistically significant ($p = 0.04$). Most investigators simply did not accept that the reclassification of these two women to be considered as part of the placebo group was scientifically valid.

There remained interest in whether or not the Smithells trial did indicate a benefit in spite of the design faults. In the case of the Laurence trial, its small size and the reclassification of the treated women to the non-treated group left the question very much still open. In addition, the trial by Smithells *et al.* (1983) had later been extended to cover over 1000 births. Pregnavite Forte F, a multivitamin/multimineral preparation, was used, thus making it difficult to recommend a specific public health response to women who were planning a pregnancy.

The questions generated by the above studies culminated in the UK Medical Research Council (MRC) funding a multicenter trial. The trial took place in 33 centers in seven countries and recruited 1817 women with a previous history of an NTD-affected pregnancy. These volunteers were divided into four groups: folic acid, folic acid plus the multivitamin/multimineral complex Pregnavite Forte F used by Smithells, the same preparation without folic acid, and a placebo group. The trial thus set out to test the preparation multivitamin/multimineral complex, which was apparently successful in reducing NTD, but looked at it both including folic acid and excluding folic acid. They organized their trial also to test the apparently positive Laurence trial. The preparation used by Smithells contained 360 μg of folic acid per day, while those used by Laurence *et al.* contained 4.0 mg per day, over 10 times as much. When the MRC trial proved successful this very high dose generated debate as to whether it was necessary or even safe. It also created a problem from the public health standpoint. Whatever the prospect of adding 360 μg of folic to the diet by way of fortification, it was clearly impossible if

the lowest target figure was 4.0 mg per day. This is about 10–20 times the recommended dietary allowance (RDA), or equivalent recommendation for normal adults, and would have safety concerns.

Nevertheless, the MRC trial showed that both treatments that contained folic reduced the prevalence of NTD-affected births. The magnitude of the reduction was calculated to be 72%. However, the design of the trial was on an intention-to-treat basis. Thus, women who entered the trial and were assigned to one of the treatment groups and who subsequently were found to be noncompliant or who had dropped out of the trial were all considered to have been fully treated. Therefore, the preventive effect of folic acid calculated in the result was an absolute minimum. It was probable that prevention was in excess of even 80%.

Simultaneously with the running of these trials, during the 1980s and 1990s, several investigations carried out case–control studies on the effectiveness of folic acid in the prevention of NTD-affected births. These studies compared the prevalence rates of NTD in women taking supplements containing folic acid with those in women in the same community who were not supplement users. By the time the MRC trial was published in 1992, reaching the conclusion that maternal periconceptional folic acid prevented most NTD, dozens of case–control studies had been completed and published. With one exception, all of these newer studies had concluded that supplements containing folic acid lowered NTD rates by the order of about 50%. Studies comparing the rate of NTD in mothers taking vitamins with the rate in those who did not suffered from the problem that these two groups may also differ with respect to their characteristics such as level of education and socioeconomic status. Such confounding makes it difficult to be certain that the benefit is due to vitamin taking and not to some other identified or unidentified benefit. Nevertheless, these studies were encouraging and helped to bring about a speedy consensus when the results of the well-designed MRC trial were positive. These case–control studies also seemed to justify that using the lower dose of 400 μg/day would be effective, because this was the level in most supplements used in the case–control studies and Smithells *et al.* (1980, 1983) had used a dose of 360 μg/day. This background swayed the UK Department of Health to come forward with the recommendation that the lower dose of 400 μg should be used to prevent the lower risk associated with NTD occurrence where there was no previous pregnancy or where the pregnancy had produced unaffected children. The risk of occurrence was between 1 and 6 per 1000 births depending on the population under study, whereas the risk of recurrence was 10–20 times higher. On the basis of a risk–benefit approach it was felt that the very high dose of 4.0 mg/day should still be used to prevent recurrence.

The MRC trial and the previous intervention trials were recurrence trials and used women who had had a previously affected pregnancy. However, while the MRC trial was underway the Hungarian trial of Czeizel and Dudas (1992) had used women with no previous history of an affected pregnancy. This occurrence trial was properly designed; although it did not contain a placebo, it compared a multivitamin preparation with a multimineral preparation, in a randomized, double-blind manner. The former contained folic acid at the intermediate to high dose of 800 μg/day. The trial found six NTD in the multimineral group and none in the group receiving the multivitamins containing folic acid. This trial was significant because although previously it could be surmised that preventing recurrence (as had been done in the MRC trial) was the same as preventing occurrence, it was not certain that this was so. This was important because the number of NTD births due to first time occurrence is by far the majority, being about 85% of all NTD births. Thus, the public health challenge has been and remains the priority of preventing first occurrence. The intervention trials examining the effect of folic acid on the prevention of NTDs are summarized in Table 17.2.

Potential roles for folate-related B-vitamins in the prevention of neural tube defects

A low status of vitamin B_{12} has been reported to be a risk factor, independent of folate status, in the etiology of NTD. This is consistent with the importance of vitamin B_{12} in the normal recycling of folate cofactors, as described earlier.

As mentioned above, new evidence suggests that optimal riboflavin status renders the effect of being homozygous for the C→T677 variant of MTHFR neutral with respect to homocysteine concentrations, implying that the impaired functioning of the variant form of this key folate-metabolizing enzyme is dependent on riboflavin status. This may explain why in some populations studies have failed to show the expected increased risk of NTD in association with this polymorphism that is seen in other populations such as

Ireland. Differences in the prevailing riboflavin status in a particular population could affect the activity of the variant form of MTHFR in cells of the closing neural tube, thereby influencing the extent to which this polymorphism is associated with the risk of NTD. In the USA, for example, mandatory fortification of flour with riboflavin for many years ensures high intakes in the whole population (irrespective of individual dietary practices), which could reduce the extent to which this polymorphism is found to carry an increased risk of NTD. The modulating effect of riboflavin on this polymorphism may have an important public health relevance with respect to NTD risk for many other countries in which the fortification of foods is not so widespread, or in countries such as Italy, Spain and Mexico, where the prevalence of this polymorphism is particularly high.

Orofacial clefts

Another common set of birth defects is grouped together as orofacial clefts (OFC) and sometimes called craniofacial anomalies. The various types of NTD are thought to have a similar etiology; however, this is not the case with OFC. There are certainly two broad divisions. The most common are cleft lip, which may also involve the palate and are thus called cleft lip plus or minus cleft palate (CL ± P). The second major type involves the palate only and is called cleft palate (CP) or sometimes isolated cleft palate. Both show a wide range of prevalence depending on the country and ethnic origin of those being investigated. The older literature suggests that the rate of CL ± P is generally higher in populations of African origin and lower in Caucasian populations. Rates per 1000 births are reported as Native American 2.7, Japanese 2.1 and African–American 0.42. A survey by the World Health Organization (WHO) showed significant variation worldwide and within Europe. A summary given by the WHO suggests that the prevalence at birth per 10 000 births is Caucasian 10, Japanese 20, Native North American 36 and African–American 3. The prevalence at birth of CP is lower and shows less variation among different racial groups, perhaps half of that of CL ± P averaged across races. As many as 30% of OFC are regarded as being syndromes. A range of conditions has specific genetic origins resulting in an identifiable syndrome that involves the lip or the palate or both, and which has frequently been associated with other congenital malformations. The most common examples, with their prevalence per

10 000 births, are Crouzon's syndrome 0.4, Treacher Collins' syndrome 0.2 and Apert's syndrome 0.15.

Since the 1970s at least eight case–control studies have compared the risk of an OFC in women taking supplements containing folic acid with the risk in those not taking supplements. Overall, the results are conflicting, with some studies showing no effect and others indicating some reduction in risk, particularly if the subclassification into CL ± P and CP was made. Perhaps one of the most discussed was a Hungarian study that seemed to show a protective effect for both types of common OFC, but only if the mother had been taking very high doses of folic acid of at least 3.0 mg/day, with levels of 800 μg/day having little effect. The latter result was supported by the evidence from a large randomized trial that found no protective effect of 0.8 μg/day.

This idea that very high doses of folic acid might be needed was attractive because a dose–response effect would explain away the most convincing piece of evidence that OFC are not prevented by increased folic acid. This evidence is as follows. In many countries, including the UK and Ireland, there was a well-documented reduction in the prevalence at birth of NTD during the 1990s. While some of this was due to elective terminations of pregnancy, it is generally agreed that this is not the complete explanation and that a real reduction in NTD prevalence occurred. Since three-quarters or more of NTD seem to be preventable by folic acid or folate, it is generally agreed that this decrease has been due to increases in intake of this vitamin. During the same time-frame well-documented studies on the prevalence of OFC showed that it has remained very constant. If folic acid and folate levels have been improving, as evidenced by the drop in NTD, and if this vitamin is protective of OFC, an obvious question is why has the prevalence of the latter not decreased? One possible explanation is that the increase in folate intake that has occurred was sufficient to reduce NTD but insufficient to reduce OFC, because the latter conditions are less responsive and would require a higher folic acid dose. Another strand of evidence has been used to try to prove or disprove a folate association with OFC. The common genetic polymorphism C→T677 MTHFR has been shown in several studies to increase the risk of NTD, presumably by interfering with folate metabolism. It would seem logical that if folate were also involved in the risk of OFC, the risk might also show a decreasing gradient in those homozygous, heterozygous or wild-type for the polymorphism. Here again, there is a lack of information. Studies in California considered that there was no increased risk either for CL + P or for isolated CP in association with this polymorphism. However, a study in Ireland found a statistically significant increase in risk for isolated CP only. More recently, this polymorphism has been suggested as being a maternal risk. The picture at the moment is thus confused. More studies involving more cases may resolve this issue, particularly where they are subdivided into the two main and apparently different etiological types of CL ± P and isolated C.P. In addition, unlike in the case of NTD, there are several other well-established circumstances where OFC risk has been established as being increased, for example maternal smoking, and solvent and drug exposure. Perhaps such causes, if not removed from the folate risk analysis, sufficiently obscure a clear-cut result and, therefore, future studies in which these confounding issues can be excluded may produce a definitive answer.

Congenital heart disease

There is some interest in the possibility that improved maternal folate status may decrease the risk of such defects.

Other adverse pregnancy outcomes

Apart from congenital birth defects, a considerable number of conditions with the potential for an adverse outcome for either the baby or the mother has been associated with low folate status. In some instances, the result may be loss of the baby (e.g. abruptio placentae or spontaneous abortion), while in others the development of the fetus (e.g. intrauterine growth retardation) or the health of the mother (e.g. preeclampsia) is affected. Some of the conditions have been linked to low folate status through the measurement of the biomarker plasma homocysteine, an elevated level of which is a sensitive indicator of low folate status. These conditions are summarized in Table 17.1, together with their approximate prevalence and an indication of the evidence linking them to low folate status.

Maternal folate deficiency and neonatal health

In general, pregnancy is a time of increased folate requirement that may or may not result in maternal folate deficiency depending on the mother's nutritional status. Thus, as pregnancy progresses, the importance of folate in maternal health becomes more evident.

Table 17.1 Adverse pregnancy outcomes associated with low folate status

Adverse outcome	Approximate prevalence (%)	Evidence linking low folate status to adverse outcome
Intrauterine growth retardation	6–10	Folic acid intervention trial supports a link
Preterm delivery	5	Elevated plasma homocysteine
Preeclampsia	5	Elevated plasma homocysteine
Recurred repeat pregnancy	5	Reduced folate stores may increase risk generally
Pregnancy-induced hypertension	3	No evidence
Abruptio placentae	1	Elevated plasma homocysteine; homozygosity for C→T677 MTHFR polymorphism

MTHFR: 5,10-methylenetetrahydrofolate reductase.

Evidence suggests that folate-responsive megaloblastic anemia occurs in up to 24% of unsupplemented pregnancies in certain parts of Asia, Africa, Central and South America, and in 2.5–5.0% of those in the developed world. Bone marrow megaloblastosis, indicative of subclinical deficiency, occurs in as many as 25% of women not receiving supplements in otherwise well-nourished societies. Serum and red blood cell folate levels decline throughout pregnancy, but this fall is not seen where folic acid supplementation is introduced or where there is sufficient dietary folate to meet the increased requirements of pregnancy. Poor maternal folate status has consequences not only for the mother's health, but also for that of the neonate. There is good evidence from the USA of a positive association between maternal folate status and birth weight. Poor maternal folate status is associated with a greater risk of an infant with LBW (defined as weighing less than 2.5 kg at birth). Infants with LBW (representing 16% of all newborn infants in developed countries and 90% of those in developing countries) are known to have a several-fold increased risk of neonatal mortality. Maternal folate deficiency has also been shown to result in neonatal folate deficiency, with important implications for the health of the neonate and infant.

Therefore, during the periconception phase and throughout pregnancy, folate plays an important role in the maintenance of maternal, embryonic, fetal and neonatal health, and in protecting against a number of potential adverse outcomes for the mother and the baby.

17.4 Prevention of folate-responsive adverse outcomes of pregnancy

Pregnancy is a complex period resulting in huge physiological and nutritional demands upon the mother.

In addition, the rapid development in going from a fertilized ovum, through implantation, embryonic and fetal development, and subsequent birth, represents perhaps the period of greatest risk to any individual. The folates, involved as they are in cell division and a wide range of methylation reactions, are bound to be important to several aspects of pregnancy.

Scale of potential reduction in neural tube defects

Incomplete closures of the neural tube are collectively called NTD. They consist of 50% spina bifida and 40% anencephaly, with the remaining 10% being made up of other abnormalities, principally encephalocele.

Spina bifida is where there is a failure in the closure of the vertebral arches. It is characterized by a protrusion of the meninges (meningocele) or of both the meninges and neural tissue (meningomyelocele).

Anencephaly is where there is a failure in the formation of the cranium and is characterized by the absence of the skull. It is a lethal condition, with death occurring either *in utero* or shortly after birth.

Encephalocele is a defect in the cranium, usually of the occipital region, through which meninges on the brain tissue protrude, usually covered by skin. Taken together, spina bifida and encephalocele account for 60% of all NTD cases. About 80% of babies born with these forms of NTD survive the newborn period, but the vast majority (85%) of those who survive have lifelong moderate or severe handicap. It was recently estimated that if mean folic acid intakes were increased by 200 μg/day, the incidence of NTD-affected pregnancies could be reduced by 41%. To put this reduction into context (based on 1997/98 NTD figures), it would be equivalent to the prevention of 38 of the 93 NTD-affected births in England and Wales, 30 of the 74 in Scotland, six of the 14 in Northern Ireland, and 31 of the 75 babies born with NTD every year in the Republic of Ireland. Although the prevalence of NTD in Ireland, as elsewhere, has fallen markedly since the 1980s, the condition remains more common in Ireland than in most other parts of the world. Apart from the 89 or so babies born with NTD every year in the Republic of Ireland and Northern Ireland, many more affected fetuses are lost as miscarriages.

Optimal folate status versus prevention of folate deficiency: current recommendations

The term optimal nutrition has evolved in recognition of the finding that, at least for some nutrients, there may be specific health benefits from optimizing status by levels of intake well above those considered adequate for the prevention of the specific disease associated with deficiency of the nutrient. Folate is perhaps one of the best examples of a nutrient for which optimal versus adequate status can be clearly understood. Traditionally, the general approach used to generate dietary folate recommendations has, as for any nutrient, involved examining data on average intake of folate among individuals with no overt signs of folate deficiency. The dietary recommendation was thus calculated on the basis of establishing the amount of folate that was adequate to prevent clinical or subclinical folate deficiency. However, scientific evidence is emerging to such an extent that there now appears to be a number of potential benefits of this vitamin at levels of intake greater than those that are adequate for the prevention of overt folate deficiency, which is itself not uncommon in pregnancy. Thus, folate is attracting major interest as having possible preventive roles against CVD, certain cancers and neuropsychiatric conditions. However, its role in the prevention of NTD is currently the only condition in which there is a proven benefit of optimal folate status. For the prevention of NTD, official bodies worldwide now recommend that women take an additional 400 μg/day folate before conception and in early pregnancy. These recommendations effectively replace any folate recommendations for women of reproductive age (such as current UK dietary reference values) which were set before the publication in 1991 of conclusive evidence linking folate and NTD.

Irrespective of the prevailing folate recommendations, what is very evident is that the diet currently consumed by women even in the most affluent and developed

countries within Europe does not provide adequate levels of folate to ensure an optimal status of the vitamin for protection against NTD and other diseases. Reported dietary folate intakes of adults in different European countries range between 168 and 326 μg/day, with many adults failing to meet even current folate recommendations, which in many cases are likely to be revised upwards in the future in an effort to aim for optimal folate status. If this is to be achieved, current dietary folate intakes will need to increase considerably in Europe. The introduction in recent years of mandatory fortification of grain foods with folic acid in the USA and Canada means that dietary folate intakes in these populations have markedly improved compared with prefortification intakes.

Strategies to achieve optimal folate status

In response to its established protective role against both recurrence and first occurrence of NTD, national committees worldwide have set almost identical folate recommendations. To prevent recurrence of NTD, the recommendation is 4 mg/day folic acid, while 400 μg/day is recommended for the prevention of first occurrence, to be commenced before conception and continued until the twelfth week of pregnancy. In the former case, the recommendation is clearly achievable only by folic acid supplementation in tablet form in women identified as being at risk. However, as stated above, the prevention of first occurrences of NTD is the more significant public health concern since these represent about 95% of all NTD cases. There are three suggested ways in which the recommendation for the prevention of first occurrences can be achieved:

- increased intake of foods naturally rich in folate
- folic acid supplementation
- folic acid fortification.

The implementation of this recommendation is proving difficult for a number of reasons which are discussed below. These include the practical consideration of achieving a three-fold increase in current folate intakes and the poor stability and bioavailability of natural food folates. In addition women tend to be poorly compliant with supplementation or may not have planned to become pregnant. They may not have access to, or necessarily choose, foods that have been fortified.

Table 17.2 Intervention trials to examine the effect of folic acid on prevention of neural tube defects (NTD)

Investigators (year)	Type of intervention	Outcome
Smithells et al. (1980)	Nonrandomized trial Pregnavite Forte F (multivitamin/mineral 360 μg/day folic acid) All given treatment Controls were those who declined or were pregnant at referral (untreated)	An apparent effect, but not accepted owing to poor study design Treated, $n = 178$: 1 recurrence (0.6%) Untreated, $n = 260$: 13 recurrences (5.0%)
Smithells et al. (1983)	Nonrandomized trial (Extension of above trial)	An apparent effect, but poor study design Subjects included in combined analysis below
Schorah and Smithells (1991)	Nonrandomized trials Combined analysis of previous trials by this group	An apparent effect, but poor study design Fully treated, $n = 1093$: 14 recurrences (1.3%) Partially treated, $n = 211$: 2 recurrences (0.9%) Untreated, $n = 486$: 24 recurrences (4.9%)
Holmes-Siedle et al. (1992)	Nonrandomized trial Design as for Smithells et al. (1980)	An apparent effect, but poor study design Treated, $n = 204$: 1 recurrence (0.5%) Untreated, $n = 28$: 3 recurrences (10.7%)
Laurence et al. (1981)	Double-blind RCT Treatment (4.0 mg/day folic acid) versus placebo	No significant effect until reclassification Treatment group, $n = 60$: 2 recurrences Placebo group, $n = 51$: 4 recurrences
MRC Vitamin Study Research Group (1991)	Double-blind RCT; four groups: 1. Folic acid (4.0 mg/day) 2. Folic acid plus multivitamins 3. Multivitamins without folic acid 4. Placebo	Significant (72%) protective effect Folic acid treatment, $n = 593$: 6 recurrences (1.0%), groups 1 and 2 combined No folic acid, $n = 602$: 21 recurrences (3.3%), groups 3 and 4 combined
Czeizal and Dudas (1992)	Double-blind RCT Multivitamin (800 μg/day folic acid) versus multimineral	Significant (100%) protective effect Vitamin treatment, $n = 2104$: no occurrence (0%) Mineral treatment, $n = 2052$: 6 occurrences (0.3%)

RCT: randomized controlled trial.
All interventions, except that of Czeizal and Dudas, involved women with a previous history of an NTD-affected pregnancy and were thus attempts to prevent recurrence of NTD. Czeizal and Dudas (1992) confirmed for the first time that folic acid was also effective in preventing the first occurrence of NTD.

Individual strategy

A major problem in implementing the recommendation of an extra 400 μg/day folate (i.e. a total of 600 μg/day, based on typical dietary intakes of about 200 μg/day) is that this level represents a three-fold increase in current folate intakes in women. Thus, achieving the recommendation through folate-rich foods alone (e.g. liver, green leafy vegetables, green beans and yeast extract) would require major dietary modifications, unlikely to be reached by most women planning a pregnancy, not to mention those not planning to become pregnant.

An even greater problem lies in the fact that even when a significant increase in food folates is achieved experimentally in intervention studies in women, it appears to be a much less effective means of optimizing folate status (as measured by the red cell folate response, the best long-term index of folate status) than equivalent intakes of the vitamin as folic acid in fortified food or supplements. The obvious explanation for the observed differences in response to intervention relates to structural differences in the vitamin, depending on whether it is present in the synthetic form (folic acid) as in supplements and fortified foods, or the natural food folate form. For example, folic acid is fully oxidized, and therefore much more stable to typical conditions of storage and preparation than the natural vitamin, which is a reduced molecule and thus may be prone to considerable losses, particularly under certain cooking conditions (e.g. boiling). Another important structural difference is that folic acid is a monoglutamate and as such is readily absorbed, whereas natural food folates are predominantly polyglutamates, which require conversion to the monoglutamate form for their absorption. A number of factors (including the food matrix and the presence in food of certain components that can inhibit intestinal folate deconjugation) may potentially reduce this process, resulting in an overall incomplete bioavailability of natural food folates. Thus, the potential to optimize folate status by means of increased consumption of foods naturally rich in folate is somewhat limited, a finding generally attributed to the poorer bioavailability of natural food folates compared with folic acid. A great deal of uncertainty still exists in our knowledge of folate bioavailability from natural food sources which, depending on the methodology used, has been reported to range anywhere between 10 and 98% relative to that of folic acid. Despite this uncertainty, current US dietary recommendations for folate are based on the differences in bioavailability between natural food folates and the synthetic vitamin, with the recent introduction of the concept of dietary folate equivalents (DFE). The definition of DFE is based on the assumption that the bioavailability of folic acid added to food is greater than that of natural food folate by a factor of 1.67. This estimation relies heavily on one metabolic study in nonpregnant women which estimated food folate bioavailability from a mixed diet to be approximately 50% that of folic acid, and other evidence indicating that folic acid added to food had about 85% of the bioavailability of free folic acid.

Given the poor bioavailability of natural food folates outlined above, folic acid supplements, which have been proven to be a very effective strategy for optimizing folate status in the individual women who receive them, are the major focus of health promotion of folate in women planning a pregnancy.

Population strategy

Although supplementation with folic acid is a very effective strategy for optimizing folate status in individual women, it is not an effective population strategy for a number of reasons. The neural tube closes in the first few weeks of pregnancy and therefore the malformations of NTD may have occurred before a woman even knows that she is pregnant. Thus, supplementation will be ineffective for women with unplanned pregnancies, which are estimated to account for 50% of all pregnancies in the UK and the USA. Even in women who have planned their pregnancy, compliance with

current folate recommendations may be poor. One study in 1997 in the UK reported that only 30% of an interviewed sample of pregnant women had followed the official folic acid recommendations correctly. Thus, for practical reasons, folic acid supplements do not offer an effective strategy for the primary prevention of NTD in the general population. Any intervention aimed at preventing NTD should be targeted not just at women planning to become pregnant, but at all women of childbearing age, to achieve optimal periconceptional folate status in the majority of those who could become pregnant. For this reason, mandatory fortification of grain products with folic acid has been introduced in the USA and certain other countries (e.g. Canada) and is under consideration elsewhere. As discussed below, the UK recommendation of the expert Committee on Medical Aspects of Food and Nutrition Policy (COMA) panel to fortify the diet with folic acid has been deferred. Informed people in the relevant government departments interpret this as rejection, certainly in the short term.

Folic acid fortification of grain foods on a mandatory basis was introduced in the USA in 1998. Because of the safety concerns surrounding this issue, the US Food and Drug Administration (FDA), which was responsible for implementing the new fortification legislation, opted for the relatively low folic acid concentration of $140 \, \mu g/100 \, g$ product, which was projected to result in a mean additional intake of $100 \, \mu g/day$ in the US population. This level of folic acid was considered low enough almost certainly to carry no risk, but some argued that it would turn out to be ineffective in preventing NTD. However, evidence published in 2001 indicated that the incidence of NTD in the USA had declined by almost 20% as a result of the new folic acid fortification policy. More recent evidence from Canada suggests that the decrease is even greater.

Mandatory folic acid fortification for the UK population was proposed by COMA in 2000. The main conclusion of the report was that "universal folic acid fortification of flour at $240 \, \mu g/100 \, g$ in food products as consumed would have a significant effect in preventing NTD-affected conceptions and births without resulting in unacceptably high intakes in any group of the population." The fortification level of $240 \, \mu g/100 \, g$ flour was estimated to increase mean folic acid intakes by $200 \, \mu g/day$ which, in turn, was predicted to reduce the incidence of NTD-affected pregnancies by 41%. Although the report focused primarily on the proven role of folic acid in the prevention of NTD, the potential benefit of folic acid in reducing the risk of CVD via homocysteine lowering was also acknowledged.

The conclusions of the COMA report were based on a detailed risk–benefit assessment. Such an assessment estimates the likely benefits of folic acid fortification in terms of NTD reduction, as well as the risk of overexposure by those with high intakes. The risk–benefit assessment requires the manipulation of a representative dietary survey database, which is sometimes referred to as dietary modeling. In the COMA report, estimates of the exposure of different groups in the population to additional folic acid were made by modeling dietary intake data from four National Diet and Nutrition Surveys for each age group, at five possible levels of fortification of flour as consumed in finished products: 140, 200, 240, 280 and 480 μg/100 g. At each of these fortification levels, an estimation was provided as to the number of NTD-affected births per year that would be prevented, as well as the percentage of people over 50 years who would be exposed to a folic acid intake greater than 1 mg/day (equivalent to the upper tolerable intake level). The concern here relates to the potential masking of the anemia (and therefore the possibility of delaying the diagnosis) of vitamin B_{12} deficiency among older people exposed to high folic acid intakes. The risk–benefit assessment performed by COMA was dependent on the availability of experimental data from which the additional folic acid intake at the various fortification levels could be related to NTD risk. For this purpose, COMA used the results of a placebo-controlled trial which estimated the potential effects on NTD risk of a 6 month folic acid intervention at 100, 200 or 400 μg/day, by measuring the response of each dose in terms of the impact on red cell folate concentrations, which have been established to relate to NTD risk in an inverse dose–response relationship. The reliability of this approach as a basis for predicting NTD risk has been confirmed by recent US evidence. The intervention study predicted a 22% reduced risk of NTD arising from the extra 100 μg/day folic acid being targeted under the US folic acid fortification program. This compares very closely with the actual US experience in which NTD reported on birth certificates fell from 37.8 per 10 000 live births before fortification to 30.5 per 100 000 live births after fortification, representing a 19% decline in NTDs. The incidence of spina bifida fell by 23%. Thus, there can be a good degree of confidence in COMA's predicted 41%

reduction in the incidence of NTD-affected pregnancies arising from the recommended folic acid fortification level of 240 μg/100 g flour (Department of Health, 2000).

Food fortification in general remains an important issue for policy makers in Europe. Current fortification policy varies considerably across different European countries, with major implications for European Union food legislation and trade. In certain countries, the fortification of food with any nutrient is forbidden, others specifically forbid fortification with folic acid, while others permit the fortification of foods with a range of nutrients including folic acid on a voluntary basis. The specific issue of mandatory folic acid fortification is a separate, more urgent case. With various governments considering the introduction of new policy in this regard, the question of fortification with folic acid is the topic of much debate. Although evidence from the USA shows a 19% decrease in the incidence of NTD since the introduction of the new policy, mandatory fortification is controversial for various reasons. Fortification, unlike supplementation, is untargeted; therefore, in order to ensure that the required nutrient levels are delivered to the target group, a proportion of the general population is inevitably exposed to high levels. The greatest concern regarding universal fortification with folic acid is that it may mask the hematological changes associated with vitamin B_{12} deficiency (which has a high prevalence among elderly people), thereby allowing the concomitant irreversible nerve degeneration to go undetected. Because of these issues, many countries are opting not to introduce mandatory folic acid fortification.

Establishing the lowest amount of folic acid that will be effective in protecting most women against an NTD-affected pregnancy is a critical question when mandatory fortification is being considered. Although folic acid is considered to be nontoxic, even at high doses, there remains some concern that its widespread, chronic use in fortification may cause some harm. Folic acid can be used to treat the anemia of vitamin B_{12} deficiency. Essentially, folic acid overcomes the methyltetrahydrofolate trap by introducing new folate cofactors into the cell which initiate new DNA biosynthesis before they become trapped as 5-methyltetrahydrofolate. Such new DNA causes a hemopoetic response and if folic acid intervention is continued, which it usually is, it will appear that the anemia has been treated. Unfortunately, such new folates do nothing to restart the methylation cycle because of its requirement for vitamin B_{12} for methionine synthase. The absence of this cycle causes a progressive neuropathology. The masking of the anemia prevents the timely diagnosis and treatment of such conditions as pernicious anemia, resulting in late detection, by which time the neuropathy of vitamin B_{12} deficiency may be partly irreversible. This is really the only potential risk known to be associated with folic acid intervention. Many consider vitamin B_{12} deficiency to be very rare and that, in most cases, it will be diagnosed even if the anemia is masked. However, there is no doubt that however small the number, some people with vitamin B_{12} deficiency will not be diagnosed as early as they might be if they were not receiving extra folic acid.

Other suggested risks are either remote or do not have any real basis. It is suggested that patients on anticonvulsants may have less control of their epilepsy, but such known cases are limited and the evidence is weak. While there is no direct evidence that extra folic acid may potentiate the risk of the progression of established cancers, it has to be said that two of the most successful anticancer drugs, methotrexate and 5-fluorouracil, act by interrupting folate metabolism. It has also been suggested that some polymorphisms, known to impair folate metabolism for example the C→T677 for MTHFR and methionine synthase 2756A→G), decrease the risk of colon and other cancers. The lower the effective dose, the lower the risk (however small) of exposure to high levels in some people. This is the basis of risk–benefit assessments such as the one performed by COMA.

Other potential health benefits of optimal folate status

The achievement of optimal folate status in the population would be beneficial in alleviating folate deficiency and suboptimal folate status arising in a variety of situations as a result of decreased folate availability, increased requirement or both. Certain drugs, alcohol and smoking are all known to compromise folate status. Poor dietary intake appears to be a contributory factor in many cases and is considered to be the most common cause of suboptimal folate status. For example, the ability of a mother to sustain the increased folate demands of pregnancy will be considerably reduced if her habitual diet is low in folate.

Apart from its role in pregnancy, the role of folate in lowering homocysteine conentrations is of greatest cur-

rent interest. An elevated level of plasma homocysteine is widely recognized as an independent risk factor for CVD. Because folate is essential for homocysteine metabolism (in its cofactor form 5-methyltetrahydrofolate it is involved in the remethylation of homocysteine to methionine), suboptimal folate status causes an elevation in plasma homocysteine, while the administration of folic acid is very effective in lowering it. Evidence suggests that approximately two-thirds of apparently healthy individuals have plasma homocysteine concentrations that can be lowered in response to folic acid. A metaanalysis of 12 randomized controlled trials of folic acid supplementation showed that folic acid can lower homocysteine by about 25%. Although folate plays the major role in preventing homocysteine accumulation, metabolically related B-vitamins (vitamin B_{12} and vitamin B_6) play additional roles, and therefore may also be protective against CVD. Other emerging roles for optimal folate status include possible protective effects against certain cancers and neuropsychiatric conditions, such as depression, dementia and Alzheimer's disease.

17.5 Perspectives on the future

The periconceptional period is a particularly vulnerable time of pregnancy. Optimal folate status has an established role in preventing NTD at this time, but will only be achieved with levels of intake of the vitamin greater than those currently provided by a typical diet as eaten in most European countries. For both practical and physiological reasons the fortification of staple foods with folic acid offers the best strategy for achieving optimal folate status in the population as a whole, for mothers who have planned their pregnancies as well as those who have not. Fortification with low-dose folic acid (which has recently been adopted on a mandatory basis in the USA) would not only be effective in the primary prevention of NTD, but also prevent folate deficiency of pregnancy in the mother, a common condition with consequences for both maternal and neonatal health. Apart from its role in pregnancy and maternal and neonatal health, the achievement of optimal folate status in the population may have other health benefits, in particular a possible protective effect against CVD. In addition, folate is attracting interest as having possible preventive roles against certain cancers and neuropsychiatric conditions. Its role in the prevention of

NTD, however, is currently the only condition in which there is a proven benefit of optimal folate status. While folate plays the major protective role, the roles of metabolically related B-vitamins are being increasingly recognized and may be particularly important in the face of a genetic predisposition to impaired folate status. The priority and challenge for public health is to achieve optimal folate status in women of reproductive age.

Further reading

Bailey LB, ed. Folate in Health and Disease. New York: Marcel Dekker, 1995.

Carmel R, Jacobsen DW, eds. Homocysteine in Health and Disease. Cambridge: Cambridge University Press, 2001.

Czeizal AF, Dudas J. Prevention of the first occurrence of neural-tube defects by periconceptional vitamin supplementation. N Engl J Med 1992; 327: 1832–1835.

Daly S, Mills JL, Molloy AM et al. Minimum effective dose of folic acid for food fortification to prevent neural-tube defects. Lancet 1997; 350: 1666–1669.

Holmes-Siedle M, Lindenbaum RH, Galliard A. Recurrence of neural tube defect in a group of at risk women: a 10 year study of Pregnavite Forte F. J Med Genet 1992; 29: 134–135.

Honein MA, Paulozzi LJ, Mathews TJ et al. Impact of folic acid fortification of the US food supply on the occurrence of neural tube defects. JAMA 2001; 285: 2981–2986.

Laurence KM, James N, Miller MH et al. Double-blind randomised controlled trial of folate treatment before conception to recurrence of neural-tube defects. BMJ 1981; 282: 1509–1511.

MRC Vitamin Study Group. Prevention of neural tube defects: results of the Medical Research Council Vitamin study. Lancet 1991; 338: 131–137.

Ray JG, Meier C, Vermeulen MJ et al. Association of neural tube defects and folic acid food fortification in Canada. Lancet 2002; 360: 2047–2048.

Schorah CJ, Smithells RW. A possible role for periconceptional multivitamin supplementation in the prevention of recurrence of neural tube defects. In: Micronutrients in Health and Disease Prevention (Bendich A, Butterworth CE, eds), pp. 263–285. New York: Marcel Dekker, 1991.

Smithells RW, Sheppard S, Schorah CJ et al. Possible prevention of neural tube defects by periconceptional vitamin supplementation. Lancet 1980; i: 339–340.

Smithells RW, Ankers C, Carver ME et al. Further experience of vitamin supplementation for prevention of neural tube defect recurrences. Lancet 1983; i: 1027–1031.

Thurnham DI, Bender DA, Scott J, Halsted CH. Water soluble vitamins. In: Human Nutrition and Dietetics; 10th edn. (Garrow JS, James WPT, Ralph A, eds). Edinburgh: Churchill Livingstone, 2000.

Wald NJ, Polani PE. Neural-tube defects and vitamins: the need for a randomized clinical trial. Br J Obs Gyn 1984; 91: 516–523.

Website

http://lpi.oregonstate.edu/infocenter/vitamins.html

18

Maternal Nutrition, Fetal Programming and Adult Chronic Disease

David JP Barker and Keith M Godfrey

Key messages

- Low birth weight is associated with increased rates of coronary heart disease and the related disorders stroke, hypertension and type 2 diabetes.
- These associations have been extensively replicated in studies in different countries and are not the result of confounding variables.
- Associations between birth size and later disease extend across the normal range of birth weight and depend on lower birth weights in relation to the duration of gestation, rather than the effects of premature birth.
- These effects may be consequences of programming, whereby a stimulus or an insult at a critical, sensitive period of early life has permanent effects on structure, physiology and metabolism.
- Programming of the fetus may result from adaptations invoked when the maternoplacental nutrient supply fails to match the fetal nutrient demand.
- Although the influences that impair fetal development and program adult cardiovascular disease are yet to be defined, there are strong pointers to the importance of maternal body composition and dietary balance during pregnancy.

18.1 Introduction

The fetal origins hypothesis proposes that alterations in fetal nutrition and endocrine status result in developmental adaptations that permanently change structure, physiology and metabolism, thereby predisposing to cardiovascular, metabolic and endocrine disease in adult life. Coronary heart disease (CHD) is now thought to be a consequence of fetal adaptations to undernutrition that are beneficial for short-term survival, even though they are detrimental to health in postreproductive life.

In fetal life the tissues and organs of the body go through critical periods of development. These may coincide with periods of rapid cell division. In common with other living creatures, humans are plastic in their early life, and are moulded by the environment. Although the growth of a fetus is influenced by its genes, studies in humans and animals suggest that it is usually limited by the environment, in particular the nutrients and oxygen it receives from the mother. There are many possible evolutionary advantages in the body remaining plastic during development, rather than having its development driven only by genetic instructions acquired at conception.

Programming describes the process whereby a stimulus or insult at a critical period of development has lasting or lifelong effects. Experimental studies in animals have documented many examples of fetal programming, with recent studies showing that alterations in maternal nutrition can have long-term effects on the offspring that are of relevance to human cardiovascular disease. These long-term effects of alterations in maternal nutrition include changes in vascular structure and function, insulin secretion, renal development, and glucose and cholesterol metabolism. For example, feeding pregnant rats a low-protein diet results in lifelong elevation of blood pressure in the offspring; rats whose mothers had been fed a diet with a low ratio of protein to energy during pregnancy also exhibited a permanently altered balance between hepatic glucose production and utilization.

Although some effects of maternal nutrition may be direct consequences of alterations in substrate availability, others are thought to be mediated by hormonal effects. Experiments in animals have shown that alterations in maternal and fetal hormonal status can have important long-term consequences. Substrate availability and hormonal milieu may alter the development of specific fetal tissues during critical periods of development, or may lead to long-lasting changes in hormone secretion or tissue hormone sensitivity. The fetal hypothalamus is implicated as a key site that can be programmed by transient changes in prenatal endocrine status.

18.2 Observations establishing the link between size at birth and later cardiovascular disease

Ecological observations

At the start of the twentieth century the incidence of CHD rose steeply in Western countries to become the most common cause of death. In many of these countries the steep rise has been followed by a fall over recent decades that cannot be accounted for by changes in adult lifestyle. The incidence of CHD is now rising in other parts of the world to which Western influences are extending, including China, India and eastern Europe.

An important clue suggesting that CHD might originate during fetal development came from studies of death rates among newborn babies in Britain during the early 1900s. The usual certified cause of death in newborn babies at that time was low birth weight (LBW). Death rates in the newborn period differed considerably between one part of the country and another, being highest in some of the northern industrial towns and the poorer rural areas in the north and west. This geographical pattern in death rates closely resembled today's large variations in death rates from CHD, variations that form one aspect of the continuing north–south divide in health in Britain. One possible conclusion suggested by this observation was that

low rates of growth before birth are in some way linked to the development of CHD in adult life. The suggestion that events in childhood influence the pathogenesis of CHD was not new. A focus on intrauterine life, however, offered a novel point of departure for research.

Cohort studies of birth weight and coronary heart disease

More direct evidence that an adverse intrauterine environment might have long-term consequences came from follow-up studies of men and women in middle and late life whose body measurements at birth had been recorded. A study of men and women born in Hertfordshire, UK, showed for the first time that those who had had low birth weights had increased death rates from CHD in adult life. Thus, among 15 726 men and women born during 1911–1930, death rates from CHD fell progressively with increasing birth weight in both men and women (Figure 18.1). A small rise in the highest birth weights in men could relate to the macrosomic infants of women with gestational diabetes. Another study, of 1586 men born in Sheffield, UK, during 1907–1925, showed that it was particularly people who were small at birth as a result of growth retardation, rather than those born prematurely, who were at increased risk of the disease.

Replication of the UK findings has led to wide acceptance that low rates of fetal growth are associated with CHD in later life. For example, confirmation of a link between LBW and adult CHD has come from studies of 1200 men in Caerphilly, South Wales, and of 70 297 nurses in the USA. The latter study found a two-fold fall in the relative risk of nonfatal CHD across the range of birth weight. Similarly, among 517 men and women in Mysore, south India, the prevalence of CHD in men and women aged 45 years or older fell from 15% in those who weighed 2.5 kg or less at birth to 4% in those who weighed 3.2 kg or more.

Body proportions at birth and cardiovascular disease

The Hertfordshire records and the Nurses and Caerphilly studies did not include measurements of body size at birth other than weight. The weight of a newborn baby without a measure of its length is as crude a summary of its physique as is the weight of a child or an adult without a measure of height. The addition of birth length allows the thin baby to be distinguished

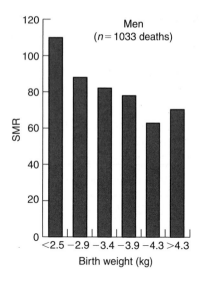 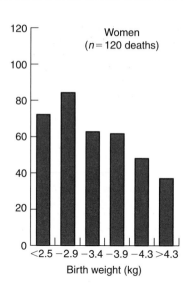

Figure 18.1 Death rates from coronary heart disease, expressed as standardized mortality ratios (SMR), in 10 141 men and 5585 women born in Hertfordshire, UK, according to birth weight. Derived from Osmond *et al.* (1993), with permission from the BMJ Publishing Group.

from the short, fat baby. With the addition of head circumference the baby whose body and trunk are small in relation to its head, as a result of brain-sparing, can also be distinguished. Thinness, shortness and a small trunk are thought to reflect differing fetal adaptations to undernutrition, hypoxia and other influences, and they have different long-term consequences.

In Sheffield, death rates for CHD were higher in men who had had a short crown–heel length at birth. The mortality ratio for CHD in men who were 47 cm or less in length was 138 compared with 98 in the remainder. Thinness at birth, as measured by a low ponderal index (birth weight/length³), was also associated with CHD. Table 18.1 shows data for a group of men born in Helsinki, Finland. While LBW was associated with raised death rates for CHD, there was a stronger association with thinness at birth, especially in men born at term. Men who had a low ponderal index had death rates that were twice those of men who had a high ponderal index.

In Finland, raised death rates from CHD were associated with low placental weight. In Sheffield, however, CHD did not vary with placental weight, but showed a U-shaped relation with the ratio of placental weight to birth weight, the highest mortality ratios being at either end of the distribution. The pattern of body proportions at birth that predicts death from CHD may be therefore summarized as a small head circumference, shortness or thinness, which reflect retarded fetal growth, and either low placental weight or an altered ratio of placental weight to birth weight. The pattern

Table 18.1 Standardized mortality ratios (SMR) for coronary heart disease in 3302 Finnish men during 1924–1933

Birth weight (kg)	SMR (no. of deaths)
≤2.5	84 (11)
2.6–3.0	83 (44)
3.1–3.5	99 (124)
3.6–4.0	76 (80)
>4.0	66 (27)
All	85 (286)
p-Value for trend	0.09

Term babies only	
Ponderal index at birth (kg/m³)	SMR (no. of deaths)
≤25.0	116 (59)
25.1–27.0	105 (88)
27.1–29.0	72 (64)
>29.0	56 (33)
All	86 (244)
p-Value for trend	<0.0001

for stroke, which has been reported in Sheffield and Helsinki, is different. Whereas stroke was similarly associated with LBW it was not associated with thinness or shortness. Instead, there were increased rates among men who had a low ratio of birth weight to head circumference. One interpretation of these associations is that normal head growth has been sustained at the cost of interrupted growth of the body in late gestation.

Table 18.2 Prevalence of type 2 diabetes (2 h glucose ≥11.1 mmol/l) and impaired glucose tolerance (2 h glucose 7.8–11.0 mmol/l) in 370 men aged 59–70 years

Birth weight (kg)	No. of men	% with 2 h plasma glucose ≥11.1 mmol/l	% with 2 h plasma glucose ≥7.8 mmol/l	OR (95% CI)[a] of type 2 diabetes or impaired glucose tolerance
<2.54	20	10	40	6.6 (1.5 to 28)
2.55–2.95	47	13	34	4.8 (1.3 to 17)
2.96–3.41	104	6	31	4.6 (1.4 to 16)
3.42–3.86	117	7	22	2.6 (0.8 to 8.9)
3.87–4.31	54	9	13	1.4 (0.3 to 5.6)
>4.31	28	0	14	1.0
All	370	7	25	

Derived from Hales *et al.* (1991) with permission from the BMJ Publishing Group.
[a] Adjusted for current body mass index.
OR: odds ratio, CI: confidence interval.

18.3 Potential confounding influences

The results of research discussed so far in this chapter suggest that influences linked to fetal and placental growth have an important effect on the risk of CHD and stroke. It has been argued, however, that people whose growth was impaired *in utero* may continue to be exposed to an adverse environment in childhood and adult life, and it is this later environment that produces the effects attributed to programming. There is strong evidence that this argument cannot be sustained. In three of the studies that have replicated the association between birth weight and CHD data on lifestyle factors, including smoking, employment, alcohol consumption and exercise, were collected. Allowance for them had little effect on the association between birth weight and CHD.

In studies exploring the mechanisms underlying these associations, the trends in CHD with birth weight were found to be paralleled by similar trends in two of its major risk factors: hypertension and type 2 (non-insulin-dependent) diabetes mellitus. Table 18.2 illustrates the size of these trends, with the prevalence of type 2 diabetes and impaired glucose tolerance falling three-fold between men who weighed 2.5 kg (5.5 lb) at birth and those who weighed 4.3 kg (9.5 lb). These associations with small size at birth were again independent of social class, cigarette smoking and alcohol consumption. Influences in adult life, however, add to the effects of the intrauterine environment. For example, the prevalence of impaired glucose tolerance is

highest in people who had low birth weight, but became obese as adults.

18.4 Findings for particular cardiovascular and metabolic disorders

Hypertension

Associations between LBW and raised blood pressure in childhood and adult life have been extensively demonstrated around the world. Figure 18.2 shows the results of a systematic review of published papers describing the association between birth weight and blood pressure; this review was based on 34 studies of more than 66 000 people of all ages in many countries. Each point on the figure with its confidence interval represents a study population and the populations are ordered by their ages. The horizontal position of each population describes the change in blood pressure that was associated with a 1 kg (2.2 lb) increase in birth weight. In almost all the studies an increase in birth weight was associated with a fall in blood pressure, and there was no exception to this in the studies of adults, which now total nearly 8000 men and women. The associations are less consistent in adolescence, presumably because the tracking of blood pressure from childhood through adult life is perturbed by the adolescent growth spurt. These associations were not confounded by socioeconomic conditions at the time of birth or in adult life. The difference in systolic pressure associated with a 1 kg difference in birth weight was around

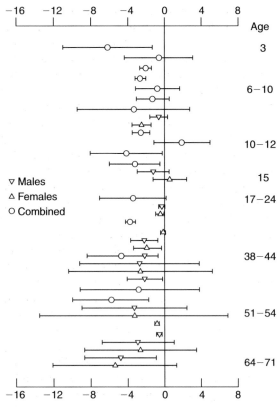

Figure 18.2 Difference in systolic pressure (mmHg), with confidence intervals, per 1 kg increase in birth weight (adjusted for weight in children and body mass index in adults) in published studies of people of different ages.

Table 18.3 Mean systolic blood pressure (mmHg) of men and women aged 50 years, born after 38 completed weeks of gestation, according to placental weight and birth weight

Birthweight (kg)	Placental weight (g)				
	≤454	455–568	569–681	>681	All
≤2.9	149 (24)	152 (46)	151 (18)	167 (6)	152 (94)
3.0–3.4	139 (16)	148 (63)	146 (35)	159 (23)	148 (137)
>3.4	131 (3)	143 (23)	148 (30)	153 (40)	149 (96)
All	144 (43)	148 (132)	148 (83)	156 (69)	149[a] (327)

Figures in parentheses are numbers of subjects.
[a] SD = 20.4.

3.5 mmHg. In clinical practice this would be a small difference, but these are large differences between the mean values of populations. Available data suggest that lowering the mean systolic pressure in a population by 10 mmHg would correspond to a 30% reduction in total attributable mortality.

The association between LBW and raised blood pressure depends on babies who were small for dates, after reduced fetal growth, rather than on babies who were born preterm. Although in these studies alcohol consumption and higher body mass were also associated with raised blood pressure, the associations between birth weight and blood pressure were independent of them. Nevertheless, body mass remains an important influence on blood pressure and, in humans and animals, the highest pressures are found in those who were small at birth, but become overweight as adults.

As has already been discussed, birth weight is a crude measure of fetal growth that does not distinguish thinness or short length, differences in head size, or variations in the balance of fetal and placental size. Analyses in Preston, UK, defined two groups of babies who developed raised blood pressures. The first group had below-average placental weight and were thin with a low ponderal index and a below-average head circumference. The second had above-average placental weight and a short crown–heel length in relation to their head circumference; such short babies tend to be fat and may have above-average birth weight. In contrast to the associations between birth size and CHD, those between birth weight and blood pressure are generally as strong as those between thinness, shortness and blood pressure. Associations between blood pressure, thinness and shortness have been found in some studies, but not in others. In a longitudinal study of young people in Adelaide, Australia, associations between blood pressure, thinness and shortness were not apparent at the age of 8 years, but emerged at the age of 20.

Placental size and blood pressure

Table 18.3 shows the systolic pressure of a group of men and women who were born, at term, in Preston, UK, in the 1950s. The subjects are grouped according to their birth weights and placental weights. Consistent with findings in other studies, systolic pressure falls between subjects with low and high birth weight. In addition, however, there is an increase in blood pressure with increasing placental weight. Subjects with a mean systolic pressure of 150 mmHg or more, a level sometimes used to define hypertension in clinical practice, comprise a group who as babies were relatively small in relation to the size of their placentas. There are similar trends with diastolic pressure. A rise in blood pressure with increasing placental weight was also found in 4-year-old children in Salisbury, UK, and among 8-year-old children in Adelaide. In studies of children and adults the association between placental enlargement and raised blood pressure has, however, been inconsistent. For example, among men and women born in Aberdeen, Scotland, after World War II, at a time when food was still rationed, raised blood pressure was associated with small placental size. As referred to later, animal studies offer a possible explanation of this inconsistency. In sheep the placenta enlarges in response to moderate undernutrition in midpregnancy. This effect, thought to be an adaptive response to extract more nutrients from the mother, is only seen in ewes that were well nourished before pregnancy.

Mother's blood pressure

In some studies the blood pressures of the mother during and after pregnancy have been recorded. They correlate with the offspring's blood pressure. However, the associations between body size and proportions at birth and later blood pressure are independent of the mother's blood pressure. Recent observations show that if the mother's blood pressure is measured throughout a 24 h period, rather than by isolated readings at antenatal clinics, there is a continuous inverse association between a woman's blood pressure and her infant's weight at birth. It could be argued, therefore, that the association between LBW and raised adult blood pressure reflects an association, possibly genetic, between a mother's ambulatory blood pressure and the blood pressure of her offspring. The demonstration that experimental undernutrition during gestation programs blood pressure in animals argues against this interpretation. One possibility is that raised blood pressure during pregnancy reflects failure of maternal cardiovascular adaptations to pregnancy; this may reduce uteroplacental blood flow and fetal nutrient supply, leading to LBW and raised blood pressure in the offspring.

Mechanisms that may underlie the programming of hypertension

There are several possible mechanisms by which restricted intrauterine growth could either initiate raised blood pressure or lead to accentuated amplification of blood pressure in later life. Studies in the USA, the UK and the Netherlands have shown that blood pressure in childhood predicts the likelihood of developing hypertension in adult life. These predictions are strongest after adolescence. In children the rise in blood pressure with age is closely related to growth and is accelerated by the adolescent growth spurt. These observations led Lever and Harrap (1992) to propose that essential hypertension is a disorder of growth. The hypothesis that hypertension is a disorder of accelerated childhood growth can be reconciled with the association with LBW by postulating that postnatal catch-up growth plays an important role in amplifying changes established in utero.

If the maternoplacental supply of nutrients does not match fetal requirements in the last trimester of pregnancy the fetus diverts blood and nutrients to maintain brain metabolism at the expense of the trunk and limbs. This adaptation acts to reduce blood flow to the fetal kidneys and may underlie the observation that the fetal renin–angiotensin system is activated during intrauterine growth retardation. While this raises the possibility that changes in the system the may underlie the programming of hypertension, a follow-up study of men and women born in Sheffield found that those who had been small at birth had lower plasma concentrations of inactive and active renin.

An alternative explanation for the low plasma renin concentrations of people who were small at birth is that they reflect a relative deficit of nephrons. Brenner (1995) has suggested that retarded fetal growth leads to reduced numbers of nephrons which, in turn, lead to increased pressure in the glomerular capillaries and the development of glomerular sclerosis. This sclerosis leads to further loss of nephrons and a self-perpetuating cycle of hypertension and progressive glomerular injury. The number of nephrons in the normal population varies widely, from 300 000 to 1 100 000 or more. Animal and human studies have shown that low rates of intrauterine growth are associated with reduced numbers of nephrons.

Animal studies have led to the hypothesis that fetal undernutrition leads to lifelong changes in the hypothalamic–pituitary–adrenal axis of the fetus which, in turn, resets homeostatic mechanisms controlling blood pressure. A study of 9-year-old children in Salisbury, UK, showed that those who had been small at birth had increased urinary adrenal androgen and glucocorticoid metabolite excretion, preliminary evidence that the hypothalamic–pituitary–adrenal axis is programmed in humans. The growth hormone– insulin-like growth factor-1 (IGF-1) axis may also be programmed *in utero*. Children who had LBW have raised plasma IGF-1 concentrations.

The content and arrangement of elastin in the aorta and large conduit arteries play an important part in minimizing the rise in blood pressure in systole and maintaining blood pressure in diastole. Elastin is only synthesized in early life and the gradual loss or fracture of elastin fibers is thought to contribute to the rise in systolic and pulse pressure with aging. These considerations have led to the hypothesis that impaired fetal development may be associated with a relative deficiency in elastin synthesis, resulting in stiffer arteries and raised blood pressure in postnatal life. This hypothesis is supported by a study of 50-year-old men and women showing that those who had a small abdominal circumference at birth tended to have a higher pulse wave velocity and decreased arterial elasticity in adult life.

Type 2 diabetes

Insulin has a central role in fetal growth, and disorders of glucose and insulin metabolism are therefore an obvious possible link between early growth and cardiovascular disease. Although obesity and a sedentary lifestyle are known to be important in the development of type 2 diabetes, they seem to lead to the disease only in predisposed individuals. Family and twin studies have suggested that the predisposition is familial, but the nature of this predisposition is unknown. The disease tends to be transmitted through the maternal rather than the paternal side of the family.

Several studies have confirmed the association between birth weight and impaired glucose tolerance and type 2 diabetes first reported in Hertfordshire, UK (Table 18.2). In the Health Professionals Study, USA, the odds ratio for diabetes, after adjusting for current body mass, was 1.9 among men whose birth weights were less than 2.5 kg (5.5 lb) compared with those who weighed 3.2–3.9 kg (7–8.5 lb). Among the Pima Indians in the USA, the odds ratio for diabetes was 3.8 in men and women who weighed less than 2.5 kg. In Preston, UK, it was the thin babies who developed impaired glucose tolerance and diabetes. Lithell and colleagues (1996) confirmed the association with thinness in Uppsala, Sweden (Table 18.4). The prevalence

Table 18.4 Prevalence of type 2 diabetes by ponderal index at birth among 60-year-old men in Uppsala, Sweden

Ponderal index at birth (kg/m^3)	No. of men	Prevalence (%) of diabetes
<24.2	193	11.9
24.2 to <25.9	193	5.2
25.9 to <27.4	196	3.6
27.4 to <29.4	188	4.3
≥29.4	201	3.5
All	971	5.7
p-Value for trend		0.001

of diabetes was three times higher (relative odds by logistic regression 4.4) among men in the lowest fifth of ponderal index at birth. This was a stronger association than that with birth weight, the prevalence of diabetes being only twice as high among men in the lowest fifth of birth weight. Among the Pima Indians diabetes in pregnancy is unusually common, and young men and women with birth weights over 4.5 kg (9.9 lb) had an increased prevalence of type 2 diabetes. The association between birth weight and type 2 diabetes was therefore U-shaped. The increased risk of diabetes among babies with high birth weights was associated with maternal diabetes in pregnancy.

Associations between LBW, or thinness or shortness at birth, and altered glucose–insulin metabolism have been found in children in Europe, India and Jamaica. These findings provide further support for the hypothesis that type 2 diabetes originates from impaired development *in utero* and suggests that the seeds of diabetes in the next generation have already been sown and are apparent in today's children.

Insulin resistance

Both insulin resistance and deficiency in insulin production are thought to be important in the pathogenesis of type 2 diabetes. There is evidence that both may be determined in fetal life. Men and women with LBW have a high prevalence of the insulin resistance syndrome, in which impaired glucose tolerance, hypertension and raised serum triglyceride concentrations occur in the same patient. Patients with the syndrome are insulin resistant and have hyperinsulinemia. Table 18.5 shows the association between birth weight and the insulin resistance syndrome for a sample of 407 men in Hertfordshire, UK. Phillips *et al.* (1994) carried out insulin tolerance tests on 103 men and women in

Table 18.5 Prevalence of the insulin resistance syndrome in men aged 59–70 years according to birth weight

Birth weight (kg)	No. of men	% with insulin resistance syndrome	OR (95% CI)[a]
≤2.50	20	30	18 (2.6 to 118)
2.51–2.95	54	19	8.4 (1.5 to 49)
2.96–3.41	114	17	8.5 (1.5 to 46)
3.42–3.86	123	12	4.9 (0.9 to 27)
3.87–4.31	64	6	2.2 (0.3 to 14)
>4.31	32	6	1.0
All	407	14	

[a] Adjusted for current body mass index.
OR: odds ratio, CI: confidence interval.

Preston, UK. At each body mass, insulin resistance was greater in people who had a low ponderal index at birth. Conversely, at each ponderal index, resistance was greater in those with high body mass. The greatest mean resistance was therefore in those with low ponderal index at birth, but high current body mass.

A study in San Antonio, Texas, USA, confirmed the association between LBW and insulin resistance in a different ethnic group. In 30-year-old Mexican Americans and non-Hispanic white people, those with lower birth weight had a higher prevalence of the insulin resistance syndrome. Among men and women in the lowest third of the birth weight distribution and the highest third of current body mass, 25% had the syndrome. By contrast, none of the people in the highest third of birth weight and lowest third of current body mass had it. A study of young adults in the city of Haguenau, France, showed that those who had had intrauterine growth retardation had raised plasma insulin concentrations when fasting and after a standard glucose challenge. They did not show any of the other abnormalities that occur in the insulin resistance syndrome. One interpretation of this is that insulin resistance is a primary abnormality to which other changes are secondary. Follow-up of men and women who were *in utero* during the Dutch famine following world war II provides direct evidence that fetal undernutrition can program insulin resistance and type 2 diabetes. Men and women exposed to famine *in utero* had higher 2 h plasma glucose concentrations than those born before or conceived after the famine. They also had higher fasting proinsulin and 2 h plasma insulin concentrations, suggesting insulin resistance.

Mechanisms that may underlie the programming of insulin resistance

The processes that link thinness at birth with insulin resistance in adult life are not known. Babies born at term with a low ponderal index have a reduced mid-arm circumference, which implies that they have a low muscle bulk as well as less subcutaneous fat. It is therefore possible that thinness at birth is associated with abnormalities in muscle structure and function which develop in midgestation and persist into adult life, interfering with insulin's ability to promote glucose uptake. Magnetic resonance spectroscopy studies show that people who were thin at birth have lower rates of glycolysis and glycolytic adenosine triphosphate (ATP) production during exercise. In response to undernutrition a fetus may reduce its metabolic dependence on glucose and increase oxidation of other substrates, including amino acids and lactate (Figure 18.3). This has led to the hypothesis that a glucose-sparing metabolism persists into adult life, and that insulin resistance arises as a consequence of similar processes, possibly because of reduced rates of glucose oxidation in insulin-sensitive peripheral tissues.

When the availability of nutrients to the fetus is restricted, concentrations of anabolic hormones, including insulin and IGF-1, fall, while catabolic hormones, including glucocorticoids, rise (Figure 18.3). Persisting hormonal changes could underlie the development of insulin resistance. Bjorntorp (1995) has postulated that glucocorticoids, growth hormone and sex steroids may play major roles in the evolution of the metabolic syndrome.

Recent advances in assay methodology make it possible to measure specifically plasma concentrations of the precursor of insulin, 32–33 split proinsulin. Higher concentrations are found in people who had LBW and low weight at 1 year. The significance of raised plasma split proinsulin concentrations remains unclear, but they are thought to indicate both insulin resistance and impaired pancreatic β-cell dysfunction.

Insulin deficiency

Infants who are small for dates have fewer β-cells. There are conflicting reports on whether the β-cell mass is reduced in patients with type 2 diabetes. As a working hypothesis it seems reasonable to propose that nutritional and other factors determining fetal and infant growth influence the size and function of the adult pancreatic β-cell complement. Whether and

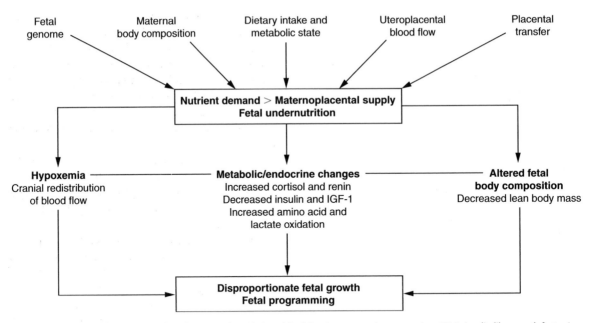

Figure 18.3 Framework for understanding the maternal regulation of fetal development and programming. IGF-1: insulin-like growth factor-1.

when type 2 diabetes supervenes will be determined by the rate of attrition of β-cells with aging, and by the development of insulin resistance, of which obesity is an important determinant.

In a sample of 103 of the men and women who took part in the Preston study, Phillips and colleagues measured insulin secretion following intravenous infusion of glucose. The insulin response was not related to birth weight or other measurements at birth. This argues against a link between reduced fetal growth and insulin deficiency in adult life. Similarly, a study of men in Stockholm, Sweden, found no association between birth weight and insulin responses to infused glucose. Birth length and other measures of birth size were not available in that study. There was, however, an association between short stature and a low insulin response. It is possible that insulin resistance in adult life changes insulin secretion and obscures associations with fetal growth. Studies of younger people may resolve this. Among men aged 21 years, Robinson *et al.* (1992) showed that those with lower birth weight had reduced plasma insulin concentrations 30 min after a glucose challenge. Another study of men of similar age showed that a low insulin response to glucose was associated with a high placental weight and a high ratio of placental weight to birth weight. This study also confirmed the association between low insulin secretion

and short stature. In contrast, among young Pima Indians those with LBW had evidence of insulin resistance, but no defect in insulin secretion.

In Mysore, south India, men and women with type 2 diabetes showed signs of both insulin resistance and insulin deficiency. The high prevalence of insulin resistance, central obesity and type 2 diabetes in people from south India living in Britain has been remarked on and was again shown in the Mysore men and women. In Mysore, those with type 2 diabetes, however, also had a low insulin increment after a standard challenge, indicating that they were insulin deficient as well as resistant. Whereas insulin resistance was associated with LBW, type 2 diabetes was associated with shortness at birth in relation to birth weight, that is a high ponderal index, and with maternal adiposity.

These findings led to a novel explanation for the epidemic of type 2 diabetes in urban and migrant Indian populations (Figure 18.4). Widespread fetal undernutrition predisposes the Indian population to insulin resistance. On moving to cities, people's levels of physical activity diminish. Young women, no longer required to do agricultural work or walk long distances to fetch water and firewood, become fatter and therefore more insulin resistant. They are therefore unable to maintain glucose homeostasis during pregnancy, even at relatively low levels of obesity, and become

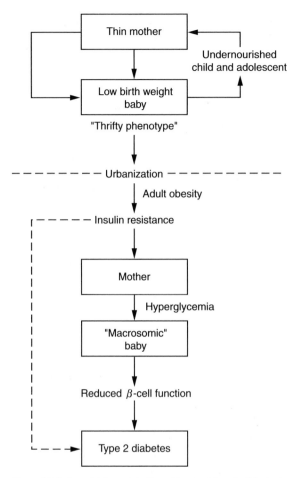

Figure 18.4 A model to explain the epidemic of type 2 diabetes in urban India.

hyperglycemic, although not necessarily diabetic. It is known that high plasma glucose concentrations within the normal range influence fetal growth and lead to macrosomia (see Section 18.6).

Serum cholesterol and blood clotting

Studies in Sheffield, UK, show that the neonate that has a short body and LBW in relation to the size of its head, although within the normal range of birth weight, has persisting disturbances of cholesterol metabolism and blood coagulation. Disproportion in body length relative to head size is thought to result from cranial redistribution of blood flow associated with hypoxemia and undernutrition in late gestation. The fetus diverts oxygenated blood away from the trunk to sustain the brain. This affects the growth of the liver, two of whose functions, regulation of cholesterol and of blood clotting, seem to be permanently perturbed. Disturbance of cholesterol metabolism and disturbance of blood clotting are important features of CHD.

The Sheffield records included abdominal circumference at birth, as well as length, and it was specifically reduction in this birth measurement, which reflects liver size, that predicted raised serum low-density lipoprotein cholesterol and plasma fibrinogen concentrations in adult life. The differences in concentrations across the range of abdominal circumference were large, statistically equivalent to 30% differences in mortality caused by CHD. The findings for plasma fibrinogen concentrations, a measure of blood coagulability, were of similar size.

Since both cholesterol and fibrinogen metabolism are regulated by the liver, one interpretation of these findings is that they reflect impaired liver growth and reprogramming of liver metabolism. Further understanding of liver programming may come more rapidly from animal than from human studies. Experiments on rats have shown that undernutrition *in utero* can permanently alter the balance of two liver enzymes, phosphoenolpyruvate carboxykinase and glucokinase, which are involved, respectively, in the synthesis and breakdown of glucose. A low-protein diet during gestation permanently changes the balance of enzyme activity in the offspring in favor of synthesis. It is thought that this reflects enhancement of cell replication in the area around the portal vein, which carries blood from the gut to the liver, at the expense of the cells around the hepatic vein. These experiments are of particular interest because they show that undernutrition after birth has no effect, and because the two enzymes are not normally synthesized until after birth, which suggests that their production can be regulated before the genes encoding them are transcribed.

18.5 Determinants of fetal growth and programming: the importance of fetal nutrition

The demonstration that normal variations in fetal size and thinness at birth have implications for health throughout life has prompted a reevaluation of the regulation of fetal development. Although the fetal genome determines growth potential *in utero*, the weight of evidence suggests that it plays a subordinate role in determining the growth that is actually achieved.

Rather, it seems that the dominant determinant of fetal growth is the nutritional and hormonal milieu in which the fetus develops, and in particular the nutrient and oxygen supply.

Evidence supporting the importance of the intrauterine environment comes from animal cross-breeding experiments and from studies of half-siblings related through either the mother or the father. For example, among half-siblings, related through only one parent, those with the same mother have similar birth weights, the correlation coefficient being 0.58; the birth weights of half-siblings with the same father are dissimilar, the correlation coefficient being only 0.1. A study of babies born after ovum donation illustrates how birth size is essentially controlled by the mother's body and the nutritional environment it affords. The birth weights of the babies were strongly related to the weight of the recipient mother, heavier mothers having larger babies. Birth weights were, however, unrelated to the weights of the women who donated the eggs. Although maternal cigarette smoking is known to also restrict fetal growth, follow-up studies have generally found that it is not related to levels of cardiovascular risk factors in the offspring in childhood.

Animal experiments have suggested that fetal undernutrition in early gestation produces small but normally proportioned offspring, whereas undernutrition in late gestation may have profound effects on body proportions but little effect on birth weight. The varying critical periods during which organs and systems mature indicate that an adverse intrauterine environment at different developmental stages is likely to have specific short- and long-term effects. A critical period for gonadal development exists, for example, very early in gestation, compared with a critical period for renal development later in gestation between 26 and 34 weeks of pregnancy. The observation that babies that were symmetrically small, short or thin at birth are predisposed to different disorders in adult life may in part reflect an adverse intrauterine environment at different developmental stages.

With respect to timing, it is important to appreciate that effects manifest late in pregnancy may originate much earlier in gestation. For example, studies of the Dutch famine of 1944–45 led to the dogma that thinness at birth results from influences operating in the last trimester of pregnancy. Outside the setting of famine, animal and human studies both indicate that fetal undernutrition late in pregnancy is, however, more commonly a consequence of an inadequate maternoplacental supply capacity set up earlier in gestation. Thus, while the short- and long-term effects of an acute severe famine are scientifically important, they could result in erroneous conclusions about timing in the nonfamine situation.

18.6 Maternal influences on fetal nutrition

Size at birth reflects the product of the trajectory of growth of the fetus, set at an early stage in development, and the maternoplacental capacity to supply sufficient nutrients to maintain that trajectory. Failure of the maternoplacental supply line to satisfy fetal nutrient requirements results in a range of fetal adaptations and developmental changes that may lead to permanent alterations in the body's structure and metabolism, and thereby to cardiovascular and metabolic disease in adult life (Figure 18.3). In Western communities, randomized controlled trials of maternal macronutrient supplementation have had relatively small effects on birth weight. These have led to the view that regulatory mechanisms in the maternal and placental systems act to ensure that human fetal growth and development are little influenced by normal variations in maternal nutrient intake, and that there is a simple relationship between a woman's body composition and the growth of her fetus. Recent experimental studies in animals and observational studies in humans challenge these concepts. These studies suggest that a mother's own fetal growth and her dietary intakes and body composition can exert major effects on the balance between the fetal demand for nutrients and the maternoplacental capacity to meet that demand.

Quite apart from any long-term effects on health in adult life, specific issues that have not been adequately addressed in previous studies of maternal nutrition include:

- effects on the trajectory of fetal growth
- transgenerational effects
- effects on placental size and transfer capabilities
- effects on fetal proportions and specific tissues
- the importance of the balance of macronutrients in the mother's diet and of her body composition.

The fetal growth trajectory

A rapid trajectory of growth increases the fetus's demand for nutrients. This reflects effects on both maintenance requirements, greater in fetuses that have achieved a larger size as a result of a faster growth trajectory, and requirements for future growth. Although the fetal demand for nutrients is greatest late in pregnancy, the magnitude of this demand is thought to be determined primarily by genetic and environmental effects on the trajectory of fetal growth set at an early stage in development. Experimental studies of pregnant ewes have shown that, although a fast growth trajectory is generally associated with larger fetal size and improved neonatal survival, it renders the fetus more vulnerable to a reduced maternoplacental supply of nutrients in late gestation. Thus, maternal undernutrition during the last trimester adversely affected the development of rapidly growing fetuses with high requirements, while having little effect on those growing more slowly. Rapidly growing fetuses were found to make a series of adaptations in order to survive, including fetal wasting and placental oxidation of fetal amino acids to maintain lactate output to the fetus.

Although the identity of the major genes determining growth potential and the fetal growth trajectory is unknown, animal studies indicate that insulin-like growth factors and their receptors may be important. While the glucose–insulin–IGF-1 axis is thought to play a central role in the nutritional regulation of fetal growth and anabolism, constitutively expressed IGF-2 has an important effect on background rates of fetal growth from early pregnancy onwards. Experiments in animals have shown that periconceptional alterations in maternal diet and plasma progesterone concentrations can alter gene expression in the preimplantation embryo to change the fetal growth trajectory. Environmental effects have been demonstrated on both embryonic growth rates and cell allocation in the preimplantation embryo. Maternal progesterone treatment can, for example, permanently alter the trajectory of fetal growth by changing the allocation of cells between the inner cell mass that develops into the fetus and the outer trophectoderm that becomes the placenta. The trajectory of fetal growth is thought to increase with improvements in periconceptional nutrition, and is faster in male fetuses. One possibility is that the greater vulnerability of such fetuses on a fast growth trajectory could contribute to the rise in

CHD with Westernization and the higher death rates in men.

Transgenerational effects

Experimental studies in animals have shown that undernutrition over many generations can have cumulative effects on reproductive performance over several generations. Thus, feeding rats a protein-deficient diet over 10–12 generations resulted in progressively greater fetal growth retardation over the generations; following refeeding with a normal diet it then took three generations to normalize growth and development.

Strong evidence for major intergenerational effects in humans has come from studies showing that a woman's birth weight influences the birth weight of her offspring. Moreover, whereas LBW mothers tend to have thin infants with a low ponderal index, the father's birth weight is unrelated to ponderal index at birth (Figure 18.5); crown–heel length at birth is, however, more strongly related to the father's birth weight than to the mother's. The effect of maternal birth weight on thinness at birth is consistent with the hypothesis that the maternoplacental supply line may be unable to satisfy fetal nutrient demand in LBW mothers. Potential mechanisms underlying this effect include alterations in the uterine or systemic vasculature, programmed changes in maternal metabolic status and impaired placentation. The strong effect of paternal birth weight on crown–heel length may reflect paternal imprinting of genes important for skeletal growth, such as those regulating the concentrations of insulin-like growth factors.

Placental size and transfer capabilities

Although the size of the placenta gives only an indirect measure of its capacity to transfer nutrients to the fetus, it is nonetheless strongly associated with fetal size at birth. Experiments in sheep have shown that maternal nutrition in early pregnancy can exert major effects on the growth of the placenta, and thereby alter fetal development. The effects produced depended on the nutritional status of the ewe in the periconceptional period. In ewes poorly nourished around the time of conception, high nutrient intakes in early pregnancy increased the size of the placenta. Conversely, in ewes well nourished around conception, high intakes in early pregnancy resulted in smaller placental size.

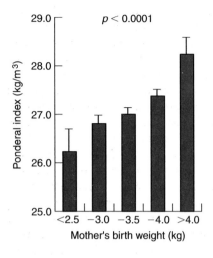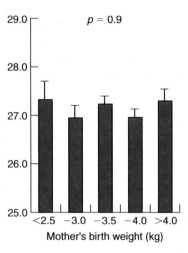

Figure 18.5 Ponderal index at birth in 492 term Southampton pregnancies according to the mother's and father's birth weights. Values are means (±SE) adjusted for gender and gestation. Data reproduced from Godfrey *et al.* (1997) with permission of Royal College of Obstetrics and Gynaecology.

Although this suppression appears paradoxical, in sheep farming it is common practice for ewes to be put on rich pasture before mating and then on poor pasture for a period in early pregnancy.

As part of a study designed to evaluate whether the normal variations in maternal diet found in Western communities could influence fetal growth and development, evidence was found of a similar suppressive effect of high dietary intakes in early pregnancy on placental growth. Thus, among 538 women who delivered at term, those with high dietary intakes in early pregnancy, especially of carbohydrate, had smaller placentas, particularly if combined with low intakes of dairy protein in late pregnancy (Table 18.6). These effects were independent of the mother's body size, social class and smoking, and resulted in alterations in the ratio of placental weight to birth weight (placental ratio). Confirmation that maternal diet can alter placental growth has come from analyses of the Dutch famine, where famine exposure in early pregnancy increased placental weight.

The U-shaped relation between the placental ratio and later CHD found in men born in the early twentieth century in Sheffield, UK, suggests that effects on placental growth could be of long-term importance. While babies with a disproportionately small placenta may suffer as a consequence of an impaired placental nutrient supply capacity, those with a disproportionately large placenta may experience fetal catabolism and wasting to supply amino acids for placental consumption. Consequent fetal adaptations may underlie the increased adult CHD death rates in those with both low and high placental ratios.

Table 18.6 Mean placental weight in 538 women delivered at term in Southampton, UK

Dairy protein intake in late pregnancy (g/day)	Carbohydrate intake in early pregnancy (g/day)			
	≤265	266–340	>340	All
≤18.5	539	507	494	516
18.6–26.5	556	546	509	540
>26.5	582	533	536	544
All	554	531	517	534[a]

Derived from Godfrey *et al.* (1996) with permission from the BMJ Publishing Group.
[a] Overall SD = 121 g.
Values are adjusted for gender and the duration of gestation at delivery.
p-Values for associations with placental weight: carbohydrate $p = 0.002$, dairy protein $p = 0.005$.

Effects on fetal proportions and specific tissues

Experimental studies in animals have shown that dietary manipulations during early development can have tissue-specific effects, resulting in alterations in an animal's proportions. For example, in pigs fed differing diets in the first year of life those fed a protein-deficient diet had a disproportionately large head, ears and genitalia compared with those fed an energy-deficient diet. Recent experiments in guinea-pigs have shown that maternal undernutrition in pregnancy resulted in offspring that not only had altered body proportions at birth, but also showed profound elevation of serum cholesterol concentrations when fed a high-cholesterol diet in the postweaning period.

In humans, few studies have examined the possibility of maternal nutrition during pregnancy having tissue-specific effects on the fetus, leading to greater alterations in neonatal proportions than in birth weight. Any such effects may be of importance as adult CHD and type 2 diabetes are more strongly associated with altered birth proportions than with birth weight. One study found that women with low dairy protein intakes in late pregnancy tended to have babies that were thinner at birth; maternal dairy protein intakes were not, however, related to birth weight. Furthermore, a recent follow-up study of children whose mothers took part in a randomized controlled trial of calcium supplementation in pregnancy found that while maternal supplementation was associated with lowering of the offspring's blood pressure in childhood, this effect was not associated with any change in birth weight.

Maternal dietary balance and body composition

Indications that the balance of macronutrients in the mother's diet can have important short- and long-term effects on the offspring has come from experimental studies in pregnant rats. These found that maternal diets with a low ratio of protein to carbohydrate and fat alter fetal and placental growth, and result in lifelong elevation of blood pressure in the offspring. Follow-up studies of men and women born during and after the Dutch famine found that while severe maternal caloric restriction was not associated with raised blood pressure in the offspring, there was evidence for an effect of macronutrient balance; maternal rations with a low protein density were associated with raised blood pressure in the adult offspring. This adds to studies from Aberdeen, UK, which found that maternal diets with either a low or a high ratio of animal protein to carbohydrate were associated with raised blood pressure in the offspring during adult life. Maternal diets with a high protein density were also associated with insulin deficiency and impaired glucose tolerance in the offspring.

While adverse effects of diets with a high protein density might appear counterintuitive, they are consistent with a review of 16 trials of protein supplementation showing that supplements with a high protein density were consistently associated with lower birth weight. Moreover, the Aberdeen findings have recently been replicated in a follow-up study of men and women in Motherwell, UK, whose mothers were advised to eat a high-meat-protein, low-carbohydrate diet during pregnancy. The blood pressure was higher in offspring whose mothers reported greater intakes of meat and fish and lower intakes of carbohydrate in late pregnancy, particularly if the mother also had a low intake of green vegetables. One possibility is that the long-term effects may be consequences of the metabolic stress imposed on the mother by an unbalanced diet in which high intakes of essential amino acids are not accompanied by the other micronutrients required to utilize them.

With respect to maternal body composition, observations linking high maternal weight and adiposity with insulin deficiency, type 2 diabetes and CHD in the offspring add to those of associations between gestational diabetes and adverse long-term outcomes. Follow-up of men in Finland born in the early twentieth century showed markedly raised CHD death rates in those whose mothers had a high body mass index in pregnancy. This effect was independent of an association between thinness at birth and increased rates of adult CHD. Modeling the data to derive contour lines of similar CHD death rates indicated that increasing maternal body mass index had little effect on the offspring's death rates in tall women, but strong effects in short women.

At the other extreme of maternal body fatness, of great importance is an increasing body of consistent evidence showing strong links between low weight and body mass index in the mother and insulin resistance and dyslipidemia in the adult offspring. In the Dutch famine studies the offspring of mothers who had low body weight had the highest plasma glucose concentrations and the greatest insulin resistance. Further evidence of an association between low maternal body mass and insulin resistance in the offspring comes from studies in Scotland and China. Preliminary studies in India found that a low maternal weight in pregnancy is associated with an increased risk of CHD in the offspring in adult life. While maternal weight and body mass index are not related to raised blood pressure in the offspring, consistent associations have been found with thin maternal skinfold thicknesses and low pregnancy weight gain. For example, in studies of Jamaican children, strong associations were found between low pregnancy weight gain and thinner maternal triceps skinfold thickness in early pregnancy and raised blood pressure in the offspring, but no significant associations with maternal body mass index.

18.7 Perspectives on the future

The links between normal variations in size at birth and health throughout life have prompted a reevaluation of the regulation of fetal development. Impetus has been added to this reevaluation by recent findings showing that a woman's diet and body composition in pregnancy are related to levels of cardiovascular risk factors and the prevalence of CHD in her offspring in adult life. These observations challenge the view that the fetus is little affected by changes in maternal nutrition, except in circumstances of famine.

The long timescale over which the effects of an adverse intrauterine environment act dictate that there is a need to progress beyond epidemiological associations to greater understanding of the cellular and molecular processes that underlie them. The complexities of fetal growth and development are such that currently available data form only a limited basis for changing dietary recommendations to pregnant women. Future work will need to identify the factors that set the trajectory of fetal growth, and the influences that limit the maternoplacental delivery of nutrients and oxygen to the fetus. There is also a need to define how the fetus adapts to a limited nutrient supply, how these adaptations program the structure and physiology of the body, and by what molecular mechanisms nutrients and hormones alter gene expression.

If a woman's own fetal growth, and her diet and body composition before and during pregnancy play a major role in programming the future health of her children, mothers will want to know what they can do to optimize the intrauterine environment that they provide for their babies. A recent technical consultation organized by the United States Department of Agriculture, the World Bank and the United Nations Children's Fund (UNICEF) concluded that a key area of focus to reduce the burden of low birth weight and its associated morbidities is to improve the nutritional status of adolescent girls and young women. Similarly, one of the two main recommendations of the Acheson Report on Inequalities in Health in the United Kingdom was that **"a high priority is given to policies aimed at improving health and reducing inequalities in women of childbearing age, expectant mothers and young children"**. A strategy of interdependent clinical, animal and epidemiological research is required to identify specific recommendations for both whole populations and vulnerable groups such as pregnant teenagers and single parents. Research is also required to identify the barriers to healthy eating among young women, whose diets are important both for their own health and for the health of the next generation. Such an approach may allow reductions in the prevalence of major chronic diseases and social inequalities in health.

Further reading

Barker DJP. Mothers, Babies and Health in Later Life, 2nd edn. Edinburgh: Churchill Livingstone, 1998.

Barker DJP, ed. Fetal Origins of Cardiovascular and Lung Disease. National Institutes of Health Monograph Series 151. New York: Marcel Dekker, 2001.

Bateson P, Martin P. Design for a Life: How Behaviour Develops. London: Jonathan Cape, 1999.

Bjorntorp P. Insulin resistance: the consequence of a neuroendocrine disturbance? Int J Obesity 1995; 19 (suppl): S6–S10.

Godfrey K, Robinson S, Barker DJP et al. Maternal nutrition in early and late pregnancy in relation to placental and fetal growth. BMJ 1996; 312: 410–414.

Godfrey KM, Barker DJP, Robinson S, Osmond C. Maternal birth-weight and diet in pregnancy in relation to the infant's thinness at birth. Br J Obstet Gynaecol 1997; 104: 663–667.

Hales CN, Barker DJP, Clark PMS, Cox LJ, Fall C, Osmond C, Winter PD. Fetal and infant growth and impaired glucose tolerance at age 64. BMJ 1991; 303: 1019–22.

Lever AF, Harrap SB. Essential hypertension: a disorder of growth with origins in childhood? J Hypertens 1992; 10: 101–20.

Lithell HO, McKeigue PM, Breglund L, Mohsen R, Lithell UB, Leon DA. Relation of size at birth to non-insulin dependent diabetes and insulin concentrations in men aged 50–60 years. BMJ 1996; 312: 406–10.

Lucas A, Bock GR, Whelen J, eds. The Childhood Environment and Adult Disease. Chichester: Wiley, 1991.

Mackenzie HS, Brenner BM. Fewer nephrons at birth: a missing link in the etiology of essential hypertension? Am J Kidney Dis 1995; 26(1): 91–8.

O'Brien PMS, Wheeler T, Barker DJP, eds. Fetal Programming – Influences on Development and Disease in Later Life. London: RCOG Press, 1999.

Osmond C, Barker DJP, Winter PD et al. Early growth and death from cardiovascular disease in women. BMJ 1993; 307: 1519–1524.

Phillips DIW, Hirst S, Clark PMS, Hales CN, Osmond C. Fetal growth and insulin secretion in adult life. Diabetologia 1994; 37: 592–6.

Robinson S, Walton RJ, Clark PM, Barker DJP, Hales CN, Osmond C. The relation of fetal growth to plasma glucose in young men. Diabetologia 1992; 35: 444–6.

Websites

http://www.mrc.soton.ac.uk/
http://www.sneha-india.org/
http://www.som.soton.ac.uk/research/foad/centre/

19

Cardiovascular Disease

Jim Mann

Key messages

- In most industrialized countries coronary heart disease (CHD) is the most common single cause of death and a major cause of admission to hospital.
- A variety of cells and lipids is involved in the pathogenesis of CHD and nutrition can influence the development of CHD by modifying one or more of these factors.
- Standard epidemiological approaches have been used to identify risk factors and their nutritional determinants.
- Attempts to explain the processes underlying CHD and to identify individuals at risk confirm that there is no single cause of the disease. It seems most likely that many potentially reversible risk factors for the development of CHD interact with each other as well as the irreversible, psychosocial and geographically related risk factors in the etiology of CHD.
- The hope of population-based public health nutrition strategies is to reduce morbidity and mortality from CHD in those who are in the prime of life.

19.1 Introduction

Cardiovascular disease is usually assumed to include coronary heart disease (CHD) [also referred to as coronary artery disease (CAD) or ischemic heart disease (IHD)], cerebrovascular disease and peripheral arterial disease. Inappropriate nutrition has most consistently been associated with CHD and this chapter therefore deals principally with the diet–CHD link. The association between diet and cerebrovascular disease will be considered briefly. Few data are available concerning the role of diet and peripheral arterial disease.

The basic pathological lesion underlying CHD is the atheromatous plaque which bulges on the inside of one or more of the coronary arteries that supply blood to the heart muscle (myocardium). In addition, a superimposed thrombus or clot may further occlude the artery. A variety of cells and lipids is involved in the pathogenesis of the atherosclerotic plaque and the arterial thrombus, including lipoproteins, cholesterol, triglycerides, platelets, monocytes, endothelial cells, fibroblasts and smooth-muscle cells. Nutrition can influence the development of CHD by modifying one or more of these factors. Two major clinical conditions are associated with these processes.

Angina pectoris is characterized by pain or discomfort in the chest that is brought on by exertion or stress, and which may radiate down the left arm and to the neck. It results from a reduction or temporary block to the blood flow through the coronary artery to the heart muscle. The pain usually passes with rest and seldom lasts for more than 15 min.

Coronary thrombosis, or myocardial infarction, results from prolonged total occlusion of the artery, which causes infarction or death of some of the heart muscle cells and is associated with prolonged, and usually excruciating, central chest pain. The terms coronary thrombosis and myocardial infarction are used to describe the same clinical condition, although they really describe pathological processes.

Standard epidemiological approaches including an examination of trends in rates over time, geographical

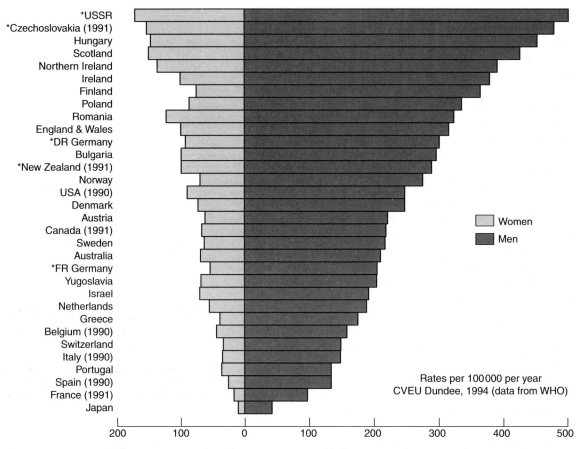

Figure 19.1 International differences in coronary heart disease rates. League table for 1992: mortality in men and women aged 40–69 years (Cardiovascular Epidemiology Unit, University of Dundee). *Former states. Reproduced with permission from Tunstall-Pedoe *et al.* (1999).

variation, migrant studies, case–control and prospective studies, and clinical trials have been used to identify risk factors and their nutritional determinants. Such studies also provide the basis of recommendations that aim to reduce the risk of developing CHD in populations where rates are high or increasing. A population-based approach is essential since, in more than half of all fatal myocardial infarctions, death occurs in the first hour after the attack. Most CHD deaths, therefore, occur too rapidly for treatment to influence the prognosis.

In most industrialized countries CHD is the most common single cause of death and a major cause of admission to hospital. However, mortality and hospital statistics appreciably underestimate the total morbidity resulting from CHD. Some cases of myocardial infarction, especially in older people, are not admitted to hospital and there are no statistics regarding the far

greater number of people who are debilitated by angina pectoris even though they may not have suffered an acute myocardial infarction.

19.2 Epidemiology

There are marked international differences in the rate of occurrence of CHD. The lower rates in communities following their traditional lifestyle than in more affluent industrialized countries has long been recognised. However, Figure 19.1 shows that even among industrialized countries, mortality rates also vary considerably. Some of the variation between countries is undoubtedly due to differences in diagnostic practice and coding of death certificates, but numerous studies using comparable methods have confirmed that real differences exist in the frequency of the disease. In Europe there is an approximately four-fold difference between France, Spain and Portugal on the one hand, and such countries as Finland, Scotland and Northern Ireland on the other, but now, eastern European countries such as Hungary, former Czechoslovakia and the former USSR are in the worst position.

These international comparisons have played an important part in the search for causes. The experience of migrants suggests that these variations between countries are likely to be the result chiefly of environmental and behavioral differences. People who have migrated from a low-risk country (e.g. Japan) to a high-risk country (e.g. the USA) tend to have rates of CHD approaching those of the host country. There is also some evidence for the reverse: Finns living in Sweden have appreciably lower rates than those in their country of origin. In the UK, where CHD rates are appreciably higher in Scotland and Northern Ireland than in England, CHD risk depends on country of residence at the time of death rather than country of birth.

There have been major changes in the CHD rates of many countries. Among men these include the increase in many European countries, Australia and New Zealand during the period 1952–1967, and the continuing increase in eastern Europe during the later period of 1970–1985, whereas in nearly all Western European countries, North American and Oceania rates have shown an appreciable decline. Figure 19.2 shows the dramatic reduction in Finland, the country that had the highest CHD mortality rates in the world in the 1960s. In most countries except for eastern Europe, the rates in women have been declining. In general, the decline has been most marked in countries where the attempt to reduce cardiovascular risk factors has been most effective. These changes over a relatively short period encourage the belief that the disease is preventable if the causes can be found and modified. They certainly argue strongly against the suggestion that the powerful genetic factors involved in CHD are likely to negate the beneficial effect of environmental change. The hope is to reduce morbidity and mortality from CHD in those who are in the prime of life.

19.3 Correlations between coronary heart disease rates and food intake

Most of the early attempts to study dietary determinants of CHD rates were based on food or nutrient

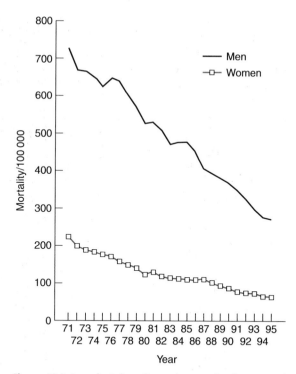

Figure 19.2 Age-adjusted cardiovascular mortality in men and women in Finland from 1972 to 1995. Source: Statistics Finland. Reproduced with permission from Pietinen *et al.* (2001). © Springer Publishing Company, Inc.

data derived from national food consumption data, the balance sheets of the Food and Agriculture Organization or, in the UK, more reliably, on household food surveys and on the national mortality statistics before 1970, during which time CHD was increasing (at least in men) in most affluent societies. The studies have either been cross-cultural comparisons at a single point in time, or an examination of increasing trends in relation to changing food consumption data in one or more countries. Positive associations with saturated fat, sucrose, animal protein and coffee, and negative correlations with flour (and other foods rich in polysaccharides) and vegetables are some of the best described. However, population food consumption data are notoriously unreliable (they are usually derived from local production figures, imports and exports, often with an incomplete account of quantities not utilized as food), and the accuracy with which mortality is recorded varies from country to country. Consequently, such data do not provide direct evidence concerning etiology, only clues for further research.

Other studies from the USA, the UK, Australia, New Zealand, Finland and Iceland have examined the downward trend of CHD rates in relation to dietary change. There are certainly associations between falling CHD rates apparent in these countries and changes in some foods and nutrients, but in view of the strong correlations (positive and negative) among different dietary constituents it is difficult to be sure which dietary factor is principally involved, or indeed whether dietary change is simply occurring in parallel with some other more important environmental factor, for example, increasing physical activity and reduction in cigarette smoking. The most recent estimate regarding the potential for lifestyle and diet modification to reduce CHD risk in the USA suggests that 82% [95% confidence interval (CI) 58 to 93%] of coronary events could be prevented by adhering to guidelines involving diet, exercise, body weight and abstinence from smoking.

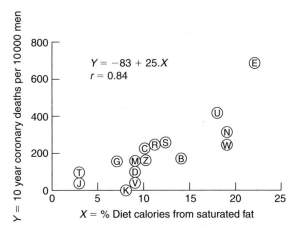

Figure 19.3 Data from the original Seven Country Study showing the association between coronary heart disease and dietary saturated fat content. B: Belgrade; C: Crevalcore; D: Dalmatia; E: East Finland; G: Corfu; J: Ushibuka, K: Crete; M: Montegiorgio; N: Zutphen; R: Rome; S: Slavonia; T: Tanushimaru; U: USA; V: Velika Krsna; W: West Finland; Z: Zrenjanin.

19.4 Prospective observation of subjects for whom diet histories are available

Measured food consumption by people in 16 defined cohorts in seven countries, and 10 year incidence rates of CHD deaths, form the basis for the correlations tested by Keys and coworkers in the classic Seven Country Study. The strongest correlation was noted between CHD and the percentage of energy derived from saturated fat (Figure 19.3). Weaker inverse associations were found between percentages of energy derived from monounsaturated and polyunsaturated fat and CHD. Total fat was not significantly correlated with CHD death. Of the other well-known risk factors for CHD investigated in this study, only cholesterol and blood pressure appeared to explain the geographical variation, leading to the suggestion that it is principally the nutrition-related factors that determine whether countries are likely to have high CHD rates. This study also provides evidence that the degree of risk conferred by factors not specifically related to nutrition is strongly influenced by nutrition-related factors. This is well illustrated by the more powerful relationship between cigarette smoking and CHD in the USA and northern Europe than in southern Europe. Saturated fat intake and mean cholesterol levels are higher in the USA and northern Europe than in southern Europe (Figure 19.4).

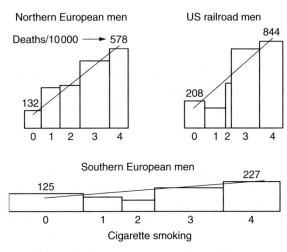

Figure 19.4 Different risks of smoking for coronary heart disease (CHD) in countries with different diets. The width of the bars is proportional to the number of men in each smoking class. Scales are the same for all three populations. The numbers above each bar indicate the number of CHD deaths per 10 000. The regression lines of death rate on smoking are shown. 0: never smoked; 1: exsmoker; 2: 2–10 cigarettes/day; 3: 10–19 cigarettes/day; 4: >20 cigarettes/day.

Several longitudinal studies have related reported intake of foods or nutrients to subsequent cardiovascular disease risk. Such studies have several potential methodological flaws, most notably the insensitivity of the instruments for measuring dietary intake in epidemiological studies and the inability of a single

Table 19.1 Associations between dietary factors and coronary heart disease: findings from the Nurses Health Study and Health Professionals Study

Food or nutrient	Protective/deleterious effect
Saturated fat (SFA)	5% en SFA vs 5% en CHO, RR = 1.17 (95% CI 0.97 to 1.41)
trans fat (TFA)	2% en TFA vs 2% en CHO, RR = 1.93 (95% CI 1.43 to 2.61)
Monounsaturated fat (MUFA)	5% en MUFA vs 5% en CHO, RR = 0.81 (95% CI 0.65 to 1.00)
Polyunsaturated fat (PUFA)	5% en PUFA vs 5% en CHO, RR = 0.62 (95% CI 0.46 to 0.85)
α-Linolenic acid (ALA)	Highest vs lowest quintile of intake, RR = 0.52 (95% CI 0.30 to 0.90)
Fish n-3 fatty acids	Weekly compared with less than weekly fish intake for sudden death, RR = 0.48 (95% CI 0.24 to 0.96)
Nuts	Eaten more than five times per week vs with rare consumption, RR = 0.65 (95% CI 0.47 to 0.89)
Whole grains	Highest vs lowest quintile of intake, RR = 0.75 (p for trend = 0.01)
Dietary fiber	Each 10 g increase in total fiber, RR = 0.81 (95% CI 0.66 to 0.99)
Carbohydrate	Highest vs lowest quintile glycemic load[a], RR = 1.98 (95% CI 1.41 to 2.77)
Antioxidants and folate	High intakes of vitamin E and folate strongly protective. Less consistent associations with other antioxidants
Protein	Highest vs lowest quintile, RR = 0.74 (95% CI 0.59 to 0.94)

[a]Glycemic load provides an indication of both amount of carbohydrate and glycemic index, i.e. the extent of blood glucose elevation produced by the carbohydrates consumed.
SFA: saturated fatty acids; TFA: *trans* unsaturated fatty acids; MUFA: monounsaturated fatty acids; PUFA: polyunsaturated fatty acids; en: total energy; CHO: carbohydrate; RR: relative risk; CI: confidence interval.

assessment to provide a representative indication of usual dietary practice. Despite these, and other causes of imprecision, a range of biologically plausible associations has been identified. Most consistent among the protective foods and nutrients are fish, whole-grain products, fruit and vegetables, nuts, garlic and moderate amounts of red wine, antioxidant nutrients (vitamins E and C, β-carotene and flavonoids), folic acid, nonstarch polysaccharides (dietary fiber) and several long-chain fatty acids (C18:2 n-6, C18:3 n-3, C20:5 n-3). In contrast, saturated fatty acids (SFA), *trans*-unsaturated fatty acids, dietary cholesterol and foods rich in these nutrients, as well as coffee, all appear to be associated with enhanced risk. While the data are not entirely consistent (e.g. in some studies the protective effect of antioxidant nutrients appears to be largely mediated via high dietary intakes, in others as a result of high intakes of supplements), the effects appear to be relatively strong. Table 19.1 summarizes the associations between dietary factors and CHD demonstrated in the Health Professionals, and Nurses, Studies carried out by the Harvard group.

In addition to these individual foods and nutrients, certain dietary patterns appear to be associated with a low CHD risk. Vegetarians appear at lower risk of CHD than meat eaters, but it has not been clearly established which attributes of the vegetarian diet might be protective, since there are many aspects other than the absence of meat which characterize these diets. Moreover, vegetarians often adopt many other lifestyle attributes that may confound comparisons with omnivores. The "prudent pattern" (high intakes of vegetables, fruit, legumes, whole grains, fish and poultry) when consumed within the context of a Western diet also appears to be protective. There has also been much publicity surrounding the relatively low CHD rates associated with traditional regional and national dietary patterns (e.g. the Mediterranean diet and the Japanese diet).

There has been considerable debate concerning which of the promoting or protective factors has the most powerful effects. However, even the most sophisticated statistical analyses cannot disentangle separate effects with certainty, and it is necessary to consider the results of longitudinal studies in conjunction with other epidemiological and experimental approaches. In particular, much helpful information has come from the study of nutritional determinants of cardiovascular risk factors.

19.5 Cardiovascular risk factors and their nutritional determinants

Attempts to explain the pathological processes underlying CHD and to identify individuals at risk confirm that there is no single cause of the disease. A wide range of potentially reversible biological characteristics has been identified as risk factors for the subsequent development of CHD in epidemiological and experimental studies. It seems most likely that these interact with each other as well as the irreversible, psychosocial and geographically related risk factors in the etiology of CHD. Some of the most important are summarized in Table 19.2. The important nutritional factors that may favorably influence risk factor level are summarized in Table 19.3. Some of the key points to note in respect of diet- and lipid-related CHD risk factors are as follows.

Low-density lipoproteins (LDL) are an atherogenic group of lipoproteins. LDL can be classified further according to density, with small dense LDL particles being the most atherogenic. However, the subfractions are not routinely measured. Rather, LDL is usually measured in terms of LDL-cholesterol, cholesterol being its main lipid fraction. Plasma levels can be lowered by reducing SFA and increasing polyunsaturated fatty acids (PUFA). LDL-cholesterol levels are increased by dietary SFA and *trans* fatty acids.

High-density lipoprotein (HDL)-cholesterol is protective against CHD and higher HDL levels are found in women, physically active people and the nonobese. HDL plays a key role in the reverse cholesterol transport pathway, which is the only route for the removal of cholesterol from the body through conversion to bile acids for intestinal secretion. HDL-cholesterol levels may be minimized by replacing some of the SFA with

Table 19.2   Risk factors for coronary heart disease

Irreversible	Masculine gender
	Increasing age
	Genetic traits, including monogenic and polygenic disorders of lipid metabolism
	Body build
Potentially reversible	Cigarette smoking
	Dyslipidemia: increased levels of cholesterol, triglyceride, low-density and very low-density lipoprotein and low levels of high-density lipoprotein
	Oxidizability of low-density lipoprotein
	Obesity, especially when centrally distributed
	Hypertension
	Physical inactivity
	Hyperglycemia and diabetes
	Increased thrombosis: increased hemostatic factors and enhanced platelet aggregation
	High levels of homocysteine
Psychosocial	Low socioeconomic class
	Stressful situations
	Coronary-prone behavior patterns: type A behavior
Geographical	Climate and season: cold weather
	Soft drinking water

Table 19.3   Nutritional manipulations that may favorably modify important cardiovascular risk factors

Risk factor	Nutritional determinants that may favorably modify risk factor
Increased LDL	↓ saturated fatty acids and *trans* unsaturated fatty acids, ↑ polyunsaturated fatty acids, ↑ soluble forms of nonstarch polysaccharide
Increased VLDL	↓ obesity, ↓ high glycemic index carbohydrate
Decreased HDL	↑ plant monounsaturated fatty acids, ↓ *trans* unsaturated fatty acids
Oxidized LDL	↑ intake of antioxidant nutrients
Hypertension	↑ fruit, vegetables and low-fat dairy products, ↓ sodium
Hyperglycemia/diabetes	↓ obesity, ↓ saturated fatty acids, use of carbohydrate foods with low glycemic index
Enhanced platelet aggregation	↑ fish sources of n-3 fatty acids
Increased hemostatic factors, especially factor VII	↓ fat intake
High homocysteine	↑ dietary folate, vitamins B_{12} and riboflavin, or folic acid supplements or fortification
Obesity	↓ energy-dense foods, rich in fat and sugars, ↑ whole grains, vegetables and fruit

LDL: low-density lipoproteins; VLDL: very low-density lipoproteins; HDL: high-density lipoproteins.

monounsaturated fatty acids (MUFA) rather than total replacement with carbohydrate. HDL exists in two sub-fractions, HDL_2 and HLD_3, and it is the former which exerts a protective effect with regard to CHD reduction. In general, changes made to dietary fat composition lead to changes in LDL rather than HDL, with the exception that *trans* fatty acids tend to lower HDL.

Triglycerides or triacylglycerols are the main vehicle for the transport of fatty acids absorbed from the gut or secreted from the liver. Whereas in the past, plasma triacylglycerol was largely ignored, current evidence suggests an independent positive contribution of plasma triacylglycerol to CHD risk. Plasma triacylglycerol is strongly linked with plasma HDL, and as the former increases the latter decreases. Thus, high-carbohydrate diets may also be associated with increased plasma triacylglycerol. However, the effect may be transient and reduce with time. Physical activity has the opposite effect. The main dietary effects on fasting plasma triacylglycerol levels are weight loss in the overweight and obese and n-3 PUFA (eicosapentaenoic and docosahexaenoic acids). An intake of about 1.0 g/day of these n-3 PUFA is sufficient to lower plasma triacylglycerol levels.

While much attention has been devoted to the effect of diet on lipoproteins, especially LDL, and the potential of reducing LDL and CHD risk by reducing saturated fatty acids, there are many CHD risk factors that may be favorably influenced by dietary manipulations. These include lowering homocysteine levels by foods rich in natural folates or fortified with folic acid, reducing oxidation of LDL by increasing intake of foods rich in antioxidants, reducing the risk of thrombogenesis by increasing very long-chain PUFA, either by increasing intake of oily fish or by supplements, decreasing blood pressure by reducing sodium intake, and increasing intake of fruit, vegetables and low-fat dairy products.

19.6 Clinical trials of cardiovascular risk reduction by dietary modification

There are irrefutable data concerning the ability of dietary modification to influence favorably risk factors for CHD and considerable epidemiological evidence to suggest that dietary change will reduce CHD risk. However, the most direct evidence for the benefits of dietary change should come from clinical trials that include a sufficient number of subjects to be able to examine whether a particular change is able to reduce morbidity and mortality from CHD, and by doing so influence total mortality.

The early studies were single-factor intervention trials where an attempt was made to modify only one risk factor – cholesterol – and the dietary manipulation was principally that of increasing the ratio of PUFA to SFA (P/S ratio). More recent studies have adopted a multifactorial approach. In these, various dietary changes were made to achieve maximum cholesterol lowering and also to influence favorably risk factors other than cholesterol. In addition, there has sometimes been an attempt to modify risk factors that are not diet related (e.g. cigarette smoking). Some of the confusion in interpreting these clinical trials has resulted from the fact that none was specifically designed to examine the effect of diet on total mortality. The trials have been reviewed in detail elsewhere (Brunner *et al.*, 1997; Holme, 1990; Hooper *et al.*, 2001). This review will describe only a few trials most relevant to current dietary recommendations and give a brief overview of the remaining primary (i.e. those carried out on people who have no evidence of preexisting CHD) and secondary trials (i.e. those carried out on people with preexisting CHD).

Los Angeles Veterans Administration Study

This was the first of the major intervention studies, in which 846 male volunteers (aged 55–89 years) were randomly allocated to experimental and control diets taken in different dining rooms. The control diet was intended to be typical of the North American diet (40% energy from fat, mostly saturated). The experimental diet contained half as much cholesterol, and predominantly polyunsaturated vegetable oils (n-6 PUFA) replaced approximately two-thirds of the animal fat, achieving a P/S ratio of 2. As a result of skilled food technology, the study was conducted under double-blind conditions.

During the 8 years of follow-up, cholesterol in the experimental group was 13% lower, and coronary events as well as deaths due solely to atherosclerotic events were appreciably reduced, compared with the controls (Table 19.4). The beneficial effect of the cholesterol-lowering diet was most evident in those with high cholesterol levels at the outset of the study. Deaths due to other and uncertain causes occurred more frequently in the experimental group, although no single other

Table 19.4   Results of selected intervention trials (confidence interval are given in brackets)

Trial	No. of subjects	Reduction in cholesterol	OR (95% CI) (experimental vs control)	
			Total mortality	Fatal and nonfatal CHD
Veterans Administration	846	13%	0.98 (0.83 to 1.15)	0.77
Oslo	1232	13%	0.64 (0.37 to 1.12)	0.56
DART				
Fat advice	2033	3.5%	0.98 (0.77 to 1.26)	0.92 (0.71 to 1.15)
Fish advice	2033	Negligible	0.74 (0.57 to 0.93)	0.85 (0.66 to 1.07)
CHAOS	2002	Negligible	3.5% (treatment), 2.7% (controls)	0.53 (0.34 to 0.83)
Lyons Heart	605	Negligble	0.30 (0.11 to 0.82)	0.70 (0.12 to 0.59)
Gissi-Prevenzione	11 324			
n-3 supplements		N/A	0.80 (0.67 to 0.94)	0.80 (0.68 to 0.95)
Vitamin E		N/A	0.86 (0.72 to 1.02)	0.88 (0.75 to 1.04)

OR: odds ratio; CI: confidence interval; N/A: not applicable; CHD: coronary heart disease.

cause predominated. The increase in non-cardiovascular mortality in the experimental group raised for the first time the suggestion that cholesterol lowering might be harmful in some respects, despite the reduction in CHD. This will be discussed in more detail later in this chapter.

Oslo trial

In the Oslo trial men at high risk of CHD (as a result of smoking or having a cholesterol level in the range of 7.5–9.8 mmol/l) were divided into two groups; half received intensive dietary education and advice to stop smoking, and the other half served as a control group.

An impressive reduction in total coronary events was observed (Table 19.4) in association with a 13% fall in cholesterol and a 65% reduction in tobacco consumption. The beneficial effect of intervention was also reflected in a significant improvement in total mortality; there were no significant differences between the two groups with regard to noncardiac causes of death. Detailed statistical analysis suggests that approximately 60% of the CHD reduction can be attributed to serum cholesterol change and 25% to smoking reduction. The composition of the experimental diet was quite different to that used in the Veterans Administration trial: total and saturated fat were markedly reduced without any appreciable increase in n-6 PUFA, and fiber-rich carbohydrate was increased. These differences could have accounted for the different results with regard to noncardiovascular diseases.

Diet and Reinfarction Trial (DART)

This was the first trial to examine the effects of diets high in n-3 PUFA. Burr *et al.* randomized 2033 men who had survived myocardial infarction to receive or not to receive advice on each of three dietary factors: a reduction of fat intake and an increase in the P/S ratio, an increase in fatty fish intake, and an increase in cereal fiber. Those unable to consume fatty fish regularly were asked to take a fish oil supplement.

Within the short (2 years) follow-up period, the subjects advised to eat fatty fish had a 29% reduction in all causes of mortality compared with those not so advised. The other two diets were not associated with significant differences in mortality, but in view of the fact that fat modification only achieved a 3–4% reduction in serum cholesterol, it is conceivable that compliance with the fat-modified and fiber diets may have been less than that on the fish diet. Furthermore, diets aimed at reducing atherogenicity are likely to take longer to show a beneficial effect than those aimed at reducing thrombogenicity. These results are of particular interest since they are the first to show that very simple advice aimed to reduce thrombogenicity (at least two weekly portions, 200–400 g, of fatty fish) can appreciably reduce mortality.

Cambridge Heart Antioxidant Study (CHAOS) study

Several early clinical trials involving supplementation with antioxidant nutrients (vitamins C and E and β-carotene) without concomitant dietary change suggested no benefit in terms of cardiovascular risk reduction despite strong evidence of a cardioprotective effect in epidemiological studies. In this study from Cambridge, over 2000 participants with preexisting cardiovascular disease were randomized to receive either placebo or α-tocopherol 400 IU or 800 IU daily. After 17 months (median follow-up 510 days) nonfatal myocardial infarction was substantially reduced in the α-tocopherol group (14 out of 1035) compared with the control group (41 out of 967). However, there were marginally more total deaths in the α-tocopherol than in the control group (36 out of 1035 compared with 26 out of 967), thus providing no justification for the widespread use of vitamin E supplements in the secondary prevention of cardiovascular disease. The much larger Heart Outcomes Prevention Study (HOPE) study confirmed the absence of benefit in terms of both fatal and nonfatal cardiovascular disease associated with supplemental vitamin E in the doses used. It is, however, conceivable that a different dosage or a combination of supplemental nutrients may confer a different outcome.

Lyons Heart Study

The Lyons Heart Study is the most recent in the series of multifactorial dietary intervention studies in the secondary prevention of cardiovascular disease. Six-hundred and five individuals with clinical ischemic heart disease received conventional dietary advice or advice to follow a traditional Mediterranean diet. The experimental diet was lower in total and saturated fat (30 and 8% total energy) than the control diet (33 and 12% total energy) and contained more oleic (13 versus 10% total energy) and α-linolenic acid (0.80 versus 0.27%). Dietary linoleic acid was higher in the control group (5.3 versus 3.6%). The Mediterranean diet included more bread, legumes, vegetables and fruit, and less meat and dairy products. Those in the experimental group were also provided with a margarine rich in α-linolenate (C18:3 n-3). The results were dramatic: a risk ratio of 0.24 (95% CI 0.07 to 0.85) for cardiovascular deaths and 0.30 (95% CI 0.11 to 0.82) for total deaths when comparing mortality experience in experimental compared with control groups. A comparable beneficial effect was found with regard to nonfatal cardiovascular events. It is interesting to note the difference in dietary composition in this and other dietary intervention studies.

The Gissi-Prevenzione Study

This recent large study examined the effect of supplementation with very long-chain n-3 fatty acids (eicosapentaenoic and docosahexaenoic acids) or vitamin E (300 mg) or both in 11 324 subjects who had had a myocardial infarction. The trial was not conducted in a double-blind manner, but was nevertheless interesting in view of its size and otherwise appropriate conduct. Supplementation with n-3 fatty acids was associated with a statistically significant 15–20% reduction in all the important end-points (nonfatal myocardial infarction, cardiovascular deaths and total mortality). A smaller reduction in event rate in association with vitamin E supplementation did not achieve statistical significance.

Overall perspective on the trials

It is inappropriate to aggregate the results of the dietary intervention trials in a formal metaanalysis in view of the wide range of interventions that have been used. Nevertheless, certain conclusions may be drawn from the results of the various studies. There is convincing evidence that cholesterol lowering by dietary means reduces coronary events in the context of both primary and secondary prevention. Indeed, there is confirmation of the rule derived from observational epidemiology that a 2–3% reduction in coronary events results from each 1% of cholesterol lowering achieved. There would seem to be reasonably strong evidence that lowering of total cholesterol (reflecting principally a reduction in LDL-cholesterol) should primarily be achieved by reducing total and saturated fatty acids. While increasing n-6 PUFA (chiefly linoleic acid, C18:2 n-6) may further decrease LDL, the clinical trials offer little support for this measure. Rather, they suggest that when substitution is required oleic acid (C18:1 n-9) or carbohydrate from whole-grain cereals, vegetables and fruit may be the most appropriate sources of replacement energy. Two trials provide strong support for the suggestion that dietary modification has the potential to reduce cardiovascular risk by means other than cholesterol lowering. DART achieved appreciable reduction in mortality associated with increased intake of fish or the use of fish oil supplements with minimal change in cholesterol, presumably because the increase in C20:5 n-3 and C22:6 n-3 in the fish or fish oil supplements resulted in a reduced tendency to thrombosis or a reduced risk of death resulting from dysrhythmias.

Similarly, the experimental diet in the Lyons Heart Study, which showed the greatest risk reduction of all trials, was not associated with appreciable cholesterol lowering. It is impossible to identify which of the many nutritional changes may have been responsible for the beneficial effects. There was undoubtedly an increase in a range of antioxidant nutrients that may have reduced oxidizability of LDL despite minimal change in cholesterol. Nonstarch polysaccharide (dietary fiber) as well as starch increased because of the increase in cereals, vegetables and fruit. Total SFA decreased, while oleic and α-linolenic acids increased. The authors of the study regarded the last mentioned change to be of particular importance. However, it would seem to be more plausible to suggest that a combination of all these factors contributed to the overall risk reduction resulting from favorable modification of several of the risk factors listed in Table 19.3. It would be helpful if an attempt could be made to replicate the Lyons Heart Study. Unfortunately, in the context of secondary prevention this may be well-nigh impossible. The vast majority of such patients are now treated with statin drugs, which dramatically reduce the risk of subsequent cardiovascular events to the extent that it may be extremely difficult to demonstrate an additional benefit of dietary modification.

The trials of nutrient supplements have generally been disappointing, apart perhaps from the Gissi-Prevenzione study, which suggests a potential benefit of supplementation with modest amounts of fish oils. There is no clear explanation as to why antioxidant nutrient supplementation trials have been generally disappointing despite strong suggestions of benefit from epidemiological data. The most likely explanation would seem to be either that a longer time-frame is necessary to demonstrate a benefit or, more likely, that a blend of these nutrients in proportions similar to those found in foods may be required to produce benefit, rather than a pharmacological dose of a single antioxidant nutrient. Trials are underway to determine whether supplementation with folic acid and other dietary determinants of homocysteine levels have the potential to reduce cardiovascular risk.

Given the importance of metaanalyses of clinical trials in establishing evidence-based dietary guidelines, it is important to be able to assess the validity of such analyses. Even prestigious journals occasionally publish analyses and conclusions that are not justified. One such example is the metaanalysis published in the

British Medical Journal by Hooper *et al.* (2001), which aggregated the findings of 27 studies involving various manipulations to reduce or modify dietary fat intake. The overall result suggested a 14% reduction in cardiovascular events (RR 0.86, 95% CI 0.72 to 1.03) which did not quite achieve conventional levels of statistical significance; nor was the reduction in cardiovascular and total mortality statistically significant. However, the metaanalysis combined many studies that were not really comparable. For example, some studies contributed fewer than 100 person-years and others as many as 10 000 person-years, and the duration of the trials was variable. Dietary manipulations ranged from extremely low-fat diets to relatively high total fat intakes with PUFA predominating. Some involved multifactorial dietary changes. An appropriate metaanalysis should include only comparable studies. It is of interest to note that in the Hooper analysis, when only trials with at least 2 years of follow-up were included a more marked and statistically significant reduction in cardiovascular events (RR 0.76, 95% CI 0.65 to 0.90) was noted.

19.7 Nutritional strategies for high-risk populations

Most early attempts at CHD risk reduction involved strategies aimed at identifying and treating high-risk individuals with appropriate diet and drug therapies. Screening those with a family or personal history of CHD for all potentially modifiable risk factors may be a worthwhile clinical aim and result in considerable benefit for the individual. Similarly, those with any one known risk factor should be screened for other risk factors. However, such approaches will not on their own produce substantial reductions in cardiovascular morbidity and mortality in the population as a whole. This is because the majority of cases are derived from that section of the population who are at mild to modest risk, simply because there are more of them. Those with extreme levels of risk factors may be at great individual risk, but contribute only a small number of cases to the totality of CHD because there are relatively few of them. Thus, for the greatest impact it is essential to reduce the risk factor level in the population as a whole. The population and individual or high-risk approaches are usually regarded as complementary, the latter helping to raise awareness in the community.

Recommendations regarding dietary fat remain the cornerstone of most sets of nutrient-based recommended intakes. These vary from one country to another; the British Dietary Reference Values are shown in Table 19.5. It is suggested that saturated and

Table 19.5 Dietary reference values for fat and carbohydrate for adults

	Individual minimum	Population average	Individual maximum
		(% total energy intake)	
Saturated fatty acids		10 (11)	
cis polyunsaturated fatty acids		6 (6.5)	10
	n-3: 0.2		
	n-6: 1.0		
cis monounsaturated fatty acids		12 (13)	
trans fatty acids		2 (2)	
Total fatty acids		30 (32.5)	
Total fat		33 (35)	
Nonmilk extrinsic sugars	0	10 (11)	
Intrinsic and milk sugars and starch		37 (39)	
Total carbohydrate		47 (50)	
Nonstarch polysaccharide (g/day)	12	18	24

Source: Department of Health (1991).
The average percentage contribution to total energy does not total 100% because figures for protein and alcohol are excluded. Protein intakes average 15% of total energy, which is above the recommended nutrient intake (RNI). It is recognized that many individuals will derive some energy from alcohol, and this has been assumed to average 5% approximating to current intakes. However, the Panel recognized that some groups chose not to drink alcohol and that for some purposes nutrient intakes as a proportion of food energy without alcohol might be useful. Therefore, average figures are given as percentages both of total energy and, in parentheses, of food energy.

trans-unsaturated fat should average 10 and 2% of total energy, respectively. While this target is less restrictive than in some countries it nevertheless represents an appreciable reduction from present intakes in many high-risk countries. At 12% total energy, on average, monounsaturated fat intake would appear to be similar to that presently consumed. However, a reasonably high proportion of these fatty acids is derived from animal sources, which are also relatively rich in saturated fat, so that compliance with advice to reduce saturated fat would inevitably mean consuming monounsaturated fats from vegetable rather than animal sources. Uncertainty remains regarding the optimal quantities and ratios of n-3 and n-6 PUFA. A population average of 6% and an individual maximum of 10% total energy for total PUFA would appear to be a reasonable compromise given, on the one hand, the potential benefits of n-6 PUFA, and on the other, the potential deleterious effects of excessive intakes. Intakes of n-3 fatty acids greater than amounts required to avoid deficiency may well confer additional benefit, with separate and additive benefit accruing from fish and plant-based sources, providing principally C20:5 n-3 and C20:6 n-3, and C18:3 n-3 respectively. The British recommendations also suggest average, minimum and maximum intakes of nonstarch polysaccharide, but not for dietary cholesterol, since dietary cholesterol is inevitably reduced when food rich in saturated fat is reduced. There are also no specific recommendations regarding optimal amounts of antioxidant nutrients or folic acid, although it seems likely that quantities greater than the recommended nutrient intakes are required to exert a cardioprotective effect. Guidelines from the USA are summarized in Table 19.6. These recommendations represent expert opinion of the American

Table 19.6 Summary of Dietary Guidelines, American Heart Association

	Population goals			
	Overall healthy eating pattern	Appropriate body weight	Desirable cholesterol profile	Desirable blood pressure
Major guidelines	Include a variety of fruits, vegetables, grains, low-fat or nonfat dairy products, fish, legumes, poultry, lean meats	Match energy intake to energy needs, with appropriate changes to achieve weight loss when indicated	Limit foods high in saturated fat and cholesterol and substitute unsaturated fat from vegetables, fish, legumes and nuts	Limit salt and alcohol; maintain a healthy body weight and a diet with emphasis on vegetables, fruits, and low-fat or nonfat dairy products

Reproduced with permission from Krauss et al. (2000). © 2000 American Heart Association

Heart Association and are therefore more specific to CHD than the British Dietary Reference Values. They also take into account the findings of more recent prospective epidemiological studies, most notably the Nurses Health Study and the Health Professionals Study. They are predominantly food based rather than nutrient based. The guidelines in Table 19.6 are intended for the general population. Separate guidelines are also provided for special populations (e.g. older adults, children) and individuals with specific medical conditions (e.g. raised LDL-cholesterol, pre-existing CHD, diabetes mellitus). There is at present no case to be made for the use of single antioxidant nutrient supplements, although it is conceivable that future research may demonstrate benefit from blends of these nutrients in appropriate quantities. The Gissi-Prevenzione and DART studies suggest possible benefit from supplementation with n-3 fatty acids, at least for those with established CHD. Thus, it may be reasonable to suggest small amounts as supplements in high-risk individuals who are not regularly consuming oily fish. However, there is no case to be made for the recommendation of such supplements at the population level.

It is beyond the scope of this chapter to attempt a detailed translation of recommendations and reference values into guidelines for the population. The basic principles underlying this translation are covered in Chapter 7, although it should be noted that several different dietary patterns are compatible with the nutrient targets suggested here.

It is extremely difficult to quantify the likely benefits of such dietary change. The benefit that accrues from cholesterol lowering (a 2–3% reduction in CHD for each 1% reduction in cholesterol) has been fairly well established. However, the additional benefit that may result from an increase in potentially beneficial unsaturated fatty acids, nonstarch polysaccharides, foods rich in antioxidant nutrients and folic acid might be appreciably greater. The findings of the Lyons Heart Study suggest that this may be the case.

Barker's fetal origin hypothesis (see Chapter 18) suggests that intrauterine malnutrition leads to small babies who are subsequently at greatly increased risk of CHD, especially when exposed to an environment in which the availability of energy-dense foods can lead to a fairly rapid catch-up in weight, but not in height. This has been taken by some to suggest that environmental manipulation later in life is likely to have little impact on risk reduction. The data presented here provide strong evidence that this is not the case. Indeed, the benefit of dietary change appears to be evident even after a relatively short time interval. It will now never be possible to undertake a formal clinical trial in which the potential benefit of the full range of dietary manipulations can be evaluated. However, periodic national surveys of dietary intake and risk factor measurement in conjunction with monitoring mortality statistics as well as CHD incident data should provide helpful clues. The North Karelia Project in Finland demonstrated many years ago the potential for an educational program involving basic nutrition information to influence favorably risk factor status and CHD mortality when comparing the intervention area with other regions of Finland that did not receive the same level of dietary advice.

19.8 Perspectives on the future

It is conceivable that therapeutic nutrition aimed at the individual in a clinical setting will begin to take on board how common genetic polymorphisms influence the responsiveness of dietary intervention to lower plasma LDL-cholesterol and influence other risk factors. Quite how that may translate into public health nutrition is uncertain. Enthusiasm for research into gene–nutrient interactions should not dilute the emphasis on population-oriented dietary advice that is of proven benefit. It will be of interest to see how soon knowledge advances to the extent to which individuals may opt to have their relevant genes screened to ascertain either their sensitivity to diet-related risk factors or their ability to respond to specific dietary therapies.

At present, many spreads are available enriched in plant sterols which lower plasma LDL and, by inference, the risk of CHD. The average scale of reduction, around 10%, is well above that which can be achieved solely by manipulating dietary fat composition. Such functional foods which influence other risk factors in addition to LDL are likely to grow in significance and may well have a considerable influence on the population risk of cardiovascular disease.

Further reading

Appel LJ, Moore TJ, Obarzanek E *et al.* A clinical trial of the effects of dietary patterns on blood pressure (DASH Collaborative Research Group). N Engl J Med 1997; 336: 1117–1124.

Brunner E, White E, Thorogood M, Bristow A, Curle D. Can dietary nterventions change diet and cardiovascular risk factors? A meta-analysis of randomized controlled trials. American Journal Public Health 1997; 87: 1415–1422.

Burr ML, Gilbert JF, Holliday RM et al. Effects of changes in fat, fish and fibre intakes on death and myocardial reinfarction: Diet and Reinfarction Trial. Lancet 1989; ii: 757–761.

Department of Health Dietary Reference Values for Food Energy and Nutrients for the United Kingdom. Report on Health and Social Subjects 41. London, HMSO, 1991.

Heart Outcomes Prevention Evaluation Study Investigators. Vitamin E supplementation and cardiovascular events in high-risk patients. N Engl J Med 2000; 342: 154–160.

Holme I. An effect of randomised trials evaluating the effect of cholesterol reduction on total mortality and coronary heart disease incidence. Circulation 1990; 82: 1916–1924.

Hooper L, Summerbell CD, Higgins JPT et al. Dietary fat intake and prevention of cardiovascular disease: systematic review. BMJ 2001; 322: 757–763.

Hu FB, Stampfer MJ, Manson JE et al. Trends in the incidence of coronary heart disease and changes in diet and lifestyle in women. N Engl J Med 2000; 343: 530–537.

Hu FB, Willett WC. Diet and coronary heart disease: findings from the Nurses' Health Study and the Health Professionals' Follow-up Study. J Nutr Health Aging 2001; 5: 132–138.

Keys A. Seven Countries: A Multivariate Analysis of Death and Coronary Heart Disease. USA, Harvard University Press, 1980.

Krauss RM, Eckel RH, Howard B et al. AHA Dietary Guidelines: revision 2000: a statement for healthcare professionals from the Nutrition Committee of the American Heart Association. Circulation 2000; 102: 2284–2299.

Pietinen P, Lahti-Koski M, Vartianen E, Puska P. Nutrition and cardiovascular Disease in Finland since the early 1970's: a success Story. J Nutr Health Aging 2001; 5: 150–154.

Stamler J. Population studies. In: Nutrition, Lipids and Coronary Heart Disease (Levy RI, Rifkind BM, Dennis BH, Ernst N, eds), pp. 25–88. New York: Raven Press, 1979.

Stampfer MJ, Hu FB, Manson JE et al. Primary prevention of coronary heart disease in women through diet and lifestyle. N Engl J Med 2000; 343: 16–22.

Stykowski PA, Kannel WB, D'Agostino RB. Changes in risk factors and the decline in mortality from cardiovascular disease. The Framingham heart study. N Engl J Med 1990; 322: 1635–1641.

Tunstall-Pedoe H, Kullasmaa K, Mahonen M et al. Contribution of trends in survival and coronary event rates to changes in coronary heart disease mortality: 10-year results from 37 WHO MONICA project populations. Monitoring trends and determinants of cardiovascular disease. Lancet 1999; 353: 1547–1557.

20
Diabetes Mellitus

Ambady Ramachandran and Chamukuttan Snehalatha

Key messages

- Diabetes mellitus (DM) is a metabolic disorder with a multifactorial etiology. It is characterized by chronic hyperglycemia and affects metabolism of carbohydrates, protein and fats.
- Long-term DM leads to a series of metabolic disturbances causing macrovascular and microvascular pathology.
- Diabetes is classified as type 1 diabetes, type 2 diabetes and gestational diabetes, impaired glucose tolerance and the metabolic syndrome or syndrome X are closely associated with diabetes.

- Type 2 DM is a multifactorial disease having equally strong genetic and environmental components contributing to its development. Some of these factors can be modified by lifestyle changes, whereas other factors cannot.
- The estimated prevalence of DM in the adult populations worldwide will rise by 35% in the two decades, affecting up to 300 million adults by the year 2025. The major part of this numerical increase will occur in developing countries.
- Now, and in the future, type 2 diabetes presents an enormous public health nutrition challenge.

20.1 Introduction

Diabetes mellitus (DM) is a metabolic disorder with a multifactorial etiology. It is characterized by chronic hyperglycemia and affects metabolism of carbohydrates, protein and fats. The pathophysiology of DM centers on impaired insulin secretion/or impaired insulin action. Subjects with DM present with varied symptoms such as polyuria, polydypsia and polyphagia with weight loss. Hyperglycemia may remain undetected as the disease may be asymptomatic causing vascular damage even before the detection of the disease. Long-term DM leads to a series of metabolic disturbances causing macrovascular and microvascular pathology. Microvascular complications associated with DM include retinopathy, nephropathy and neuropathy. People with DM are at an increased risk of cardiovascular, cerebrovascular and peripheral vascular diseases.

20.2 Classification of diabetes

The recent classification encompasses both clinical stages and etiological types of DM and other categories of hyperglycemia. The terms insulin-dependent diabetes mellitus (IDDM) and noninsulin-dependent diabetes mellitus (NIDDM) are no longer used. The etiological classification is shown in Table 20.1.

Impaired glucose tolerance

The class impaired glucose tolerance (IGT) is a stage of impaired glucose regulation, since it can be observed in any hyperglycemic disorder, and is itself not DM.

Type 1 diabetes

Type 1 DM is characterized by reduced insulin levels (insulinopenia) due to β-cell destruction. Patients require insulin for survival. In the absence of exogenous insulin, they develop ketoacidosis, coma and death.

Type 2 diabetes

Type 2 DM is the most common form of DM and is characterized by impaired insulin action and insulin secretion. Both of these defects are present in clinical

Table 20.1 Etiological classification of disorders of glycemia

Type 1	Characterized by partial or total failure of insulin production by the β-cells of the pancreas. Causative factors remain poorly understood, but certain viruses, autoimmune disease and genetic factors may all contribute
Type 2	Characterized by insulin resistance, where insulin is produced but in amounts that are insufficient or in an ineffective form. Strong genetic links with this form of diabetes and its development are closely linked with obesity
Other specific types	Genetic defects of β-cell function Genetic defects in insulin action Diseases of the exocrine pancreas Endocrinopathies Drug or chemical induced Infections Uncommon forms of immune-mediated diabetes Other genetic syndromes sometimes associated with diabetes
Gestational diabetes	A form of diabetes that develops during pregnancy. Most, but not all, cases resolve after delivery

DM. Multiple and varied reasons for the development of these abnormalities have been identified.

Type 2 DM also has a multifactorial etiology. The majority of patients are noninsulin dependent and mostly have adult-onset DM. In type 2 DM insulin resistance is common, with relative insulinopenia and occasionally requiring insulin in times of stress. Obesity and central obesity are commonly seen in type 2 diabetics. Ketoacidosis is uncommon and, if seen, is related to stress or other intercurrent illness. Patients are also prone to microvascular and macrovascular complications. Etiological factors include genetic factors, age, obesity and lack of physical activity.

Gestational diabetes

Gestational DM is carbohydrate intolerance resulting in hyperglycemia of variable severity with onset or first recognition during pregnancy. The definition applies irrespective of whether or not insulin is used for treatment or the condition persists after pregnancy. The glucose intolerance may precede pregnancy, but has been previously unrecognized.

The metabolic syndrome or syndrome X

A cluster of abnormalities, namely hyperglycemia, hypertension, central obesity, dyslipidemia and insulin resistance, occurs frequently. This clustering of risk factors for cardiovascular diseases is termed syndrome X, the insulin resistance syndrome or the metabolic syndrome. Epidemiological studies confirm that this syndrome occurs commonly in a wide variety of ethnic groups, including Europeans, African–Americans, Mexican Americans, Asian Indians and Chinese, Australian Aborigines, Polynesians and Micronesians. The management of people with hyperglycemia and other features of the metabolic syndrome should not only focus on blood glucose control, but also include strategies for reduction of the other cardiovascular disease risk factors.

20.3 Diagnosis of diabetes

Standardization of the criteria for diagnosis and classification of DM proposed by the National Diabetes Data Group of the USA (NDDG) and the World Health Organization (WHO) expert committee brought in a certain degree of uniformity to the global studies on this metabolic disorder. An oral glucose tolerance test (OGTT) with a 75 g glucose load is used to distinguish between DM and non-DM. Table 20.2 shows the diagnostic criteria.

There is an underestimation of DM prevalence when the fasting plasma glucose (FPG) criterion is used. In the US National Health and Nutrition Examination Survey (NHANES) III population study, the prevalence of undiagnosed DM was 6.34% by the WHO criteria (2 h), but only 4.4% if diagnosis was based only on the FPG cut-off of 126 mg/dl (7.0 mmol/l) or above. The Diabetes Epidemiology: Collaborative Analysis of Diagnostic Criteria in Europe (DECODE) study group, which analyzed the data from 16 European countries, found that there was an underestimation of DM if the FPG criterion was used, with a concordance of only 28%. Sensitivity of the FPG for diagnosis of diabetes was also low in Asian populations.

Mode of diagnosis

- Symptoms of DM, such as thirst and polyuria, and a random plasma glucose ⩾ 200 mg/dl (11.1 mmol/l)
- or FPG ⩾ 126 mg/dl (7.0 mmol/l)
- or 2 h plasma glucose ⩾ 200 mg/dl (11.1 mmol/l) during an OGTT

Table 20.2 Values for diagnosis of diabetes mellitus and other categories of hyperglycemia

	Glucose concentration, mmol/l (mg/dl)		
	Whole blood		Plasma (Venous)
	Venous	Capillary	
Diabetes mellitus			
Fasting	≥6.1 (≥110)	≥6.1 (≥110)	≥7.0 (≥126)
or			
2 h postglucose load or both	≥10.0 (≥180)	≥11.1 (≥200)	≥11.1 (≥200)
Impaired glucose tolerance			
Fasting concentration (if measured) and	<6.1 (<110)	<6.1 (<110)	<7.0 (<126)
2 h postglucose load	≥6.7 (≥120) and <10.0 (<180)	≥7.8 (≥140) and <11.1 (<200)	≥7.8 (≥140) and <11.1 (<200)
Impaired fasting glycemia			
Fasting	≥5.6 (≥100) and <6.1 (<110)	≥5.6 (≥100) and <6.1 (<110)	≥6.1 (≥110) and <7.0 (<126)
2 h (if measured)	<6.7 (<120)	<7.8 (<140)	<7.8 (<140)

Source: WHO (1998). Reproduced with permission from the WHO.

- for population screening purposes, the fasting or 2 h value after 75 g oral glucose may be used.

Pregnant women who meet the WHO criteria for DM or IGT are classified as having gestational DM. Screening for gestational DM is unnecessary in women younger than 25 years of age who are at low risk. Glucose tolerance should be reclassified by a 75 g load OGTT, 6 weeks or more after delivery. The American Diabetes Association (ADA) recommends a screening by measuring plasma glucose concentration 1 h after a 50 g oral glucose load between 24 and 28 weeks of gestation. If the glucose concentration is at least 7.8 mmol/l (140 mg/dl), a full 3 h OGTT should be performed. Any two of the four plasma glucose values obtained during the test meeting or exceeding the values shown below indicate a diagnosis of gestational DM:

Time	mg/dl	mmol/L
fasting	95	5.3
1 h	180	10.0
2 h	155	8.6
3 h	140	7.8

The glycosylated hemoglobin (HbA_{Ic}) measurement is an index of glycemic status over the past 2–3 months. It is recommended as a tool for monitoring glycemic control.

20.4 Risk factors for the development of diabetes

Type 2 DM is a multifactorial disease with equally strong genetic and environmental components contributing to its development. Some of these factors can be modified by lifestyle changes, other factors cannot.

Genetic factors

Evidence for a genetic component comes from the increased concordance of DM in monozygotic twins, a high prevalence in the offspring of diabetic parents and a high prevalence in certain ethnic groups. Associations of DM with many candidate genes have been identified in different populations, but none has been shown to be the major gene involved in the development of the disorder. Type 2 DM is a polygenic disorder, and no clear relationship is described with human leukocyte antigen (HLA) genes. Maturity-onset diabetes in the young (MODY) is a monogenic form of type 2 DM with an early age of onset, less than 25 years. It has an autosomal dominant inheritance and mutations have been described in at least five genes. Another genetic variant is maternally inherited deafness in diabetes mellitus (MIDDM), which has characteristics of both type 1 and type 2 DM. Sensory neural deafness is associated with an early onset of DM and this form is characterized by a strict maternal inheritance. Only a daughter can transfer the disease to her progeny, although both genders are affected equally.

Thrifty genotype and thrifty phenotype

The thrifty genotype hypothesis was put forward by Neel in 1962, and proposes that certain populations exposed to cycles of starvation and times of plenty have been benefited by a thrifty gene which has helped them to store a high proportion of energy intake as fat during times of plenty. It could be used during times of famine. This was proposed to be common among the hunter–gatherer populations. During the process of modernization, when these individuals with a thrifty genotype are confronted with a continuous supply of energy and reduced physical activity, the condition is favorable for development of DM and IGT. Hyperinsulinemia is considered to be a mechanism of preferential energy storage, which has become a disadvantage in modern populations. Such a phenomenon is observed in cases of Pacific islanders, Native Americans and Asian Indians.

In recent years a different hypothesis of a thrifty phenotype has gained significant importance. Barker's hypothesis (see Chapter 18) states that fetal and childhood malnutrition, by programming metabolism, predisposes to chronic diseases in adulthood such as hypertension, coronary heart disease and type 2 DM. A thrifty phenotype has been proposed in which inadequate fetal nutrition programs lead to the development of insulin resistance in adulthood. It may well be that such a phenomenon is more relevant in the developing countries where malnutrition is a major health problem.

Environmental risk factors

Epidemiological studies from different parts of the world have shown that the major environmental risk factors for DM are:

- age
- obesity and central obesity
- insulin resistance
- dietary factors
- physical inactivity
- urbanization and modernization.

Age

Aging is an important risk factor for DM. In all of the epidemiological studies in different populations, the prevalence of DM shows an age-specific increase. In the European population, the age of onset of DM is generally in the region of 50–60 years, but it is significantly lower in the Native American and Asian Indian populations, who have a high prevalence of DM.

Obesity and central obesity

Obesity is a major risk factor for DM. Its relationship with type 2 DM is complex. Although the rates of obesity measured by the body mass index (BMI) is generally low in Indians, it has been strongly associated with glucose intolerance in both urban and rural populations. Even within an acceptable body weight range, weight gain could increase the risk of DM, especially in the presence of a familial predisposition. This may be due to the adverse effect of age and body weight on the high degree of insulin resistance in populations such as Asian Indians. Body fat distribution may be more valuable as a predictor of DM than obesity. Upper body adiposity measured by the waist/hip ratio (WHR) has been more closely associated with DM in a number of cross-sectional and prospective studies. Studies from India have consistently shown that despite lower rates of general obesity an average Indian has high upper body adiposity. The upper cut-off value for normal BMI for an Asian Indian is $23 \, \text{kg/m}^2$.

Insulin resistance

Defects in insulin secretion and action are the two major pathogenic factors in DM. A subnormal action of insulin on insulin-mediated tissues results in decreased glucose disposal even in nondiabetic subjects. This would result in a compensatory hyperinsulinemia. Therefore, it is extremely difficult biologically to differentiate between insulin resistance and compensatory hyperinsulinemia in nondiabetic subjects. Asian Indians have higher plasma insulin responses during fasting and in response to stimulation compared with Europeans and other ethnic groups. This is an indication of a state of insulin resistance in Indians. Prospective studies in several high-risk populations have produced evidence to show that insulin resistance precedes the development of hyperglycemia. In addition, Asian Indians display a tendency for a clustering of related abnormalities: central adiposity, obesity, hyperinsulinemia, dyslipidemia, hypertension and glucose intolerance.

Dietary factors

Diet is an important determinant of obesity and also influences insulin resistance, and thus has an important role in the development of type 2 DM. With urbanization, changes in lifestyle and food habits occur. The consumption of high-energy, high-fat diets, as well as low levels of physical activity, lead to a change in energy balance with a conservation of energy as depot fats, which are rarely used. Excess energy intake per se promotes insulin resistance even before significant weight gain occurs. A high-calorie, high-fat and low-carbohydrate diet has an association with type 2 DM. A diet rich in energy and low in fiber promotes weight gain and insulin resistance, even in such low-risk populations as Europeans (see Chapter 10).

Physical inactivity

Several cross-sectional studies in Pacific, Polynesian and Micronesian populations show a strong association between the prevalence of type 2 DM and physical inactivity. The impact of physical inactivity is manifested more markedly in populations who have been accustomed to habitual heavy physical activity.

Progression of IGT to DM can be prevented by increased physical activity, which may protect against the development of type 2 DM both directly and through its effects on obesity and fat metabolism (see Chapter 4).

Exercise improves insulin sensitivity and increases glucose uptake by the muscles, and in this way has a beneficial effect on carbohydrate metabolism in both diabetic and nondiabetic subjects. It also has favorable effects on lipid metabolism and contributes to weight loss. An analysis among US nurses has also shown a benefit of exercise in the form of brisk walking in reducing the risk of DM and coronary artery disease. A 6 year follow-up study from China showed a 40% reduction in the risk of progression from IGT to DM in subjects assigned to an exercise program.

Urbanization and modernization

A transition from a traditional to a modern life by urbanization has produced severe health hazards in many populations, including the Asian Indians, Pacific Islanders, Chinese, North Africans, Native Americans and Australian Aborigines. The impacts of urbanization are particularly evident from the epidemiological data from Mauritius. Urbanization is associated with increasing obesity, decreasing physical activity and other risk factors associated with DM development. Recent epidemiological data indicate that migration from a traditional to urban lifestyle, whether within a country or to a more developed country, produces similar adverse environmental effects. A rural to urban migration within the country is associated with massive increases in the prevalence of type 2 DM in Asian Indians (Figure 20.1).

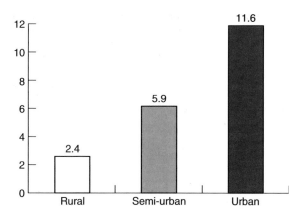

Figure 20.1 Impact of urbanization on the prevalence of diabetes: southern Indian data. Reprinted from Ramachandran *et al.* (1999) with permission from Elsevier.

Gestational diabetes

Risk factors for the development of gestational diabetes include:

- older women
- previous history of glucose intolerance
- history of large-for-gestational-age babies
- women from certain high-risk ethnic groups
- any pregnant woman who has elevated fasting or postprandial blood glucose levels.

20.5 Diabetes as a public health issue

Type 1 diabetes

Type 1 DM occurs worldwide. It typically develops abruptly with severe hyperglycemia and there is usually the presence of ketonuria or ketosis at diagnosis. The age of onset is generally in children and young adults, but it may occur at any age. A lifelong dependence on insulin is universal. Although type 1 DM is the most extreme form of the disease, it is not prevented by dietary intervention, so the remainder of this chapter will deal with the public health implications and management of type 2 DM.

Type 2 diabetes

A worldwide epidemic of DM is likely to occur in the first quarter of the twenty-first century. The estimated prevalence of DM in the adult populations worldwide will rise by 35% from 4.0% in 1995 to 5.4% in 2025. The WHO report states that the number of adults with DM in the world will rise from 135 million in 1995 to

Table 20.3 Prevalence, numerical estimates and projections of diabetes

	World		Developed countries		Developing countries	
	1995	2025	1995	2025	1995	2025
Diabetes prevalence %	4.0	5.4	6.0	7.6	3.3	4.9
% Increase		35		27		48
Number with diabetes (millions)	135	300	51	72	84	228
% Increase		122		42		170

Adapted from WHO (1998). Reproduced with permission from the WHO.

300 million in the year 2025. The major part of this numerical increase will occur in developing countries. There will be a 42% increase, from 51 to 72 million, in the developed countries, and a 170% increase, from 84 to 228 million, in the developing countries (Table 20.3). It has been estimated that more than 75% of the people with DM will be in developing countries. The highest increases in prevalence between 1995 and 2025 will be for China (68%) and India (59%). The Middle East countries would experience a 30% increase, and for Latin America and the Caribbean islands a 41% increase is projected. Table 20.4 illustrates the scale of the problem of rising levels of type 2 DM in Asia.

Although these internal comparisons give an indication of changing patterns, it should be noted that particularly vulnerable ethnic groups exist. The highest prevalence of type 2 DM is seen among the Pima Indians of Arizona, and in Nauru in the Pacific Basin. The Native American tribes have a high prevalence rate, ranging from 15 to 41% in the age group above 45 years, unlike the Alaskan Indians who are less Westernized and have only 3% of DM. In the Pacific Islands, the Melanesians of Papua New Guinea have a prevalence of 37%, while in Kiribati and Western Samoa the prevalence ranges between 11 and 16% in subjects aged 30–64 years. In the USA, the African–American population (10%) and Mexican Hispanics (14%) have higher susceptibility to DM than the Caucasian population (6%).

There is increasing evidence to show that urbanized Asian Indians have a high risk of DM, both within the homeland and in various countries to which they have migrated. Figure 20.2 is an example of the temporal changes occurring in the prevalence of DM in urban southern India. The effect of urbanization is apparent in the southern Indian community by people in urban

Table 20.4 Prevalence of type 2 diabetes in south-east Asia

	Year	Urban	Rural
India	1972	2.3	
	1979	3.0	1.3
	1988	5.0	
	1992	8.2	2.4
	1997	11.6	
Singapore Chinese	1984	4.0	
	1992	8.0	
Malays	1984	7.6	
	1992	9.3	
Migrant Indians	1984	8.9	
	1992	12.8	
Phillipines	1992	8.4–12.0	3.8–9.7
Malaysia	1984	3.3	
	1988	6.6	
	1994	12.2	
Thailand	1971	2.5	
	1986	6.0	6.0
	1989	6.7	
Sri Lanka	1994		5.0
	1995	8.1	

locations having a much higher rate of DM than their rural counterparts.

Impaired glucose tolerance

The ratio of the prevalence of IGT to DM varies in different populations and usually is around 1 (i.e. equal prevalence of IGT and DM). This observation of a high prevalence of IGT assumes great significance because about 35% of people with IGT become diabetic during a mean period of 5 years. Moreover, people with IGT also carry a high cardiovascular risk. In certain races such as the Africans in Cameroon (urban and rural), the prevalence of DM is still low, yet the prevalence of IGT appears to be increasing.

Complications of diabetes

Type 2 DM and hypertension are commonly associated conditions. The presence of both together accentuates the risk of cardiovascular, renal and retinal complications in DM. Screening for retinopathy and microalbuminuria should be done at the time of diagnosis of type 2 DM and annually thereafter. Two recent landmark studies, the Diabetes Control and Complications Trial (DCCT) in type 1 DM and the United Kingdom Prospective Diabetes Study (UKPDS) in type 2 DM have conclusively shown that the tight control of glycemia

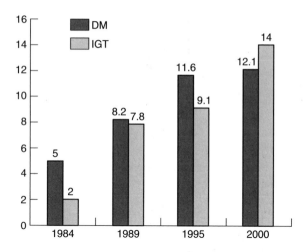

- Prevalence of diabetes is increasing gradually
- IGT showed a sharp increase in the last five years
- IGT to diabetes ratio is >1 in 2000

Figure 20.2 Increasing prevalence of diabetes (DM) and impaired glucose tolerance (IGT) in south India.

and blood pressure reduces the vascular complications of DM significantly. Several factors that contribute to the development of DM and coronary heart disease, such as obesity, physical inactivity and inappropriate diet, are amenable to modification. Guidelines are now available for modification of these risk factors based on several long-term prospective studies.

20.6 Prevention and management of diabetes

The primary route to managing type 1 DM is the provision of exogenous insulin. The dietary management of both type 1 and type 2 DM is almost identical. Current recommendations for macronutrient distribution in the DM diet are summarized in Table 20.5. Given the central role of obesity and physical inactivity in the etiology of type 2 DM, public health nutrition has a large role to play in its prevention.

Goals of diabetes management

The goals of management of DM are to make a patient symptom free and to allow him or her to lead a normal life without the burden of the vascular complications associated with the disease. A multifaceted team approach is essential to achieve these goals. The components of the treatment regimen include:

- nutritional therapy including dietary modification
- exercise
- drug management
- DM education.

Nutritional therapy and dietary modification

The goals of nutrition therapy are:

- to attain and maintain optimal metabolic outcomes, including normal glucose levels, favorable lipid profile and acceptable blood pressure levels, to reduce the risk of macrovessel and microvessel disease
- to prevent and treat chronic complications of DM by modifying nutrient intake and lifestyle as appropriate for the prevention and treatment of obesity, dyslipidemia, cardiovascular disease, hypertension and nephropathy
- to improve health through healthy food choices and physical activity
- to give specific advice necessary for minority groups such as:
  - young people with type 1 or type 2 DM
  - pregnant and lactating women
  - older adults
  - individuals treated with insulin
  - those at risk of developing DM.

Medical nutrition therapy is an integral component of DM management. The following paragraphs outline the rationale for nutrition recommendations for the person with DM. Current recommendations for macronutrients are summarized in Table 20.5.

Carbohydrate

A number of factors influence glycemic responses to foods, including the amount of carbohydrate, type of sugar, nature of the starch, cooking and food processing,

Table 20.5 Current recommendations for macronutrient distribution

Nutrient	Unit	Diabetes UK (2003)	NCEP II 1994	ADA 2002	EASD 2000	ALFEDIAM 1996
Protein	% Energy	Not > 1 g per kg body weight	±15	15–20	10–20	10–20
Fat	% Energy	<35%	<30	60–70 for CHO + MUFA (individually tailored)	≤35%	30–40 (individually tailored)
SFA	% Energy	<10	8–10	<10	<10	<10
MUFA	% Energy	60–70 for CHO + MUFA	≤15	60–70 for CHO + MUFA	60–70 for CHO + MUFA individually tailored	10–20
PUFA	% Energy	<10	≤10	≈10	≤10	±10
Cholesterol	mg/day	≤300	≤300	<300	<300	<300
Carbohydrates (CHO)	% Energy	60–70	≥55	Total amount of CHO in meals/snacks more important than source or type	cis-MUFA and CHO 60–70	40–55 (individually tailored)
CHO fraction					Foods with lower glycemic index or rich in fibre	Foods with lower glycemic index
Sucrose	% Energy	Up to 10		Taken in context of a healthy diet	<10	<10
Fructose				No restrictions	Use not encouraged	
Complex CHO		Preferred		As for normal population		Preferred

Adapted from (1998) with permission from Elsevier.

BDA: British Diabetic Association; NCEPII: National Cholesterol Education Program Step II Diet; ADA: American Diabetes Association; EASD: European Association for the Study of Diabetes; ALFEDIAM: French Language Association for the Study of Diabetes and Metabolism; SFA: saturated fatty acids; MUFA: monounsaturated fatty acids; PUFA: polyunsaturated fatty acids; CHO: Carbohydrate; LDL: low-density lipoprotein.

and food form, as well as other food components. Many studies examining this area conclude that the total amount of carbohydrate in meals and snacks is more important than the source or the type. In people with type 2 DM with normal body weight, replacing some carbohydrate with monounsaturated fat reduces postprandial glycemia and triglyceridemia. However, there is concern that increased fat intake in *ad libitum* diets may promote weight gain. Therefore, the contributions of carbohydrate and monounsaturated fat to energy intake should be individualized based on nutrition assessment, metabolic profiles and treatment goals.

Glycemic index

Carbohydrate foods are digested and absorbed at different rates, so similar amounts of carbohydrate do not have similar effects in terms of glycemia, insulin production or blood lipid concentration. The effect of carbohydrate on glycemia is complex. In general, refined sources of sugars are absorbed more rapidly than carbohydrate from starchy or fiber-containing foods such as cereals and fruit. However, there is considerable variability in glycemic effect between foods of seemingly similar composition, and this can be quantified in terms of the glycemic index (GI). The GI provides a means of comparing quantitatively the blood glucose responses following ingestion of equivalent amounts of digestible carbohydrate from different foods, and is defined as the glycemic effect of 50 g of a particular food in relation to 50 g glucose or another carbohydrate standard. Encouraging low rather than high GI food choices is therefore an important aspect in diabetes management and may also have an application in the management of hypertriglyceridemia and hyperinsulinemia associated with obesity.

Fiber

As for the general population, people with DM are encouraged to choose a variety of fiber-containing foods such as whole grains, fruit and vegetables, because they provide vitamins, minerals, fiber and other substances important for good health. In subjects with type 2 DM, it seems that the ingestion of very large amounts of fiber is necessary to confer metabolic benefits on glycemic control, hyperinsulinemia and plasma lipids, the volume of which may be unacceptable to most people.

Protein

In people with controlled type 2 DM, ingested protein does not increase plasma glucose concentrations, although protein is just as potent a stimulant of insulin secretion as carbohydrate. There is no evidence to suggest that usual protein intake (15–20% of total daily energy) should be modified if renal function is normal.

Fat

The primary dietary fat goal in people with DM is to limit saturated fat and dietary cholesterol intake. Saturated fat is the principal dietary determinant of plasma low-density lipoprotein (LDL)-cholesterol. Furthermore, people with DM appear to be more sensitive to dietary cholesterol than the nondiabetic population. Including exercise results in greater decreases in plasma total and LDL-cholesterol and triglycerides, and prevents the decrease in high-density lipoprotein (HDL) cholesterol associated with low-fat diets. To achieve the cardioprotective benefits of n-3 fatty acids, two or three servings of fish per week are recommended. The intake of *trans*-unsaturated fatty acids (formed when vegetable oils are hydrogenated) should be minimized owing to their adverse effects on plasma LDL-cholesterol.

Alcohol

People with DM should follow the same precautions regarding the use of alcohol that apply to the general population. Alcohol can have both hyperglycemic and hypoglycemic effects in DM. These effects are determined by the amount of alcohol acutely ingested.

Physical activity and exercise

Physical exercise in the management of DM is as important as dietary modifications. While assessing the physical activity of an individual, activity at work, activity while traveling to and from the workplace, and activity in domestic chores should be considered. Additional physical exercise is recommended for individuals with sedentary lifestyles. Exercise leads to an increase in glucose uptake by the muscles, which is the source of maximum glucose oxidation. Regular exercise improves carbohydrate metabolism and insulin sensitivity. It also improves blood pressure and blood lipid profile. Exercise enhances weight loss in overweight individuals and helps to maintain normal weight when used in combination with dietary modification. To combat or avoid chronic or acute hypoglycemia, the patient should be educated on appropriate self-monitoring, intake of additional carbohydrates and dose adjustment of glucose-lowering drugs, such as insulin secretagogues or insulin.

Drugs

Oral hypoglycemic agents (OHA) are required in the treatment of type 2 DM when lifestyle intervention with diet and exercise is inadequate to control hyperglycemia. OHA are mainly of two types, insulinotropic and insulin sensitizers. Insulin therapy is the only mode of controlling hyperglycemia in type 1 diabetic patients who have absolute insulinopenia. Insulin therapy is indicated in type 2 diabetic patients with OHA failure, presence of significant complications, acute problems such as severe infection, injury, ketosis, tuberculosis, and during surgery and pregnancy; contraindications for oral drugs are present in underweight patients with symptoms, to reduce the severity of DM owing to severe insulin resistance or glucose toxicity. A combination of insulin with OHA helps to achieve glycemic control in patients showing a suboptimal response with OHA alone.

20.7 Scope for primary prevention of diabetes

Prevention is the most important strategy in the crusade against DM. Prevention of type 2 DM is possible with changes in lifestyle. Genetic and environmental factors are of equal importance in the causation of DM, and so primary prevention strategies including genetic counseling and health promotion are necessary.

Detection of early biochemical abnormalities

In the natural history of DM, several subclinical stages are present before it finally manifests as clinical DM. Definite abnormalities of glucose tolerance and hormonal secretion and action, especially of insulin, have been detected in genetic prediabetic individuals, several years before clinical DM is detected.

The identifiable biochemical markers are:

- elevated plasma insulin with normoglycemia
- fasting glucose and glucose in the upper limit of normal: higher than control subjects
- low insulin to glucose ratio at 2 h in subjects with IGT
- low incremental insulin to glucose ratio at 30 min (insulinogenic index).

With proper screening procedures, early detection of these abnormalities can be achieved. Measures to improve insulin sensitivity would help to prevent or postpone the development of hyperglycemia.

Identification of impaired glucose tolerance

Individuals with IGT have a high potential to deteriorate to DM. Up to 50% of IGT cases may develop DM in 2–12 years. IGT can be easily identified by an OGTT and individuals with IGT should be advised on preventive measures. Two major prospective studies on IGT, one in the USA and the other in Finland, have shown a definite beneficial role for lifestyle modification in the prevention of diabetes. The US study also showed a role for the insulin-sensitizing drug metformin in preventing the deterioration of IGT to diabetes.

Correction of environmental diabetogenic factors

While the genetic component for the development of diabetes cannot be corrected, the environmental factors can be modified to varying extents. These factors include:

- obesity
- diet
- physical inactivity.

The interaction of diet and exercise influences the body fat pattern, which has a significant role in determining insulin sensitivity.

The intervention methods involve:

- dietary modification: avoidance of excess calories and high-fat diet; consumption of complex carbohydrates and fresh fruit and vegetables
- increased physical activity
- maternal nutrition: *in utero* malnutrition and low birth weight increase the risk of type 2 DM in adult life; improved maternal nutrition would help to prevent DM in the offspring (see Chapter 18).

Traditional lifestyles characterized by a diet including less saturated fat and more complex carbohydrates, and by greater physical activity, may protect against the development of cardiovascular risk factors, obesity and type 2 DM, even in the presence of a potential genetic predisposition.

Efficacy of physical activity in the prevention and management of type 2 diabetes

The metabolic abnormalities associated with abdominal obesity may be improved by physical training. One in four cases of type 2 DM may be prevented by moderate physical activity, that is, 30 min of moderate physical activity on most days of week. As less than 10% of the adult population currently meet this level of physical activity, methods of effective behavior modification need to be evolved to achieve the desired efficacy goal. Education regarding DM should involve not only diabetic patients, but also their families and the community in general. Regular follow-up and constant motivation are required to ensure that the preventive measures are put into practice over a number of years.

20.8　Perspectives on the future

Noncommunicable diseases such as DM, cardiovascular disease and cancer are on the increase, especially in developing countries where lifestyles are changing rapidly. The prevalence of type 2 DM is increasing all over the world, especially in the developing countries. According to the WHO, by 2025 there will be 84–224 million diabetic subjects in the developing countries, and the highest numbers of diabetics will be in India (57 million), China and the USA. Recent epidemiological studies in urban native Indians showed a 40% increase (8.2 to 11.6%) in its prevalence during a 5 year period. Considering the magnitude of the population, the number likely to suffer from morbidity due to the disorder would be very high. DM is a chronic disorder requiring lifelong modifications in lifestyle and medication. Although this is an inconvenience to the patients, the availability of new forms of treatment associated with a reduction in complications provide hope that they can lead a healthy and normal life.

Further reading

Alberti KGMM, Zimmet PZ, for the WHO Consultation. Definition, diagnosis and classification of diabetes mellitus and its complications. Part 1: Diagnosis and classification of diabetes mellitus. Provisional Report of a WHO Consultation. Diabet Med 1998; 15: 539–553.

American Diabetes Association. Nutrition recommendations and principles for people with diabetes mellitus. Diabetes Care 2000; 23 (Suppl 1): S43–S46.

American Diabetes Association Position Statement. Evidence based nutrition principles and recommendations for the treatment and prevention of diabetes and related complication. Diabetes Care 2002; 25: S50–S60.

Diabetes and Nutrition Study Group of the European Association for the Study of Diabetes. Recommendations for the nutritional management of patients with diabetes mellitus. European Journal of Clinical Nutrition 2002; 54: 353–355.

King H, Aubert RE, Herman WH. Global burden of diabetes 1995–2025; prevalence, numerical estimates, and projection. Diabetes Care 1998; 21: 1414–1431.

Nutrition recommendations for the person with diabetes. Clin Nutr 1998, 17: 2.

Nutrition Sub-committee of the Diabetes Care Advisory Committee of Diabetes UK. The implementation of nutritional advice for people with diabetes. Diabetes Medicine 2003; 20: 786–807.

Ramachandran A, Snehalatha C, Latha E, et al. Impacts of urbanisation on the lifestyle and on the prevalence of diabetes in native Asian Indian population. Diabetes Res Clin Pract 1999; 44: 207–213.

Shaw JE, De Courten M, Zimmet PZ. The epidemiology of diabetes: a world-wide problem. In: Diabetes in the New Millennium, (Turtle JR, Kaneko T, Osato S, eds), pp. 1–10. Mumbai, India: Suketu Kothari, Kothari Medical Subcription Service, 1999.

Stern MP. The insulin resistance syndrome. In: International Textbook of Diabetes Mellitus, 2nd edn (Alberti KGMM, Zimmet P, DeFronzo RA, eds), pp. 255–283. Chichester: Wiley, 1997.

Wing RR, Polley BA, Venditti E et al. Lifestyle intervention in overweight individuals with a family history of diabetes. Diabetes Care 1998; 21: 350–359.

21
Cancer and Diet

Lenore Arab and Susan Steck-Scott

Key messages

- Cancer is not a single disease; it is a term that summarizes a variety of entities. The dietary behaviors associated with the risk and the prevention of specific cancers therefore are diverse. The role of diet is greater in some instances than in others.
- Dietary constituents can influence carcinogenesis at various stages in the process, under a variety of mechanisms.
- The study of diet and cancer places special demands on epidemiological study designs.
- Although little is known about the actual mechanisms by which cancer can be prevented, a number of food patterns, specific foods and some nutrients are believed to be particularly chemopreventive.
- Food preparation and food preservation practices or the lack thereof can contribute to cancer risk.
- Dietary influences are believed to be second only to tobacco elimination in the potential for prevention of avoidable cancer.
- Policy initiatives involving governments, international agencies, industry, health professionals, consumers, interest groups and the media have tremendous potential for reducing the burdens of cancer.

21.1 Introduction

The global burden of cancer, as illustrated in Figure 21.1, is substantial. Mortality from cancer is greatest worldwide from lung cancer and stomach cancer in men, and breast cancer in women. These mortality data are reasonably good, but are still subject to misdiagnoses and underreporting in countries where cause of death is not completely reported. The incidence rates presented in Figure 21.1(b, c) show the estimated occurrence of new cancers in developing countries and in developed countries. As true incidence data depend on complete registration of new cases of cancer, and this is done in very few countries, the incidence data are less reliable than the mortality data. The figure shows incidence per year to be greater than mortality and, contrary to expectations, that the majority of incident cancers arise from developing countries. This is a function of the disease rates and the size of the populations at risk. Survival is not addressed by these figures, and may also be impacted by diet,

although this has hardly been addressed to date. Cancer survivors are particularly motivated to change their diets, but there is little available evidence to provide a foundation for good advice on what diets might best prevent cancer recurrence and enhance quality of life.

21.2 Mechanisms of effect of diet

A tumor occurs when cells within a tissue grow in an uncontrolled and progressive fashion. If the tumor is malignant, that is, if it is growing rapidly and invading adjacent normal tissue, and the cells are becoming irregular in appearance, it is called a cancer. Cancer is a genetic disease. It requires the development of rogue cells with functionally altered DNA. The sources of these alterations can be due to inheritance, damage by radiation or chemicals, and hypermethylation or hypomethylation of DNA resulting in the loss of an essential protein or the production of a harmful protein. In addition, other alterations in expression of genes or

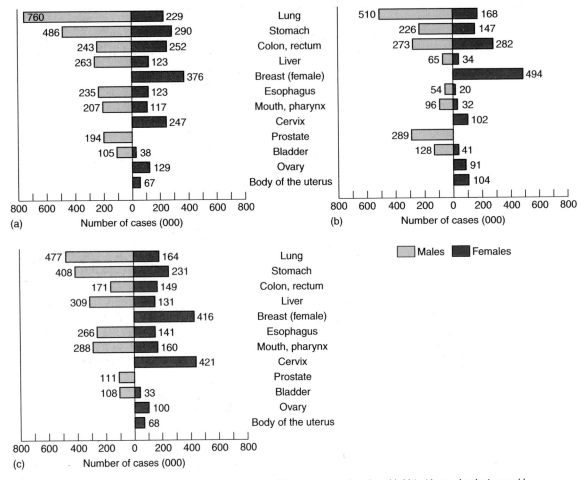

Figure 21.1 The burden of cancer, 1996: (a) mortality, worldwide; (b) incidence, developed world; (c) incidence, developing world.

proteins can influence the risk of the disease at the promotion or progression stage. Consequently, an understanding of the ways in which nutrition and food intake can influence carcinogenesis requires knowledge of molecular biology. This includes understanding the process of cancer initiation, from procarcinogen activation to adduct formation, from DNA repair to DNA replication, from cell cycling to cell apoptosis and tumor growth.

Undoubtedly our diets, as major exposures in our lives, can influence cancer occurrence and growth. Experimental models of chemically induced carcinogenesis have shown the macronutrients, various vitamins (folic acid, vitamin B_{12}, riboflavin, retinol, β-carotene and α-tocopherol) and some minerals, including selenium, zinc, magnesium and calcium, to modulate cancer risk. Other foodborne nonnutrients

such as resveratrol and lycopene also appear to influence carcinogenesis pathways. Numerous epidemiological research findings ranging from ecological comparisons of differences in risk between countries, to migrant studies of change in risk within populations, and including observational data from case–control and cohort studies as well as intervention studies, provide evidence which in part supports these and in part is contradictory to these premises from animal and cell models. The relationship between diet and cancer has only recently begun to unfold, and as the research develops, the attention on the role of diet is being drawn more away from the initiating event in cancer to the multiple roles of foods and nutrients in cell signaling, growth and apoptosis that influence tumor growth and cancer survival.

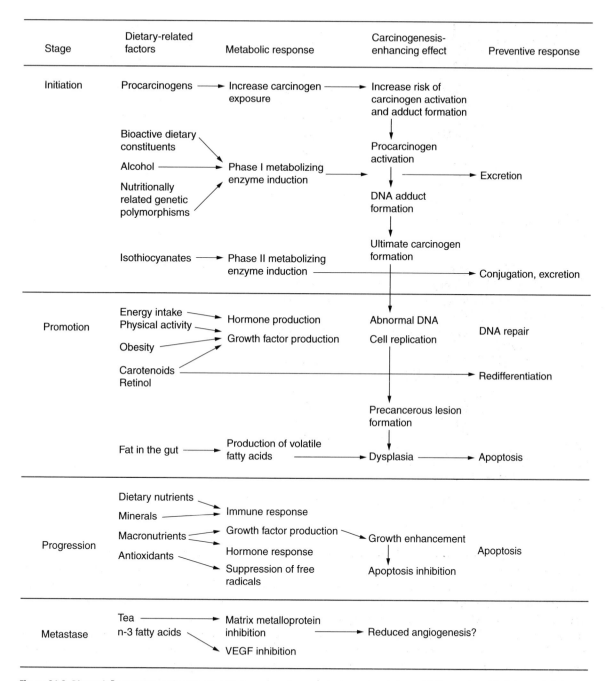

Figure 21.2 Dietary influences on carcinogenesis: initiation, promotion, progression and metastases. VEGF, vascular epithelial growth factor.

21.3 Carcinogenesis: initiation, promotion and progression to metastases

Figure 21.2 integrates the known and suspected role of diet on the carcinogenesis pathway from initiation, through promotion and progression. It illustrates where dietary components can act as the carcinogen or procarcinogen themselves, and where bioactive dietary constituents can influence the enzymes that activate procarcinogens (phase I) or the enzymes that metabolize carcinogens (phase II). Figure 21.2 simplifies the story and suggests pathways that underlie a single disease. However, cancer is not a single disease, but really a term that covers a large set of cancers that differ not only in the afflicted organ, but also in the risk factors involved. Very many dietary factors have been studied for their putative role in the causation, promotion and prevention of cancers. Many of these are summarized in Table 21.1. Readers should not presume that just because these factors have been the focus of study, they are proven carcinogens or otherwise. Much of this research is epidemiological, where true cause and effect cannot be proven. This can only be achieved by intervention studies, that for practical reasons, are rarely initated to study diet and cancer etiology. Foods contain potent mutagens and carcinogens, such as aflatoxins and heterocyclic amines, which are carried on or created within foods and are known mutagens. These activities relate to the stage of initiation of carcinogenesis. This is the part of the process during which alterations in the genetic make-up of cells are induced through the production of DNA adducts. Such adducts can result in DNA mutations or deletions if the adduct causes faulty translation or replication of the DNA, or even DNA breakage. Alterations to protooncogenes (such as *ras* or *myc*) resulting in transformations can result in unregulated cell growth or damage to tumor suppressor genes (such as *p53*, *Rb* or *APC*). Some nutrients, such as fatty acids, are believed to affect gene transcription directly.

This model also shows the potential of dietary factors to have an impact on hormones, growth factors and the immune system in ways that can influence promotion and progression. Promotion is the stage during which initiated cells are transformed into populations of altered cells. Tumor promoters do not affect DNA directly. Instead, they enhance cellular replication and cell growth. Pathways through which dietary constituents can enhance redifferentiation, or affect growth factor levels or cell apoptosis (programmed cell death) may also affect promotion.

Progression is the expansion of a population of initiated and promoted cancer cells to an invasive tumor mass. This is characterized by a variety of abnormalities in the DNA. This may be held in check by immune responses such as through dendritic and killer T-cells. Hormone levels can enhance tumor growth. Excessive amounts of antioxidants can theoretically inhibit apoptosis. Any dietary factors that influence the balance of cellular proliferation or mitosis to cell death can impact tumor progression. Metastases occur when these cells are no longer encapsulated and migrate to distant sites. The influence of dietary factors on metastases has been studied to some extent in animal models of clinical carcinogenesis. Among other dietary factors, tea and n-3 fatty acids appear to be modulators. The possible dietary influences on each stage are presented in Figure 21.2. As a single cancer may involve multiple initiations and the alterations of multiple genes, it should be remembered that these stages do not represent a linear progression. In fact, it is likely that all cancers result from multiple initiation and promotion cycles.

Foods can also stimulate activation of procarcinogens. The stimulatory influence of different foods on phase I enzymes, such as the cytochrome P450s, is well documented. More attention is being addressed to the multiple mechanisms by which our diets can protect against carcinogenesis by trapping singlet oxygen (carotenoids), stabilizing free radicals (as with chlorophyll) and enhancing the excretion of harmful products by stimulating conjugation.

An especially high risk of cancer results from nutrient-induced damage to protooncogenes. The activation of these genes through DNA mutation can produce growth signals to cells, resulting in uncontrolled cell growth. Once the damage is done, defensive responses include stimulation of DNA repair enzymes, a slowing of cell turnover and enhancement of apoptosis to minimize the risk of procreation of this altered DNA.

As initiation is a random, rapid and likely event, the prevention of morbidity and mortality from cancer in humans may be more strongly impacted by dietary influences that slow tumor growth. Study of the impact on growth hormones of dietary nutrients is currently actively being pursued.

21.4 Gene–nutrient interactions in carcinogenesis

Different disciplines start with different conceptual frameworks for gene–nutrient interactions. A model of levels of interaction between genes and nutrients, including the perspectives of the toxicologist (food as a carcinogen or anticarcinogen), the nutritionist (inborn errors of metabolism) and the epidemiologist (genetic polymorphisms that can determine susceptibility to nutritional influences) is presented in Box

21.1. Gene–nutrient interactions can reflect the role of genes in responding to nutrients or the role of nutrients in genetic expression. Box 21.1 emphasizes the bidimensionality of the gene–nutrient relationship. Genetic predispositions can determine the effectiveness

of nutrients. Genetic susceptibility can modulate the activity and metabolism of foodborne substances. This can range from the severe and acute effects of dietary components on preconditions such as phenylketonuria to the more subtle effects of genetic polymorphisms of enzymes that influence the metabolism of procarcinogens and anticarcinogens, such as the cytochrome P450s, the *N*-acetyltransferases and the glutathione-*S*-transferases. The presence or absence of specific nutrients can precipitate the onset of disease (as with phenylketonuria) in the presence of specific genetic polymorphisms. The presence of the polymorphism, in turn, affects the rate at which a nutrient, or a foodborne toxin, is metabolized. At the other end of the spectrum, nutrients can directly affect genetic integrity and expression in ways that can enhance or inhibit carcinogenesis.

Box 21.1 Potential gene–nutrient interactions in carcinogenesis

Genes determine the effects of nutrients
- Inborn errors of metabolism
- Genetic polymorphisms of metabolic enzymes (fast and slow acetylators)

Nutrients impact genetic expression
- Nutrient-induced DNA damage (aflatoxins)
- Nutrient-enhanced DNA protection (chlorophyll, antioxidants)
- Nutrient-related tumor growth or growth suppression (retinol)
- Nutrient impact on apoptosis

Table 21.1 Dietary factors that have been studied for their possible role in the cause or prevention of specific cancers[a]

Cancer sites, sorted by relative frequency worldwide	Risk factors	Preventive factors
Lung	Possibly total fat, saturated/animal fat, cholesterol, alcohol	Fruit and vegetables, carotenoids, possibly vitamin C, vitamin E, selenium, physical activity
Breast	Rapid growth greater adult height, high body mass, adult weight gain, alcohol, possibly total fat, saturated/animal fat, meat	Possibly fruit and vegetables, physical activity, nonsoluble polysaccharides/fiber, carotenoids
Stomach	Salt, possibly starch, grilled and barbecued meat and fish	Fruit and vegetables, refrigeration, possibly carotenoids, allium compounds, whole-grain cereals, green tea
Cervix		Possibly fruits and vegetables, carotenoids, vitamin C, vitamin E
Colon, rectum	Red meat, alcohol, possibly high body mass, greater adult height, frequent eating, sugar, total fat, saturated/animal fat, processed meat, eggs, heavily cooked meat	Vegetables, physical activity, possibly nonsoluble polysaccharides, fiber, starch, carotenoids
Prostate	Possibly total fat, saturated/animal fat, meat, milk and dairy products	Possibly vegetables
Mouth and pharynx	Alcohol, meat	Fruit and vegetables, possibly vitamin C
Liver	Alcohol, probably aflatoxins	Possibly vegetables
Ovary		Possibly fruit and vegetables
Esophagus	Alcohol, possibly meat, very hot drinks, *N*-nitrosamines	Fruit and vegetables, possibly vitamin C, carotenoids
Endometrium	High body mass, possibly saturated/animal fat	Possibly fruit and vegetables
Bladder	Possibly coffee	Fruit and vegetables
Larynx	Alcohol	Fruit and vegetables
Pancreas	Possibly high energy intake, cholesterol, meat	Fruit and vegetables, possibly nonsoluble polysaccharide, fiber, vitamin C
Kidney	High body mass, possibly meat, milk and dairy products	Possibly vegetables
Nasopharynx	Cantonese salted fish	

[a] These dietary factors have been the subject of study, but ranking in the above table should not be taken to indicate their true role relative to one another.

21.5 Epidemiological studies of diet and cancer

Cancer is not a rare disease. Although the risk of any single cancer is relatively low for an individual, the lifetime risk of developing some cancer in populations with life expectancies above 55 years is 30% or greater. The result is over 10 million new cases of cancer occurring yearly at a global level (not including skin cancer) and over 7 million cancer deaths per year. This is the result of the accumulation of risk over time. Familial risk factors for specific cancers also play an important role in risk in many individuals. Migrant studies have, however, proven that the environment plays an equally strong, if not a stronger role, in the expression of cancer within a population.

Although the relationship between diet and cancer was not widely appreciated in the 1970 and 1980s, a strong foundation of epidemiological research now exists. Research published before 1997 has been reviewed in the World Cancer Research Fund (WCRF) expert reports on "Food, Nutrition and the Prevention of Cancer: A Global Perspective". Epidemiology of diet and cancer, as the study of human populations, rely primarily on observational data, although a few well-controlled, double-blind, randomized intervention trials on dietary constituents and cancer occurrence have been conducted. The strengths and weaknesses of various epidemiological studies in the context of the study of diet and cancer are reviewed below, along with examples of various types of nutritional epidemiological studies that have contributed to our knowledge in this field.

Ecological studies

Rather than examining dietary data at the level of the individual, ecological or correlation studies examine population-wide exposures and disease rates to ascertain disease risk based on dietary intakes of groups or nations. These studies can be used to examine differences in risk across countries, but are severely limited by the potential for confounding. Ecological studies cannot examine whether the individual with low exposure is the one at higher risk. They also cannot separate out the effects of diet from those of the correlates of certain diets: drinking, smoking and consumption of other foods concurrently. However, they can be powerful indicators of strong trends across nations or over time. Examples of the illumination of possible diet and cancer relationships through ecological exploration are the strong association between dietary fat intake and breast cancer (Figure 21.3), and the close relationships between nonstarch polysaccharides and colon cancer risk (Figure 21.4). Although these associations look promising, they can be confounded by numerous other risk factors that are impossible to control for in these types of study, such as in the case of breast cancer, age at menarche, parity, age at first birth and age at menopause, all of which may vary considerably across different populations.

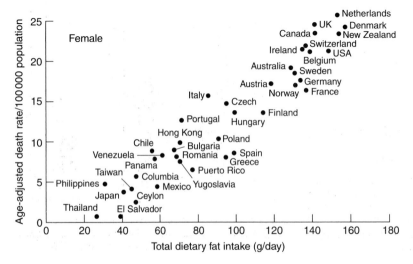

Figure 21.3 Ecological association between breast cancer incidence and total dietary fat intake.

Migrant studies

A major impetus to the acceptance of the fact that cancers are avoidable and influenced strongly by the environment has been provided by migrant studies that compare a set of individuals in their home countries with individuals of the same origin who have moved elsewhere. Populations who migrate to new countries tend to develop the cancer rates of the local populations, usually within one or two generations. Examples of insight gained from these studies come from the studies of Chinese men who moved to Los Angeles and Hawaii, where stomach cancer rates decreased dramatically and prostate cancer rates increased 10–15-fold, and studies of Japanese women who in migrating to Hawaii reduced their stomach cancer rates by 50% within a generation, and increased their breast cancer rates three-fold in the first generation and four- to five-fold in the second generation (Figure 21.5). This suggests that diet and other environmental factors play a larger role than genetics in the etiology of cancer.

Intervention studies of diet and cancer

Randomized, double-blind, placebo-controlled intervention trials are considered the gold standard in providing evidence of a causal or protective effect of specific food components or whole diets on cancer occurrence. To study cancer, such studies need to be large in scale, with individuals assigned randomly into one intervention arm, in a design in which a placebo is administered that is indistinguishable from the active product intervention. Trials are very expensive and require long periods of follow-up. Often, the focus has been on high-risk groups, such as in the intervention studies conducted to test whether supplementation with β-carotene (and α-tocopherol in some cases) prevents lung cancer occurrence. Two of these, the Alpha-tocopherol Beta Carolene Study (ATBC) and Beta-carotene and Retinal Efficacy Trial (CARET) trials, were designed this way, recruiting only long-term smokers or individuals previously exposed to asbestos, to minimize the length of time needed for follow-up.

Few of the intervention trials conducted since the late 1980s to prove preventive effects of dietary interventions on the incidence of lung, skin or esophageal cancer showed a reduction in risk of lung or any other cancer. So, for example, of the three trials of β-carotene supplementation over a 5–8 year period in people at risk of lung cancer, the two conducted among smokers and asbestos workers

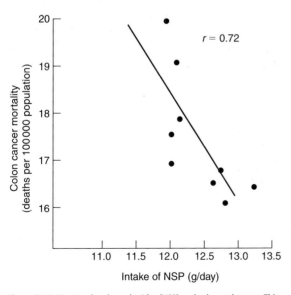

Figure 21.4 Nonstarch polysaccharides (NSP) and colorectal cancer. This figure shows the ecological relationship between the intake of NSP and the risk of colorectal cancer across regions of the UK between 1969 and 1973. There is evidence that increased intakes of NSP are associated with a lower risk of colon cancer. The usual caveats about ecological data apply. Reproduced from Bingham (1988).

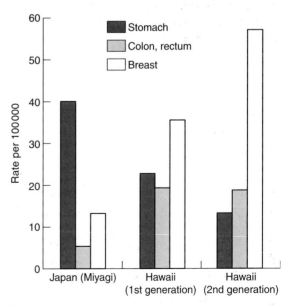

Figure 21.5 Cancer incidence for selected cancers in Japanese women by generation in Hawaii and Japan, 1968–1977. Data are age adjusted to the World Standard Population. From Kolonel *et al.* (1980).

resulted in increased risks of lung cancer, whereas the third showed no protective and no detrimental effects by the end of the intervention. Other trials of selenium-enriched yeast and α-tocopherol found no effect of these agents on the cancer of interest. This was also the case in the Linxian multifactorial intervention addressing nutritional status and esophageal cancer. Secondary analyses from each of these have, however, shown interesting results that have prompted other clinical trials. The focus is now turning to trials of subjects who are not necessarily already at high risk of disease.

A few issues hinder the ability of intervention trials in the area of diet and cancer to answer central questions regarding prevention. The first of these is the period of interest. Cancer develops slowly over time, and diet can have various influences at various phases in the process of carcinogenesis. Thus, the ideal intervention would begin in early life and monitor the effect of lifelong diets on cancer development in adult life. These studies have never been conducted because of the cost, size and difficulty in carrying out long-term dietary interventions. Another problem is that of diet-versus supplement-based interventions. It is much easier to administer a supplement than for individuals to accept and comply with random assignments into long-term dietary interventions. Therefore, most of the interventions have been supplement based, despite the fact that the evidence leading to these trials has been food based. The concern here is that the active ingredient may be wrong in the preparation.

Yet another problem with diet and cancer trials relates to the potentially different effects of dietary ingredients on cancer initiation, promotion and progression. So, for example, a substance may prevent initiation but stimulate promotion, and its administration early in the process may be beneficial, but later in the process may be detrimental. The rapid increase in lung cancer after administration of β-carotene in the ATBC and CARET trials was likely to be an effect during a later carcinogenesis stage in individuals with previous initiation. Since interventions rarely run for longer than 10 years and cancers often have etiologies believed to be 20 years or longer, intervention trials will only show late-stage impact.

Most of the clinical trials conducted to date on diet and cancer have involved administration of a nutrient in isolation, as a supplement. These are inherently easier than, although not necessarily as relevant as food-based interventions. A major problem associated with diet-based intervention trials, as noted in the Multiple Risk Factor Intervention Trial (MRFIT) and the Women's Health Initiative, is the drift of the control population towards diets more like those being administered as an intervention. This reduces the power of the intervention to detect an effect of the proposed diet.

Finally, clinical trials are costly and are rarely designed to test multiple doses and combinations. They do not provide for the variation in dose, frequency of consumption and food combinations and preparations that are seen among free-living individuals.

Cohort studies of diet and cancer

Prospective cohort studies are often considered the strongest type of observational study of diet and cancer, as there is little risk of differential recall bias as influenced by disease status. Dietary intakes are assessed at the beginning of the study, and preferably at various time-points throughout the study to obtain an integrated measure of usual intake. In this design, dietary intake is assessed before case ascertainment and cannot be biased by case status. If the cohort is followed for long enough, it can also provide for dietary assessment many years in advance of the cancer diagnoses. Cohort studies of cancer in free-living populations require extraordinarily large numbers of individuals. This is because the risk of any individual cancer is relatively low, and cancers are studied at the level of specific sites of origin. Because of large study sizes and the cost of assessment of total diets, compromises are often made in the assessment tools being applied. They tend to be semiquantitative at best and do not capture total energy intake and therefore do not capture all foods consumed. The simplified methods are also subject to results biased towards social desirability, and these biases may be related to body weight status (see Chapter 3). They also make assumptions about usual intakes, standard portions of foods and stability in the relative consumption of related foods that impact the nutrient database values strongly.

Careful attention needs to be paid to the validity of the instrument used in assessing the food or nutrient under study in that particular population at that point in time. It should be recognized that when correlation coefficients are used to assess validity, these generally derive from especially adherent subpopulations and tend to be overestimations because of correlated errors. Coefficients less than 0.5 indicate that three-quarters or more of the variance in the dietary parameter of interest is not being captured by that instrument. Such instruments may be too inaccurate to detect important associations. Of equal concern in both cohort and case–control studies is the effect of biased dietary estimates on study findings. Dietary instruments that result in underreporting of specific nutrients such as fat contribute nondifferential bias to estimates of disease effects. Dietary results can also be biased differentially when, for example, overweight individuals underreport fat more than normal weight individuals, and can lead to incorrect study conclusions. Cancer studies are particularly vulnerable to these biases because weight status can be part of the etiology of many cancers.

Often energy-adjusted nutrients are presented in diet and cancer risk estimates. These do not test the hypothesis that the nutrient under study contributes quantitatively to cancer risk or prevention. Instead, they examine whether consumption of the nutrient in amounts greater than expected for the reported energy intake are associated with greater risk. Consideration of the difference in hypotheses being tested when energy adjustment is used, compared with when absolute nutrient intakes are examined, is important in the interpretation of the findings. Cohort studies also present the challenge of capturing change in diet over time. This can be achieved by using repeat dietary assessments during the course of the study. The use of these data can then be as an average, as a ranking or in relation to the change in intake over time. There is little or no consensus about which of these is most appropriate for the study of cancer. Another characteristic of cohort studies in general is the selection of populations based on the need for stability. Attrition out of the cohort can strongly impact the internal validity of the study findings. Cohort studies also often select populations to study based on the ability of large groups of individuals to provide reliable data on exposures and disease development in inexpensive fashions. Examples of cohort studies are the Nurses Health Study and the Health Professionals Follow-up Study, which are profession-based cohorts in the USA that have followed large numbers of married nurses (sample size of approximately 90 000) or dentists, physicians and other health professionals (sample size of approxi-

mately 47 000) in adulthood for two decades. These populations are considered rather homogeneous in their lifestyles, risk factor profiles and dietary intakes, which limits the external generalizability of the findings of these studies. However, some important associations between diet and cancer have been detected within these groups, such as a reduced risk of prostate cancer in men consuming the highest amounts of tomato products compared with men consuming the lowest amounts, and a reduced risk of colon cancer in men and women consuming the most calcium compared with those consuming the least. These studies base their dietary assessments on simple, semiquantitative food frequency questionnaires. The Netherlands Cohort study is similar in design but drawn from a larger population base and includes over 120 000 subjects. The European Prospective Investigation into Cancer (EPIC) study is a large trans-European cohort of over 400 000 individuals using various dietary assessment techniques and calibration in subsets of their populations to examine diet and the risk of rare cancers in seven countries in Europe. The study makes optimal use of the wide range of exposures to many dietary dimensions seen within a relatively small geographical area with a strong infrastructure. The cohort is expected to contribute adequate cases to study rare cancer by 2010.

Case–control studies

Most of the epidemiological reports on diet and cancer are based on case–control studies as these are often the easiest and least costly study designs to implement. Case–control studies are a type of observational study in which selection into the study is based on disease status, and prior exposures are assessed either at the time of diagnosis or afterwards. These are selected as the most efficient approach to assembling a population of individuals with the rare disease of interest (a specific cancer, freshly diagnosed). They are strongest and most widely generalizable when both the cases and the controls are drawn from a population base: the cases are all those diagnosed within a defined geographical area, as opposed to from a specific hospital, and the controls are drawn at random from the population base from which the cases are derived.

One limitation of case–control studies is that it is difficult to obtain accurate dietary intake data for the appropriate time of exposure because subjects may have difficulty remembering dietary habits several years before diagnosis or the control interview. When dietary exposures are assessed using retrospective reports of prior diet, the study becomes vulnerable to recall bias, as well as recent disease-related changes in diet. When attempts are made to assess diet retroactively, many years before diagnosis, the assessments are susceptible to telescoping, differentially biased recall of diet and the artifact of bringing recent dietary behaviors into the recall of prior diet. When valid biomarkers of dietary exposure are available and not influenced by the disease process, this limitation may be overcome.

Case–control studies require less data collection than cohort studies because of the smaller sample size required, and therefore resources can be better invested in higher quality quantitative assessments of dietary intakes. Multicenter case–control studies designed to make use of the advantage of having diverse populations and diverse diets are more powerful in detecting diet and disease associations than cohorts with equal numbers of cases that are derived from more homogeneous population groups.

Case-only studies

Case-only studies are a recent development in epidemiological study designs that are attractive because of their power and efficiency profiles, and their ability to study interactions. Fewer cases are needed to study interactions in case-only studies than in case–control studies, and the effort and expense of recruiting suitable controls are bypassed. There are at least two situations in which cases may be studied without controls in the study of diet and cancer. The first is when the outcomes of interest are survival, recurrence or quality of life among cancer patients or tumor characteristics. In this situation, diet and nutrient use before and/or after diagnosis are studied in relation to these outcomes. This is analogous to a cohort study of cases only, recruited upon diagnosis. The second instance is when the interest is not in main effects of diet, but rather the interaction among dietary constituents or between diet and genetic factors in the cause of disease. However, since no controls are used, the results of case-only studies cannot be used to study the main effects of exposures on the incidence of disease. Instead, these studies provide hypothesis-generating results regarding the interactions under study. A major assumption is that the exposure and the gene under study are independent in the control group. Even small levels of dependence can bias the findings considerably. Case-only studies cannot be used

to study the effects of nutrient intakes and the genetic factors when the diet under study differs by ethnic group and the gene is differentially expressed within that ethnic group. A third use of case-only designs is when the object of study is the relationship between diet and therapeutic factors in disease development. This can be a combination of the two previous approaches.

21.6 Dietary constituents of interest

In the study of diet and cancer, many dimensions of dietary exposure may be of interest. The food patterns, frequency of eating and cycles of dieting are a few at the macrolevel. Within the diet, frequency of consumption of individual foods, the amounts consumed and the foods with which they may be consumed concurrently may be of interest. Beyond that, specific vitamins and nutrients are studied in relationship to cancer, and as well as nonnutrients such as polyphenols and flavonoids, and components on foods (pesticides, fungi), in foods (preservatives) and produced during preparation (heterocyclic amines).

Dietary patterns and vegetarian diet

In general, as well as it can be studied observationally, vegetarian diets that are otherwise nutritionally adequate appear to be associated with lower cancer rates. This is seen for vegan, lactoovovegetarian and lactovegetarian diets. The reasons for this are not well known, although it is important to point out that other concurrent characteristics of vegetarians need to be considered in evaluation of risk differentials, such as smoking, alcohol consumption and other health-related behaviors and exposures. Red meat (particularly well-done or charred meat) consumption is associated with increased colon and rectal cancer risk, and higher intakes of fruit and vegetables are associated with lower rates of many cancers. Beyond this, there are inadequate data to evaluate the possible roles of seeds, nuts, pulses, roots or tubers. Cereals and grains are not strongly associated with cancer risk.

Carcinogens associated with food consumption

Microbial contaminants

Fungal growth on grains and nuts can result in contamination of these foods with aflatoxins. These potent toxins are metabolites from *Aspergillus* that can cause acute death, tissue necrosis, hemorrhage, and degeneration of the liver and liver cancer. The formation of guanine adducts in human DNA has been demonstrated in response to this exposure. A specific mutation arises in response to this, resulting in a transversion of guanine to thymine in the codon 249 of the *p53* tumor suppressor gene.

Naturally occurring pesticides

In reaction to the concern about possible cancer-causing properties of industrial pesticides, an assessment of the mutagenicity and carcinogenicity of naturally occurring pesticides was undertaken. These are the substances that plants produce to prevent their consumption. High levels are present in many herbs, such as basil. When the human exposure averages were combined with the rodent potencies [human exposure/rodent potency (HERP) index] it was shown that the carcinogenic potential of these substances is 1000-fold greater than that of the industrially produced pesticides.

Food preparation and heterocyclic amines

The heating of meat including amino acids and creatinine under high temperatures can result in small amounts of heterocyclic amines. These substances have been known since 1977 to arise from charred surfaces and to be highly mutagenic. Although several epidemiological studies have addressed the consumption of heterocyclic amines and cancer risk, no risk consistent with the expectations has been found.

Polycyclic aromatic hydrocarbons (PAH) are known mutagens that are carcinogenic in laboratory animals and are present in tobacco smoke. They are also formed during grilling or broiling of fish, meat or other foods over intense heat, from the fat dripping into the flame. PAH such as benzo[a]pyrene adhere to the surface of the food. They are known to induce p450 enzymes and phase II enzymes, but the mechanism of action in carcinogenesis remains to be determined. Cancers of the stomach, colon and rectum are associated with the consumption of grilled and barbecued meats, possibly through exposures to these substances. An interaction of heterocyclic amines with polymorphisms of *NAT1* and *NAT2* is suggested in many epidemiological studies, such that fast acetylators who consume higher amounts of well-done meat

are at an increased risk for colorectal cancer compared with slow acetylators who consume less well-done meat.

Foods of particular interest as chemopreventives

Tea and coffee

Numerous epidemiological studies have examined the relationship between coffee drinking and cancer risk, including 17 studies addressing colorectal cancer, 25 addressing breast cancer, 10 addressing stomach cancer and 36 studies of pancreatic cancer. No strong relationships were detected. Smoking is correlated with coffee drinking in many countries, making this a confounder for those cancers with a tobacco-related etiology, such as pancreatic and bladder cancer. Bladder cancer was the only cancer for which the WCRF expert group considered the relationship with coffee consumption possible. Green coffee beans stimulate the activity of glutathione-S-transferase six-fold in animals, but this magnitude of effect is not seen from roasted coffee beans.

Camellis sinensis, the source of green, oolong and black teas, has been shown to inhibit experimentally induced tumors at various sites, and to inhibit mutagenicity. Few epidemiological studies have been able to replicate the chemopreventive effects of regular tea consumption in humans. The strongest evidence is for a protective effect of tea consumption on the incidence of stomach and rectal cancer. Tumor growth and metastases have been reportedly reduced in animal models of prostate cancer through tea infusion consumption. The relationship of tea consumption to recurrence and tumor growth in men with prostate cancer has not been studied to date.

Cruciferous vegetables

Cruciferous vegetables, such as broccoli, cabbage and cauliflower, horseradish and mustard seed contain very active isothiocyanates that are freed from glucosinolates by the enzyme myrosinase. When released in the body, they are conjugated and rapidly excreted in the urine. Intake of foods rich in isothiocyanates results in induction of phase II enzymes, which enhance the conjugation and excretion of these and other substances. The net effect of consumption of diets rich in cruciferous vegetables appears to be a reduction in the risk of cancer of the colon and rectum. Animal studies have shown diets rich in these substances, when provided before chemical carcinogens, to be preventive. When they are administered after the carcinogen they appear to increase tumorigenesis.

Allium vegetables

Garlic and onions are allium vegetables. They have been extensively studied as anticarcinogens in animal models and appear to be preventive against stomach cancer. This may be due to their antibacterial properties, high selenium content and contribution to selenoproteins. Part of the chemopreventive activities of onion may also be attributed to its being a primary source of quercetin in some populations.

The macronutrients and vitamins of interest

Macronutrients and specific fatty acids

Restriction of total caloric intake is related to life extension in various species. Whether this is true for humans remains to be tested, although the test may remain impossible. Studies of cancer incidence among children of the Dutch famine (1944–45) may provide some information on this, but the cohort is still too young for the effective study of cancer.

A long-standing controversy has revolved around whether dietary fat intakes increase cancer risk or whether it is the contribution of fat to energy intakes that impacts cancer risk. The expert panel of the WCRF panel concluded that diets high in total fat probably increase the risk of lung, colorectal, breast and prostate cancers. As fat intake, owing to its high caloric density, increases risk of obesity, it also serves as an indirect risk factor for endometrial, postmenopausal breast and renal cancers.

There are also reasons to believe that the families of fat [saturated, monounsaturated, and the two families of polyunsaturated fats, conjugated linolenic acids (CLA) and *trans* fatty acids] may influence carcinogenesis, aside from their contributions to caloric intakes. Saturated fats are derived primarily from animal fat and therefore are difficult if not impossible to separate from one another in epidemiological studies. They are associated with greater risk of each of the cancers associated with total fat intakes. Monounsaturated fat intakes have been hypothesized as protective against breast cancer, but the evidence is not strong that this is the case, and appears to be limited to populations in which the primary source is olive oil. Among the polyunsaturated fats, the n-3 fatty acids are present in much smaller quantities and are derived largely from fatty fish. They can compete with n-6 fatty acids as eicosanoid precursors and result in different products than are derived from the n-6 precursors. In animal studies they appear to have a chemopreventive effect, but this has not been confirmed in epidemiological studies. *trans* fats can also compete for the δ6 desaturase enzyme in the prostaglandin pathway and have been demonstrated in one study to be associated with breast cancer risk, but have not been adequately studied.

The only fatty acids consistently associated with strong chemopreventive effects are the CLA acid. These are fatty acids with adjacent double bonds (often at the 9 and 11, or 13 and 15 positions) that are found in milk and cheeses and may be formed during cooking of meat. Animal experiments show that topical application as well as diets with 1% or less CLA can prevent chemical carcinogens. As the amounts in foods are not well documented in food composition tables, and the amounts in milk depend on meadow grazing, season and sunlight exposure, human exposures are still difficult to quantify in epidemiological studies, and are often made synonymous with dairy fat intake. This makes it difficult to separate the effects of CLA from those of saturated fats.

As for the other macronutrients, protein intake has not been consistently associated with increases in cancer risk. Carbohydrates differ in their physiological effects, including their ability to induce a blood glucose response (glycemic index) and are generally studied as sugars, fiber and starch. Starch may increase the risk of stomach cancer and appears to decrease the risks of colon and rectal cancers, which are increased with increased sugar intakes (Figure 21.6). Closer examination of starch-rich foods as a function of their glycemic index may shed more light on these relationships. High-fiber diets are associated with a lower risk of pancreatic cancer and cancers of the colon, rectum and breast.

Alcohol is the macronutrient with the strongest carcinogenicity. Consumption of alcoholic beverages increases the risk of cancers of the mouth, pharynx, larynx, esophagus and liver. Associations with colorectal and breast cancer are also seen at high intakes.

Vitamin D and calcium

Ecological studies of sunlight and cancer occurrence suggest that rates of cancers of the prostate, colon and breast may be lower in people exposed to greater sunlight. Although these associations have not been

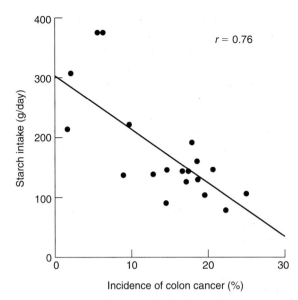

Figure 21.6 Starch and colon cancer. This figure shows the relationship between the intake of starch and the risk of colon cancer, from an international correlation study of 12 populations, using data on actual intakes, and adjusted for intakes of fat and protein. The usual caveats about ecological data apply. Reproduced from Cassidy *et al.* (1994) with permission of Nature Publishing Group.

proven, clinical trials of high-dose vitamin D in the prevention of prostate cancer recurrence are underway. Clinical trials have shown calcium to affect colorectal epithelial cell proliferation. Human breast cells have vitamin D receptors, and serum levels of vitamin D metabolites have been associated with lower breast cancer risk.

Folic acid

Epidemiological studies have found significant associations of higher intake of folic acid with reduced risk of colon cancer primarily, as well as cervix, lung, breast and esophageal cancers. Associations tend to be stronger in subjects who are not heavy alcohol drinkers, as alcohol alters normal folate metabolism. The mechanism by which folic acid may be working has been examined in experimental studies which have found that folate depletion results in alterations in DNA methylation and aberrations in DNA. These disruptions in DNA integrity can lead to enhanced carcinogenesis through alterations in the expression of tumor suppressor genes and protooncogenes. Several small clinical trials have found promising effects of folate on colorectal cancer. An interaction between a common polymorphism in the methylenetetrahydrofolate reductase (MTHFR) gene and folate status in relation to colon cancer risk has been found in epidemiological studies. MTHFR is responsible for catalyzing the reaction that diverts folate to either biological methylation or nucleotide synthesis.

Nonnutrients of interest in chemoprevention

Isoflavones (see also Chapter 14 in *Nutrition and Metabolism*)

Isoflavones are phytoestrogens present in high quantities in soy products. Because of their hormone-like activities, they are actively being studied in relation to breast and prostate cancers. The hormonal influence of isoflavones can be either competitive at the estrogen receptor level or as an additional source of estrogenic compound which may be detrimental. Epidemiological studies show neither a consistent protective nor a harmful relationship between the postmenopausal occurrence of breast cancer and the consumption of soy or isoflavones. Dietary interventions have shown an enhancement of mammary cell proliferation in women on high-isoflavone diets. However, a protective relationship between intake of soy and breast cancer occurrence in premenopausal women is suggested by the epidemiological data on Asian women with high dietary intakes.

Antioxidants

Dietary antioxidants include vitamin C, vitamin E, the carotenoids and selenium, as the limiting factor in some antioxidant functioning enzymes. An abundance of data suggests that consuming diets high in fruit and vegetables, and thus antioxidants, results in a decreased risk for many cancers, including colorectal and lung. However, it is not known whether it is the antioxidants or other factors such as fiber, folate or phytochemicals in fruit and vegetables that may be protective. Vitamin C intake has been associated with a reduced risk of many types of cancer, but the evidence is strongest for stomach cancer. As mentioned previously, the intervention trials have not supported an effect of high-dose supplementation with vitamin E and β-carotene on lung cancer, although an ancillary effect of the ATBC trial was a decreased risk of prostate cancer in men taking vitamin E. Similarly, a trial designed to decrease skin cancer recurrence with selenium supplementation as enriched yeast did not affect that specific cancer, but did result in a reduction in prostate cancer and overall cancer mortality. A follow-up trial based on both of these findings, the Selenium and Vitamin E Cancer Prevention Trial (SELECT), is underway and will supplement men with vitamin E or selenium, or both, to examine the effect of this intervention on prostate cancer risk in the USA.

Some antioxidants can be assessed objectively using biomarkers of prior intake. These rely on plasma concentrations, adipose tissue levels (for fat-soluble nutrients) and toenails (for selenium) as indicators of prior exposure. These values will not be synonymous with actual intake and are influenced by individual differences in metabolism and absorption, as well as cofounders such as smoking.

Resveratrol

Resveratrol (trans-3,4′,5-trihydroxystilbene) is a polyphenolic phytoalexin found in grapes and other fruits. It is an antioxidant and has been shown to exhibit strong antiinflammatory, cell growth-modulatory and anticarcinogenic effects in animal models and cell culture. The mechanism of effect remains unknown. There is evidence that it inhibits nuclear factor-κB, a nuclear transcription factor that regulates the expression of various genes involved in inflammation, and carcinogenesis.

21.7 Prevention: preventive potential

Until 1970 there was not a widespread belief that cancer could be prevented through dietary interventions. Before then, there was concern about carcinogens in the food supply, both naturally occurring and in the form of additives and preservatives, but little belief in associations between food and nutrient consumption and cancer. The seminal report in 1970 by Doll and Peto on "Avoidable causes of cancer" was the first indication that a large proportion of cancers (they estimated 35% with a confidence interval of 10 to 70%) might be related to diet. Since then, based on more recent knowledge, an attempt has been made to estimate the preventive potential of diet in relation to specific cancer sites on a global basis. This is summarized in Table 21.2.

These data represent crude estimates of the magnitude of effect of the totality of all dietary behaviors. They show that in many cases 33–66% of individual cancers might be prevented by appropriate dietary practices, which translates into the prevention of 3–4 million cases of cancer per year. The largest impact is likely to be increasing fruit and vegetable consumption, which is projected to prevent 20% of all cancers. Reducing alcohol intake alone could eliminate one-fifth

Table 21.2 Percentages of specific cancers related to diet and estimates of the preventable numbers of cancers worldwide in 1997

Cancer	Ranking of global incidence in 1997	Preventable by diet Low estimates (%)	High estimates (%)	Preventable by diet worldwide using the low estimate
Lung	1	20	33	264 000
Stomach	2	66	75	670 000
Breast	3	33	50	300 000
Colon, rectum	4	66	75	578 000
Mouth, pharynx, nasopharynx	5	33	50	190 000
Liver	6	33	66	178 000
Cervix	7	10	20	53 000
Esophagus	8	50	75	240 000
Prostate	9	10	20	40 000
Bladder	11	10	20	31 000
Pancreas	13	33	50	66 000
Larynx	14	33	50	63 000
Ovary	15	10	20	19 000
Endometrium	16	25	50	43 000
Kidney	17	25	33	41 000

of the cancers of the aerodigestive tract, colon, rectum and breast.

Attempts have also been made to determine the impact of realistic expectations of dietary and behavioral change on the total burden of cancer worldwide. This comparison shows that the single most effective cancer-reducing intervention would be to eliminate tobacco. The second most potent intervention would be dietary change, which in 1995 was estimated as having the potential for reducing the burden of cancer by 3–4 million cases per year. As can be seen in Table 21.2, the greatest preventive potential through diet is a function of both the frequency of cancer and the preventive proportion. Stomach and colorectal cancers add up to 1.2 billion per year, estimated conservatively, as caused by and therefore theoretically preventable through diet. Cancers of the breast, lung and esophagus follow, with approximately 240 000–300 000 of each being preventable through diet, followed by cancers of the upper digestive tract and cancer of the liver, at about 180 000 each being caused annually.

21.8 Prevention guidelines for individuals and populations

Based on the most recent evaluation of the evidence regarding diet and cancer, recommendations to prevent cancer in individuals suggest that populations consume diets of plant origin, diets that are varied and nutritionally adequate, and diets that maintain both a normal body mass index and active lifestyles. At least 7% of energy should come from fruit and vegetables, and 45–60% from starch and protein-rich foods of plant origin. Excessive intakes of salt, alcohol, heavily cooked meats and hydrogenated fats should be avoided. In addition, fungal contamination should be minimized. This preventive approach, if widely implemented by international agencies, national governments, industry, health professionals, consumer and public interest groups, might reduce the global incidence of cancer by 10–20% within 10–25 years.

21.9 Perspectives on the future

Government, industry, medical and public health can work alone and together with consumers and the media to strive for implementation of cancer prevention strategies. More specifically, the partners in prevention should include international agencies and national, state and local governments; multiple industrial groups involved in food and nutrition in various ways, including agriculture, manufacturing, retail, catering and those involved in food processing, distribution and storage; the medical and public health communities; consumer and public interest groups; and the media.

The international agencies that play important roles towards these ends are the United Nations (UN), the Food and Agriculture Organization (FAO) of the UN, the World Trade Organization (WTO) and the World Health Organization (WHO) along with the United Nations Children's Fund (UNICEF) and the International Bank for Reconstruction and Development (World Bank). National governments and individual states need to implement coherent food and nutrition policies, of which cancer prevention should be a part. Policy initiatives towards preventing cancer that have been proposed include making prevention of cancer a key policy, estimating the economic impact of diet-related cancers and providing adequate funding for the necessary prevention activities. Appropriate agriculture and production of foods that contribute to disease prevention need to be encouraged. Price support systems that encourage production of land animals as food sources are detrimental to this goal. Setting targets for prevention, establishing dietary goals in the short and long term, developing programs designed to achieve these goals and evaluating the effectiveness of the programs are logical steps towards this goal.

The media already play an important role that can be enhanced by focusing on primary prevention rather than treatment, employing health correspondents to cover public health, prevention and nutrition, sponsoring campaigns designed to encourage healthy lifestyles and devoting more time, space and resources to well-informed information on the topic of health maintenance and cancer prevention through dietary choices.

The medical and public health communities can collaborate more actively with other groups and be promoters of prevention by lobbying and media campaigns, and through the education of practitioners. They can direct more research and funding to this area, and enhance the training of professionals as researchers, practitioners and community leaders, and they can take a more active role in the review and translation of findings into accessible messages for policy makers and the public. Public health nutritionists in particular can serve as advocates, sources of information, educators of the public and of the other partners mentioned above, developers of policies of cancer prevention through diet at various levels, and developers of the goals, aims and targets that are central to this. They are also particularly suited to serve as the implementers of programs and evaluators of programs in this area.

Further reading

Alpha-Tocopherol, Beta Carotene Cancer Prevention Study Group. The effect of vitamin E and beta-carotene on the incidence of lung cancer and other cancers in male smokers. N Engl J Med 1994; 300: 1029–1035.

American Cancer Society. Dietary Guidelines on Diet, Nutrition and Cancer Prevention: Reducing the Risk of Cancer with Healthy Food Choices and Physical Activity. Washington, DC: ACS, 1996.

Ames BN. Dietary carcinogenesis and anticarcinogens, oxygen radicals, and degenerative diseases. Science 1983; 221: 1256–1264.

Ames BN, Magaw R, Gold LS. Ranking possible carcinogenic hazards. Science 1987; 236: 271–280.

Bingham SA. 1988. Meat, starch and nonstarch polysaccharides and large bowel cancer. Am J Clin Nutr 1988; 48 (3 Suppl): 762–767.

Bingham SA, Nelson M. Assessment of food composition and nutrient intake. In: Design Concepts in Nutritional Epidemiology (Margetts BM, Nelson M, eds), pp. 153–191. Oxford: Oxford Medical Publications, 1991.

Blot WJ, Li JY, Taylor PR et al. Nutrition intervention trials in Linxian, China: supplementation with specific vitamin/mineral combinations, cancer incidence, and disease-specific mortality in the general population. J Natl Cancer Inst 1993; 85: 1483–1492.

Cassidy A, Bingham SA, Cummings JH. Starch intake and colorectal cancer risk: an international comparison. Br J Cancer 1994; 69: 937–942.

Doll R, Peto R. The causes of cancer. J Natl Cancer Inst 1981; 66(6): 1191–1308.

Fearon ER, Vogelstein B. A genetic model for colorectal tumorigenesis. Cell 1990; 61: 759–767.

Knekt P. Role of vitamin E in the prophylaxis of cancer. Ann Med 1991; 23: 3–12.

Kolonel LN. Cancer patterns of four ethnic groups in Hawaii. J Natl Cancer Inst 1980; 65: 1127–1139.

Kolonel LN, Hinds MW, Hankin JW. Cancer patterns among migrant and native-born Japanese in Hawaii in relation to smoking, drinking, and dietary habits. In: Genetic and Environmental Factors in Experimental and Human Cancer (Gelboin HV, MacMahen B, eds), pp. 327–340. Matsushima, Japan Scientific Societies Press, 1980.

Rothman KJ. The proportion of cancer attributable to alcohol consumption. Prev Med 1980; 9: 174–179.

Trichopoulos D, Li F, Hunter DJ. What causes cancer? Sci Am 1996; 50–57.

World Cancer Research Fund and American Institute for Cancer Research (1997). Food, Nutrition and the Prevention of Cancer: a global perspective. American Institute for Cancer, pp. 50, 71, 380, 542.

Website

www.wcrf.org/publications/

22
Disease Prevention: Osteoporosis and Hip Fracture

Nicholas Harvey and Cyrus Cooper

Key messages

- Osteoporosis is a major public health problem through morbidity, mortality and costs associated with resultant fractures.
- Altered calcium homeostasis, with a secondary hyperparathyroid response, is an important risk factor for osteoporotic fracture.
- Dietary calcium intake is only weakly associated with bone density and risk of hip fracture in Western populations.

- Calcium and vitamin D supplements in the frail elderly reduce the risk of hip fracture significantly.
- At present, secondary prevention with calcium and vitamin D appears the most appropriate public health measure.

22.1 Introduction

Falls and fractures in older people are a major and increasing public health issue, affecting 150 000– 200 000 people each year in the UK and about 3 million people worldwide. A bone's tendency to fracture depends on the strength of the bone and the amount of trauma applied to it. In the majority of cases in the elderly, these fractures are attributable at least in part to structural weakness of the skeleton referred to as osteoporosis. The roots of this problem lie many years before it becomes manifest as a fracture, and involve growth and nutrition across the whole lifespan, starting *in utero*. This chapter describes the epidemiology of osteoporosis, the personal and social impact of the disease process, the biology of bone growth and repair, and the major nutritional elements involved in the maintenance of bone health.

22.2 Definition

The term osteoporosis (literally porous bone) describes a systemic skeletal disorder characterized by

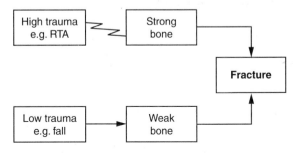

Figure 22.1 Bone strength and trauma. RTA: road traffic accident.

low bone mass and microarchitectural deterioration of bone tissue, leading to increased propensity to fractures (Figure 22.1). Recognition of increased fragility of the bones in older women dates back to surgical accounts in the nineteenth century literature, but it is only since the mid-twentieth century that osteoporosis has been described as a specific entity and its importance as a cause of fracture appreciated. Much of the impetus for our developing understanding of the condition has been linked to the development of radiological

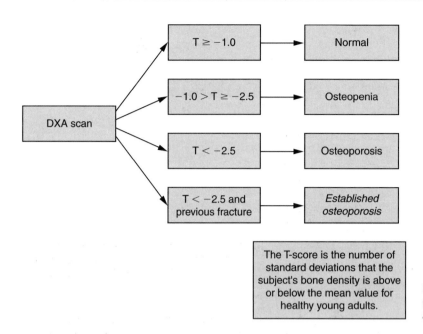

Figure 22.2 WHO (1994) definition of osteoporosis by T-score. DXA: dual-energy X-ray absorptiometry.

techniques that allow identification of osteoporosis without the highly invasive procedure of bone biopsy. Once a workable clinical definition of osteoporosis based on radiological techniques had been established by the World Health Organization (WHO) it became practicable to conduct clinical studies including pharmaceutical trials of treatments for osteoporosis (Figure 22.2). It is important to realize, however, that although the WHO definition is based on bone density measurement, bone density is just one risk factor for susceptibility to fracture.

22.3 Epidemiology: the scale of the problem

It is clear from large population studies in North America and Europe that osteoporosis-related fracture is common in both genders throughout the developed world. Analysis of hospital discharge records shows that there are now more than 150 000 osteoporosis-related fractures in the UK each year, of which over 60 000 are hip fractures. In the USA, more than 1.2 million osteoporosis-related fractures are reported annually. A reasonable estimate of the current annual incidence of hip fractures worldwide would be 6 million, extrapolating from known rates in populations of various ethnic and social compositions. The incidence of osteoporotic fracture has been increasing since the condition

was first recorded, and although the most influential factor has been change in the age distribution of the populations studied, there has been a separate and rather worrying increase in age-specific rates as well. Various explanations have been put forward; the most credible is the decrease in daily weight-bearing physical exertion resulting from the general movement away from agriculture and heavy industry. The incidence of osteoporosis has not been widely studied among agrarian societies (whose people often have more pressing health concerns). Future projections show a worrying increase: the predicted annual incidence of hip fractures in Europe and North America will be over 1.3 million by the year 2025.

So far, osteoporosis has been very much a disease of Western and Westernized societies of white European origin, but this is certain to change as a result of increased longevity, cultural change and growth of other risk factors among black and Asian people. Such populations have not been studied as diligently, and fracture risk estimates are often based on fairly small and perhaps unrepresentative samples. Nonetheless, it is reasonable to accept that non-European races are relatively protected against osteoporosis, partly because of a higher average bone density in people of black African descent, but mostly because of a lower fracture rate at any given bone density in both Africans and Asians. The explanation for this latter finding is

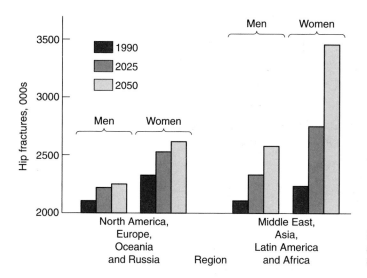

Figure 22.3 Predicted increase in osteoporosis worldwide over the next 50 years. Reproduced with permission for Cooper *et al.* (1992). © Springer Publishing Company, Inc.

unclear, but if it relates to cultural rather than racial factors (physical exertion, low rates of smoking, etc.) then one would expect the same increase in age-specific rates already seen in white Westerners to show up in due course. Population expansion is a factor in this as in all other public health issues, but changes in age distribution may have a greater effect on the impact of osteoporosis on a society. As life expectancy increases and birth rates fall – the pattern associated with accession to "developed" status – the majority of fractures in 2025 will be in the developing world (Figure 22.3).

Etiology

A low bone mass may result from a failure to achieve normal bone accrual during development, or from excessive loss. Peak bone mass is reached in the early twenties, and there is evidence that factors such as lack of exercise, poor intake of vitamin D and calcium, delayed puberty, smoking and excess alcohol consumption adversely affect bone mineral accrual. Importantly, recent work has shown that maternal factors can influence bone growth *in utero*, and it is becoming apparent that influences in early life are also an important determinant of later fracture risk (see Intrauterine programming in Section 22.4). In women estrogen protects against bone loss, so the rate of bone resorption increases after the menopause, leading to postmenopausal osteoporosis. A late menarche increases the risk of fracture in later life. Genetic factors play a role, but only account for up to 60% of variance in bone mineral density (BMD). There is no one

gene that account for this: several genes, such as the vitamin D receptor, collagen 1A1 and insulin-like, growth factor-1 (IGF-1), play a part, but studies have demonstrated only a small effect. Recent work suggests an interaction between polymorphisms in the vitamin D receptor gene and the early life environment, influencing bone mass in later life. Drug treatment with corticosteroids is an important cause of secondary osteoporosis. Systemic diseases that lead to low bone mass are listed in Table 22.1.

Presentation

Osteoporosis is asymptomatic until fractures occur. There are three ways in which the possible diagnosis of osteoporosis may be raised: incident low-trauma fracture, radiological evidence of osteopenia and presentation with risk factors. Diagnosing osteoporosis on the basis of a fracture is rather like diagnosing hypertension on the basis of a stroke; much of the damage has been done and intervention can only ameliorate the effects of established disease. In a perfect world, osteoporosis would be detected at a presymptomatic stage and fractures prevented, but until recently the diagnosis was often not considered even after a fracture. People with osteoporosis are at risk of fractures at any site exposed to trauma, and will suffer a fracture at a lower level of transmitted energy than people who do not have osteoporosis.

The most widely recognized osteoporotic fractures are those of the hip, wrist and vertebral body, but in adults osteoporosis is a principal or contributory

Table 22.1 Risk factors for osteoporosis in late life

Untreatable	Treatable	Associated diseases
Age	Hysterectomy/oophorectomy	Hyperthyroidism
Female gender	Low peak bone mass	Hyperparathyroidism
Family history	Low calcium/vitamin D intake	Myeloma
Previous fracture	Prolonged immobilization	Inflammatory arthritis
Early menopause	Gonadal failure (men)	Malabsorption
Low peak bone mass	Corticosteroid use	Celiac disease
	Smoking	Inflammatory bowel disease
	Excess alcohol	Chronic renal failure
		Anorexia nervosa

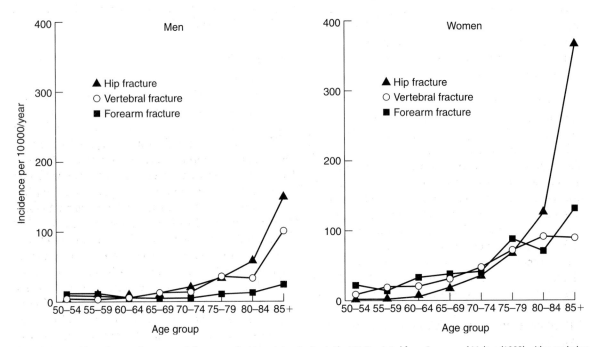

Figure 22.4 Incidence by age of osteoporotic fracture at the hip, wrist and spine in the UK. Reprinted from Cooper and Melton (1992) with permission from Elsevier.

factor in the majority of fractures at all sites other than the facial bones and skull. The relative contribution of trauma and bone fragility in any given fracture is often difficult to estimate, although in circumstances such as road traffic accidents or falls out of bed one can be fairly clear where the problem lies. The classic sites for osteoporosis-related fracture have a higher than average percentage of trabecular bone, and fractures at such sites are associated with conditions causing rapid bone turnover, the most important of which is the menopause. The slowly progressive involutional osteoporosis of late life has no particular association with specific fractures, but it has been estimated that osteoporosis is associated with over 90% of hip fractures in the elderly (Figure 22.4).

Vertebral fracture

Vertebral fractures are often silent, but may present with acute onset of severe back pain in the midthoracic or upper lumbar region, associated with heavy lifting or a fall. There are many other causes of back pain and the diagnosis is often missed, particularly in men. However, in postmenopausal women it is very likely that such symptoms are due to osteoporotic fracture.

Pain is typically severe for 6–8 weeks, subsiding to a dull ache and remitting completely after a few months. Subsequent fractures are associated with progression to chronic pain, height loss and kyphosis. In some cases, however, symptoms may be minimal until several vertebrae have collapsed, leading to the characteristic "dowager's hump". Height loss may exceed 20 cm in severe cases, compromising respiratory function and leading to repeated chest infections. Early mortality from vertebral fractures is negligible, but sufferers have a persistent excess in all-cause mortality which reaches almost 20% at 5 years. This is partly due to a combination of underlying diseases that predispose to osteoporosis, and subsequent high-mortality fractures (for which vertebral fractures are a risk factor). Treatments for vertebral osteoporosis reduce fracture risk at all sites, but have not been shown to reduce mortality.

Nonvertebral fractures

The diagnosis of nonvertebral fractures is usually straightforward, although many doctors would admit to having missed a femoral neck fracture in a confused elderly person at least once. Most fractures present to medical attention promptly, but the importance of osteoporosis as a causal factor is still often overlooked. Although fractures of the distal radius and proximal femur are most clearly linked to bone fragility, virtually all fractures other than those of the facial bones and skull are markers of osteoporosis. As this is now well recognized, there are medicolegal implications for failing to investigate and treat appropriately after a first fracture.

Other presentations: risk factors and the worried well

Many conditions are associated with osteoporosis, and these are shown in Table 22.1. Most are detectable by taking a careful clinical history, and this is essential to the management of any patient with low-trauma fracture. By contrast, the diagnostic yield from physical examination is fairly limited. The general population is becoming much more aware of osteoporosis, partly through the excellent work of several nongovernmental organizations, and thus are requesting screening from their general practitioners. This should start with assessment of risk factors, and then further investigation should be offered if clinically justified, as bone density is just one component of risk; if it is not used in the context of other risk factors, much needless anxiety for the patient may result.

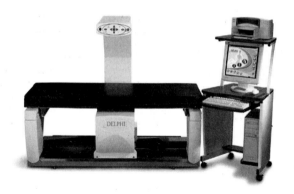

Figure 22.5 A dual-energy X-ray absorptiometry (DXA) scanner. With permission from Hologic, Inc.

Diagnosis

Plain X-rays

The role of plain radiography is to demonstrate the presence of a fracture. Osteoporosis is asymptomatic until fractures occur, so if a patient with back pain has no vertebral fractures on spine X-rays then the patient's symptoms are not due to osteoporosis. Sometimes a working diagnosis of osteoporosis based on clinical history and fracture type is sufficient for managing the patient, but this is the exception. In some cases the possibility of osteoporosis may be suspected if plain radiographs show reduced contrast between bone and soft tissues. Abnormal bone texture may be apparent, and scoring systems such as the Singh grade have been used to assess bone fragility. However, in the absence of a fracture the predictive value of radiographic osteopenia is low unless other risk factors are present, and it should definitely not be regarded as synonymous with osteoporosis.

Bone mineral density measurement

Of the characteristics of bone that determine its strength, mineral content is the easiest to measure. Several techniques are available, with dual-energy X-ray absorptiometry (DXA) the best established (Figure 22.5). DXA uses two X-ray beams of different energies to image a region of interest such as the spine or hip, and then corrects for differences in soft-tissue attenuation to calculate BMD. DXA is the accepted standard for the WHO's definition of osteoporosis in women (Figure 22.2). There is much evidence for the use of DXA to guide therapy for osteoporosis. However, very few drug trials have included patients over 75 years old, and none has related treatment efficacy to BMD measurement in this age group. Nonetheless, it seems reasonable to use BMD in the elderly as one important factor in deciding risk of fracture. Population screening for asymptomatic osteoporosis is not justified in the absence of proven treatments, and it is important to remember that a low BMD is only one risk factor for osteoporotic fracture.

Other radiological investigations
Other techniques for estimating bone strength include quantitative computed tomography (QCT) and various ultrasound-based devices. QCT is accurate and informative, but delivers a relatively high radiation dose, whereas ultrasound measurements involve no ionizing radiation but lower precision. Ultrasound techniques combine BMD with an ill-defined quality termed "bone stiffness". The best predictor of fracture risk appears to be broadband ultrasound attenuation (BUA). This variable is a measure of the rate of change of ultrasonic attenuation with increasing frequency, and the relationship between BUA and the physical properties of bone is complex. Ultrasound measurement has been shown to predict fracture risk in postmenopausal women, but its use in other groups is unvalidated. Unfortunately, ultrasound machines are appearing increasingly in high-street shops for walk-in screening, where a false positive may produce much needless anxiety in healthy young subjects.

Bone turnover markers
Markers of bone resorption and formation are present in blood and urine, and may give useful information about bone turnover. They are produced by the action of osteoblasts and osteoclasts during bone remodeling, and their serum or urine levels relate with varying accuracy to the rate of turnover. Markers of resorption are mostly degradation products of collagen, particularly the pyridine cross-links that are released by proteolysis of mature type I collagen. Some of these are present in any collagenous tissue and are therefore affected by the patient's diet, making them too nonspecific for diagnostic use; others are mainly or wholly restricted to bone. Of these, deoxypyridinoline (DPD) or the N-terminal collagen fragment attached to it (N-telopeptide) are the breakdown products for which the most reliable assays are currently available. Markers of bone formation include fragments cleaved from the procollagen molecule such as procollagen I C-terminal peptide (P1CP), the enzyme

alkaline phosphatase which participates in mineralization, and osteocalcin.

In research settings these agents are able to give useful information on the rate of bone turnover and on any imbalance between formation and resorption (uncoupling), but in clinical use correlations with bone density are modest. A particular difficulty is that all markers are increased for several months after a fracture, making it impossible to assess bone turnover at the time when patients are most likely to come to medical attention. Nonetheless, turnover markers have been shown to be an independent predictor of fracture risk in otherwise healthy postmenopausal women. Combining BMD measurement with a resorption marker such as DPD may improve the ability to identify those most at risk of fracture, but this dual technique remains experimental and marker assays have no current place in the routine management of osteoporosis or fracture.

Fractures and falls
Fracture risk is a composite of risk of injury, efficiency of protective responses and bone strength. Evidence from epidemiological studies suggests that the most important risk factors can be grouped into factors that predispose to falls (Table 22.2) and factors that affect the rate of bone turnover in the mature skeleton (Table 22.1). In the context of older adults, randomized trials have shown that secondary falls prevention, involving collaborative multiprofessional assessment and intervention by physicians, physiotherapists and occupational therapists, can reduce the rate of injurious falls. However, this type of multimodality intervention is somewhat cumbersome and costly; efforts have been made to isolate the most critical parts of the package, but have not so far been convincing. There is a substantial group of patients in whom it is apparent that an incident fracture is part of a more general physical decline and in whom preventive measures may have little effect. This suggests that intervention could

Table 22.2 Risk factors for falls

Intrinsic	Extrinsic
Poor mobility	Steps, loose rugs, carpets
Poor eyesight/hearing	Medication
Alcohol excess	Unfamiliar surroundings
Dementia	High winds
Parkinson's disease	Slippery surfaces

most efficiently be targeted at subgroups within the overall at-risk population.

Consequences of osteoporosis

There are no symptoms of osteoporosis unless and until an affected person suffers a fracture. Osteoporotic fractures cause pain, loss of mobility, loss of confidence and increased mortality. The effects of femoral neck fractures, which carry a 15–20% mortality risk in the first year, dominate the morbidity of osteoporosis. Of the survivors, 50% can no longer walk unaided, 20–40% require formal care in the community or in residential or nursing homes, and many others depend on informal carers. Not surprisingly, these fractures are associated with the bulk of resource consumption, accounting for four million bed-days in UK hospitals each year, 20% of all orthopedic bed occupancy and 87% of the total economic cost of osteoporosis. However, other fractures may have equally devastating effects, through excess mortality (other lower limb and pelvic fractures) or impairment of quality of life. For example, forearm fractures have a negligible mortality, but continuing pain, loss of function and loss of confidence are common and long lasting. Many otherwise well older people become effectively housebound after such fractures, their own loss of confidence compounded by overprotectiveness on the part of relatives and professional carers. The economic costs of managing osteoporosis are very large, with estimates of £942 million per year in the UK and $13.8 billion per year in the USA.

Therapeutic interventions

Treatment of established osteoporosis is directed at the relief of immediate symptoms and the prevention of further fracture.

Symptom control after fracture

The first principle of treatment is that symptom relief has priority over attempts to influence bone density. Osteoporotic long-bone fractures are as painful as any other, and strong analgesia is usually required. Reduction and immobilization of a fracture, by splinting or fixation, is an important modality of pain control, and permits early mobilization of the patient. This reduces the risks of prolonged hospitalization such as pneumonia and pressure sores. The unsatisfactory situation whereby elderly patients sometimes wait for prolonged periods for operative fixation of their fractures can be avoided by good coordination of services across specialties and professional groups.

Some patients develop chronic intractable pain in association with vertebral fractures, and combined-modality treatment with analgesics, drugs for neuropathic pain, physical therapies and transcutaneous electrical nerve stimulation (TENS) may be necessary. Investigation for the causes of secondary osteoporosis mentioned above may be helpful, and unrelated causes of back pain should be kept in mind. Vitamin D and parathyroid hormone (PTH) should always be measured, as vitamin D insufficiency is very common and easily treatable. Treatment of an underlying disease is likely to be more effective than specific antiosteoporosis therapy.

Prevention of falls and impact deflection

Based on epidemiological evidence and the limited clinical trial data available, it seems reasonable to focus attention on the prevention of falls and on relevant lifestyle factors. Falls prevention is too large a topic to be included in this article, but it is worth stressing the very large part that drug toxicities play in the etiology of injurious falls in the elderly. This is one area in which every health-care professional who interacts with older people can make an immediate difference, by always reviewing the need for the medication prescribed to patients, and trying to keep it to the minimum necessary.

The recent development of hip protectors offers a useful alternative to drug therapy in high-risk groups. These plastic shields are worn in an unobtrusive undergarment which maintains their position over the greater trochanters; in the event of a fall they disperse impact force away from the trochanters into the soft tissue. They are extremely effective when worn, but compliance tends to be poor, mainly because they can look unsightly and they make toileting difficult. They probably work best in very well-motivated, cognitively sound people, and in demented patients who live institutional care, who are not concerned about the appearance and cannot remove them unaided.

22.4 The biology of bone health

Calcium balance: vitamin D, parathyroid hormone and calcitonin

Approximately 97% of the total body calcium in a healthy human is deposited in the skeleton in the form

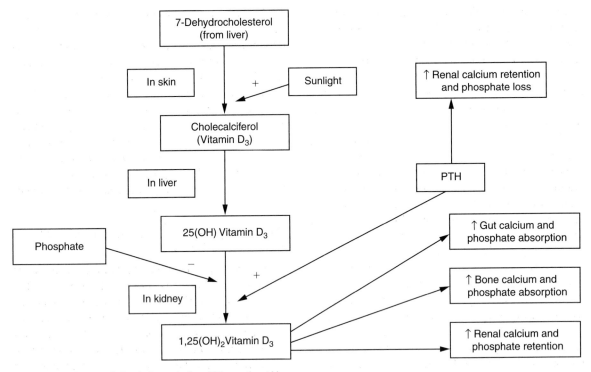

Figure 22.6 Calcium and vitamin D metabolism. PTH: parathyroid hormone.

of insoluble hydroxyapatite. The remaining small fraction is critically important in a vast range of metabolic activities ranging from muscle contraction to cell death. The regulation of calcium balance is therefore one of the most important processes in human metabolism (Figure 22.6). Calcium is present in many foodstuffs, in a variety of forms of differing bioavailability, and its absorption is subject to a wide range of physiological variability. For a full review of dietary calcium handling refer to Chapter 9 in *Introduction to Human Nutrition*.

Vitamin D

This is not strictly a vitamin at all; adequate levels can be generated in the body by the action of sunlight on skin without any dietary intake, although most people in northern latitudes do not receive enough sunlight exposure to achieve this. Figure 22.6 shows the synthesis of vitamin D_3 in the skin and conversion to $25(OH)D_3$ in the liver and then to $1,25(OH)_2D_3$ (calcitriol) in the kidney. The $1,25(OH)_2$ form is around 1000 times more active than the $25(OH)$ form, and historically has been known as activated vitamin D. However, the concentration of $1,25(OH)_2$ is 1000 times less than $25(OH)D_3$, so the overall activity may be similar.

For further information on vitamin D absorption, synthesis and metabolism, refer to Chapter 8 in *Introduction to Human Nutrition*.

Calcitriol, like other steroid hormones, is taken up into target tissues by nonreceptor-mediated pathways and interacts with a nuclear receptor, in this case the vitamin D receptor. This causes synthesis of new messenger RNA for a variety of proteins, including calcium binding protein (CaBP) in intestinal cells and osteocalcin in osteoblasts. The major effects of this process are an increase in calcium absorption in the proximal small intestine, an increase in bone turnover (both formation and resorption) and possibly an increase in resorption of calcium by renal tubular cells. The net result is an increase in whole-body calcium and an increase in the fraction of ionized calcium available for nonbone metabolic processes. Calcitriol also exerts strong negative feedback on its own synthesis and induces an enzyme pathway that hastens its own metabolic inactivation.

Parathyroid hormone

PTH is a single-chain polypeptide hormone of 84 amino acids, with a highly conserved sequence across vertebrate species.

The secretion of PTH is stimulated by a fall in the plasma ionized calcium. Chronic stimulation of parathyroid cells by hypocalcemia (or high phosphate levels) leads to secondary hyperparathyroidism (see below) and eventually to loss of regulatory control, leaving the parathyroid glands permanently switched on even if calcium levels are too high (tertiary hyperparathyroidism).

The actions of PTH are predominantly on kidney and bone, and are mediated through binding to a membrane receptor coupled to G-protein. In the kidney, PTH stimulates the resorption of calcium, inhibits the absorption of phosphate and stimulates the conversion of 25-hydroxycalciferol to calcitriol. The resulting increase in calcitriol leads to increased calcium absorption from the gut.

The action of PTH on bone is less straightforward, mainly because it is indirect and inherently complex. Osteoblasts have receptors for PTH, whereas mature osteoclasts do not, yet it is increased osteoclast activity that causes the rapid turnover of bone mineral calcium induced by PTH. It is likely that osteoblasts respond to PTH by producing a cell-surface protein called osteoclast differentiating factor (ODF). This, in turn, induces any osteoclast precursors in direct contact to mature and begin bone resorption. Taken together, the various actions of PTH serve to increase the available ionized calcium levels in the blood and extracellular fluid. The drawback of this essential process is its tendency to demineralize bone in the absence of sufficient dietary calcium absorption.

Calcitonin

Calcitonin is a single-chain peptide, produced in the thyroid gland by cells of neuroendocrine lineage known as C-cells. Secretion is triggered by rising levels of extracellular calcium, detected by the same calcium receptor present on parathyroid cells. However, unlike PTH secretion, sustained hypercalcemia seems to exhaust the calcitonin-producing capacity of the C-cells rather than inducing cell proliferation, so calcitonin levels are unpredictable in this situation. The principal action of calcitonin is to stop bone resorption by osteoclasts, a highly specific receptor-mediated process that rapidly reduces osteoclast activity and may lead to programmed cell death. As osteoblasts are unaffected, this causes bone mineral formation to outstrip resorption, leading to net movement of calcium from the extracellular fluid into the skeleton.

The major unanswered question about calcitonins is: do we actually need them? No syndrome of calcitonin deficiency has been reported, and the gross excess produced by calcitonin-secreting tumors such as medullary thyroid carcinoma does not seem to cause hypocalcemia. It has even been proposed that calcitonin is an evolutionary remnant with no physiological role in higher vertebrates. Conversely, it has been suggested that calcitonin may be critical in fetal growth and development, where it may have additional actions not detectable in adults. Regardless of its uncertain physiological function, calcitonin is an effective drug treatment for osteoporosis.

Calcium and vitamin D supplements for fracture prevention

While there is good evidence for the efficacy of newer drugs (such as bisphosphonates) for the prevention and treatment of osteoporosis, evidence relating to calcium and vitamin D supplementation is often conflicting.

Epidemiological studies confirm that in both northern and southern hemispheres, and from latitudes from 35 to 60 degrees, hip fracture incidence is greater in the winter months. This may be associated with seasonal variation in vitamin D and PTH levels, which are reflected in BMD. Hip fracture patients have lower vitamin D levels than controls. Supplementation with, and high dietary intake of, calcium have also been associated in epidemiological studies with lowered risk of hip and appendicular fractures.

Vitamin D may be administered orally or by injection. A single injection given at the onset of winter will prevent the seasonal increase in PTH concentrations. In some but not all studies, high or supplemented dietary intake of calcium is associated with lowered risk of hip and appendicular fractures, but the interaction with vitamin D is strong. Many elderly people in the UK do not have an adequate intake of either nutrient, but it remains unclear whether increasing intake will reduce fracture risk. In a prospective, semirandomized study from Finland, a single annual injection of vitamin D 150 000 or 300 000 U was associated with a reduced incidence of fracture in a mixed population of institutionalized and free-living elderly people. A larger, fully randomized study of oral vitamin D_3 at a dose of 400 U daily found no beneficial effect in healthy older people. However, two trials of combined oral vitamin D_3 700–800 U and calcium showed a significant protective effect against hip and other fractures in elderly participants who lived in residential care and sheltered accommodation.

The economic cost per unit health gain varies enormously according to the prior risk of fracture and the cost of the treatment. In a cost-effectiveness analysis, Torgerson and Kanis (1995) calculated costs per hip fracture prevented using either daily oral vitamin D_3 with calcium or annual injection of vitamin D_3 in both low- and high-risk groups. They concluded that vitamin D injection therapy offered to the general elderly population was likely to result in substantial net savings to the health-care services.

Overall, the differences in results from studies probably reflect the differing study populations, their risk of vitamin D deficiency and differential prevalence of other fracture risks. Since calcium and vitamin D supplements are very cheap and there is no evidence that they cause harm in normal doses, it seems reasonable to recommend them to the majority of elderly patients, institutionalized or not.

Calcium and vitamin D intake and bone health

Optimum calcium and vitamin D intake and synthesis throughout life is important for bone health, but again the evidence regarding levels of intake is scanty. The clinically important end-point of osteoporosis is fracture, and unless an intervention reduces the risk of fracture, it is not likely to be clinically useful. There have been two major reports on calcium and vitamin D intake; one from the USA (consensus.nih.gov/cons/097/097_statement.htm) and one from the UK (www.info.dh.gov.uk/home/fs/en). The two reviews interpret the available evidence rather differently, with the UK report looking at evidence regarding fractures and the US report basing recommendations at various ages on studies with non-fracture end-points. The American report gave optimal calcium intake required to:

- maximize peak adult bone mass
- maintain adult bone mass
- minimize bone loss in later years.

However, the available evidence is insufficient to draw these conclusions safely. For the sake of clarity only the recommendations of the British report are shown below.

- A healthy lifestyle should be followed, with varied diet, weight-bearing exercise and adequate sunlight exposure.
- Optimum body weight should be maintained.
- The recommended nutrient intake (RNI) in the elderly is 700 mg/day for calcium and 10 µg/day for vitamin D.
- Ideally, calcium should come from the diet.
- High-risk groups (elderly, housebound, Asians) may need vitamin D supplementation.

It is important to bear in mind that these values are recommendations based on the available evidence, and that this evidence is far from conclusive. It is still unclear whether both vitamin D and calcium are required for benefit, what dosage of each is ideal and which subgroups (if any) within the whole elderly population have the most to gain. Several larger randomized trials, which should answer most of these questions, are in progress.

Noncalcium nutrition and bone health

It is tempting to think of the skeleton as wholly calcium based and therefore dependent only on factors relating to mineral content. However, although the mineral component of the skeleton makes up 85–90% of the whole there is ample evidence that other nutritional factors affect bone health and fracture risk at every stage from conception to advanced old age.

Protein–energy nutrition

Protein and energy intake affects bone growth in childhood and fracture risk in later life. In childhood, maintenance of adequate protein intake is necessary for osteoid synthesis; in individuals who are chronically malnourished there is a tendency for bones to be thinner in cross-sectional area. However, taller people have a higher risk of hip fracture owing to greater mechanical loading of bone during a fall, so nutritional stunting of growth may in fact reduce fracture risk. This surprising (and somewhat perverse) conclusion is supported by the rapidly rising incidence of hip fractures seen in Caucasian populations worldwide during the latter half of the twentieth century, which persists after correction for increasing population age and other variables known to affect bone strength. This finding should not be overinterpreted, as the effect of protein–energy nutrition on the skeleton is probably a dynamic process which varies over time. For the present it is not justifiable to promote an increase in protein–calorie intake in childhood to improve bone health. In older adults, the situation is confounded by the interaction between bone health and the risk of falls. Adults who are well nourished tend to retain musculature and subcutaneous fat into later life, and muscle weakness is a strong risk factor for falling in the elderly. The role of subcutaneous fat is two-fold: first, a thick fat pad cushions the hip on impact, and secondly, adipose tissue contains the sex hormone converting enzyme aromatase, which is responsible for production of estradiol in men and in postmenopausal women. Relative estradiol deficiency due to ovarian failure is the major cause of rapid bone loss at the menopause, and the lower levels present after the menopause and in older men seem to be active regulators of bone turnover.

Magnesium

Magnesium levels influence mineral metabolism in hard and soft tissues indirectly through hormonal and other modulating factors, and by direct effects on bone turnover. Chronic magnesium deficiency often occurs in malabsorption syndromes such as gluten-sensitive enteropathy, in chronic diarrheal syndromes such as inflammatory bowel disease, and in conditions associated with persistent vomiting, notably bulimia. Patients with hypomagnesemia have hypocalcemia resistant to calcium supplementation. Magnesium deficiency is known to impair PTH secretion and action in humans, and leads to osteopenia and increased skeletal fragility in animal models.

Clinically, patients with moderate to severe magnesium depletion are resistant to exogenously administered PTH and also to calcium and vitamin D_3 therapy. Resistance to vitamin D_3 is primarily due to impaired conversion to calcitriol, although it is unclear whether this is a direct consequence of hypomagnesemia or is due to reduced PTH levels. Replenishment of magnesium usually by injection or infusion in a hospital setting, results in a prompt rise in PTH secretion within minutes of commencing treatment, but serum calcium levels do not recover for several days. This delay presumably reflects the slower recovery of intracellular magnesium levels; until this is achieved bone cells will remain PTH resistant.

Hypermagnesemia is much less common and is almost always due to excess magnesium intake, most frequently by consumption of magnesium-based antacids or laxatives, in patients with moderate to severe renal impairment. It should be noted that older people almost all have mild to moderate renal impairment owing to the decline in glomerular number and function which is an inevitable feature of aging. Older people are also most likely to be taking laxatives and other drugs that impair renal function, such as antihypertensives and nonsteroidal antiinflammatory drugs. Although mild hypermagnesemia is probably quite common, it is little studied, and effects on bone metabolism are not well characterized. More severe degrees of hypermagnesemia are associated with hypocalcemia and PTH suppression, but the clinical picture is usually dominated by other effects on the heart and nervous system.

Phosphate

This is the "shadow partner" of calcium in bone metabolism. The amount of phosphate ion in the circulation is only 1–2% of bodily stores and, apart from its role in bone mineralization, phosphate ions are central to the major biological processes of life such as transfer of energy from foodstuffs to cell metabolism. Perhaps surprisingly, physiological control of phosphate levels is not nearly as rigorous as for calcium; there are no regulatory hormones specific to phosphate handling and extracellular levels are kept in a rough equilibrium by balancing dietary intake with renal excretion. In consequence, renal impairment is the usual cause of hyperphosphatemia. Other causes or contributory factors include excess intake of phosphate, usually iatrogenic, and hypoparathyroidism, which impairs renal excretion.

Hyperphosphatemia induces hypocalcemia through two mechanisms: first, a rise in phosphate leads to deposition of calcium phosphate at nonskeletal sites (ectopic calcification) to maintain a constant calcium–phosphate product in the extracellular fluid; secondly, high phosphate levels inhibit renal conversion of 25-hydroxyvitamin D_3 to calcitriol, which impairs intestinal calcium absorption and induces skeletal resistance to the actions of PTH. These effects result in most of the features of renal bone disease.

Hypophosphatemia is associated with starvation (including anorexia nervosa), persistent vomiting, alcohol abuse, overuse of phosphate-binding antacids and some genetic disorders affecting bone mineral metabolism. Its effects are complex and diverse, and are covered in detail in Chapter 9 in *Introduction to Human Nutrition*.

Iron

Excess iron, in association with genetic hemochromatosis, has been shown to result in loss of bone; this effect is mediated mainly by associated hypogonadism, but there does appear to be some direct suppression of bone formation. It is increasingly recognized that genetic hemochromatosis is underdiagnosed, so may account for a small proportion of "idiopathic" osteoporosis. Other causes of iron excess are rare; the best characterized is Bantu siderosis associated with the brewing of beer in large cast-iron pots in South African villages. Because vitamin C deficiency and other nutrient imbalances are common in this population, it is not at all certain that the osteoporosis seen in this condition is genuinely related to iron excess. In addition, the association may be related to excess consumption of the beer in the pots, rather than iron from the pot walls.

Other vitamins and minerals

Vitamin C is necessary for the synthesis and maturation of type I collagen, which is the main structural protein in bone matrix; it might therefore be anticipated that a higher vitamin C intake would protect against fracture. Unfortunately, in the largest epidemiological study completed to date, vitamin C emerged as a fairly strong risk factor for fracture. This result is unexplained and has been hotly debated. Vitamin K is involved in the maturing of osteocalcin, a small protein invariably associated with osteoblast activity; undercarboxylated osteocalcin is known to be associated with deficient bone mineralization. Evidence from knockout mice in which the osteocalcin gene has been deleted suggests that osteocalcin inhibits bone formation, implying that it is part of a negative feedback pathway to control osteoblast activity. The exact function in humans is unclear. Osteocalcin does, however, provide a potentially useful, if expensive, way to measure bone formation in clinical practice.

Trace elements

The role of trace elements in bone metabolism is only now being elucidated. Zinc, copper, boron and manganese have been evaluated both in population studies and in small randomized controlled trials, with mixed results; there is clearly room for further research in this area.

Caffeine

Caffeine, for example in coffee, increases urinary calcium output, is associated with accelerated bone loss in postmenopausal women and has been implicated as a risk factor for nonvertebral fracture. However, the results of studies in this area conflict; one suggestion is that regular milk consumption offsets the calcium-wasting action of caffeine, but no study has yet demonstrated a difference in effect between black and white coffee.

Other lifestyle issues

Factors other than diet have an effect on fracture risk. Smoking has been shown to reduce bone density, and also may make hormone replacement therapy less effective. A moderate alcohol intake may be beneficial, but excess alcohol seems to increase the risk of fracture. This may related to the increased risk of falls with higher intakes. Beer seems to increase risk more than wine consumption, and the reason for this is not clear. Weight-bearing exercise appears to increase bone density at the proximal femur: impact is necessary to have this beneficial effect, so nonweight-bearing exercise, such as swimming, is not helpful in this context. However, too much exercise, if not balanced by adequate nutrient intake, may have an adverse effect. Elite athletes and ballet dancers are at risk of spinal osteoporosis, probably as a result of low fat mass and insufficient diet consumption.

Intrauterine programming

Just as nutrition in adult life is important, it is becoming increasingly apparent that nutrition in early life has crucial long-term consequences for bone health. Evidence is accruing that nutritional influences *in utero* affect bone mass and risk of fracture in later life. The concept of programming describes "persisting changes in structure and function caused by an environmental stimulus at a critical period in early development". Epidemiological studies have demonstrated that low birth weight (a marker of fetal undernutrition) and low weight at 1 year predict lower bone mass in adulthood. Risk of hip fracture in the seventh decade is increased by lower birth size and poor childhood growth. Evidence has emerged that factors underlying these observations may relate to maternal influences in the intrauterine period. Maternal smoking during pregnancy, low maternal birth weight, vigorous activity in late pregnancy and low maternal fat stores all predict lower bone mass in the neonate. Both the calcium–vitamin D axis and the growth hormone–IGF-1 axis seem to be involved in this process. 1,25 Vitamin D levels in adulthood are inversely correlated with birth weight, as is calcium absorption in the gut, and it seems logical that if the fetus is undernourished vitamin D levels will be up-regulated,

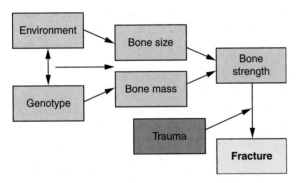

Figure 22.7 Interaction between the environment, genotype and bone mass. Adapted from Harvey and Cooper (2003) with permission from Current Science.

to try to scavenge all the available calcium. Levels of IGF-1 in childhood are predicted by current size, but correlate inversely with birth weight and may relate to catch-up growth in childhood. Work is underway to elucidate possible strategies to maximize peak bone mass, using the window of opportunity presented by the intrauterine period, and it is possible that interventions here could reduce later fracture risk by up to 25%.

22.5 Perspectives on the future

Osteoporosis is a common, serious and sometimes life-threatening disorder, which will affect at least one-sixth of the population of developed countries. Over the next 50 years the burden is set to increase dramatically in the developing world, with enormous cost to the world economy. Strategies to decrease this burden fall into two groups: those that decrease the population risk (e.g. by moving the population BMD upwards) and those that target those at most risk (e.g. by looking for risk factors). A mixture of the two approaches is likely to lead to the most cost-effective interventions. These may include ensuring adequate calcium and vit-

amin D for the population, increasing exercise levels, and reducing smoking and excess alcohol. This may be via education or food supplementation. The interaction between the environment, genotype and bone mass (Figure 22.7) will be better understood in the future. Family doctors may be able to recognize those most at risk and these people could be sent for BMD measurement. Newer research suggests that addressing factors in early life (such as optimizing vitamin D intake in pregnancy) may help to maximize peak bone mass and thus also help to reduce the burden of this devastating disease.

Further reading

Chapuy MC, Arlot ME, Delmas PD, Meunier PJ. Effect of calcium and cholecalciferol treatment for three years on hip fractures in elderly women. BMJ 1994; 308: 1081–1082.

Cooper C. Osteoporosis. In: Epidemiology of the Rheumatic Diseases (Hochberg M, Silman A, eds), pp. 422–464. Oxford: Oxford University Press, 1993.

Cooper C, Melton, LJ III. Epidemiology of osteoporosis. Trends Endocrinol Metab 1992; 314: 224–229.

Cooper C, Campion G. Melton LJ III. Hip fractures in the elderly: a worldwide projection. Osteoporos Int 1992; 2: 285–289.

Cooper C, Javaid MK, Taylor P et al. The fetal origins of osteoporotic fracture. Calcif Tissue Int 2002; 70: 391–394.

Harvey N, Cooper C. Determinants of fracture risk in osteoporosis. Curr Rheumatol Rep 2003; 5: 75–81.

Heaney RP, Recker RR. Estimation of true calcium absorption. Ann Intern Med 1985; 103: 516–521.

Nutrition and Bone Health: with particular reference to calcium and vitamin D, p. 49. Report of the Subgroup on Bone Health, Working Group on the Nutritional Status of the Population of the Committee on Medical Aspects of Food and Nutrition Policy, London, 1998.

Torgerson DJ, Kanis JA. Cost-effectiveness of preventing hip fractures in the elderly population using vitamin D and calcium. QJM 1995 Feb; 88(2): 135–9.

Websites

www.nos.org.uk
www.info.dh.gov.uk
consensus.nih.gov

Appendix

Common features of fad slimming diets and reasons why they should not be recommended for the treatment of obesity

Fad diets	Common features	Why they should not be used
Food combining	The rationale dictates that macronutrients, such as protein and carbohydrate should not be eaten at the same meal. This is based on the misconception that the activity of acid and alkaline digestive enzymes simultaneously, causes stress and that acid-producing nutrients are unhealthy.	Compliance results in a restrictive diet due to the presence of both nutrients in many staple foodstuffs. Furthermore the beneficial effects of the interaction of these nutrients is lost, e.g. the sparing effect of carbohydrates on protein requirements.
Foods eaten before a meal	The misconception here is that foods eaten before a meal can induce weight loss, e.g. the acid in grapefruits gets rid of body fat.	Any weight loss is due to these lower energy foods displacing calories and has nothing to do with any intrinsic 'fat burning' component of the food itself.
Certain foods only up to a particular time each day	This is based on the misconception that certain components in these foods will aid weight loss, e.g. the "enzymes in fruit". It is claimed that "after this activity" other foods eaten will have a reduced energy value.	Weight loss will be due to the combined effects of the lower energy content of recommended foodstuffs compared to those usually consumed during the set time period every day; and to the appetite-suppressing effects of higher intakes of these lower energy foods.
Single low-calorie food diets or fasting	The only fortunate aspect of these diets is that they are generally only recommended for very limited time periods whereupon it is claimed they aid detoxification of the body, e.g. "the cabbage diet".	These diets represent a starvation regime and thus carry significant health risks. In addition to the loss of the body's energy stores, muscle mass will be depleted including cardiac muscle which can lead to fatal arrythmias. At best these diets are deficient in a wide range of nutrients and should be avoided at all costs.
Mutivitamin and herbal supplements, teas and sprays	These are usually recommended as an adjunct to a weight-reducing diet or liquid formula. It is claimed that they contain components to boost energy, rejuvenate cells, provide micronutrients and eliminate cellulite and "detoxify".	These supplements and remedies are expensive and unnecessary.
Single food or beverage diets	Nutritionally complete diets that are based on a single food or drink, may be effective at reducing energy intake as they are so monotonous and may cause "sensory-specific satiety".	These diets tend to be very low in energy, it is recommended that their use is medically supervised, restricted to the treatment of obesity only and not used for more than 4 weeks. Any other approach represents a "fad" in that it fails to meet needs of the dieter.

Fad diets	Common features	Why they should not be used
Ketogenic diets	Hailed as the method whereby one can eat unlimited calories and still lose weight as long as carbohydrate intakes are severely restricted.	Initial rapid weight loss on very low carbohydrate diets is due to excessive water loss which is associated with depletion of liver and muscle glycogen stores. The severe restriction of carbohydrate intake results in a net reduction in energy intakes. Vitamin and mineral intakes are often inadequate. Side-effects include ketosis, dehydration nausea (ketosis), calcium depletion, weakness and exacerbation of gout. Long-term use may increase risk of coronary heart disease. Finally the basis of this diet runs contrary to evidence that high-fat intakes may be an aetiological factor in the development of obesity.
Hypoallergenic diets	The rationale for this approach suggests that overweight and obesity are the result of food allergies. Blood, hair or skin samples are collected for "analysis" and a list of offending food items are drawn up for exclusion. Foods commonly implicated include staples such as wheat and dairy products.	The tests used are not established immunological techniques. Individuals on these diets will lose weight as a result of restricted energy intakes due to the limited range of foods that can be eaten. There is a significant risk of nutritional deficiencies because entire food groups are often excluded without provision for the adequate replacement of lost nutrients.
Water	Drink at least eight 200 ml (8 oz) glasses of water per day and take at least one glass with each meal. It is claimed that "for each 20 pounds you want to lose, add a glass of water".	Water contains no energy, therefore drinking excessive amounts of water will only be effective at reducing fat stores through suppression of appetite. There is no basis for a prescription of an amount of water for the achievment of a certain amount of weight loss.
Skipping meals	The rationale is simple – by skipping one or two meals per day total energy intakes will be reduced.	This is very popular among teenagers. The misconception lies in the fact that over-eating and bingeing are often the sequelae to such dietary restraint. Also the nutrients missed out on at meals may not be adequately compensated for during periods of snacking or bingeing.

Index

Note: page numbers in *italics* refer to figures, those in **bold** refer to tables and boxes